Cricket Sports Medicine

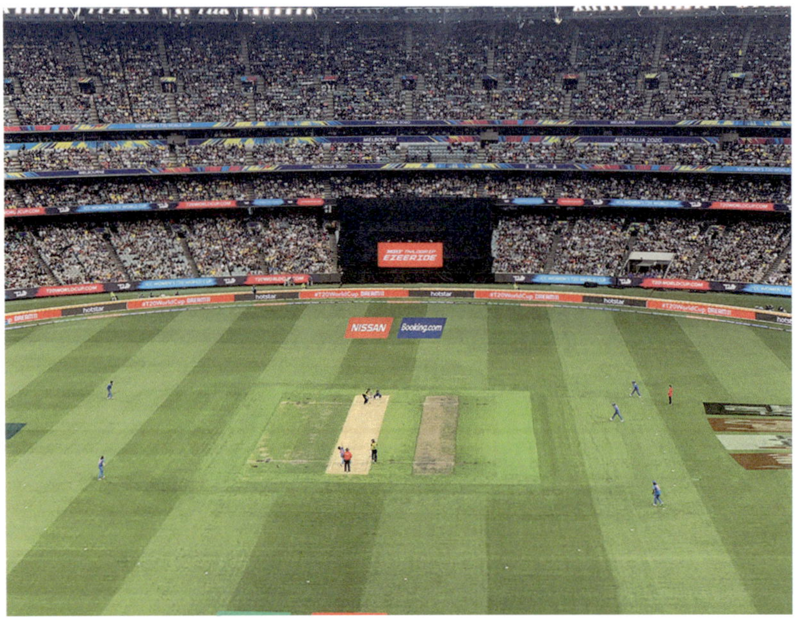

The women's T20 World Cup final at the MCG in 2020 between Australia and India, before a crowd of 86,174 people

Benita Olivier • John W. Orchard
Editors

Cricket Sports Medicine

Springer

Editors
Benita Olivier
Centre for Healthy Living Research,
Oxford Institute of Applied Health
Research, Faculty of Health,
Science and Technology
Oxford Brookes University
Oxford, UK

John W. Orchard
School of Public Health
University of Sydney
Sydney, NSW, Australia

ISBN 978-981-96-6320-0 ISBN 978-981-96-6321-7 (eBook)
https://doi.org/10.1007/978-981-96-6321-7

This Springer imprint is published by the registered company Springer Nature Singapore Pte Ltd.
The registered company address is: 152 Beach Road, #21-01/04 Gateway East, Singapore 189721, Singapore

Foreword

'What's been the biggest change in cricket since you played?' I asked the ex-Australian cricket captain.

Without hesitation, and before my last syllable dropped, came the reflex answer: 'Helmets'.

The answer was delivered decisively, like a yorker aimed at the base of the stumps. I was curious.

'Helmets?' I fished for an explanation.

My companion, now a slight man in his mid-70s, leaned back and focused on a distant past, when a cloth baggy green cap was the only protective partition between a skull and a red-rock ball; I was aware of entering a part of his mind that was part-pleased, part-fearful of where it was going.

'When I went out to bat and the bowler was at the far end of his run, my first thought was always "don't get hit, watch the ball". In that split moment between knowing I was safe, and needing to make runs, that's when I decided what shot to play. If you watch a batsman today, they skip the middleman. There's no thought of safety. They assume they'll never get hurt … because of the helmet. Their first instinct is to hit the ball. My first instinct was "don't get hit".'

I was sitting in a coffee shop in Bowral when this conversation took place just over 10 years ago. Next to me sat Ian Craig, Australia's youngest-ever cricket captain. Burdened by expectation (as the next Bradman) and compromised by illness, his shooting star skied heavenwards in the 1950s, faded, spluttered and was soon extinguished. By 26 years of age, he was out of the First-class game.

A lot has happened since my conversation with Ian Craig. As I write this foreword, it is only days since the tenth anniversary of the death of Phillip Hughes, felled by a cricket ball on the Sydney Cricket Ground. The death of a young man in full public view has left a sensitivity and concern about the welfare of players that shows no sign of diminishing and has altered the mood of the game. Head injury in cricket is not new, but the response is new, shaped by a sense of medical and legal responsibility, and an overriding moral sentiment that we must care for those who play the game of cricket. The list of players seriously injured by ball smashing into bone and flesh is long: Bert Sutcliffe struck in the head while batting for New Zealand against South Africa (1953), Nari Contractor (Indian captain) also brutally struck in the head while batting in the West Indies (1962) and Rick McCosker batting with a shattered jaw and disfigured face in the Australia-England Centenary Test (1977). There are many others.

Fortunately, life-threatening injuries and illnesses in cricket are rare. This important book on *Cricket Sports Medicine*, edited by Benita Olivier and John Orchard—both distinguished researchers in the field—is the first attempt to draw the experiences of expert clinicians and academics into a single volume. It ranges over and explores the varied physical injuries suffered by players; the erosive changes in the body as years of wear and tear take their toll; the illnesses commonly afflicting cricketers; and it documents studies from epidemiology to biomechanics.

If there is any signature injury in cricket, it is lower back bone stress suffered by fast bowlers, and this book delves into the history and treatment of this breakdown of the body's frame. The history of fast bowling and its associated injuries can be traced to the nineteenth century. In 1864, the Marylebone Cricket Club (MCC) ordained that bowlers were permitted to bowl by raising their arm above the horizontal plane. Prior to that, if a bowler raised his arm above the horizontal as his arm swung into action, he would be no-balled. In a flash, the modern biomechanics of fast bowling was sealed by the MCC.

To see a young fast bowler with stress fractures of the lower vertebrae is to see much more than a physical injury. They are bedevilled by troubling thoughts of insecurity, and the dual fears of performance failure and that of recurring fractures. Coupled with the sometimes-unbearable expectations of those around them, it is hardly surprising that dissatisfaction, anger and depression are common bedfellows of chronic back pain in the fast bowler. The assessment of mental state and treatment of any associated psychiatric disorder is a crucial component of the care and treatment of all cricketers in the twenty-first century.

If I were to ask Virat Kohli, or Alyssa Healy in 50 years' time, the same reflective question I asked Ian Craig: 'What's been the biggest change in cricket since you played?' they might touch upon the commercial or legal aspects of the game, but I suspect part of their answer would focus on the advances in physical and psychological care for the cricketer of 2074. This new book is a step along this path.

Consultant Psychiatrist
for Cricket Australia
and Cricket New South Wales
Westmead Hospital
Sydney, NSW, Australia
Gregory.deMoore@health.nsw.gov.au

Gregory De Moore

Preface

Cricket is played in 104 countries and enjoyed by over 2.5 billion people worldwide. Keeping our cricketers safe, healthy and happy is essential. It is, therefore, our pleasure and pride to have edited the first book on Cricket Sports Medicine.

The book was born from the recognised need to consolidate practical knowledge in one place. The chapters were identified through a co-production process, where professionals, cricketers and even parents from around the world shared their thoughts on what should be included. The project evolved into a global collaboration among experts. We are thrilled at the depth of both nations and professions represented amongst the contributors. Sports Science Sports Medicine (SSSM) requires a team approach, and the team has participated in this text. We are deeply grateful for the time, energy and dedication every author has contributed to this book. Each author has brought their unique expertise, professional background and perspective, enriching the book's impact through these diverse contributions.

We've also succeeded in having a book that is 'cricket-specific', with the section on lumbar stress fractures, the signature injury in cricket fast bowlers, a great example. There are 39 chapters, illustrating a very broad coverage of the field. We are aware that there are still some potential chapters that have been left out. There are some injuries we haven't covered, including the hip joint, testicular trauma, facial fractures and neck pain. There are some missing topics that may, in hindsight, be still traumatic, such as learnings from the COVID pandemic, or the even sadder topic of deaths in cricket. There is the potential for a second edition to cover additional relevant material—watch this space!

While each chapter has been written by experts in medical and scientific research and practice, the ultimate beneficiary of our knowledge and efforts is the cricketer. Cricketers strive to perform at their highest potential, and maintaining their health and well-being is essential for optimal performance.

The perspective of cricketers themselves matters in ensuring that we practise medicine and science ‘with’ rather than ‘for’ them. Therefore, we have included a chapter written by a cricketer, sharing his lived experience with injury and its impact on performance and quality of life.

This book is dedicated to those passionate about cricket and those who work tirelessly behind the scenes to keep our cricketers safe, healthy and happy. Enjoy it!

Oxford, UK Benita Olivier
Sydney, NSW, Australia John W. Orchard

Contents

Part I
Foundations of Cricket Sports Medicine and Performance Science

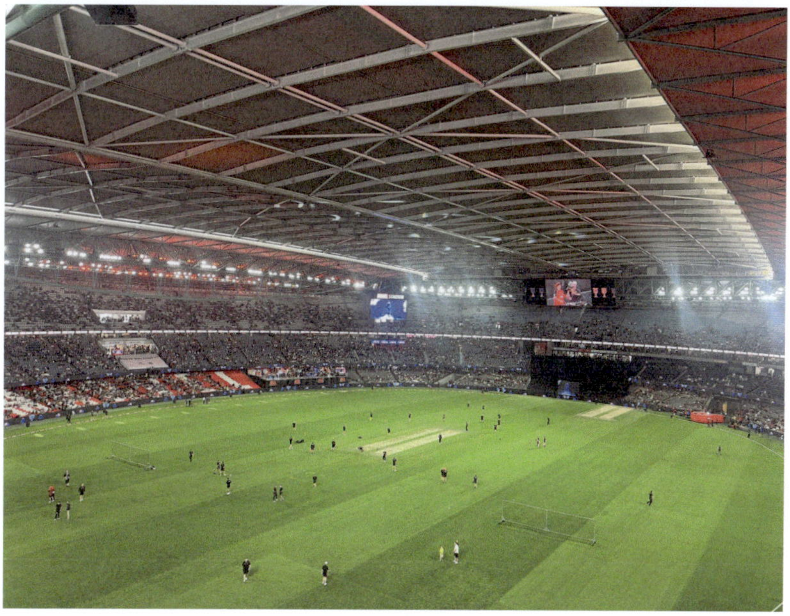

Warm-up for a BBL cricket match at Docklands (Marvel) Stadium

1 Injury Epidemiology in Cricket

Benita Olivier, Akshai Mansingh, John W. Orchard, Mandeep S. Dhillon, and Sibi Walter

1.1 Introduction

Injury epidemiology refers to the quantification and analysis of the frequency, type and nature of injuries. Knowing how and how many injuries occur in a sport and the different roles within a sport helps us better plan our injury prevention, treatment and rehabilitation approaches. As the game continues to evolve, new injury patterns may arise with the rising popularity of shorter formats and greater physical demands. Ongoing monitoring and analysis of injury data will be crucial for developing targeted preventive strategies, optimising medical support and safeguarding cricketers' health and longevity at all levels.

This chapter will give an overview of the prevalence and incidence of injuries in cricket, including injury prevalence in the different playing positions and activities of cricket, namely bowling, batting, fielding and wicketkeeping. Injury predisposition by body areas and injury patterns per activity will also be provided.

1.2 Injury Incidence and Prevalence

1.2.1 Overall Injury Rates

The prevalence of injury in cricket has been a concern in published research since early 1965 [1]. Cricketers are playing cricket with the primary purpose of performing well and enjoying the game, not remaining injury-free as a purpose in itself. A reduction in injury rates seems to be associated with a positive effect on the perfor-

B. Olivier (✉)
Centre for Healthy Living Research, Oxford Institute of Applied Health Research, Faculty of Health, Science and Technology, Oxford Brookes University, Oxford, UK

Wits Cricket Research Hub for Science, Medicine and Rehabilitation, Department of Physiotherapy, School of Therapeutic Sciences, Faculty of Health Sciences, University of the Witwatersrand, Johannesburg, South Africa
e-mail: Benita.olivier@brookes.ac.uk

A. Mansingh
Faculty of Sport, The University of the West Indies, Kingston, Jamaica
e-mail: akshai.mansingh@uwi.edu

J. W. Orchard
School of Public Health, University of Sydney, Sydney, NSW, Australia
e-mail: john.orchard@sydney.edu.au

M. S. Dhillon
Orthopaedics and Sports Medicine, FORTIS Hospital Mohali, Lamba, Punjab, India

S. Walter
Faculty of Health, University of Canterbury, Christchurch, New Zealand
e-mail: sibiboycott.noelwalter@canterbury.ac.nz

B. Olivier, J. W. Orchard (eds.), *Cricket Sports Medicine*,
https://doi.org/10.1007/978-981-96-6321-7_1

mance of a cricket team [2]. Remaining injury-free is, therefore, a means to achieve good performance and enjoyment of the game, as well as an opportunity to draw on the health benefits of sports participation.

The epidemiology of cricket injury has been explored amongst males and females and at various levels of play, from grassroots to elite. Injury rates are often presented as incidence or prevalence. While we are tempted to use these terms interchangeably, they have two different meanings (Box 1.1).

> **Box 1.1 Definitions of Prevalence and Incidence**
>
> *Incidence*: "…the number of new injuries (or new plus recurrent) occurring over a given time period"
>
> *Prevalence*: "…the average number of squad members not available for selection through injury or illness for a given time period, divided by the total number of squad members. Injury prevalence should be expressed as a percentage, representing the percentage of players missing through injury on average for that team for the season in question." [3, p. 1248]

1.2.2 Injury Rates Among Elite Male Cricketers

Let's start by looking at injury rates among male cricket players. When Soomro et al. [4] combined data from 15 studies involving 12,511 able-bodied male players and 7627 injuries, the overall injury rate was approximately 53 injuries per 10,000 hours of play. Injuries at the community level are far lower than at the elite level [5, 6]. However, injury rates among elite male players can vary considerably between countries. For instance, a nine-season review from 2010 to 2018 found that English and Welsh players sustained 102 injuries per 1000 days of play [7]. Among elite senior male Australian cricketers, a study found an injury rate of 155 injuries per 1000 days of play, with an annual injury incidence of 64 injuries per 100 players per season [8]. In New Zealand, the total new match injury incidence rates for domestic and international male cricketers ranged from 37.0 to 58.0 injuries per 10,000 player hours, depending on the level of play [9]. In contrast, a study on one elite North Indian male cricket team reported a lower rate of 3.27 injuries per 10,000 hours of play [10].

1.2.3 Injury Rates Among Elite Female Cricketers

While research on women's cricket is significantly less than research on their male counterparts, an increasing number of studies are being published on injuries among female players. The pooled injury rate among female players was 71.9 injuries per 1000 player hours [11]. For female players participating in elite cricket, injury trends described in a study from Australia revealed 600 medical-attention injuries sustained over two seasons, with 77.7% of players sustaining at least one injury. Of the injuries sustained that warranted medical treatment, around one-fifth (20.2%) caused the athletes to have some time away from the sport, while over one-third (34.7%) resulted in missed match time specifically [12]. In the United Kingdom (UK), a four-year study tracked injuries among female players enrolled in the England and Wales Cricket Board's international development academy squads. It revealed a rate of seven match time-loss injuries per 1000 player match days. Additionally, around 8.4% of players were affected by injury or illness over the course of a year. On any given day, 2.3% of players were completely unavailable due to injury or illness [13].

1.2.4 Comparing Injury Rates in Male and Female Cricketers

Comparing injury rates between males and females across different studies can be challenging due to variations in how researchers calculate and analyse the data. However, one study by Orchard et al. [14] directly compared injury rates between elite Australian male and female cricketers. The study looked at data from 453 and 297 unique male and female elite players in Australia, respectively, over seven seasons, considering that many players were involved in more than one season in their data analyses.

Some notable differences in injury patterns between the sexes were observed. Male players had a higher incidence of injuries compared to females, averaging 136 injuries per 1000 match days for males versus 101 injuries per 1000 match days for females. Additionally, a higher percentage of male players experienced match time-loss injuries, with an average of 10.4% being unavailable compared to 6.5% of female players. However, when considering all medical-attention injuries, regardless of time loss, the overall incidence was similar between male and female elite cricketers. These findings may mean that males tend to sustain more severe injuries, which leads to not being available for selection in matches, while both males and females sustained the same number of overall documented injuries (time-loss and non-time-loss injuries combined). In a separate study, researchers analysed injury data from eight men's and women's teams participating in 'The Hundred' competitions from 2021 to 2023. They described higher injury rates among males for both time-loss and non-time-loss injuries. Specifically, the study revealed that the incidence of time-loss injuries among men was 10.0 per 100 players per tournament compared to 7.9 for women. Similarly, the incidence of non-time-loss injuries among men was 26.6 per 100 players per tournament, whereas for women, it was 24.6 [15].

1.2.5 Injury Rates in Different Formats of the Game

Injury rates also seem to vary depending on the format of cricket being played. A study by Goggins et al. [7] in the UK found that more injuries occurred during One-Day matches (254 injuries per 1000 days of play), followed by T20 matches (136 injuries per 1000 days) and then First-Class Cricket (68 injuries per 1000 days). In the West Indies [16], the mean match injury rate among international and domestic male cricketers was 48.7 per 10,000 player hours in Test cricket and 40.6 per 10,000 player hours in one-day international matches. For elite Australian female players, Perera and colleagues [12] reported that the match injury rate per 10,000 player hours was highest in Twenty20 matches (600.4), followed by One-day matches (341.0) and lowest in Multi-day matches (186.5). Orchard et al.'s study [8] among elite senior male Australian cricketers over 10 seasons also found the highest match injury rates occurred in 50-over cricket, followed by 20-over matches and then First-Class matches.

1.2.6 Injury Rates in Different Levels of Play in Cricket

Injury rates differ at different levels of play. The New Zealand study by Dovbysh et al. [9] found that male cricketers in the domestic circuit had a total new match injury rate of 37.0 per 10,000 player hours, while the rate was higher at 58.0 per 10,000 player hours for international-level male players. In addition to elite and domestic levels, researchers have examined injury rates across all levels of play combined, including community and recreational cricket. To do this, some researchers have used data from emergency department or accident compensation fund records to gain insights into cricket-related injuries occurring at all levels of play, including elite, community and recreational. Injury rates at community-level cricket are lower than at the elite level (Fig. 1.1). In New Zealand, data from the national Accident Compensation Corporation (ACC) between 2005 and 2016, combining all age groups and levels, revealed that males had a higher cricket injury incidence of 64.1 per 1000 participants, compared to 36.1 injuries per 1000 female participants [17]. For Australian female cricketers across all ages and levels, Perera et al. [18] found an overall participation-adjusted injury rate of 1.5 emergency department presen-

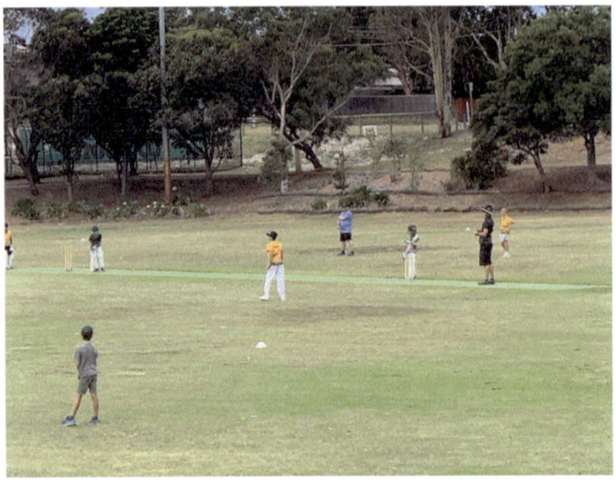

Fig. 1.1 Injury rates at community-level cricket are lower than at the elite level

tations per 1000 participants and 0.3 hospital admissions per 1000 participants. No fatalities were reported in this study. These findings are interesting as they portray the more serious incidents requiring a visit to the emergency department or leading to an accident compensation fund claim. Table 1.1 shows the injury incidence and prevalence rates amongst elite cricket players in different countries.

When looking at a comparison between injuries in junior players versus adults, the average injury incidence for junior players is 129.7 injuries per 10,000 hours of play and for adults, it is 98.2 injuries per 10,000 hours of play. While the findings come from a systematic review, one should exercise caution in interpreting them because the meta-analyses included a limited number of studies on junior participants (only three), whereas a larger number of studies (ten) focused on adult participants [4].

1.2.7 Injury Rates During Specific Cricket Tournaments

Some studies have specifically examined injury rates during major cricket tournaments and events instead of injury surveillance over a season. This data provides valuable insights into the injury risks players face in these high-intensity competition environments. For instance, during a professional women's T20 tournament in 2016 and 2017, researchers prospectively recorded injuries across 68 matches involving six teams of 15 players each [19]. They found a rate of 2.1 time-loss injuries and 12.2 non-time-loss injuries per 100 match days. On average, 4.6% of players were unavailable for match selection due to injuries during this tournament. Injury prevalence rates in tournaments will automatically be lower than year-round surveillance as players with chronic injuries who are unavailable will be excluded from tournament selection. A different study examined the injuries during the 2013 Asian Cricket Council (ACC) Under-19 Elite Cup. Among the 28 players who sustained 31 injuries throughout the tournament, seven occurred during practice sessions. The overall injury incidence rate was 292.0 per 10,000 player hours [20]. During the 2011 ICC Cricket World Cup for male players, there were 23 injuries resulting in time loss and 97 injuries without time loss, leading to an overall injury rate of 3.7 per 100 player-days (0.7 injuries with time loss and 3.0 injuries without time loss) [21]. When a research team from New Zealand realised that no formal injury surveillance was being planned for the 2015 ICC Cricket World Cup, they decided to prospectively quantify the number and type of media-reported injuries on the tournament website, official team web pages and major news websites. The media reported that 23 of the 219 players (11%) sustained injuries during the tournament [22].

1.2.8 Injury Rates in Terms of Different Roles and Activities in Cricket

Different positions and activities carry unique demands and injury risks in cricket, whether you're bowling, batting or keeping wicket. Pooled data from a systematic review [4] show that male bowlers, for instance, face a higher risk, with an average injury rate of 188.38 per 10,000 hours of play, compared to the overall rate of 53.7 hours of play. English and Welsh players tend to sustain the most injuries while bowling (41.6 injuries per 1000 days of play), followed by

Table 1.1 Injury incidence and prevalence rates amongst elite cricket players in different countries

Country	Population	Incidence	Prevalence
Australia [12]	Elite senior female players	Total match injury incidence: 424.7 injuries per 10,000 player hours	77.7% players reporting ≥1 injury
Australia [8]	Elite senior male cricketers	Match time-loss injuries: 155 injuries/1000 days of play. Annual injury incidence: 64 injuries per 100 players per season	Annual injury prevalence: 12.5%
England and Wales [13]	Female pathway players registered to an academy squad on the England and Wales Cricket Board (ECB)	Match time-loss injuries: 7 per 1000 player match days	2.3% of players unavailable for selection on any given day
England and Wales [7]	Male players from the 18 First-Class County Cricket (FCCC) clubs	Match injury incidence: 102 injuries per 1000 days of play	7.5% of players were unavailable on any given day during the domestic season when all injuries were considered (match and training)
India [10]	One elite North Indian male cricket team	'Significant' injury: 3.27 injuries per 10,000 hours of play	10.14% of players not available for selection during match and training
New Zealand [9]	Domestic and international-level male cricketers	Total new match injury incidence rates - Domestic: 37 injuries per 10,000 player hours; International: 58.0 injuries per 10,000 player hours	Domestic: 7.6% International: 10.0% not available for selection
South Africa [23]	International male cricket players	Match injury incidence: 90 injuries per 10,000 hours of matches	Match injury prevalence: 3.8%
West Indies [16]	International and domestic male cricket players	Mean match injury Incidence: Test cricket: 48.7 per 10,000 player hours One day; International cricket: 40.6 per 10,000 player hours	Test cricket: 11.3%; One-day international cricket: 8.1%

fielding (26.8 injuries per 1000 days of play) and batting (22.3 injuries per 1000 days of play) [7].

For Indian players, most lower limb injuries occur during bowling, with equal numbers during batting and fielding and fewer during wicket-keeping [10]. Among T20 female players in the World Cup, fielding has been shown to have the highest incidence of injuries (5.2 injuries per 100 match days), followed by the category 'other activities and sports' (3.5 injuries per 100 match days), fast bowling (2.5 injuries per 100 match days), batting (1.5), slow bowling (0.6) and wicketkeeping (0.3) [19].

In Australian male elite players, injury prevalence has been shown to vary by player position: Bowlers experience the highest at 20.6%, followed by batters at 7.4%, wicketkeepers at 4.7% and spinners at 6.7%. In addition, fast bowlers also tend to have more time-loss injuries [8]. Conversely, a study in the West Indies found that batters and bowlers lose an equal number of days due to injury [16].

1.2.9 Injury Rates in Terms of Body Regions and Types of Injuries

Orchard et al. [14] analysed the injury data from elite Australian male and female cricket players contracted to play for a national and/or state/ter-

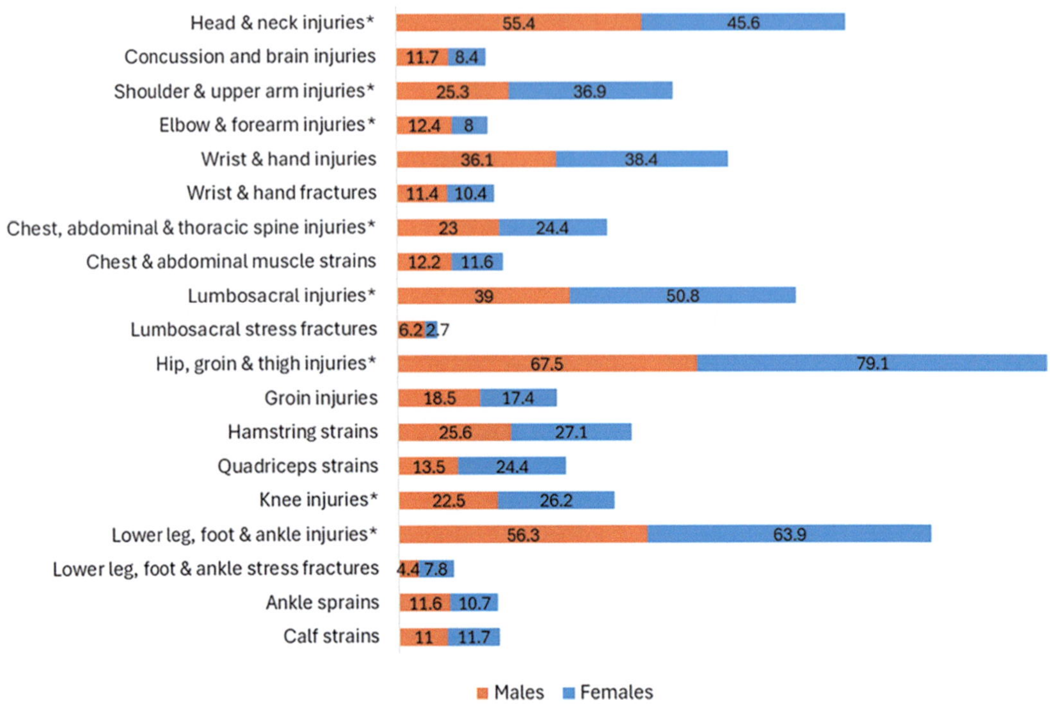

Fig. 1.2 Incidence of all injuries (incl. non-time loss) per 100 players per season by injury category (Orchard et al. [14]). (*Overarching injury category)

ritory team and/or T20 franchise between 2015–16 and 2021–22 (i.e. over seven seasons). Injury incidence per 100 players per season is categorised by injury category in Fig. 1.2, for both male and female players, hip, groin and thigh injuries were the most common, followed by lower leg, foot and ankle injuries.

1.2.9.1 Injury Rates by Body Region in Male Cricketers

Injury epidemiology studies have identified the body areas most commonly affected by injuries in cricketers across different levels and regions. Among elite male players in England and Wales, thigh injuries had the highest incidence rate at 7.4 injuries per 100 players per season. However, lumbar (lower back) injuries resulted in the highest prevalence, with 1.3% of players being unavailable on any given day during the season due to such injuries [7]. For elite male Indian players, lower limb injuries were the most frequent, followed by upper limb injuries and then back and trunk injuries. Within lower limb injuries, the ankle was the most commonly affected area, followed by the lower leg, knee and foot [10].

In the West Indies, finger injuries followed by lumbar spine were the most frequent site of injury overall [16]. Across all levels and age groups of male cricketers in New Zealand, the highest injury rates were for the hand and fingers (10.0 per 1000 participants), followed by the lumbar spine (9.1 per 1000), shoulder (7.8 per 1000), knee (7.5 per 1000) and head (7.4 per 1000) [17].

In a study on domestic and international male New Zealand cricketers, lumbar spine injuries caused the most domestic match days lost. In contrast, groin injuries resulted in the most international match days lost. Hamstring injuries were the most common during domestic play, while groin injuries were the most frequent in international cricket [9].

Among elite senior male Australian cricketers, the most common injuries were hamstring strains (8.7 per 100 players per year), followed by side and abdominal strains (6.1), wrist and hand fractures (4.7), groin injuries (4.5), lumbar injuries other than stress fractures (4.0) and lumbar stress fractures (3.2) [8].

1.2.9.2 Injury Rates by Body Region in Female Cricketers

Studies have revealed some common patterns in the body areas most prone to injuries among female cricketers across different levels of play. A systematic review by Jacobs et al. [11] found that the shoulder and knee were the body regions with the highest prevalence of injuries in female players. However, hand, wrist and fingers injuries had the highest incidence rates. In New Zealand, data from female cricketers of all ages and levels showed the highest injury rates were to the head (6.0 per 1000 participants), hand and fingers (5.1 per 1000), knee (4.2 per 1000), lower back or lumbar spine (3.6 per 1000) and ankle (3.5 per 1000) [17]. During the women's T20 World Cup, shoulder injuries were the most common (12.4% of all injuries, 1.8 per 100 match days), closely followed by lower back and knee injuries (each accounting for 11.7% of all injuries, 1.7 per 100 match days) [19]. For female cricket injuries requiring emergency department visits or hospital admissions in Australia, the head was the most frequently affected area (27.8% of emergency department visits and 28.1% of hospital admissions), followed closely by the wrist and hand (27.8% of emergency department visits and 17.4% of hospital admissions) [18]. Among elite Australian female cricketers, the most frequently injured body regions were the thigh (14.0%), wrist (12.8%), knee (11.3%), shoulder (11.0%) and lower back or lumbar spine (10.5%) [12].

1.2.9.3 Injury Rates by Body Region in Terms of Role or Activity

Among elite Australian female cricketers, the most common injury sustained during bowling was to the lower back or lumbar spine, while batters were most prone to thigh injuries. For both fielders and wicketkeepers, wrist and hand injuries were the most frequent [12]. In a study on elite male Indian cricket players, Dhillon et al. [10] found that bowling was more likely to cause lower limb injuries, while fielding was associated with a higher risk of upper limb injuries. Furthermore, they observed that fast bowlers were more prone to lower back injuries. A study on male West Indies cricketers revealed that most injuries affected either the fingers of batters or the lower backs of fast bowlers. Of the 10 lower back injuries reported in their study, four were stress fractures, with one occurring in a spin bowler. Two fast bowlers had symptomatic prolapsed intervertebral discs, and another two had facet joint inflammation. In addition, one fast bowler and one wicketkeeper had muscle strains in the lower back region [16].

1.2.10 Injury Rates for the Various Injury Types

Looking at injury types across all ages and levels of play, soft tissue injuries were the most common in both male (54.0 per 1000 participants) and female (30.2 per 1000 participants) cricketers. Fractures and dislocations were the second most frequent, occurring at rates of 7.5 per 1000 male participants and 3.3 per 1000 female participants [17]. Data from cricket-related injuries treated at emergency departments in the United States between 2000 and 2019 showed that lacerations were the most common type reported, followed by strains, sprains and then fractures. This data captures more serious injuries across all ages and levels [24]. In Australia, a study of female cricket injuries requiring emergency care found that dislocations, sprains and strains accounted for 36.4% of cases. While fractures made up a lower percentage (17.2%) of emergency department visits, they were the most common cause (19.9%) of hospital admissions [18]. Regarding injury occurrences, the vast majority (80%) were first-time injuries. Around 10% were recurrences from the same season, while the remaining 10% were recurring injuries initially sustained in previous seasons. Most (76%) were acute injuries, 16% were acute-on-chronic and 8% were chronic overuse injuries [16].

1.2.11 Injury Rates of Contact and Non-contact Injuries

When looking at the mechanisms of cricket injuries across all ages and levels of play, contact-related injuries were the most common cause for both male (48.2 per 1000 participants) and female (28.6 per 1000 participants) players. Non-contact mechanisms accounted for substantially fewer injuries, with rates of 21.3 per 1000 male participants and 10.4 per 1000 female participants [17]. However, a different pattern emerged at the elite level during the Women's T20 World Cup. Gradual onset or overuse injuries had the highest incidence at 7.9 per 100 match days, while impact or traumatic injuries occurred less frequently at 2.0 per 100 match days [19]. Among developmental- and community-level cricket contact-type injuries are more prevalent, but as the playing level increases more non-contact-type injuries are prevalent. Also, contact-type injuries are more frequent in the hand and wrist among all levels of play in comparison to lumbar and thigh injuries which are due to overuse mainly among higher levels of competition.

References

1. Pye DW. Physiotherapy in Cricket. Physiotherapy. 1965;51:121–4.
2. Goggins L, Peirce N, Stokes K, Williams S. Negative association between injuries and team success in professional cricket: a 9-year prospective cohort analysis. J Sci Med Sport. 2021;24(2):141–5. https://doi.org/10.1016/j.jsams.2020.07.007.
3. Orchard JW, Ranson C, Olivier B, Dhillon M, Gray J, Langley B, et al. International consensus statement on injury surveillance in cricket: a 2016 update. Br J Sports Med. 2016;50(20):1245–51. https://doi.org/10.1136/bjsports-2016-096125.
4. Soomro N, Strasiotto L, Sawdagar T, Lyle D, Mills D, Ferdinands R, et al. Cricket injury epidemiology in the twenty-first century: what is the burden? Sports Med. 2018;48(10):2301–16. https://doi.org/10.1007/s40279-018-0960-y.
5. Soomro N, Redrup D, Evens C, Strasiotto LP, Singh S, Lyle D, et al. Injury rate and patterns of Sydney grade cricketers: a prospective study of injuries in 408 cricketers. Postgrad Med J. 2018;94(1114):425–31. https://doi.org/10.1136/postgradmedj-2018-135861.
6. McLeod G, Murphy M, Gianotti S, Orchard JW, Fortington LV. Cricket injury in New Zealand: a study of injury insurance claims from 2008 to 2018. J Sci Med Sport. 2023;26(2):109–13. https://doi.org/10.1016/j.jsams.2022.12.001.
7. Goggins L, Peirce N, Ranson C, McCaig S, Newman D, Langley B, et al. Injuries in England and Wales elite men's domestic cricket: a nine season review from 2010 to 2018. J Sci Med Sport. 2020;23(9):836–40. https://doi.org/10.1016/j.jsams.2020.03.009.
8. Orchard JW, Kountouris A, Sims K. Incidence and prevalence of elite male cricket injuries using updated consensus definitions. Open Access J Sports Med. 2016;7:187–94. https://doi.org/10.2147/OAJSM.S117497.
9. Dovbysh T, Reid D, Shackel D. Injury incidence within male elite New Zealand cricket from the early T20 era: 2009-2015. BMJ Open Sport Exerc Med. 2021;7(4):e001168. https://doi.org/10.1136/bmjsem-2021-001168.
10. Dhillon MS, Soni RK, Aggarwal S, Dhillon H, Prabhakar S. Epidemiology of orthopedic injuries in Indian cricket: a prospective one year observational study. J Postgrad Med Edu Res. 2015;49(4):168–72.
11. Jacobs J, Olivier B, Dawood M, Perera NKP. Prevalence and incidence of injuries among female cricket players: a systematic review and meta-analysis. JBI Evid Synth. 2022;20(7):1741–90. https://doi.org/10.11124/JBIES-21-00120.
12. Perera NKP, Kountouris A, Kemp JL, Joseph C, Finch CF. The incidence, prevalence, nature, severity and mechanisms of injury in elite female cricketers: a prospective cohort study. J Sci Med Sport. 2019;22(9):1014–20. https://doi.org/10.1016/j.jsams.2019.05.013.
13. Goggins L, Warren A, Smart D, Dale S, Peirce N, McKay C, et al. Injury and player availability in women's international pathway cricket from 2015 to 2019. Int J Sports Med. 2020;41(13):944–50. https://doi.org/10.1055/a-1192-5670.
14. Orchard JW, Inge P, Sims K, Kountouris A, Saw AE, Saw R, et al. Comparison of injury profiles between elite Australian male and female cricket players. J Sci Med Sport. 2023;26(1):19–24. https://doi.org/10.1016/j.jsams.2022.12.002.
15. Williams A, Peirce N, Griffin S, Langley B, Warren A, Wedatilake T, et al. A similar injury profile observed in franchise men's and women's cricket in England and Wales: injury surveillance analysis from the first three 'the hundred' competitions. BMJ Open Sport Exerc Med. 2024;10(1):e001815. https://doi.org/10.1136/bmjsem-2023-001815.
16. Mansingh A, Harper L, Headley S, King-Mowatt J, Mansingh G. Injuries in West Indies cricket 2003–2004. Br J Sports Med. 2006;40:119–23.
17. Walter S, King D, Hume P. New Zealand cricket injury analysis based on 12 years of Accident Compensation Corporation data. BMJ Open Sport Exerc Med. 2022;8(3):e001340. https://doi.org/10.1136/bmjsem-2022-001340.

18. Perera NKP, Kemp JL, Joseph C, Finch CF. Corrigendum to "epidemiology of hospital-treated cricket injuries sustained by women from 2002–2003 to 2013-2014 in Victoria, Australia. [J. Sci. Med. Sport. 22 (2019) 1213–1218]". J Sci Med Sport. 2020;23(9):790–1. https://doi.org/10.1016/j.jsams.2020.04.009.
19. Warren A, Dale S, McCaig S, Ranson C. Injury profiles in elite women's T20 cricket. J Sci Med Sport. 2019;22(7):775–9. https://doi.org/10.1016/j.jsams.2019.01.018.
20. Das NS, Usman J, Choudhury D, Abu Osman NA. Nature and pattern of cricket injuries: the Asian cricket council Under-19, Elite Cup, 2013. PLoS One. 2014;9(6):e100028. https://doi.org/10.1371/journal.pone.0100028.
21. Ranson C, Hurley R, Rugless L, Mansingh A, Cole J. International cricket injury surveillance: a report of five teams competing in the ICC Cricket World Cup 2011. Br J Sports Med. 2013;47(10):637–43. https://doi.org/10.1136/bjsports-2012-091783.
22. Walter S, Petersen C, Basu A. International cricket injury surveillance: A media- based injury report on the ICC men's Cricket World Cup 2015. J Sport Exer Sci. 2020;4:84–9
23. Stretch R, Raffan R. Injury patterns of South African international cricket players over a two-season period. SAJSM. 2011;23(2):45–9.
24. Forrester MB. Cricket-related injuries treated in United States emergency departments. Am J Emerg Med. 2021;45:389–91. https://doi.org/10.1016/j.ajem.2020.09.010.

Injury Surveillance in Cricket: Imperatives and Challenges

2

Benita Olivier, Candice MacMillan, Oluchukwu Loveth Obiora, Akshai Mansingh, John W. Orchard, Mandeep S. Dhillon, and Sibi Walter

2.1 Introduction

Injury surveillance plays a vital role in identifying injury patterns, understanding risk factors and informing the development of targeted injury prevention strategies. Implementing an effective injury surveillance system is crucial for monitoring the prevalence and incidence of injuries across all levels of cricket, from the elite ranks down to the grassroots community-level. However, establishing such a system poses significant challenges, including issues related to resources, compliance, standardisation and data quality. This chapter delves into the importance of injury surveillance in cricket, outlining its key benefits and exploring the obstacles that must be overcome to ensure successful implementation and long-term sustainability of these initiatives. Additionally, it discusses the essential components of an effective injury-tracking system, emphasising the need for standardised injury definitions, systematic data collection processes and user-friendly platforms to facilitate accurate and comprehensive injury reporting.

Supplementary Information The online version contains supplementary material available at https://doi.org/10.1007/978-981-96-6321-7_2.

B. Olivier (✉)
Centre for Healthy Living Research, Oxford Institute of Applied Health Research, Faculty of Health, Science and Technology, Oxford Brookes University, Oxford, UK

Wits Cricket Research Hub for Science, Medicine and Rehabilitation, Department of Physiotherapy, School of Therapeutic Sciences, Faculty of Health Sciences, University of the Witwatersrand, Johannesburg, South Africa
e-mail: Benita.olivier@brookes.ac.uk

C. MacMillan
Faculty of Health Sciences, Department of Physiology, University of Pretoria, Pretoria, Gauteng, South Africa
e-mail: Candice.macmillan@up.ac.za

O. L. Obiora
College of Nursing, Texas Woman's University, Houston, TX, USA
e-mail: oobiora1@twu.edu

A. Mansingh
Faculty of Sport, The University of the West Indies, Kingston, Jamaica
e-mail: akshai.mansingh@uwi.edu

J. W. Orchard
School of Public Health, University of Sydney, Sydney, NSW, Australia
e-mail: john.orchard@sydney.edu.au

M. S. Dhillon
Orthopaedics and Sports Medicine, FORTIS Hospital Mohali, Lamba, Punjab, India

S. Walter
Faculty of Health, University of Canterbury, Christchurch, New Zealand
e-mail: sibiboycott.noelwalter@canterbury.ac.nz

B. Olivier, J. W. Orchard (eds.), *Cricket Sports Medicine*,
https://doi.org/10.1007/978-981-96-6321-7_2

2.2 The Importance of Injury Surveillance

Injury surveillance is the ongoing and systematic collection, analysis, interpretation and dissemination of data related to injuries occurring in a sport or athletic population. It involves monitoring the incidence, severity, causes and patterns of injuries to identify risk factors, detect clusters or trends and inform the development and evaluation of injury prevention and treatment strategies.

The Translating Research into Injury Prevention Practice (TRIPP) model, shown in Fig. 2.1, emphasises the importance of injury surveillance as a crucial first step towards effective injury prevention. Finch [1] proposed the TRIPP model, which is a framework that outlines the systematic process of developing and implementing effective injury prevention strategies in sports.

The key steps involved are as follows:

- Step 1: Injury surveillance: The ongoing and systematic collection of injury data to establish the extent of the injury problem, identify risk factors and inform subsequent prevention efforts.

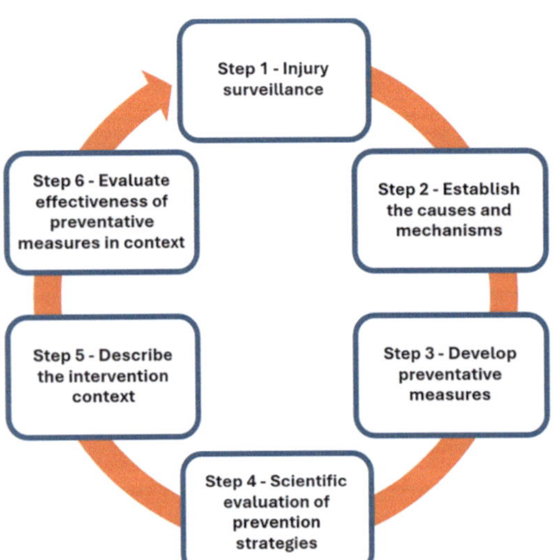

Fig. 2.1 The key steps involved in the Translating Research into Injury Prevention Practice (TRIPP) model

- Step 2: Establish the causes and mechanisms of injury: Using injury surveillance data to investigate and understand the causes and mechanisms underlying the injuries.
- Step 3: Develop preventative measures: Based on the knowledge gained from the previous steps, designing and implementing preventive measures or interventions tailored to the specific injury problem.
- Step 4: 'Ideal conditions'/scientific evaluation of prevention strategies: Rigorously evaluating the effectiveness of the implemented prevention strategies through further injury surveillance and research.
- Step 5: Describe the intervention context to inform the implementation strategies: Examine the facilitators and barriers to adopting and implementing the prevention strategies in the real-world.
- Step 6: Evaluate the effectiveness of the preventative measures in the implementation context: Ongoing monitoring, evaluation and refinement of prevention strategies implemented in the real-world based on the feedback loop provided by injury surveillance data.

The TRIPP model emphasises the crucial role of injury surveillance as the foundation for developing evidence-based, targeted and effective injury prevention approaches in sports. Injury surveillance has helped us identify the types of injuries more common to the sport and has led to many reductions in incidence. For example, the severity of lumbar stress fractures in young fast bowlers has decreased over the past decades due to the emphasis on early detection [2] and the advances in treatment techniques [3]. This is due to the clear identification of prevalence and incidence, as well as causative factors (body strength, style of bowling and bowling demands) and their correction or control. Close monitoring of the changes in injury trends may lead to reductions in these new injuries with similar interventions.

There are several significant benefits of implementing injury surveillance systems for cricket teams (see Box 2.1 for a summary):

- Identify injury patterns and trends: Systematic injury data collection quantifies the impact of injuries through metrics like injury incidence rates and time lost from the sport. It allows for recognising common injury types, body regions affected and patterns over time.
- Determine injury risk factors: With detailed data on athlete exposures (training/competition loads) and contextual factors, risk factors like playing positions, training loads, equipment issues, etc., can be investigated.
- Develop targeted prevention plans: The insights from injury surveillance inform the design of evidence-based preventive interventions tailored to the specific injury problem in that sport/team. This leads to the evidence-based design of position-specific strength and conditioning programmes and bowling and throwing workload guidelines for developmental stage cricketers.
- Evaluate prevention effectiveness: Continued surveillance after implementing preventive measures tracks changes in injury rates over time, evaluating the real-world impact of the interventions.
- Facilitate research: The centralised injury database enables further epidemiological studies on injury causation and mechanisms to guide future prevention strategies.
- Benchmark and compare to learn: Standard injury definitions allow comparing injury rates/patterns across teams, leagues and regions to identify best practices and areas for improvement.

Box 2.1 The Benefits of a Functional Injury Surveillance System

- Identify injury patterns and trends.
- Determine injury risk factors.
- Develop targeted prevention plans.
- Evaluate prevention effectiveness.
- Facilitate research.
- Benchmark and compare to learn.

Overall, implementing injury surveillance provides the critical data-driven foundation for a practical sports injury prevention cycle, from problem identification to intervention design, implementation and evaluation.

2.3 Challenges of Injury Surveillance

Implementing a structured, standardised injury-tracking system is the optimal thing to do but does not come without challenges. Many of these challenges are more pronounced at lower resourced levels, such as the community-level of play, which involves clubs and schools.

Ekegren et al. [4] identified several obstacles that can hinder the successful implementation and long-term sustainability of an injury surveillance system:

- Personal factors: Injury surveillance may not be considered a priority or essential task by those involved.
- Social and contextual factors: staff turnover, injuries not being reported consistently, lack of support from leadership and lack of dedicated staff.
- System-related factors: the time-consuming process of uploading injury data, technical issues with the system, extensive data requirements and the adjustment period needed to get used to a new system.

Making an injury-tracking system work by overcoming these barriers largely depends on having enough financial and operational resources [5]. This includes costs like purchasing software licenses, getting technical support, ensuring people comply with the system and providing training on data collection [6]. Community-level cricket organisations, especially, often lack the resources or expertise to implement and maintain an ongoing injury surveillance system.

Injury data collection in community sports often relies on volunteers, and tracking injuries is not considered mandatory [4]. Many community-level teams don’t have a dedicated sports physician or physiotherapist. When an injury-tracking system is in place, the coaching staff are expected to record injuries since they are the closest and most consistent members working with the team. However, capturing injury data is not part of a coach's typical responsibilities, and it's not mandatory for them to do so, which makes them less likely to comply [4]. In contrast, at the elite level, there's often a contractual obligation for team medical staff, like sports physicians or physiotherapists, to report injuries as part of their job duties. They understand and accept this responsibility as part of their role.

These hurdles in injury-tracking can lead to unreliable data. This makes it hard to create targeted prevention plans, assess their effectiveness over time, or compare them to other sports. Data issues can stem from unclear injury definitions, missing information, misdiagnoses, missed cases and entry errors. Having a transparent system with consistent injury definitions is one way to enhance data quality and usefulness.

In the absence of a cricket-specific injury surveillance system, alternative data sources may be helpful, although not ideal. In New Zealand, residents of all age groups can claim treatment and rehabilitation costs for any sporting injury through the Accident Compensation Corporation (ACC) [7]. The ACC maintains these longitudinal sports injury records. The ACC records specific to cricket injuries can be used to understand cricket-related injury information. Even though these records provide valuable injury information, they have limitations, as important injury information such as cricket playing position, cricket-specific injury onset activity, specific injury diagnosis and time loss due to injury are not recorded. Therefore, national cricket boards are recommended to implement a rigorous injury surveillance system for community-level cricketers. If national boards do not oversee community-level cricket, it may be more realistic to request that any insurers for community cricket need to conduct injury surveillance and periodically publicly release the results.

Overcoming the various personal, social, operational and resource barriers remains a significant challenge when implementing a standardised injury surveillance system, especially at the community-level, where dedicated staffing and budgets are limited. However, recognising and proactively addressing these potential obstacles is crucial for successfully implementing and sustaining an effective injury-tracking programme across all levels of cricket. In the next section, we'll discuss the key characteristics a cricket injury-tracking system must have to succeed.

2.4 Effective Injury Surveillance Implementation

An injury-tracking system aligned with global consensus standards is crucial for elite and community cricket. Clear, standardised and systematic data collection processes and standard definitions of injuries help ensure the data gathered is accurate and useful. It also enables meaningful comparisons across communities, countries and regions by ensuring consistent injury definitions and data collection methods.

One initiative to promote consistency has been the development of an international consensus statement with standard injury definitions and surveillance methods [8]. While already implemented at the elite level in some nations, community cricket should adopt these internationally accepted standards for optimal data sharing and analysis. This chapter includes supplementary material, which is a downloadable injury report form.

Injury definitions can be more easily implemented at the elite or professional level since the sports medicine staff have medical training. However, at the community-level, the injury definition shouldn't rely on a healthcare professional's diagnosis since they may not be readily available. A consistent player-reported injury definition should be used to ensure all injuries are captured and enhance the system's effectiveness [8] (see Box 2.2). It's ideal to record both injuries requiring time off and those not, as non-time-loss injuries often progress to time-loss injuries; however, reporting of non-time-loss injuries is often less complete [9]. If only time-loss injuries are recorded, this leads to underreporting of overall injuries. Also, at the developmental and community-levels of cricket, athletes might play multiple sports and injuries might not be solely due to cricket. It is ideal to record injuries that occur when playing other sports but which impact participation and performance in cricket.

An injury classification system in sports medicine is a standardised framework or taxonomy used to accurately categorise and code different types of injuries. It serves two primary purposes:

- To classify diagnoses into broader parent categories allows for easy tabulation and summarisation of injury data from various studies or sources. This promotes clarity and consistency when reporting overall injury patterns or trends.
- To create a comprehensive database from which specific injury cases can be extracted for detailed research. Here, the level of diagnostic detail is fundamental to enable in-depth analysis of certain injury types.

The Orchard Sports Injury and Illness Classification System (OSIICS) [10] is an example of a system designed to meet these objectives. It offers a comprehensive taxonomy to consistently code and organise sports injury data, enabling clear communication of overall injury patterns and detailed analysis of particular injury types for research purposes in sports medicine.

Online injury-tracking can work well if thorough data collection processes are followed [11]. Moreover, making the system and platform user-friendly is key to success, encouraging participation and accurate reporting [4, 6]. One challenge is that players may have recall bias, struggling to accurately remember injuries after a long period [1]. Using a weekly injury questionnaire can help limit this bias.

2.5 Research-Practice Partnerships toward Successful Injury Surveillance

Establishing a purposeful collaboration between a research institution, such as a university, and a community cricket entity, such as a high school or cricket club, could serve as an effective approach to surmount common obstacles and yield reciprocal advantages [12]. During the planning phase of their cricket injury research, researchers encounter obstacles in pinpointing the pressing real-world issues, translating them into relevant research questions and securing access to research participants. Furthermore, research entities critically require a platform where research findings can be applied in a sports context to catalyse positive change. Conversely, schools and clubs often lack the necessary resources to design or implement an evidence-based injury surveillance system and may even be unaware of its advantages. By working closely together, practice-informed research can be generated which has the potential for vast impact.

Implementing a user-friendly system with clear injury definitions and systematic data collection processes is vital for capturing comprehensive, high-quality injury data that can inform prevention and management strategies across all levels of cricket.

Box 2.2 Injury Definitions

Match time-loss injury: 'Any injury or other medical condition that either: (1) prevents a player from being fully available for selection for a major match or (2), during a major match, causes a player to be unable to bat, bowl or keep wicket when required by either the rules or the team's captain'.

General time-loss injury: 'A general time-loss injury is any injury (or illness) that would have resulted in a player being considered unavailable for match-play, irrespective of whether a match or training was actually scheduled'.

Medical attention injury: 'A medical attention injury (or illness) is any health-related condition that required medical (or medical staff) attention and had the potential to affect cricket training or playing. It therefore includes time-loss and non-time-loss injuries'.

Player-reported injury: 'A player-reported injury is any condition which was considered to represent an injury by a player who is under survey'. [8]

2.6 Supplementary Material: Recommended Variables and Example Injury Report Form

2.6.1 Recommended Variables to Include in an Injury Report Form

Use these variables to create a basic online or hard copy data capture form to monitor injuries in cricket. Add more variables to this form based on your context's needs. The definition of injury needs to be defined beforehand, and guidance can be found in Orchard et al. [8]. The Injury Consensus paper of Orchard et al. [8] will be a helpful guide in creating an injury report form.

Player name and surname.
Date of injury.
Injury captured by.
Date injury resolved.
Date cleared to play.

Diagnoses: Use the Orchard Sports Injury and Illness Classification System (OSIICS) [10].

If it is not practical to use the OSIICS, add the following to the injury report form:

Injury type.
Injury region/body area.
Dominant/non-dominant.
Impact/non-impact.
First-time/recurring.

Injury significance:

- Time-loss.
- Non-time-loss.

Activity of onset:

- Bowling.
- Batting.
- Fielding.
- Wicket keeping.
- Other.

2.6.2 Example Injury Report Form

The following injury report form was used by Benita Olivier as part of the Fearless Fast Bowling project. The form was built in REDCap, and branching logic was used to ensure that only the relevant questions were shown. Download the Microsoft Word version or the exported REDCap form as Electronic Supplementary Material.

References

1. Finch C. A new framework for research leading to sports injury prevention. J Sci Med Sport. 2006;9(1–2):3–9; discussion 10. https://doi.org/10.1016/j.jsams.2006.02.009.
2. Saw A, Eales B, Jones N, Obst A, Smith M, Kountouris A, et al. Lumbar bone stress injuries and nonunited defects in elite Australian cricket players. Clin J Sport Med. 2023;34:44. https://doi.org/10.1097/jsm.0000000000001132.
3. Pardiwala DN, Rao NN, Varshney AV. Injuries in cricket. Sports Health. 2018;10(3):217–22. https://doi.org/10.1177/1941738117732318.
4. Ekegren CL, Donaldson A, Gabbe BJ, Finch CF. Implementing injury surveillance systems alongside injury prevention programs: evaluation of an online surveillance system in a community setting. Inj Epidemiol. 2014;1(1):19. https://doi.org/10.1186/s40621-014-0019-y.
5. Ekegren CL, Gabbe BJ, Finch CF. Sports injury surveillance systems: a review of methods and data quality. Sports Med. 2016;46(1):49–65. https://doi.org/10.1007/s40279-015-0410-z.
6. Finch CF, Goode N, Shaw L, Salmon PM. End-user experiences with two incident and injury reporting systems designed for led outdoor activities – challenges for implementation of future data systems. Inj Epidemiol. 2019;6:39. https://doi.org/10.1186/s40621-019-0214-y.
7. Walter S, King D, Hume P. New Zealand cricket injury analysis based on 12 years of Accident Compensation Corporation data. BMJ Open Sport Exerc Med. 2022;8(3):e001340. https://doi.org/10.1136/bmjsem-2022-001340.
8. Orchard JW, Ranson C, Olivier B, Dhillon M, Gray J, Langley B, et al. International consensus statement on injury surveillance in cricket: a 2016 update. Br J Sports Med. 2016;50(20):1245–51. https://doi.org/10.1136/bjsports-2016-096125.
9. Olivier B, Lala B, Gillion N. The cricketer's shoulder and injury: asymmetries in range of movement and muscle length. S Afr J Physiother. 2020;76(1):a754. https://doi.org/10.4102/sajp.v76i1.754.

10. Orchard JW, Rio E, Crossley KM, Orchard JJ, Mountjoy M. Orchard Sports Injury and Illness Classification System (OSIICS) version 15. J Sport Health Sci. 2024;13(4):599–604. https://doi.org/10.1016/j.jshs.2024.03.004.
11. Ebrahimi Varkiani M, Alizadeh MH, Rajabi R, Minoonejad H. Comparing two sports injury surveillance systems: a novel systematic approach. Phys Treat Spec Phys Ther. 2020;10(3):135–44. https://doi.org/10.32598/ptj.10.3.421.1.
12. Olivier B, Obiora OL, MacMillan C, Finch C. Injury surveillance in community cricket: a new innings for South Africa. S Afr J Physiother. 2022;78(1):1756. https://doi.org/10.4102/sajp.v78i1.1756.

Injury Risks Associated with Match Conditions in Cricket

3

John W. Orchard, Akshai Mansingh, and Benita Olivier

3.1 Introduction

Many outdoor sports have the delightful aspect of varying environmental conditions, making them less monotonous and predictable. They include tennis with varying court surfaces and the football codes, where play proceeds in sunny, rainy or even snowy conditions. There is an argument that multi-day (red ball) cricket has greater variation in play due to environmental conditions than any other sport, based on the varying effect that pitch conditions will have on the bounce of the ball. This is a particular contrast between cricket and its sister sport of baseball, where the ball doesn't bounce before being hit and where weather conditions have little effect on the game. Plenty has been written on the tactical relevance of variation in cricket pitch conditions over the years, including the regular complaints from visiting teams about pitch conditions favouring the home side.

By understanding the intricate relationships between playing conditions, demands and injury risks, the cricket community can work towards creating a safer and more sustainable environment for this beloved sport. The focus of this chapter will be to consider the extent to which injuries result from the inevitable variation in style of play depending on the prevailing conditions.

There are three main forms of cricket, with the shorter formats becoming more popular in the last decade. First Class and Test cricket are four- and five-day matches, respectively. Each day typically lasts 6–7 hours. Much of the early data on injury rates is based on this form of cricket. One-day cricket is a 50 over-per-side format which is played over 6–7 hours, whereas the most common short format, T20 comprises 20 overs per side and lasts 3–4 hours. Shorter formats still are also evolving, such as T10 and The Hundred. The intensity and frequency of matches are likely to impact injury types and rates.

J. W. Orchard
School of Public Health, University of Sydney, Sydney, NSW, Australia
e-mail: john.orchard@sydney.edu.au

A. Mansingh
Faculty of Sport, The University of the West Indies, Kingston, Jamaica
e-mail: akshai.mansingh@uwi.edu

B. Olivier (✉)
Centre for Healthy Living Research, Oxford Institute of Applied Health Research, Faculty of Health, Science and Technology, Oxford Brookes University, Oxford, UK

Wits Cricket Research Hub for Science, Medicine and Rehabilitation, Department of Physiotherapy, School of Therapeutic Sciences, Faculty of Health Sciences, University of the Witwatersrand, Johannesburg, South Africa
e-mail: Benita.Olivier@brookes.ac.uk

B. Olivier, J. W. Orchard (eds.), *Cricket Sports Medicine*,
https://doi.org/10.1007/978-981-96-6321-7_3

3.2 Limited Overs Cricket Protects Against Injury in Fast Bowlers but May Increase Injury Risks for Batters and Fielders

Cricket has traditionally been considered a low-injury-risk sport in general, with the exception of being a high-injury-risk for pace bowlers at the elite level [1, 2]. Higher injury prevalences were reported in pace bowlers than in other positions, particularly studies in the 2000s and early 2010s, which had a focus on red ball men's cricket [3–5]. Tournament injury prevalence, involving limited overs cricket where all bowlers have personal bowling limits (Fig. 3.1), is consistently lower than red ball cricket [6–8]. The major concern for fast bowlers with limited overs cricket is deconditioning if and when they drop from or return to red ball (unlimited over) cricket [9, 10]. The injury prevalence of fast bowlers in women's cricket—where red ball (unlimited overs) play is uncommon—is lower than for male fast bowlers and much closer to the other positions in women's cricket [11].

Anecdotally, male pace bowlers who retire from red ball cricket and concentrate on bowling for T20 franchises around the world (with a match day limit of 24 balls) suffer far fewer injuries than those playing red ball cricket.

Not only are the shorter formats (T20 in particular) becoming more popular, but the demands on and expectations from players are also changing. Additionally, leagues with multinational players are springing up globally, increasing the time played by most players. In this format especially, players are diving acrobatically to take catches or to stop balls going to the boundary. Fielders are expected to throw the ball at full speed to prevent runs. Bowlers tend to bowl flat and fast (even spin bowlers) when compared to other formats. As they only bowl four overs per match, the intensity of each over is full effort. And batters are not only swinging to hit more boundaries but are now trying to hit the ball as far as they possibly can as the sixes are being measured and projected as a quasi-competition.

The rates of certain injuries are likely to increase. For example, shoulder injuries from falling on the shoulder, attempting to take difficult catches, throwing the ball from the deep repeatedly, or trying to hit the ball as far as possible many times and over are likely to increase. Even spin bowlers who quicken rotation of their shoulders with each delivery could potentially have increased impingement. Hamstring and quadriceps strains from sprinting for runs for batsmen or to stop runs by fielders are likely to increase. A few instances of a relatively new injury are being reported—that of complete tears of intercostal muscles of the ribs in players who swing hard and miss the ball completely. The force generated in trying to hit the ball as far as possible engages the intercostal muscles, which become susceptible to tearing, especially if contact with the ball is not made. As the ball is being hit harder and more catches are attempted in the deep, finger injuries including fractures are likely to increase.

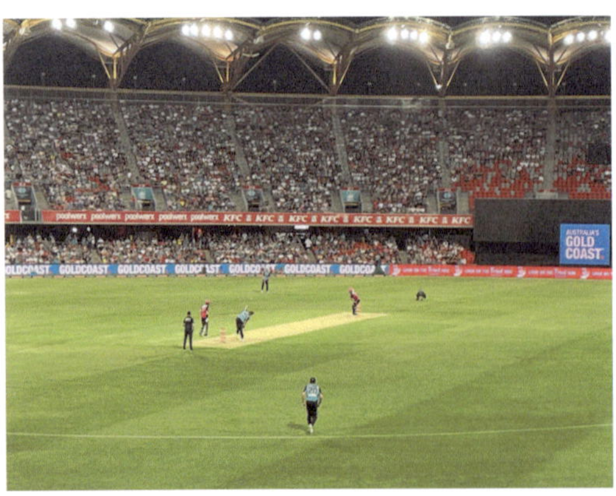

Fig. 3.1 Limited over cricket leads to less over-bowling of the injury-prone pace bowlers, but fielding athleticism may lead to more injuries

3.3 Spin-Friendly Conditions Protect Fast Bowlers

Bibliometric analysis of cricket injury research has found that authors from Australia and England have published far more than those from India [12], a finding not in keeping with India being the major financial powerhouse of the modern cricket world. One explanation is that red ball cricket in India has traditionally had *far less* of a problem with injuries due to a focus on spin-friendly bowling conditions. Spin-friendly conditions involve dry pitches with very little grass (Fig. 3.2). The seam of the new ball (which leads to pace bowlers getting both swing and deviation off the seam) is blunted very quickly in dry conditions, rendering pace bowling less effective than in well-grassed conditions. However, a dry pitch is prone to wear, which leads to uneven bounce. The wear occurs away from the stump-to-stump line, which is where pace bowlers need to pitch the ball to be effective. Spin bowlers can threaten the stumps with wider deliveries, as greater deviation is available after bouncing from spin (slow) deliveries than pace deliveries, making spin bowling particularly effective on worn pitches after a few days of play. Spin bowlers, with a slower run-up, are also less prone to injury because they generate less force through the legs and back than pace bowlers. Because spin bowlers are able to resist injury and they bowl a far higher percentage of overs in red ball cricket in spin-friendly conditions (due to their greater efficacy), pace bowlers (the higher risk position) are spared from overuse injury.

In red ball cricket, spin-friendly conditions may lead to a higher risk of contact injury (including concussion) in the fielders. Fielding positions close to the bat (short leg, silly mid-off, short cover) are much more commonly used to try to take catches off spin bowlers. The designation 'silly' for a fielding position probably makes some sense that you might be considered 'silly' to field there. Protective equipment, other than gloves, including helmets, are allowed in these close-in fielding positions.

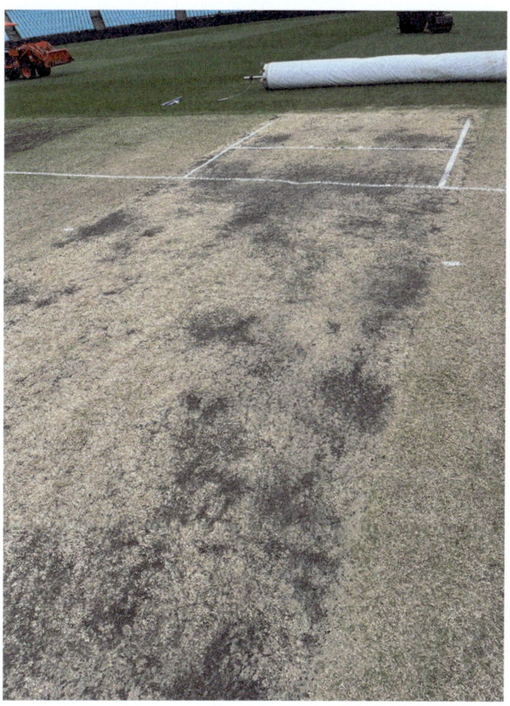

Fig. 3.2 A worn or dry cricket pitch is most likely to favour spin bowling

3.4 Seam-Friendly Conditions Also Protect Fast Bowlers

There is such a pitch as 'seam-friendly' or pace bowler-friendly. It shouldn't be considered the opposite of a 'spin-friendly' pitch, as both these types are bowler-friendly as opposed to batter-friendly. It is just that the type of bowler who benefits most is different. In terms of moisture, seam-friendly conditions are perhaps the opposite of spin-friendly. Whereas the Indian subcontinent is the home of spin-friendly batting conditions (which are maximal late in a red ball match when the pitch is worn), England is the traditional home of the seam-friendly pitch (which is often most so on the opening morning of a red ball match). This is partially due to the higher moisture content of the pitch, perhaps partially due to the grass type and humidity, and also partially due to the chosen ball for First Class cricket in the UK. English pitches typically use ryegrass (a cool-season grass), which is a non-branching grass that holds together with rhizomes (below the surface) that retain moisture. Traditionally, a generous coverage of grass is left on the pitch at the start of the red ball game, making the conditions even softer early in the match. Finally, Duke's ball (Fig. 3.3) is used for matches in England, which has a more pronounced seam than other balls that retain their elevation for longer, and hence the 'new ball' swings for longer.

Whilst it would appear that if pace bowlers have to bowl more often in seam-friendly conditions, they would bowl more overs and might suffer more injuries, they have the benefit of bowling fewer overs if they can quickly dismiss the opposition. Matches in England are more likely to be finished quickly if wickets fall in rapid succession, which itself can limit over-bowling.

There may also be a trend towards fewer contact batting injuries (hand injuries and concussions) in matches played on seam-friendly pitches (Fig. 3.4).

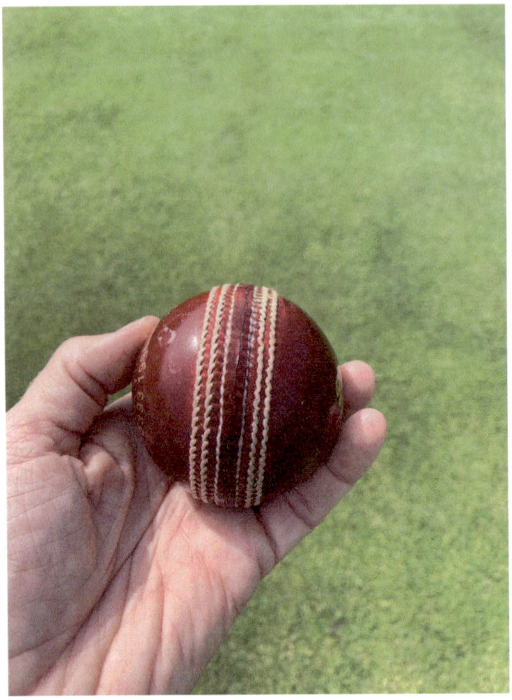

Fig. 3.3 The Dukes ball with a very pronounced seam

Because of the extra ball movement, it encourages bowlers to 'pitch the ball on a fuller length', as all bowled, LBW and caught by the keeper or slips cordon are in play.

3.5 Batting-Friendly Conditions in Red Ball Cricket Probably Lead to Greater Injuries

The triangular opposite of the spin-friendly and seam-friendly pitch is the batting-friendly pitch, with an even but short cut of grass (Fig. 3.5). The new ball quickly flattens out and does not swing for long, and there are minimal areas of uneven soil that might be helpful to spin bowlers. Most white ball (limited overs) matches have the pitch prepared in a way that will be helpful to the batters on the basis that the limited overs would not lead to boring play. For a red ball match, the ground staff are encouraged to avoid the extremes,

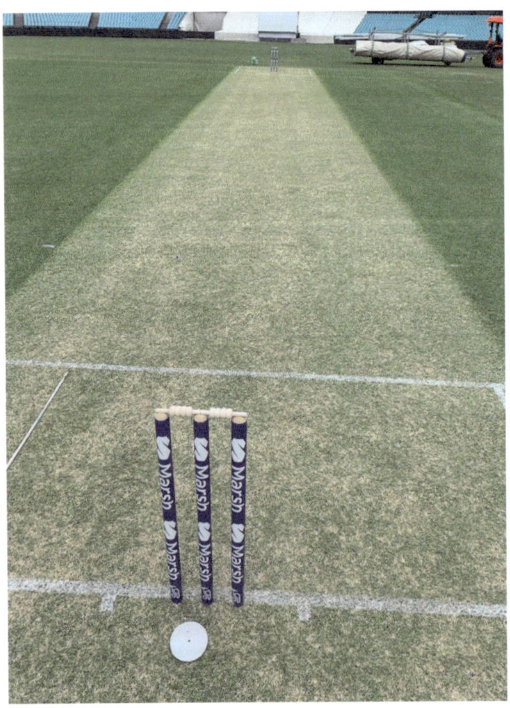

Fig. 3.4 A well-grassed pitch that would be expected to favour pace-bowling early in the match

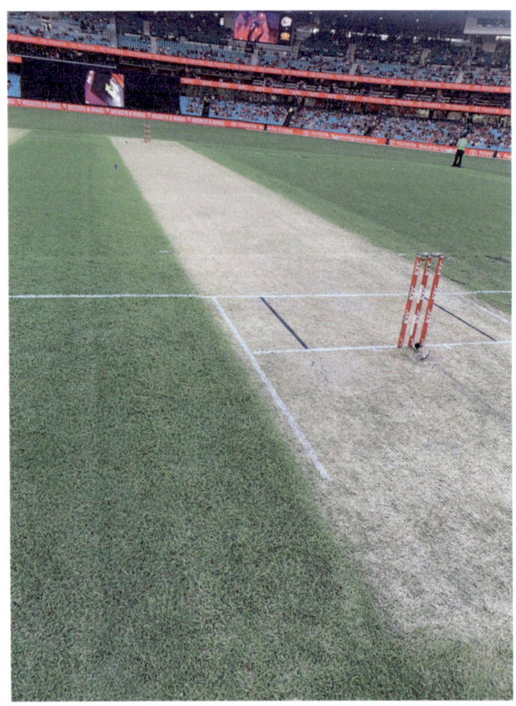

Fig. 3.5 A minimally grassed but even pitch which would be expected to lead to helpful conditions for batters

giving the pace bowlers some encouragement with the new ball, especially on day 1; the batters good conditions to bat in, especially on day 2; and the spin bowlers good conditions to bowl in late in the match. Overcast and humid conditions might lead to the grass staying fresher for longer early in the game. In contrast, sunny and windy conditions might dry the grass out more quickly and initially favour batters.

If a pitch does favour batters in a red ball match, scoring may be higher, and innings will tend to last longer. The primary increase in injury risk might be to the pace bowlers on the bowling team, who might be called upon to bowl higher numbers of overs if wickets are not forthcoming. There have been studies showing higher workloads leading to more injuries in bowlers [2, 13–15]. A secondary concern is that a non-responsive pitch might lead to more 'short-pitched bowling'. If the ball is not moving at all off the seam, then full-pitched balls can more easily be scored from by the batters. Short-pitched bowling can slightly slow the scoring rate if the batters are on top. It means that balls hit to the outfield are usually in the air for longer. If a batter is less likely to be out bowled or LBW and slips are not in place, then the major mode of dismissal becomes the catch in the infield or outfield, which is slightly more common off short-pitched bowling. However, short-pitched bowling can lead to a higher risk of concussion and hand injuries [16, 17]. When protective equipment was not as advanced, it was considered unsporting to resort to short-pitched bowling due to injury risk to the batters (most famously in the 'Bodyline' Ashes series of the 1930s). However, due to much better protective equipment, it is now considered to be within the spirit of the game to bowl short unless the batter is, say, a particularly poor no. 11.

3.6 Other Pitch and Field Considerations

Drop-in pitches (used at cricket venues where the ground is shared with other sports, like the various football codes), on grounds which regularly use them, have a reputation for being batter-friendly. The pitches must be moved in on a solid block, which may be less likely to crumble under dry weather conditions. In the 2024 ICC Men's T20 World Cup, drop-in pitches were used for the first time in the United States, which conversely led to variable bounce and subsequent injury fears as well as curtailed free batting, which lowered scores.

The Eden Park ground in Auckland has a drop-in pitch (Fig. 3.6) with a dual personality. Because the drop in the block is very small, the turf on either side of the pitch is very soft and lush, and the new ball does not lose its seam quickly, meaning that new ball conditions strongly favour seam bowling for an extended period. However, as soon as the ball loses its traditional swing, there is little further wear on the ball and little ability to develop reverse swing. Being a ground which is also of small dimensions (and also a rugby stadium), after the new ball conditions have ceased, it often then becomes a very batter-friendly venue.

In some grounds practice pitches are used for the 'nets' if space is unavailable outside (Fig. 3.7). This can sometimes be a separate square wide of the centre-wicket block (Fig. 3.8). This might lead to additional fielding injuries diving on the harder surface. It also might help the bowlers achieve 'reverse swing' later in an innings. The hard surface increases the natural wear on the ball if one side is kept polished and the other deteriorates hitting the harder surface.

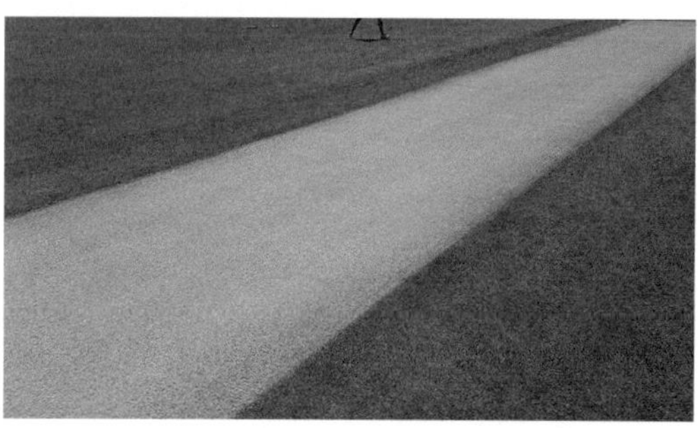

Fig. 3.6 A drop-in pitch at Eden Park in Auckland with lush grass coverage immediately on either side of the pitch

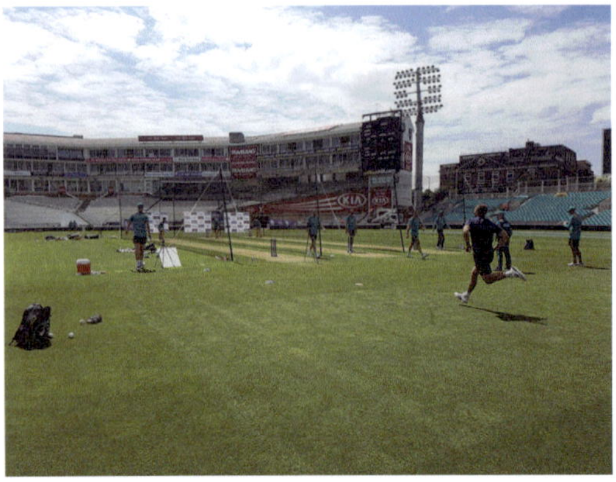

Fig. 3.7 Warm-up nets on the actual playing field at The Oval, London

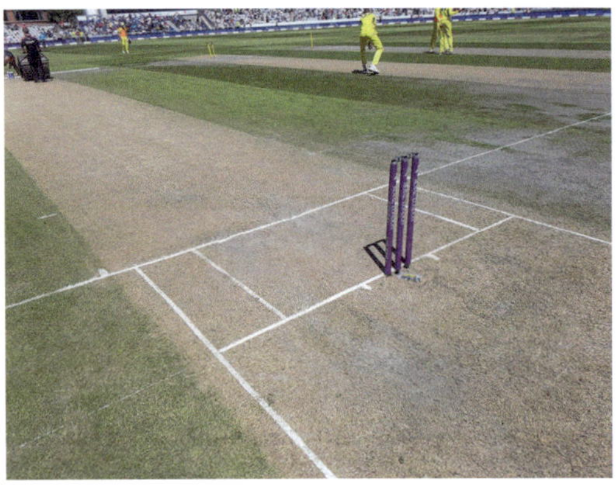

Fig. 3.8 A series of hard-surface additional pitches adjacent to the actual match pitch at Old Trafford ground, Manchester, the opposite scenario to the Eden Park pitch in Fig. 3.6

In First Class matches played in a day-night format using a hybrid 'pink ball', conditions tend to be highly variable. The pink ball becomes flatter than the traditional red ball in less time, making daytime batting more friendly than usual to the batting team. Batting under lights, particularly in twilight, appears to be more difficult than usual, perhaps less due to excessive seam movement and more due to the pink ball being less easy to see than a white ball under lights. Concerns about whether reduced vision might lead to more fielding or batting injuries when playing in pink ball conditions have been raised. Because these matches are less common, there is not much data to assess whether any of these concerns are valid.

Cricket is a summer sport which has a low tolerance for playing in the rain. Although injury risk is cited as one of the reasons for ceasing play when it is raining (due to the risk of players slipping over), it is at least as important that the conditions change markedly when it rains, possibly making the contest unfair. It is considered important to cover the pitch in longer matches to keep it from becoming moist or flooded. Many years ago, when pitches were left uncovered when it rained, conditions tended to strongly favour spin bowling on what were called 'sticky wickets'.

3.7 Large Grounds Lead to More Running-Related Injuries

Cricket grounds around the world vary in size, another factor which delights cricket fans, again leading to variations in the style of play. The biggest grounds in the world tend to be in Australia. Part of this is due to ample available space in Australia in the late 1800s when cricket grounds were becoming established. However, an even greater influence has been the sport of Australian Football. Australian Football was originally construed as a means to keep cricketers fit during the winter months, but it has become the football code with the largest grounds and highest number of players on the field (18 per team) [18]. All major Test match cricket venues in Australia also host Australian Football games in the winter, making them all larger than grounds in most other countries. The largest cricket ground (playing field wise) in the world is reputed to be the Melbourne Cricket Ground. In matches in Australia, the players tend to run more in the field and when batting. The count of boundaries (4 s and 6 s), where batters and fielders stop running, is lower on the larger Australian grounds, whereas there are more 2 s and 3 s where both batters and fielders need to sprint for up to 10 seconds. Many years ago, overs in Australia had eight balls (rather than six), possibly due to the larger grounds leading to a thought that there should be fewer changes of ends. All countries agreed to six ball overs in the 1970s. There is no doubt both batters and fielders run and sprint more during a typical day's play in the larger grounds of Australia, which leads to a higher rate of hamstring and other muscle strains [19].

In the recently created competition in England called The Hundred, six ball overs have been replaced by 10 ball overs to speed the game up. However, it also leads to less running, as there are fewer changes of ends (and the games are shorter than even T20 matches). Early indications are that The Hundred competition has low injury rates for both men's and women's matches [8].

3.8 Heavier Density of Matches and Greater Variation in Match Types Lead to Greater Injuries

Apart from the characteristics of individual matches themselves, the schedule of matches can increase the risk of injury if either more matches are played in a short period of time or if the format of matches changes more often [14, 15, 20]. This is seen in other sports as well [21, 22].

Players from older eras complain that bowlers break down in red ball cricket 'more than they used to, back in my day'. Some of this may be selective memory (as injury surveillance was not performed in cricket until the very end of the twentieth century). However, it is clear that it was easier to bowl higher workloads in red ball cricket when red ball was the only form of cricket. Although the modern fast bowler does not reach the same seasonal workloads of Test match and First Class bowlers of the past, it is probably a more difficult task to 'move between formats' [5]. An analogy can be made that it is easier for a marathon runner to cope with running over 100 km in training to concentrate on marathon races than it would be to spend half the year running marathons and the other half requiring speed work to compete in 800 m middle-distance sprints. The future may see red ball and white ball players specialise and no longer try to undertake the various formats. However, players in the current era are more likely than not to try to play multiple formats, which increases the physical challenge for pace bowlers in particular.

References

1. Foster D, John D, Elliott B, Ackland T, Fitch K. Back injuries to fast bowlers in cricket: a prospective study. Br J Sports Med. 1989;23(3):150–4.
2. Orchard J, James T, Portus M, Kountouris A, Dennis R. Fast bowlers in cricket demonstrate up to 3- to 4-week delay between high workloads and increased risk of injury. Am J Sports Med. 2009;37:1186–92.
3. Frost WL, Chalmers DJ. Injury in elite New Zealand cricketers 2002-2008: descriptive epidemiology. Br J Sports Med. 2014;48(12):1002–7. https://doi.org/10.1136/bjsports-2012-091337.
4. Orchard J, James T, Alcott E, Carter S, Farhart P. Injuries in Australian cricket at first class level 1995/1996 to 2000/2001. Br J Sports Med. 2002;36(4):270–4. discussion 5
5. Orchard J, James T, Kountouris A, Portus M. Changes to injury profile (and recommended cricket injury definitions) based on the increased frequency of Twenty20 cricket matches. Open Access J Sports Med. 2010;1:63–76.
6. Ranson C, Hurley R, Rugless L, Mansingh A, Cole J. International cricket injury surveillance: a report of five teams competing in the ICC Cricket World Cup 2011. Br J Sports Med. 2013;47(10):637–43. https://doi.org/10.1136/bjsports-2012-091783.
7. Warren A, Dale S, McCaig S, Ranson C. Injury profiles in elite women's T20 cricket. J Sci Med Sport. 2019;22(7):775–9. https://doi.org/10.1016/j.jsams.2019.01.018.
8. Williams A, Peirce N, Griffin S, Langley B, Warren A, Wedatilake T, et al. A similar injury profile observed in franchise men's and women's cricket in England and Wales: injury surveillance analysis from the first three 'The Hundred' competitions. BMJ Open Sport Exerc Med. 2024;10(1):e001815. https://doi.org/10.1136/bmjsem-2023-001815.
9. Dovbysh T, Reid D, Shackel D. Injury incidence within male elite New Zealand cricket from the early T20 era: 2009-2015. BMJ Open Sport Exerc Med. 2021;7(4):e001168. https://doi.org/10.1136/bmjsem-2021-001168.
10. Orchard J, Kountouris A, Sims K, Orchard J, Beakley D, Brukner P. Changes to injury profile of elite male cricketers in the T20 era. New Zealand J Sports Med. 2015;42(1):13–7.
11. Orchard JW, Inge P, Sims K, Kountouris A, Saw AE, Saw R, et al. Comparison of injury profiles between elite Australian male and female cricket players. J Sci Med Sport. 2023;26(1):19–24. https://doi.org/10.1016/j.jsams.2022.12.002.
12. Dhillon MS, Patel S, Sharma S. Beyond the boundary: a bibliometric analysis of the published research on injuries in cricket. Indian J Orthop. 2023; https://doi.org/10.1007/s43465-023-00973-9.
13. Dennis R, Farhart R, Goumas C, Orchard J. Bowling workload and the risk of injury in elite cricket fast

bowlers. J Sci Med Sport. 2003;6(3):359–67. https://doi.org/10.1016/s1440-2440(03)80031-2.
14. Hulin B, Gabbett T, Blanch P, Chapman P, Bailey D, Orchard J. Spikes in acute workload are associated with increased injury risk in elite cricket fast bowlers. Br J Sports Med. 2014;48:708–12.
15. Orchard J, Blanch P, Paoloni J, Kountouris A, Sims K, Orchard J, et al. Fast bowling match workloads over 5-26 days and risk of injury in the following month. J Sci Med Sport. 2015;18:26–30.
16. Brooks K, Orchard JW, Saw AE, Kountouris A. Hand fractures and return to play in elite Australian cricketers. J Orthop. 2020;22:100–3. https://doi.org/10.1016/j.jor.2020.03.039.
17. Hill T, Orchard J, Kountouris A. Incidence of concussion and head impacts in Australian elite-level male and female cricketers after head impact protocol modifications. Sports Health. 2019;11(2):180–5. https://doi.org/10.1177/1941738118811315.
18. De Moore G. Tom Wills: The insubordinate life of an Australian sporting legend. Sydney: Allen & Unwin; 2023.
19. Orchard JW, Kountouris A, Sims K. Risk factors for hamstring injuries in Australian male professional cricket players. J Sport Health Sci. 2017;6(3):271–4. https://doi.org/10.1016/j.jshs.2017.05.004.
20. Hulin B, Gabbett T, Lawson D, Caputi P, Sampson J. The acute:chronic workload ratio predicts injury: high chronic workload may decrease injury risk in elite rugby league players. Br J Sports Med. 2015;50(4):231–6. Oct 28 [online first]
21. Bengtsson H, Ekstrand J, Hagglund M. Muscle injury rates in professional football increase with fixture congestion: an 11-year follow-up of the UEFA Champions League injury study. Br J Sports Med. 2013;47:743–7.
22. Dellal A, Lago-Penas C, Rey E, Chamari K, Orhant E. The effects of a congested fixture period on physical performance, technical activity and injury rate during matches in a professional soccer team. Br J Sports Med. 2013; https://doi.org/10.1136/bjsports-2012-091290.

Fast Bowling Biomechanics and Associated Injury in Cricket

4

Peter Alway, Jolandi Jacobs, Sarah Worsdale, and Alison Facey

4.1 Introduction

Cricket bowling is a unique, dynamic, asymmetrical movement pattern that requires coordinated, sequential whole-body movements to achieve ball speed, spin rate and ball trajectory outcomes. Bowlers manipulate these characteristics, along with deception, with the aim of taking wickets and decreasing opportunities to score runs. Fast bowlers suffer more injuries than any other players due to the incredible demands imposed on them by the technique of bowling. Understanding the techniques that may influence the risk of sustaining an injury is critical to developing a holistic injury prevention strategy.

P. Alway (✉)
Department of Science and Medicine, England and Wales Cricket Board, London, UK

School of Sport, Exercise and Health Sciences, Loughborough University, Loughborough, UK
e-mail: Peter.Alway@ecb.co.uk

J. Jacobs
School of Health, Medical and Applied Sciences, Central Queensland University, Queensland Cricket, Rockhampton, Australia

S. Worsdale
School of Sport, Exercise and Health Sciences, Loughborough University, Loughborough, UK
e-mail: S.C.Worsdale@lboro.ac.uk

A. Facey
University of the West Indies, Kingston, Jamaica

This chapter will provide a description of the bowling action, the technical characteristics associated with lumbar bone stress injury, the physical characteristics that underpin the bowling technique, how to reduce the risk of lumbar bone stress injury and associations between technique and other common injuries observed in bowlers, including hamstring strains and side strains.

4.2 What Is Cricket Bowling?

According to the laws of cricket, the elbow must not extend more than 15 degrees during the bowling action, specifically between the upper arm horizontal (where circumduction of the bowling arm crosses a horizontal plane in line with the shoulder) and ball release [1]. Simply put, throwing the ball is not permitted while bowling. The bowling technique can be separated into distinct phases: run-up, pre-delivery stride (Fig. 4.1a, b), back foot contact (Fig. 4.1b, c), front foot contact (Fig. 4.1c, d) and follow-through (Fig. 4.1d, e).

The run-up phase is initiated by the whole-body acceleration of the bowler at the start of their run-up and ends with the initiation of the pre-delivery stride. Bowlers typically achieve run-up speeds in excess of 20 kph. The aim of this phase is to generate linear momentum.

The pre-delivery stride (also known as the jump-gather) is defined as the stride that occurs prior to back foot contact. In this phase, the

B. Olivier, J. W. Orchard (eds.), *Cricket Sports Medicine*,
https://doi.org/10.1007/978-981-96-6321-7_4

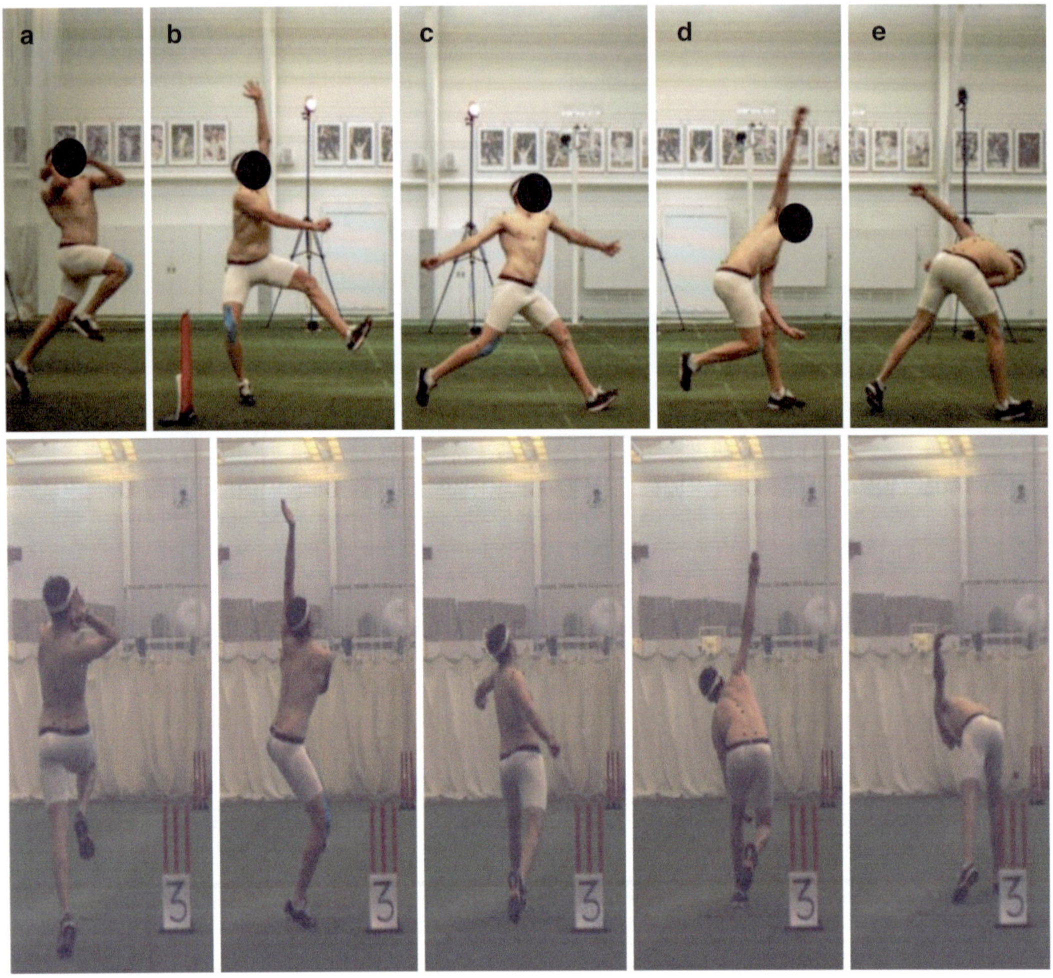

Fig. 4.1 Fast bowling technique from the side (top) and rear (bottom) views at instances of (from left to right): delivery stride take-off (**a**), back foot contact (b), front foot contact (**c**), ball release (**d**) and follow-through (**e**)

bowler bounds up and forwards, typically off the opposite leg to their bowling arm (front leg), at a magnitude much greater than their usual running stride. The aim of this phase is to position the body into a mechanically advantageous position to generate ball speed and/or spin rate and to conserve the linear momentum generated in the run-up (Fig. 4.1a, b).

The back foot contact phase begins when the back foot (on the same side as their bowling arm) contact and ends with front foot contact. The rear hip and knee flex to absorb the forces associated with landing, stabilise the position of the pelvis and redirect the centre of mass towards the target. The front hip flexes to position the leg ahead of the body. The pelvis and trunk rotate towards the bowling arm, and the trunk extends while the bowling arm begins to circumduct. The aim of this phase is to conserve linear momentum from the run-up and to continue to position the body into a mechanically advantageous position (Fig. 4.1b, c).

The front foot contact phase is initiated by the impact of the front foot (opposing side to their bowling arm) with the ground and ends with ball release. The aim of this phase is to convert the linear momentum generated during the run-up into angular momentum that can be transferred to the ball. This is achieved through rapid deceleration of the lower body upon front foot contact, coupled with powerful, coordinated proximal-to-distal rotations of the torso and bowling arm segments. In this phase, the pelvis and then trunk rapidly rotate and laterally flex away from the bowling arm and flex towards the target. Meanwhile, the bowling arm rapidly circumducts towards the target before the wrist flexes and the ball is released (Fig. 4.1c, d). Any sidespin applied to the ball is achieved through movements of the fingers (abduction and adduction), wrist (radial and ulnar deviation), forearm (pronation and supination) or shoulder (internal and external rotation) during this phase.

The follow-through phase begins with ball release and ends with the bowler completing the movement by coming to a stop. The aim of this phase is to safely decelerate the body and to potentially be in a position to field the ball (Fig. 4.1d, e).

4.2.1 Fast Bowling Technique and Lumbar Bone Stress Injury

Bowlers can generally be categorised into two types: fast bowlers and spin bowlers. Fast bowlers intend to bowl the ball at high ball release speed to decrease the time in which batters have to respond to the trajectory of the delivery. Male fast bowlers can achieve ball release speeds in excess of 41.7 m/s^{-1} (150 kph, 93 mph), whereas female fast bowlers can achieve ball release speeds in excess of 33.3 m/s^{-1} (120 kph, 75 mph). Ball release speed has consistently been linked to:

- Faster run-up speeds [2–7].
- Greater deceleration of the lower body following front foot contact [4, 8, 9].
- Delayed circumduction of the bowling arm [2, 7, 10, 11].
- Less flexion of the front knee at ball release [2, 5, 12, 13].
- Greater magnitude of trunk flexion between front foot contact and ball release [2].

In multi-day cricket, the majority of the deliveries bowled by fast bowlers will be bowled at high ball release speed to limit the amount of time batters have to react, often in conjunction with swing and seam, which allows the ball to laterally deviate. In shorter formats of the game, in particular 20-over cricket, there is a greater focus on varying pace to challenge batters. Bowlers seek to deceive batters through small alterations to their bowling action, which result in significant reductions in ball release speed, particularly to the bowling arm or position of the ball in the hand. Examples include cutters, where side spin is applied to the ball; the back of the hand, where the ball is delivered with the back of the hand facing the batter; and split-finger, where the ball is positioned deeper into the hand.

Lumbar bone stress injury is the most prevalent injury in male cricketers [14], despite the vast majority occurring to fast bowlers only [15]. Lumbar bone stress injuries describe a group of overuse bone injuries that include stress reactions, incomplete stress fractures and complete stress fractures. These injuries occur when the rate of accumulation and propagation of microdamage within bone exceeds the rate at which the microdamage can be repaired. In cricket, both fast and spin bowlers typically experience these injuries in the pars or pedicle of the lower three vertebrae, on the opposing side to the bowling arm [16]. The risk factors for lumbar bone stress injury are multifactorial, with risk factors being grouped into three categories [17] (Fig. 4.2).

- Factors influencing external load per delivery.
- Factors influencing the strength and resilience of bone.
- Factors related to workload.

The incidence of lumbar bone stress injury is lower in female fast bowlers [14], likely due to the lower bowling volumes achieved by female fast bowlers. However, as female cricket continues to increase the number of fixtures, and with further inclusion of multi-day cricket, it is possible that the incidence of lumbar bone stress injury will increase in female fast bowlers. In other activities, female athletes sustain bone stress

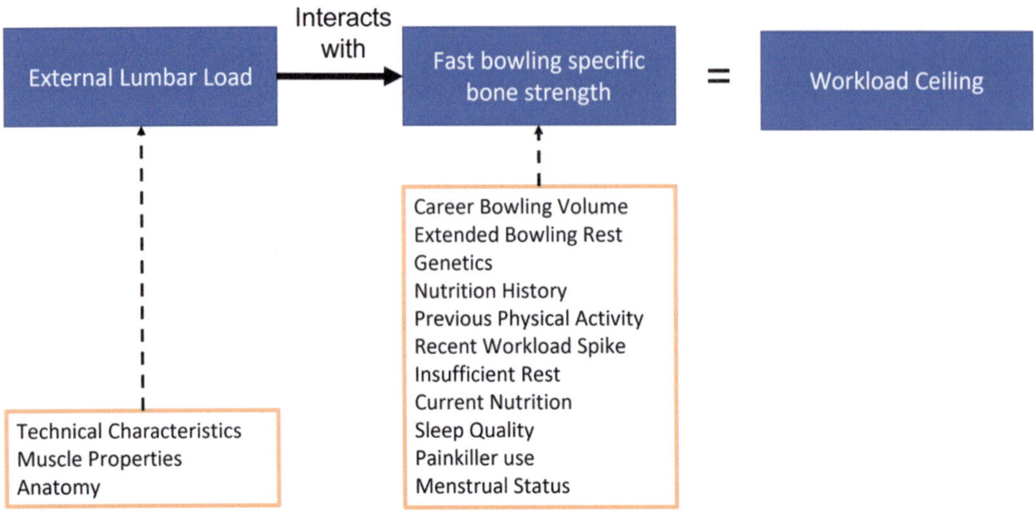

Fig. 4.2 The relationship between external loading, bone strength, workload ceiling and lumbar bone stress injury, along with the factors influencing each

injuries at greater than double the incidence of male athletes [18].

While lumbar bone stress injuries are multifactorial, the technique underpins the load experienced by the bone per delivery. Therefore, for a given bone strength and resilience, a technique associated with a lower lumbar load results in a higher safe bowling volume threshold for lumbar bone stress injury than a higher lumbar load technique.

The importance of technique in lumbar bone stress injuries has been highlighted in recent research, which demonstrated technical differences in young elite fast bowlers who did and did not sustain lumbar bone stress injuries across 2-years [19]. This study found multiple differences between groups and highlighted that fast bowlers who sustain lumbar bone stress injuries have the following technical characteristics:

- Greater rear hip flexion at back foot contact.
- Less lumbar flexion at front foot contact.
- Greater maximum contralateral (away from bowling arm) lumbar lateral flexion.
- Less maximum contralateral thoracic side flexion.
- Greater contralateral thoracic rotation at back foot contact.
- Greater anterior pelvic tilt at front foot contact.
- Greater front hip flexion at front foot contact.
- Greater rear knee flexion at back foot contact.

Further analysis in this study revealed that rear hip flexion at back foot contact and lumbopelvic flexion at front foot contact together have been demonstrated to predict 88% of future lumbar bone stress injuries (Fig. 4.3). This study also provided odds ratios (how likely a player is to sustain a lumbar bone stress injury compared with the mean uninjured player) that increase exponentially with the magnitude of hip flexion and the magnitude of lumbopelvic extension. For rear hip flexion at back foot contact, angles of 156 (24 degrees of hip flexion), 146, 136 and 126 give an odds ratio of 1.0, 3.7, 13.5 and 49.4 (Fig. 4.4), respectively. Similarly, lumbopelvic angles of 172 (8 degrees of flexion), 177, 182 and

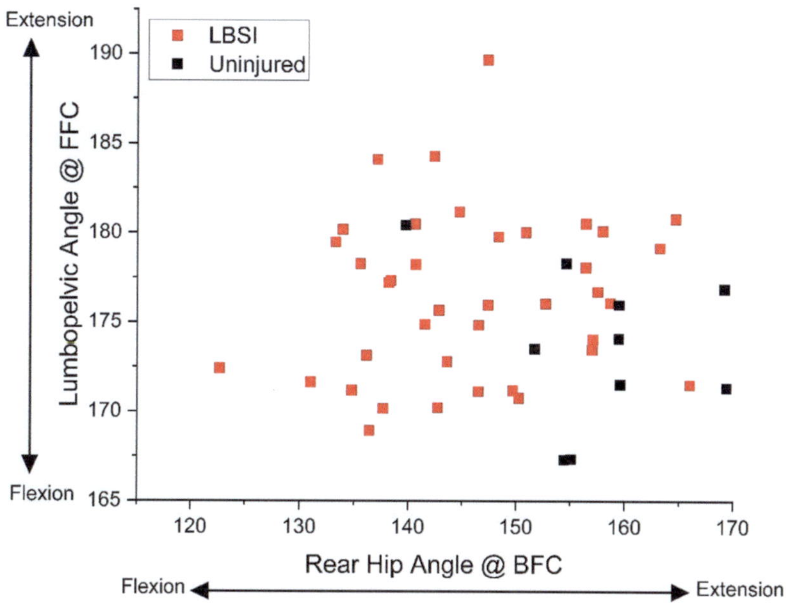

Fig. 4.3 Technique characteristics of fast bowlers who prospectively sustained lumbar bone stress injury (red squares) and those who remained uninjured and played more than 150 match days (black squares) over 2 years. Please note that only 1 player with a hip angle of less than 150 degrees (30 degrees of flexion) did not sustain a lumbar bone stress injury, and only 2 players with a lumbopelvic angle of greater than 177 degrees (3 degrees of flexion) did not sustain a lumbar bone stress injury (BFC: back foot contact; FFC: front foot contact)

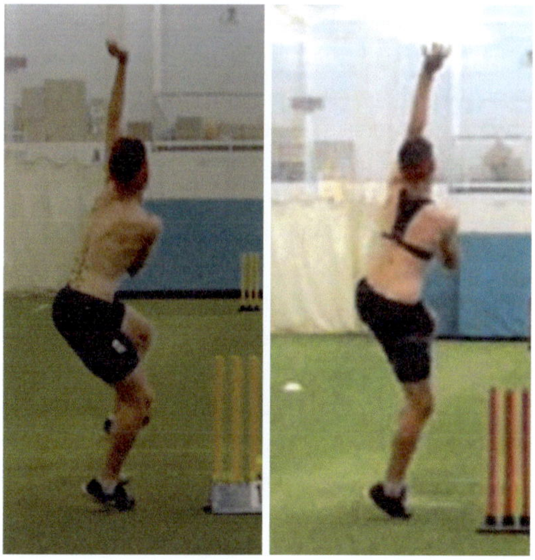

Fig. 4.4 Rear hip angle at back foot contact for a player (left) with an odds ratio of sustaining lumbar bone stress injury of 29 (130 degrees, 50 degrees flexed) and a player (right) with an odds ratio of sustaining lumbar bone stress injury of 1 (156 degrees, 24 degrees flexed)

187 degrees provided odds ratios of 1.0, 3.2, 10.0 and 31.5 (Fig. 4.5).

Excessive rear hip flexion at back foot contact is likely related to the ability of the hip musculature to provide sufficient extensor torques to stabilise the pelvis and conserve momentum generated from the run-up. Therefore, the factors which may influence rear hip flexion at back foot contact include those that may influence the amount of torque required at the hip. This includes the bowler's mass, relative run-up velocity, relative jump-gather height, horizontal change in direction of the centre of mass between jump-gather and back foot contact (e.g. moving towards or away from the stumps) and strength and power of the surrounding musculature. Furthermore, greater rear hip flexion at back foot contact has been associated with less shoulder external rotation and total rotational arc of rotation [20], worse lumbopelvic control and muscular endurance at the trunk [21].

To ensure that the trunk remains in a mechanically advantageous position to produce a high ball release speed, fast bowlers may compensate for anterior pelvic tilt at front foot contact by extending the lumbar spine. Furthermore, fast

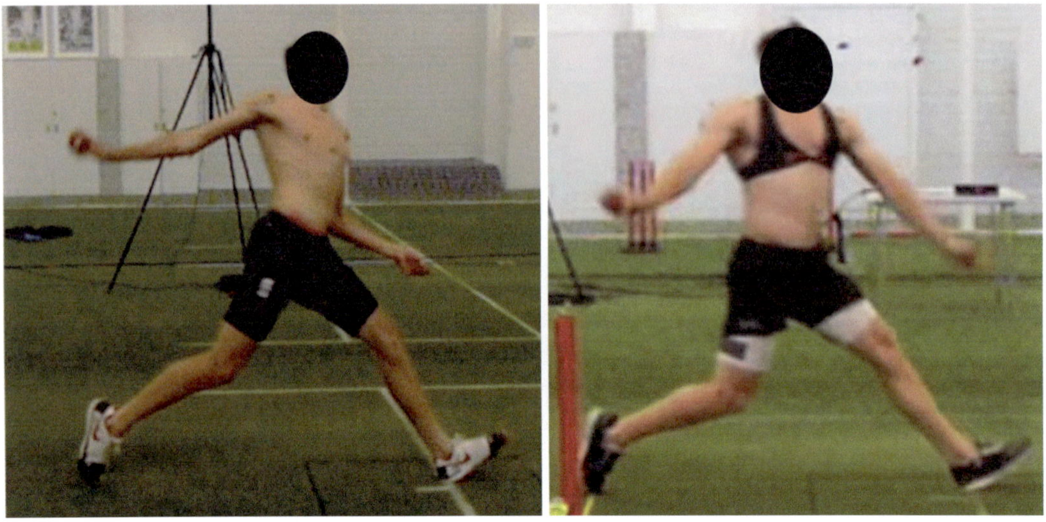

Fig. 4.5 Lumbopelvic angle at front foot contact for a player (left) with an odds ratio of sustaining lumbar bone stress injury of 19 (185 degrees, 5 degrees of extension) and a player (right) with an odds ratio of sustaining lumbar bone stress injury of 1 (172 degrees, 8 degrees of flexion)

bowlers with greater lumbar extension at front foot contact have been associated with decreased range of motion in hip flexion, extension and internal and external hip rotation, lumbopelvic control [21] and shoulder internal rotation [20]. Lumbar bone stress injury is prevalent in sports with repetitive lumbar extension, such as gymnastics, platform diving and volleyball [22], suggesting a common aetiology of lumbar bone stress injury in athletic populations.

To produce a high ball release height during bowling, players must laterally flex their trunk away from their bowling arm (contralaterally). Recent findings suggest that the source of lateral flexion is important, where fast bowlers who rely more on their lumbar spine than their thoracic spine for overall trunk lateral flexion are more likely to sustain lumbar bone stress injury [19]. This may be a consequence of impaired lumbopelvic control, a change of centre of mass direction earlier in the action, and the strength, power and endurance of the surrounding musculature.

Bowlers who sustained lumbar bone stress injuries were in a more contralaterally trunk-rotated position at back foot contact compared with their uninjured peers. This may indicate a greater reliance on trunk rotation to generate ball speeds through the subsequent need for greater magnitude and/or intensity rotation of the subsequent ipsilateral and contralateral trunk rotations.

While the vertical ground reaction forces are high (mean peak: males 4.5–6.7 body weights [5, 23]; females: 5.3 body weights [24]) and are likely to cause compression of the spine, there is limited evidence to associate this with lumbar bone stress injury. No significant differences have been observed in the magnitude or loading rate of vertical ground reaction forces between groups of uninjured fast bowlers and those with lumbar bone stress injury [19]. Further recent studies have demonstrated that only 20% of the accelerations associated with front foot contact in fast bowlers were experienced at the lumbar spine, suggesting that most of the vertical ground reaction forces are dissipated in the lower limb [25]. Further bony adaptation of the lumbar spine in fast bowlers is not associated with vertical ground reaction forces. Rather, muscular forces from trunk rotations have been associated with bone adaptation at the lumbar spine in male fast bowlers [26], suggesting greater loading from muscular forces rather than ground reaction forces. In addition, computer simulation studies have suggested that the combination of compression, extension, rotation and lateral flexion of the lumbar spine has been demonstrated to put the greatest stress upon the pars interarticularis [27, 28], part of the neural arch where lumbar bone stress injuries typically occur [16].

Mixed bowling actions, defined by the magnitude of shoulder counterrotation at back foot contact, between back foot contact and its maximum value, or by the magnitude of hip–shoulder separation, have often been associated with lumbar bone stress injury. However, recent research found no differences between fast bowlers with and without lumbar bone stress injuries in the magnitude of shoulder counterrotation, amount of hip–shoulder separation or orientation of the shoulders at back foot contact [19] and are not representative of spinal motion during fast bowling [29]. Therefore, classifying bowlers by action classification has little basis for preventing lumbar bone stress injuries.

It is plausible to suggest that excessive rear hip flexion at back foot contact consequently leads to a cascade of movements that increase the magnitude of lumbar loading, including anterior pelvic tilt, lumbar extension, contralateral lumbar lateral flexion and trunk rotation. It may also be possible that excessive rear hip flexion is a symptom of inadequate strength, power, flexibility and control of the musculature of the lumbo–pelvic–hip complex to resist the demands imposed upon it by the run-up and jump-gather characteristics.

4.2.2 Spin Bowling Technique and Lumbar Bone Stress Injury

Spin bowlers impart high spin rates on the ball to maximise the interaction between the ball and the surface of the pitch upon landing, often resulting in a significant degree of turn away or towards the batter. Spin bowlers can achieve spin rates in excess of 2000 rpm, with ball release speeds typically varying between 17.9 and 26.8 m/s [1] (64–97 kph, 40–60 mph). Spin bowlers typically have shorter and slower run-up speeds than fast bowlers. Spin bowlers are categorised as either finger spinners (e.g. right-handed finger spin bowlers turn the ball towards a right-handed batter) or wrist spinners (e.g. right-handed wrist spin bowlers turn the ball away from the right-handed batter). To date, research has linked ball spin rate and performance level with the following technical characteristics:

- Greater contralateral (more front-on) orientation of the pelvis and shoulder at front foot contact and ball release [30, 31].
- Greater and earlier timing of maximum angular velocities of the rear hip, pelvis and upper body [31, 32].
- In finger spin bowlers, a greater magnitude of pelvis rotation, trunk rotation, elbow extension [33] and forearm pronation [30] between front foot contact and ball release.

While the majority of lumbar bone stress injuries are sustained by fast bowlers, the risk to spin bowlers should not be overlooked. While the loading experienced at the lumbar spine during spin bowling is likely significantly less than in fast bowling, the volume of deliveries is substantially greater. In particular, wrist-spin bowlers who use high (relative) run-up speeds to deliver the ball may have a similar risk of lumbar bone stress injuries to fast bowlers, particularly when coupled with high magnitudes of lumbar extension, contralateral side flexion and rotation.

4.3 How Can I Decrease the Risk of Lumbar Bone Stress Injuries?

Firstly, practitioners should identify bowlers at risk of lumbar bone stress injury through the use of 3D motion analysis or 2D video analysis. By positioning a camera perpendicular to the position of the rear hip at back foot contact, it is possible to identify players who demonstrate a high magnitude of rear hip or knee flexion at the instant of back foot contact, which are highly correlated to one another. Bowlers at high risk of lumbar bone stress injury should have their workload carefully monitored, avoiding any short-term spikes in bowling volume and encouraging multi-day rest between bowling bouts.

A holistic approach should be taken to any change in fast bowling technique that requires a multidisciplinary team with expertise in fast bowling coaching, medicine and strength and conditioning. It has been previously demonstrated that fast bowling techniques can be improved through the use of strength and conditioning [34] and coaching-based [35] interventions. Fast bowlers should seek to improve their hip and shoulder flexibility, lumbopelvic control and endurance of trunk musculature, as these appear to be the physical underpinnings of safe technique.

4.4 Other Injuries and Fast Bowling Technique

Fast bowlers are at the greatest risk of injury of any of the playing roles in cricket [15]. While further research is needed to discern links between bowling technique and other injuries, there is research from other sports that can be applied to cricket.

Hamstring strains have the highest injury incidence in male and female cricket [14], with fast bowlers having the highest incidence [36], likely related to the greater number of high-intensity running efforts performed and distance covered at high velocity [37]. In addition, there are a significant number of fast bowlers who sustain this injury during the delivery stride and follow-through phases of bowling [38]. Interestingly, it has been shown in other sports that a combination of hip flexion, knee extension and trunk flexion during running at high speed increases the risk of injury (through lengthening the hamstrings) [39], a similar position to what is observed in elite fast bowlers between front foot contact and ball release [11].

The next most common injury sustained by fast bowlers is the side strain, typically presenting contralateral to the bowling arm at the internal oblique, spanning from the ninth to 12th ribs but can also present at the external oblique and rectus abdominis [40]. The mechanism of injury is suggested to be due to a combination of rapid non-bowling arm extension coupled with contralateral trunk side flexion [40]; however, further prospective studies are required to further understand the relationship between bowling technique and injury.

References

1. ICC. ICC men's test match playing conditions. Rules and Regulations; 2018.
2. Worthington P, King M, Ranson C. Relationships between fast bowling technique and ball release speed in cricket. J Appl Biomech. 2013;29:78–84.
3. Feros SA, Young WB, O'Brien BJ. Relationship between selected physical qualities, bowling kinematics, and pace bowling skill in club-standard cricketers. J Strength Cond Res. 2019;33:2812–25.
4. Glazier PS, Worthington PJ. The impact of centre of mass kinematics and ground reaction forces on ball release speeds in cricket fast bowling. Sports Technol. 2014;7:4–11.
5. Middleton KJ, Mills PM, Elliott BC, Alderson JA, Middleton KJ, Mills PM, Elliott BC, Alderson JA. The association between lower limb biomechanics and ball release speed in cricket fast bowlers: a comparison of high-performance and amateur competitors. Sports Biomech. 2016;3141:1–13.
6. Bailey D, Saw AE, Crowther RH, Sims K. Run faster, bowl faster: in-match analysis of elite female cricket pace bowlers. J Sport Exerc Sci. 2023;7 https://doi.org/10.36905/jses.2023.01.03.
7. Lyons C, Felton PJ, McCabe C. Female cricket pace bowling: kinematic and anthropometric relationships with ball release speed. S Afr J Sports Med. 2023;35 https://doi.org/10.17159/2078-516X/2023/v35i1a15080.
8. Ferdinands R, Marshall RN, Kersting U. Centre of mass kinematics of fast bowling in cricket. Sports Biomech. 2010;9:139–52.
9. King MA, Worthington PJ, Ranson CA. Does maximising ball speed in cricket fast bowling necessitate higher ground reaction forces? J Sports Sci. 2016;34:707–12.
10. Felton PJ, Shine KJ, Yeadon MR, King MA. Optimal initial position and technique for the front foot contact phase of cricket fast bowling : commonalities between individual-specific simulations of elite bowlers. J Biomech. 2023;158:111765.
11. Felton PJ, Lister SL, Worthington PJ, King MA. Comparison of biomechanical characteristics between male and female elite fast bowlers. J Sports Sci. 2019;37:665–70.
12. Wormgoor S, Harden L, McKinon W. Anthropometric, biomechanical, and isokinetic strength predictors of ball release speed in high-performance cricket fast bowlers. J Sports Sci. 2010;28:957–65.
13. Portus MR, Portus MR, Mason BR, Elliott BC, Pfitzner MC, Done RP. Cricket: technique factors

related to ball release speed and trunk injuries in high performance cricket fast bowlers. Sports Biomech. 2004;3:263–84.
14. Orchard JW, Inge P, Sims K, Kountouris A, Saw AE, Saw R, Beerworth K. Comparison of injury profiles between elite Australian male and female cricket players. J Sci Med Sport. 2023;26:19–24.
15. Orchard J, Kountouris A, Sims K. Incidence and prevalence of elite male cricket injuries using updated consensus definitions. Open Access J Sports Med. 2016;7:187–94.
16. Alway P, Brooke-Wavell K, Langley B, King M, Peirce N. Incidence and prevalence of lumbar stress fracture in English County Cricket fast bowlers, association with bowling workload and seasonal variation. BMJ Open Sport Exerc Med. 2019;5:e000529. https://doi.org/10.1136/bmjsem-2019-000529.
17. Hughes JM, Popp KL, Yanovich R, Bouxsein ML, Matheny RW. The role of adaptive bone formation in the etiology of stress fracture. Exp Biol Med. 2017;242:897–906.
18. Rizzone KH, Ackerman KE, Roos KG, Dompier TP, Kerr ZY. The epidemiology of stress fractures in collegiate student-athletes, 2004-2005 through 2013-2014 academic years. J Athl Train. 2017;52:966–75.
19. Alway P, Felton P, Brooke-Wavell K, Peirce N, King M. Cricket fast bowling technique and lumbar bone stress injury. Med Sci Sports Exerc. 2021;53:581–9.
20. Felton PJ, McCaig S, King MA. Cricket fast bowling: the relationship between range of motion and key performance and injury technique characteristics. J Sports Sci. 2023;41:112–20.
21. Worsdale S, King M, Brooke-Wavell K, Ahmun R, Griffin S, Etherington C, Alway P. Physical characteristics associated with lumbar bone stress injury related technique in male fast bowlers. International Society of Biomechanics in Sports; 2024.
22. Hoenig T, Ackerman KE, Beck BR, Bouxsein ML, Burr DB, Hollander K, Popp KL, Rolvien T, Tenforde AS, Warden SJ. Bone stress injuries. Nat Rev Dis Primers. 2022;8 https://doi.org/10.1038/s41572-022-00352-y.
23. Worthington P, King M, Ranson C, Worthington P, King M, Ranson C. The influence of cricket fast bowlers ' front leg technique on peak ground reaction forces reaction forces. J Sports Sci. 2013;31(4):434–41. https://doi.org/10.1080/02640414.2012.736628.
24. Stuelcken MC, Sinclair PJ. A pilot study of the front foot ground reaction forces in elite female fast bowlers. J Sci Med Sport. 2009;12:258–61.
25. Lamb M, McErlain-Naylor S, Felton P, King M. Relationship between lower limb joint compliance and acceleration transmission during cricket fast bowling. XIX international symposium on computer simulation in biomechanics. 2023.
26. Keylock L, Felton P, Alway P, Brooke-Wavell K, Peirce N, King M. Lumbar bone mineral adaptation: the effect of fast bowling technique in adolescent cricketers. Med Sci Sports Exerc. 2021;54:438. https://doi.org/10.1249/mss.0000000000002820.
27. Chosa E, Totoribe K, Tajima N. A biomechanical study of lumbar spondylolysis based on a three-dimensional finite element method. J Orthop Res. 2004;22:158–63.
28. Terai T, Sairyo K, Goel VK, Ebraheim N, Biyani A, Faizan A, Sakai T, Yasui N. Spondylolysis originates in the ventral aspect of the pars interarticularis: a clinical and biomechanical study. J Bone Joint Surg Br. 2010;92:1123–7.
29. Senington B, Lee RY, Williams JM. Are shoulder counter rotation and hip shoulder separation angle representative metrics of three-dimensional spinal kinematics in cricket fast bowling? J Sports Sci. 2018;36:1763–7.
30. Sanders L, Felton PJ, King MA. Kinematic parameters contributing to the production of spin in elite finger spin bowling. J Sports Sci. 2018;36:2787–93.
31. Spratford W, Elliott B, Portus M, Brown N, Alderson J. The influence of upper-body mechanics, anthropometry and isokinetic strength on performance in wrist-spin cricket bowling. J Sports Sci. 2020;38:280–7.
32. Beach AJ, Ferdinands RED, Sinclair PJ. The relationship between segmental kinematics and ball spin in Type-2 cricket spin bowling. J Sports Sci. 2018;36:1127–34.
33. Chin A, Elliott B, Alderson J, Lloyd D, Foster D. The off-break and "doosra": kinematic variations of elite and sub-elite bowlers in creating ball spin in cricket bowling. Sports Biomech. 2009;8:187–98.
34. Forrest MRL, Hebert JJ, Scott BR, Dempsey AR. Modifying bowling kinematics in cricket pace bowlers with exercise-based injury prevention: a cluster-randomised controlled trial. J Sci Med Sport. 2020;23:1172–7.
35. Ranson C, King M, Burnett A, Worthington P, Shine K. The effect of coaching intervention on elite fast bowling technique over a two year period. Sports Biomech. 2009;8:261–74.
36. Orchard JW, Kountouris A, Sims K. Risk factors for hamstring injuries in Australian male professional cricket players. J Sport Health Sci. 2017;6:271–4.
37. Petersen CJ, Pyne D, Dawson B, Portus M, Kellett A. Movement patterns in cricket vary by both position and game format. J Sports Sci. 2010;28:45–52.
38. Goggins L, Langley B, Griffin S, Peirce N, McKay C, Stokes K, Williams S. Hamstring injuries in England and Wales elite men's domestic cricket from 2010 to 2019. J Sci Med Sport. 2022;25:474–9.
39. Danielsson A, Horvath A, Senorski C, Alentorn-Geli E, Garrett WE, Cugat R, Samuelsson K, Hamrin Senorski E. The mechanism of hamstring injuries- a systematic review. BMC Musculoskelet Disord. 2020;21:641. https://doi.org/10.1186/s12891-020-03658-8.
40. Nealon AR, Kountouris A, Cook JL. Side strain in sport: a narrative review of pathomechanics, diagnosis, imaging and management for the clinician. J Sci Med Sport. 2017;20:261–6.

5 Throwing and Fielding Biomechanics and Associated Injury in Cricket

Megan Dutton and T. J. Malherbe

5.1 Introduction

The art of fielding has become increasingly more evident since the inception of the shorter, more explosive T20 format of cricket in 2003 [1]. Notably, all cricketers are required to field in order, primarily to limit the number of runs scored by the opposing team [2–4]. This can be achieved by collecting a batted ball prior to it reaching the boundary and returning it to either the wicketkeeper or bowler. Further, a fielder may dismiss a batter by either catching a batted ball or throwing a ball to strike the stumps to affect a run-out [2–4]. Optimal fielding performance is thus multifaceted and requires the refined execution of catching, sliding, diving and throwing with both speed and accuracy.

M. Dutton (✉)
Optimal Physio: Megan Dutton Physiotherapists, Pinehurst, Cape Town, South Africa

University of Cape Town, Department of Health and Rehabilitation Sciences, Division of Physiotherapy, Cape Town, South Africa

T. J. Malherbe
T-J Malherbe & Associates, Claremont, Cape Town, South Africa

5.2 Fielding Positions

The proximity of fielders to the batter on strike may influence the choice in hand position and type of slide or dive executed to collect or catch a ball, as well as the throwing technique utilised to return the ball to the wicket. It is, therefore, informative to understand the various cricket field areas and positions.

The ICC Standard Playing Conditions (Law 19.1.3) [5] require an international cricket field (irrespective of match format) to be 59.43-82 m in diameter, as measured from the centre of the pitch, for men and 54.86–64.01 m in diameter for women. The cricket field is further marked as close-infield (denoted by a dotted line), infield (dashed line) and outfield (boundary line) (Fig. 5.1a). It is important to note that close-in fielders are positioned within a 14 m radius of the batter and include the slips, gully, silly point, silly mid-on and -off and short leg (Fig. 5.1b). Infield fielders are slightly more removed from the batter, positioned within an oval with an approximate radius of 27 m from the centre of each wicket. Refer to Fig. 5.1b for a detailed understanding of the primary fielding positions that can be utilised in any match. Note that variations in these positions occur and are named with the terms highlighted in the fielding glossary found in Box 5.1.

B. Olivier, J. W. Orchard (eds.), *Cricket Sports Medicine*,
https://doi.org/10.1007/978-981-96-6321-7_5

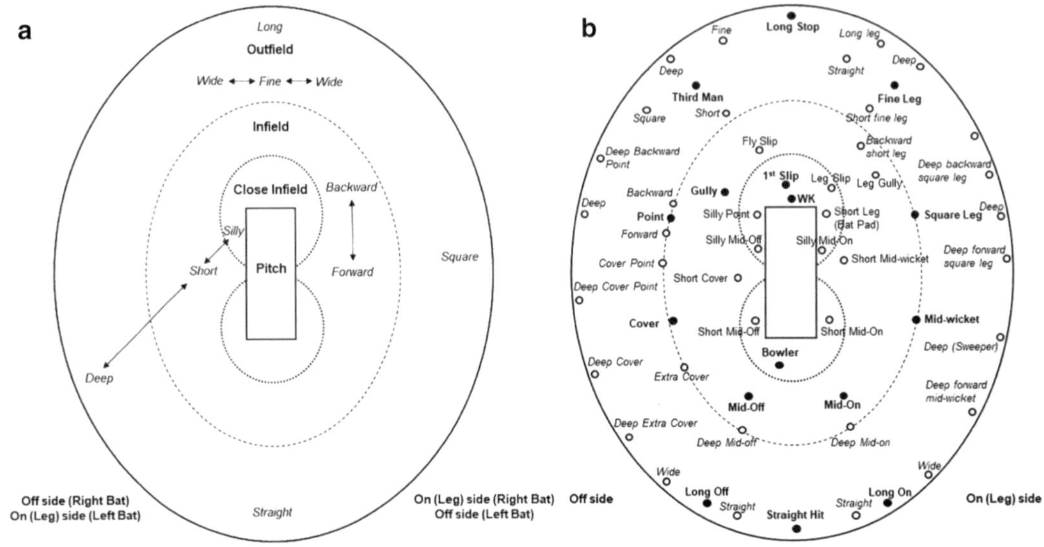

Fig. 5.1 (**a**) A standard cricket field. (**b**) The fielding positions for a right-handed batter. Primary fielding positions are indicated in bold, whilst variations are italicised. WK refers to the wicketkeeper [6]

Box 5.1 Fielding Glossary [6]

Leg- or On-side: The half of the field that corresponds to the batter's non-dominant hand from the batter's wicket and perspective. These fielders will be positioned behind the batter as he/she awaits the bowler.

Off-Side: The half of the field that corresponds to the batter's dominant hand from the batter's wicket and perspective. These fielders face the batter as he/she awaits the bowler.

Silly: Exceptionally close to the batter.

Short: Near the batter.

Deep: Furthest away from batter.

Wide: Further away from the line of the pitch.

Fine, Straight: Nearer to the line of the pitch.

Square: Nearer to the line of the batter's crease.

Front: In front of the batter's crease.

Back: Behind the batter's crease.

5.3 Catching

One of the oldest sayings in cricket is "Catches win Matches". Although seemingly simple, catching in cricket requires a range of skills including concentration, agility, quick reflexes, speedy reaction time and the anticipation of ball trajectory, amongst others [7]. Unbeknown to many, cricketers use various hand positions to execute catches effectively in specific fielding areas.

The orthodox hand or cup position (Fig. 5.2a) is characterised by palms facing upward with all fingers extended so that the little fingers are in contact with each other. This catching technique is predominantly used in the close-infield and infield to catch balls at or below chest height when the fingers are positioned downward, with palms away from the body (Fig. 5.2b). However, when running in to catch a high ball from the outfield, the orthodox cup is adjusted so that palms face the body, and fingers radiate upwards (Fig. 5.2c). Conversely, the reverse cup (Fig. 5.2d) in which the thumbs and index fingers are interlaced, and palms face upward, away from the body, is preferred when making catches overhead or above chest height in the outfield.

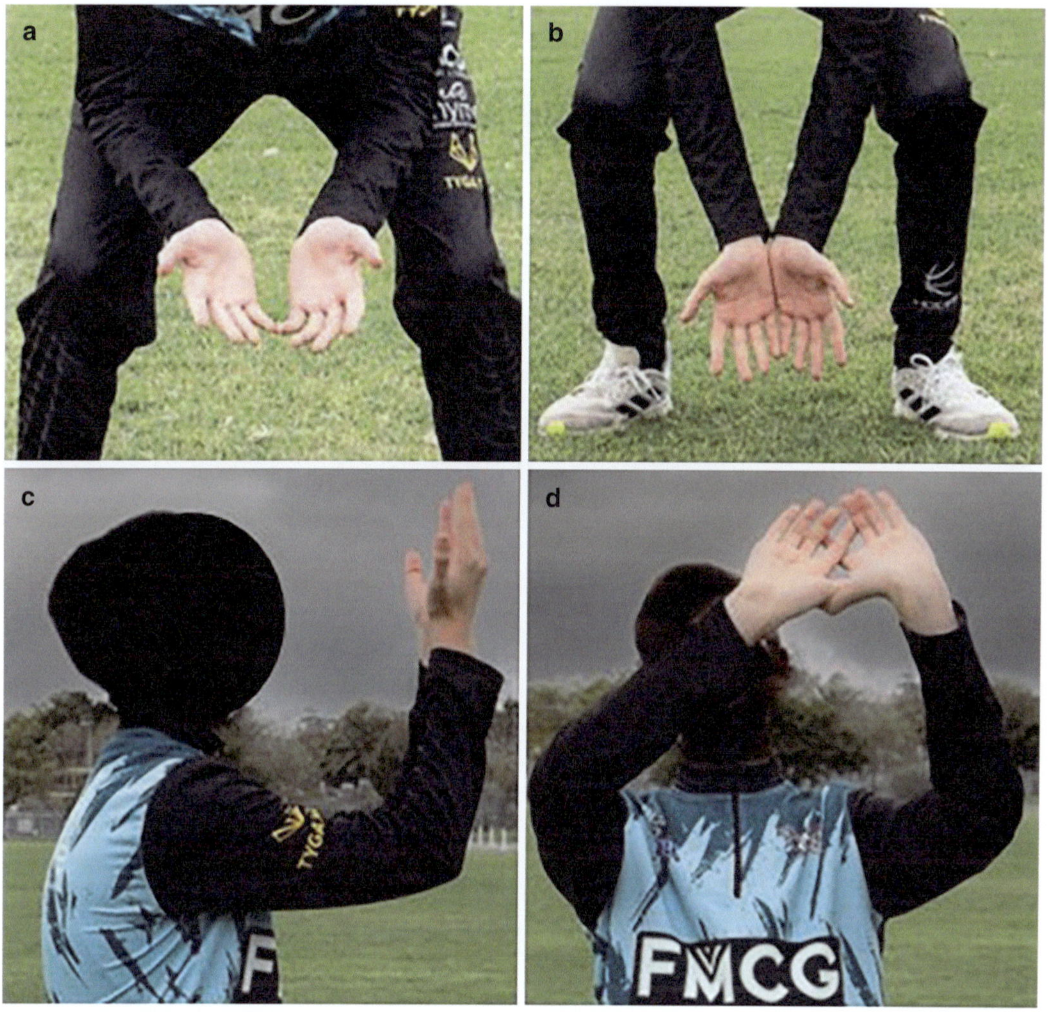

Fig. 5.2 The various hand positions used in catching including the (**a**) orthodox cup, (**b**) close-in & infield orthodox cup, (**c**) high catch orthodox cup and (**d**) reverse cup

Irrespective of hand position, cricketers should aim to catch the ball at the base of their fingers to reduce the risk of acute hand injuries. e.g. fractures and split webbing. In addition, all catches should be drawn toward the body to absorb momentum, maintain control and avoid dropping the ball.

5.4 Ground Fielding

When a batted ball is not in flight, it will be fielded off the ground by a cricketer either running towards or chasing after it, collecting the ball and returning it to the pitch. Occasionally, when a fielder is under pressure to prevent the ball from hitting the boundary rope, limit the number of runs completed by the batsmen or effect a run-out, a slide may be executed.

The two sliding techniques commonly used by cricketers are the hip or front slide [8]. The hip slide (Fig. 5.3a) is the most economical as it allows a fielder to slide past, retrieve and throw the ball in a single motion. This technique is characterised by the formation of a figure four with the lead leg, so that the fielder's hip and thigh take the impact of the slide and is heavily dependent on running speed to reduce friction. When executing a hip slide, cricketers are encouraged to avoid planting or anchoring the foot and

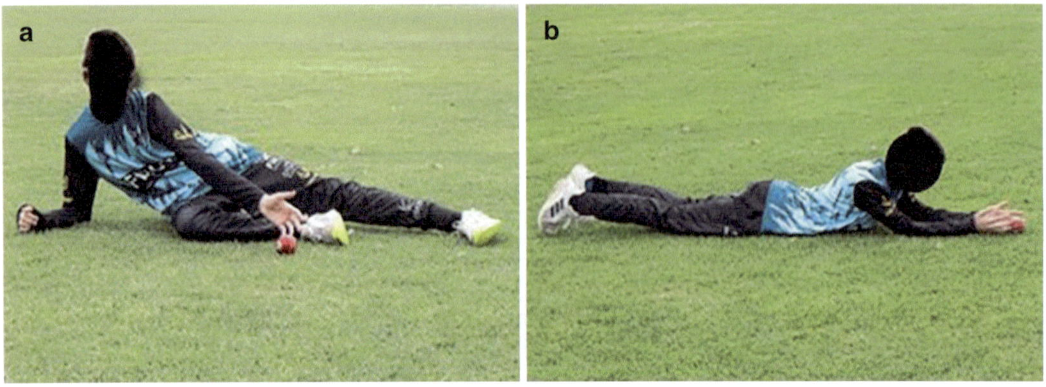

Fig. 5.3 Sliding techniques in cricket including the (**a**) hip slide and (**b**) front slide

knee of the lead leg into the ground due to the inherent risk of sustaining acute ankle (lateral ligament complex) and knee (meniscal) injuries, respectively.

Conversely, the more challenging front slide (Fig. 5.3b) requires substantial horizontal energy so that the fielder dives forward with their head up, arms extended and core braced. Initial contact with the ground is absorbed by the chest, belly and thighs. This is imperative to protect the shoulder joint and reduce the risk of labral injuries associated with landing directly on fully outstretched arms. Notably, female cricketers may choose not to front slide if they have large breasts and/or premenstrual discomfort.

Generally, a fielder will dive to stop or catch an airborne ball when out of reach. To minimise injury, it is recommended that fielders open the hip, lead with the head and hands and reduce impact and momentum by rolling (dive to the side or backwards) or sliding (dive forward) once in contact with the ground [8].

5.5 Throwing

The nature of fielding requires a cricketer to approach a batted ball from various angles and execute a throw, often in unbalanced positions. This results in substantial throwing technique variability [9]. Nonetheless, all cricketing throws can be characterised by various phases and points in movement, including the preparatory arc, point of maximum external rotation (cocking), acceleration, point of ball release, deceleration, point of maximum internal rotation and follow-through (Fig. 5.4) [9]. This cycle of movement is completed in 0.68–0.73 s [9, 10] and supports the notion that throwing is one of the fastest athletic gestures [11].

It is thought that the culminative kinematics of the lower limb generate 51–55% of the energy required to throw overhead [12]. Through the systematic activation of the kinetic chain, a lag effect is created which allows each segment of the throwing arm to accelerate past the next, in a proximal to distal pattern [13]. Consequently, a cricketer's throwing arm moves into a position of approximately 90° shoulder elevation, 75° shoulder external rotation and 95° elbow flexion from fielding a ball to cocking. The throwing arm continues to elevate slightly as shoulder internal rotation and elbow extension is initiated to provide the acceleration required for ball release. Thereafter, shoulder internal rotation, horizontal adduction and elbow flexion facilitate arm deceleration and follow-through [9, 10].

Typically, an overhead throw (shoulder elevation > 100°) performed at 75–85% maximal velocity is preferred for optimal accuracy [14, 15]. However, it has been found that cricketers tend towards a side-arm throwing technique (90–100° elevation) [9, 10]. Furthermore, the time constraints and pressures of fielding often require rapid ball release, and consequently, the throwing technique may be compromised. Within

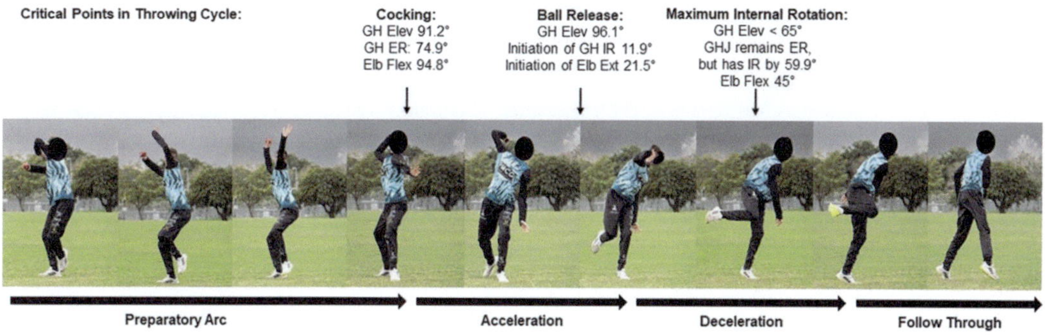
Critical Points in Throwing Cycle:
Cocking:
GH Elev 91.2°
GH ER: 74.9°
Elb Flex 94.8°
Ball Release:
GH Elev 96.1°
Initiation of GH IR 11.9°
Initiation of Elb Ext 21.5°
Maximum Internal Rotation:
GH Elev < 65°
GHJ remains ER,
but has IR by 59.9°
Elb Flex 45°
Preparatory Arc
Acceleration
Deceleration
Follow Through

Fig. 5.4 The phases and points in the cricket throwing cycle

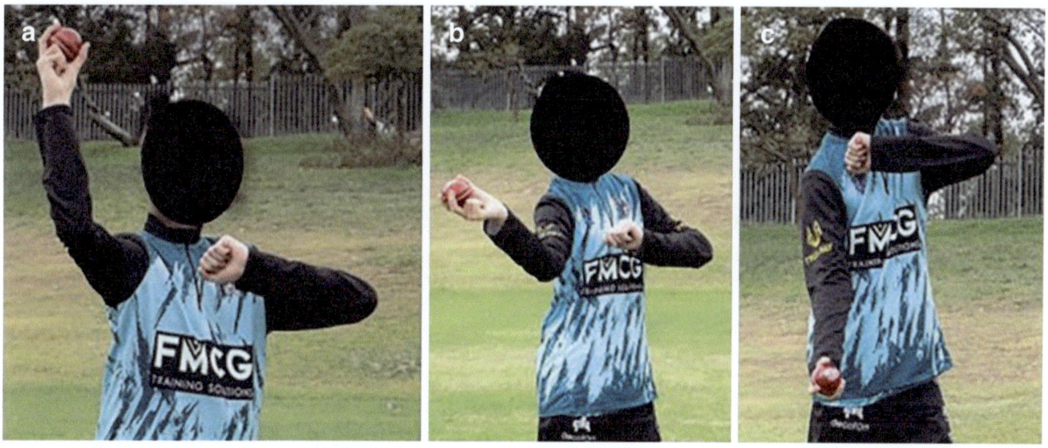
a
b
c

Fig. 5.5 Shoulder elevation categorising the (**a**) overhead, (**b**) sidearm and (**c**) submarine throwing techniques

a single match, a cricketer could throw utilising an overhead, sidearm or submarine (underarm) technique (Fig. 5.5) whilst moving in a variety of directions or possibly airborne. Table 5.1 provides a summary of the forces subjected to the shoulder and elbow during overhead, sidearm and submarine throwing from a stationary position, running towards and chasing after a ball to field it and return it to the wicket, in elite South African cricketers [9, 10, 16]. Notably, the greatest dynamic shoulder stability (compression and superior force at cocking) is provided by the overhead throw, which also imposes the greatest distractive forces on the shoulder during arm deceleration and follow-through. These forces may be attenuated when fielding a ball in motion, i.e., forward approach towards the batted ball or chasing after a ball, turning and throwing. Interestingly, dynamic shoulder stability at cocking wanes incrementally with the side arm and submarine throwing techniques. Conversely, the valgus force about the elbow escalates substantially through the techniques of overhead, sidearm (double that of overhead) and submarine (sextuple that of overhead) throwing at cocking [16]. It is therefore postulated that the injured throwing arm can be protected or off-loaded by encouraging cricketers to adopt an overhead or submarine throw, in the event of elbow or shoulder pain, respectively.

Numerous factors have been found to increase seasonal injury risk to the throwing arm in elite cricketers including:

1. Performing more than 75 throws per week and/or 40 throws per day [17].
2. Increased number of throwing days and subsequently a reduced number of rest days [17].

Table 5.1 The average shoulder and elbow forces (N) at critical points in the cycle of three throwing techniques, with a variety of approaches in male South African cricketers

	Overhead			Sidearm		Submarine/underarm	
	Stationary [9]	Running towards ball [10]	Chasing after ball & turning [16]	Stationary [16]	Running towards ball [16]	Stationary [16]	Running towards ball [16]
Shoulder							
Maximum external rotation							
Distraction (+)/ compression (−)	−102.2	−129.3	−115.5	−83.7	−108.1	−83.7	−89.0
Superior (+)/ inferior (−)	156.4	207.9	162.2	112.5	145.3	56.9	61.4
Anterior (+)/ posterior(−)	−7.2	−21.8	−20.0	6.8	−0.3	5.1	9.1
Ball release							
Distraction (+)/ compression (−)	−22.3	−4.4	−33.9	−2.1	5.2	−33.5	−32.5
Superior (+)/ inferior (−)	119.8	53.1	100.8	127.7	58.1	160.8	113.4
Anterior (+)/ posterior(−)	7.1	6.6	−0.5	3.9	−0.05	−0.4	1.8
Maximum internal rotation							
Distraction (+)/ compression (−)	61.4	68.6	61.8	47.9	66.0	12.7	15.7
Superior (+)/ inferior (−)	119.7	145.9	158.1	130.6	141.9	134.1	138.9
Anterior (+)/ posterior(−)	−62.2	−74.7	−60.3	−49.7	−58.7	−30.4	−27.7
Elbow							
Maximum external rotation							
Compression (+)/ distraction (−)	88.1	99.6	100.6	85.7	93.0	68.6	69.7
Superior (+)/ inferior (−)	27.8	31.0	37.4	19.0	17.5	48.7	50.0
Medial (+)/ lateral (−)	19.0	31.4	40.6	33.0	43.4	53.2	61.0
Ball release							
Compression (+)/ distraction (−)	22.2	4.0	17.8	8.8	6.2	−1.4	2.1
Superior (+)/ inferior (−)	39.5	10.9	30.6	31.9	7.2	71.8	48.6
Medial (+)/ lateral (−)	52.7	25.8	42.6	51.0	22.8	50.9	39.7

3. A history of previous shoulder injury increases the risk of sustaining another injury by 1.91 times [18].
4. Dominant supraspinatus tendon thickness of ≥5.85 mm (sensitivity: 72%, specificity: 63%) as measured on musculoskeletal ultrasound [19].
5. Non-dominant pectoralis minor length ≤ 12.85 mm (sensitivity: 83%, specificity: 55%) as measured from the coracoid process to the fourth costosternal junction [19].

Table 5.2 Musculoskeletal factors correlated with throwing performance in elite and amateur cricketers

	Elite Cricketers [20]		Amateur Cricketers [21]	
Performance Parameter	*Musculoskeletal Parameter*	*Effect*	*Musculoskeletal Parameter*	*Effect*
Speed	Dominant shoulder horizontal adduction ROM	1° increase in ROM increases throwing speed by 0.46 km/h	Non-dominant hip abduction strength	10 N increase in strength improves speed by 0.60 km/h
Accuracy	Dominant shoulder internal rotation strength	10 N increase in strength improves accuracy by 0.34 points	Non-dominant pectoralis minor length	1 cm increase in length improves accuracy by 0.633 points

Interestingly, not only are musculoskeletal factors predictive of seasonal shoulder injury (point 4 and 5 above) but many have been found to impact the performance of throwing speed and accuracy. Based on the level of participation of cricketers, these musculoskeletal factors, are summarised in Table 5.2 and highlight the necessity to include an assessment of the hips and non-dominant shoulder when assisting cricketers with treatment, pre- and rehabilitation of the throwing arm.

5.6 Fielding Injury Incidence

In elite men's cricket, the annual fielding (including wicketkeeping) injury incidence is 28.6% [22]. This is approximately half the fielding injury incidence of 45.8% occurring in an elite male u19 tournament held over a 1-month period [23]. In the men's game, the primary mechanisms of injury whilst fielding include running, diving, sliding, catching and throwing [23, 24]. Further, fielding injuries tend to occur at a rate of 40.6% and 42.9% to the upper and lower limbs, respectively [24]. These percentages differ slightly from those of elite u19 men, where the injury rate has been found to be 45.4% to the upper limb and 36.4% to the lower limb [23].

Conversely, in elite women's cricket, fielding is associated with the highest injury rate across all formats of the game [25]. Throwing and catching have been found to account for 10.7% of all fielding injuries, followed by diving (9.2%) [25, 26]. Approximately 22.8% of injuries occur to the upper limb (hand and wrist: 13.7%, shoulder 9.1%) and 7.7% to the lower limb (thigh: 4% and knee 3.7%) [26]. Of all fielding injuries in the women's game, 24.9% can be classified as sudden-onset non-contact injuries and 17.1% as traumatic/impact injuries [26].

Although fewer injury epidemiological studies have been conducted in women's cricket, there seems to be a trend that elite women have a lower match injury incidence in T20 and one-day cricket compared to their male counterparts [27]. However, the prevalence of injuries is known to escalate with increased match schedules and reduced rest days, irrespective of age, gender, race, format, era, country and player speciality [28].

5.7 Lower Limb Injuries

Notably, soft tissue injuries to the lower limb sustained whilst fielding account for more than half of the annual acute, first-time cricket injuries [28]. This is evidenced by the high frequency of hamstring injuries (50-over international matches: 13.4 injuries per 1000 team days; 50-over domestic matches: 10.2 injuries per 1000 team days), which most commonly result in a loss of match time (8.7 injuries/100 players per season) in elite men's cricket [29, 30]. Further, the daily hamstring injury rate has been shown to be highest in limited 50-over matches, followed by T20 and first-class matches. An unexpected risk factor for hamstring injury is the size of the cricket playing field, with Australia, whose cricket fields are approximately 40 m longer than the rest of the world, posing the greatest injury risk in men's cricket [30]. In addition, hamstring injuries account for approximately one-third (35.7%) of all thigh injuries in women's cricket, where the sudden acceleration and deceleration required when sprinting to chase a ball whilst fielding is thought to be a causative mechanism of injury [26]. Interestingly, the percentage of soft tissue injuries has been found to increase in consecutive seasons for both men and women [28].

Other common lower limb injuries sustained whilst fielding in both men's and women's cricket include acute knee (meniscal) and ankle (lateral ligament complex sprains) injuries [26, 31, 32]. These occur as a result of sprinting, sliding or diving at full length to retrieve a ball whilst fielding.

5.8 Upper Limb Injuries

The incidence of shoulder injury varies between 15–36% in elite men's cricket [18, 33–35], where throwing is the primary mechanism of injury [18]. Interestingly, fielding performance can be maintained by either modifying throwing technique or fielding position [18]. Consequently, these injuries rarely result in a loss of match time for both men and women [18, 26]. In addition, it is important to consider the secondary mechanism of shoulder injury, diving, which tends to be more prevalent in the T20 match format. Subsequently, most of the fielding shoulder injuries tend to be non-traumatic tendinopathies or traumatic muscle strains to the rotator cuff (specifically supraspinatus and biceps tendon), which can lead to humeral translation and SLAP lesions [18, 31]. Secondary injuries to the throwing arm include medial elbow apophysitis in adolescent cricketers or valgus extension overload syndrome with associated intra-articular degeneration in mature cricketers, which occur as a result of the repetitive valgus strain on the elbow [31].

Acute hand and wrist injuries in cricket vary between 11–13% of total annual injuries [31]. Finger fractures, dislocations or fracture -dislocations, and mallet finger injuries occur mostly in amateur cricket when attempting to execute a catch [31]. Similarly, hand and wrist injuries tend to be more common in female cricket players than in their male counterparts [26]. Finally, these injuries tend to be associated with the most time lost to training and matches. Box 5.2 summarises the most common injury areas when fielding in men's and women's elite cricket.

Box 5.2 Top Peripheral Injury Areas for Men's and Women's Cricket Fielding

Men:

1. Hamstring.
2. Ankle (specifically lateral ligament sprains).
3. Shoulder.
4. Hand.

Women:

1. Wrist and Hand.
2. Shoulder.
3. Thigh (specifically hamstring).
4. Knee.
5. Ankle.

5.9 Concussion

Although injury surveillance studies have extensively documented the above-mentioned peripheral injuries, increasing consideration of the effect of cervical spine whiplash injuries and associated concussion is required in the discipline of fielding [29, 36, 37]. Currently, 32% of concussions are diagnosed in fielders who contact the ground, through diving or sliding, or another player [36, 37]. Interestingly, both men and women have demonstrated a higher incidence of musculoskeletal injuries post-concussion [38]. This necessitates the need to include physical, cognitive and neuromuscular screening of the risk factors associated with concussion before returning to the field of play.

References

1. Brown P. A T20 merry-go-round, and a jelly-bean investigation. 2016.
2. MacDonald D, Cronin J, Mills J, McGuigan M, Stretch R. A review of cricket fielding requirements. S Afr J Sports Med. 2013;25(3):87–92. https://doi.org/10.7196/SAJSM.473.
3. MacDonald Wells DC, Cronin JB, Macdam P. Key match activities of different fielding positions and categories in one-day internal cricket. Int J Perform Anal Sport. 2018;18:609. https://doi.org/10.1080/24748668.2018.1501994.
4. Lim J, Wong S, McErlain-Naylor S, Scanlan A, Goggins L, Ahmun R, Comfort P, Weldon A. Strength and conditioning for cricket fielding: a narrative review. Strength Condition J. 2023;45(5):509–24. https://doi.org/10.1519/SSC.0000000000000758.
5. Cricket Rules and Regulations | ICC Rules of Cricket. https://www.icc-cricket.com/about/cricket/rules-and-regulations/playing-conditions. Accessed 12 June 2024.
6. Kanaujia A. All cricket fielding positions explained better to understand the commentary next time. 2023.
7. Bhole AM, Mittal RK. Cricket Catching Drills – application of a redundantly actuated 2-DOF-3-UPS parallel platform to increase the efficacy of providing catching drills in cricket. In: 3rd international congress on sport sciences research and technology support (icSPORTS 2015). Science and Technology Publications, Lda; 2015. p. 190–7.
8. CricFit: Athletic fielding's guidde to ground based cricket fielding: Rolling, sliding and diving. 2023. https://www.cricfit.co.uk/post/athletic-fieldings-guide-to-ground-based-cricket-fielding-rolling-sliding-diving. Accessed 19/06/2024.
9. Dutton M, Gray J, Prins D, Divekar N, Tam N. Overhead throwing in cricketers: a biomechanical description and playing level considerations. J Sports Sci. 2020;38:1096. https://doi.org/10.1080/02640414.2020.1741973.
10. Dutton M, Gray J, Divekar N, Prins D, Tam N. Overhead throwing biomechanics in cricketers: the effect of a run-up approach. Eur J Sport Sci. 2021;22:1686. https://doi.org/10.1080/17461391.2021.1979103.
11. Medina G, Bartolozzi AR, Spencer JA, Morgan C. The thrower's shoulder. J Bone Joint Surg. 2022;10(3) https://doi.org/10.2106/JBJS.RVW.21.00194.
12. Sundaram B, Skn B, Karuppannan S. Glenohumeral rotational range of motion differences between fast bowlers and spin bowlers in elite cricketers. Int J Sports Phys Ther. 2012;7(6):576 85.
13. Whiteley R. Baseball throwing mechanics as they relate to pathology and performance – a review. J Sports Sci Med. 2007;6(1):1–20.
14. Camp CL, Tubbs TG, Fleisig GS, Dines JS, Dines DM, Altchek DW, Dowling B. The relationship of throwing arm mechanics and elbow Varus torque: within-subject variation for professional baseball pitchers across 82,000 throws. Am J Sports Med. 2017;45(13):3030–5. https://doi.org/10.1177/0363546517719047.
15. Freeston JF, Ferdinands R, Rooney K. Throwing velocity and accuracy in elite and sub-elite cricket players: a descriptive study. Eur J Sport Sci. 2007;7(4):231–7. https://doi.org/10.1080/17461390701733793.
16. Leondiris J. Comparison of cricketer's shoulder and elbow loads in a variety of throwing techniques and fielding scenarios. Division of exercise science and sports medicine. Department of Human Biology, Faculty of Health Sciences: University of Cape Town; 2020.
17. Saw RD, Dennis RJ, Bentley D, Farhart P. Throwing workload and injury risk in elite cricketers. Br J Sports Med. 2011;45(10):805–8. https://doi.org/10.1136/bjsm.2009.061309.
18. Dutton M, Tam N, Gray J. Incidence and impact of time loss and non-time-loss shoulder injury in elite south African cricketers: a one-season, prospective cohort study. J Sci Med Sport. 2019;22:1200. https://doi.org/10.1016/j.jsams.2019.05.006.
19. Dutton M, Tam N, Brown JC, Gray J. The cricketer's shoulder: not a classic throwing shoulder. Phys Ther Sport. 2019;37:120–7. https://doi.org/10.1016/j.ptsp.2019.03.014.
20. Ahmed S. The influence of musculoskeletal variables on throwing performance in amateur and elite South African cricketers. Division of exercise science and sports medicine. Department of Human Biology, Faculty of Health Sciences: University of Cape Town; 2020.
21. Ahmed S, Brown J, Gray J. Predictors of throwing performance in amateur male cricketers: a musculoskeletal approach. Eur J Sport Sci. 2020;21:1119. https://doi.org/10.1080/17461391.2020.1819434.
22. Pardiwala DN, Rao NN, Varshney AV. Injuries in cricket. Sports Health. 2018;10(3):217–22. https://doi.org/10.1177/1941738117732318.
23. Das NSU, Usman J, Choudhury D, Osman NAA. Nature and pattern of cricket injuries: the Asian cricket Council Under-19, Elite Cup, 2013. PLoS One. 2014;9(6):e100028. https://doi.org/10.1371/journal.pone.0100028.
24. Stretch RA. Cricket injuries: a longitudinal study of the nature of injuries to South African cricketers. Br J Sports Med. 2003;37:250–3. https://doi.org/10.1136/Fbjsm.37.3.250.
25. Warren AD, Dale S, McCaig S, Ranson C. Injury profiles in elite women's T20 cricket. J Sci Med Sport. 2019;22(7):775–9.
26. Perera NKP, Kountouris A, Kemp JL, Joseph C, Finch CF. The incidence, prevalence, nature, severity and mechanisms of injury in elite female cricketers: a prospective cohort study. J Sci Med Sport. 2019;22:1014–20. https://doi.org/10.1016/j.jsams.2019.05.013.
27. Williams AP, Peirce N, Griffin S, Langley B, Warren A, Wedatilake T, Goggins L, McKay CD, Stokes KA, Williams S. A similar injury profile observed in

franchise men's and women's cricket in England and Wales: injury surveillance analysis from the first three "the hundred" competitions. BMJ Open Sport Exerc Med. 2024;10(1):e001815. https://doi.org/10.1136/bmj-sem-2023-001815.
28. Soomro N, Strasiotto L, Sawdagar T, Lyle D, Mills D, Ferdinands R, Sanders R. Cricket injury epidemiology in the twenty-first century: what is the burden? Sports Med. 2018;48:2301–16. https://doi.org/10.1007/s40279-018-0960-y.
29. Orchard JW, Kountouris A, Sims K. Incidence and prevalence of elite male cricket injuries using updated consensus definitions. Open Access J Sports Med. 2016;7:187–94. https://doi.org/10.2147/OAJSM.S117497.
30. Orchard JW, Kountouris A, Sims K. Risk factors for hamstring injuries in Australian male professional cricket players. J Sport Health Sci. 2017;6:271–4. https://doi.org/10.1016/j.jshs.2017.05.004.
31. Shafi M. Cricket injuries: an Orthopaedist's perspective. Orthop Surg. 2014;6(2):90–3. https://doi.org/10.1111/os.12104.
32. Oliver BN, Naude J, Mnguni N, Thotse M, Phalandwa P, Ferrao P, Saragas NP. Foot and ankle injuries in elite south African cricketers: a descriptive analysis of injury surveillance data. Indian. J Orthop. 2023;57:1592–9. https://doi.org/10.1007/s43465-023-00934-2.
33. Green RA, Taylor NF, Watson L, Ardern C. Altered scapula position in elite youngcricketers with shoulder problems. J Sci Med Sport. 2013;6:22–7. https://doi.org/10.1016/j.jsams.2012.05.017.
34. Giles KMI. A survey of glenohumeral joint rotational range and non-specific shoulder pain in elite cricketers. Phys Ther Sport. 2008;9:109–16. https://doi.org/10.1016/j.ptsp.2008.03.002.
35. Ranson C, GPSiipcPTS. Shoulder injury in professional cricketers. Phys Ther Sport. 2008;9:34–9. https://doi.org/10.1016/j.ptsp.2007.08.001.
36. Hill TO, Orchard J, Kountouris A. Incidence of concussion and head impacts in Australian elite-level male and female cricketers after Head impact protocol modifications. Sports Health. 2019;11:180–5. https://doi.org/10.1177/1941738118811315.
37. Saw AEH, Howard DJ, Kountouris A, McIntosh AS, Orchard JW, Saw R, Hill T. Situational factors associated with concussion in cricket identified from video analysis. J Concussion. 2020;4:4. https://doi.org/10.1177/2059700220947197.
38. McPherson ALN, Nagai T, Webster KE, Hewett TE. Musculoskeletal injury risk after sport-related concussion: a systematic review and meta-analysis. Am J Sports Med. 2019;47(7):1754–62. https://doi.org/10.1177/0363546518785901.

Wicketkeeping Biomechanics and Associated Injury in Cricket

6

Danielle C. MacDonald and Georgia Redmayne

6.1 Introduction

Whilst all players in a cricket team must field, the wicketkeeper has the highest probability of involvement in each delivery. The skills and attributes of a good wicketkeeper are unique to the position. Wicketkeepers can often be excellent at fielding in other positions, but it is highly unusual for another fielder to be able to keep wicket without prior training for the position. Despite this, there is a paucity of scientific literature relating to wicketkeeping; fielding already being the least investigated component of the game compared to batting and bowling [1]. This scarcity of research, ironically, may be attributable to the fact that the wicketkeeper *is* a specialist position, and therefore teams will only have a handful (at most) within their squad, and thus there is a small sample size for researchers to draw robust conclusions about [2]. This certainly seems to be the case for female wicketkeepers; despite the growing numbers of female participation in cricket, little to no research investigates female wicketkeepers.

Five components have been previously identified as contributors to wicketkeeping performance: technical, mental, physiological, physical and tactical [1]. Historically, the wicketkeeper was seen as a truly specialist position, with a player selected in a team based on their wicketkeeping skills alone, batting low down the order as bowlers do. However, the advent of limited overs cricket has seen the role evolve, as has fielding in general, and today's wicketkeepers are expected to be competent batters, usually batting in the top or middle order. The scores now seen in limited-over cricket are increasing; in 2022, England defeated the Netherlands in a One Day International match (50 overs each) by a monumental 232 runs by scoring 498 batting first [3]. In the 2024 Indian Premier League, the world's most lucrative T20 competition, there were 8 innings scores of greater than 250, meaning a run rate of more than 12 runs per over [4]. Such high scores as these mean that fewer deliveries are going through to the wicketkeeper.

The demand for all-round capability of wicketkeepers has seen tactical changes by teams, often choosing to use a player known more for their batting but who can keep wicket to a sufficient standard. This continues to be a topic of debate within coaching and commentary circles: does the players' proficiency with the bat outweigh the cost of potential poor wicketkeeping

D. C. MacDonald (✉)
England and Wales Cricket Board, National Cricket Performance Centre, Loughborough University, Loughborough, Leicestershire, UK

Tecnológico de Monterrey, Monterrey, N.L., Mexico
e-mail: danielle.macdonald@ecb.co.uk

G. Redmayne
Queensland Cricket, Allan Border Field, Albion, QLD, Australia

B. Olivier, J. W. Orchard (eds.), *Cricket Sports Medicine*,
https://doi.org/10.1007/978-981-96-6321-7_6

where, indeed, the few deliveries that do go through to the keeper often are wicket opportunities?

6.2 Skills and Attributes

The wicketkeeper is covered by Law 27 of the Laws of Cricket [5]; the law covers personal protective equipment, wicketkeeping gloves, their position in the field, their movement and restrictions on their actions. The wicketkeeper is the only fielder permitted to wear gloves and external leg guards; this right is forfeit if their actions and position in the field mean that they will not be able to carry out the normal duties of a wicketkeeper [5].

The wicketkeeper's role is to 'take' the ball, should the batter not play at the ball, to prevent the delivery from going for extras known as byes. If the batter plays a shot and the ball is fielded, the return throw is almost always to the wicketkeeper. Wicketkeepers can dismiss batters in several ways; they can catch the ball should the batter make contact with the ball in a way which causes it to travel behind the wicket; they can get a player out 'stumped' by taking the ball and breaking the wicket when the batter is out of their ground, and they can 'run out' the batter by receiving a throw from another fielder and either removing the bails from the stumps with the ball in hand or throwing the ball at the stumps. Wicketkeepers, therefore, must have 'good hands', to repetitively catch the ball and throw accurately, both overarm and underarm. Wicketkeepers may remove a glove to improve throw accuracy. Additionally, they must be agile and have excellent anticipation and reaction times to get into the best position to execute their skills.

Few studies have used notational analyses to investigate the frequency of fielding activities at a position-specific level in different formats of cricket, finding that differences exist between position in the field and format in cricket [6, 7]. A recent investigation of T20 matches from the Australian Big Bash League found that the wicketkeeper accounted for the highest number of primary fielding instances [8], but the absolute percentage of involvement of the wicketkeeper is lower than in previous studies of multiday [7] and One Day (50 over) cricket [6]. This difference is likely to be attributed to the fact that batters in T20 cricket play at a higher scoring shot percentage, and fewer balls are likely to travel through to the wicketkeeper.

Whilst their role within the match is, of course, the same as their male counterparts, the skills required of female wicketkeepers have a different emphasis. Due to the comparatively lower speeds bowled by female bowlers and the higher prevalence of spin bowlers, female wicketkeepers spend more time standing up to the stumps for spin and medium-pace bowlers.

Law 23 of the Laws of Cricket states that 'the ball becomes dead when it is finally settled in the hands of the wicketkeeper or bowler' [5]. Therefore, the wicketkeeper must have excellent physical stamina and mental concentration. Other fielders can generally 'switch off' mentally once they see that the ball has been hit to a different area of the field; wicketkeepers must be prepared to receive the ball from all other fielders and potentially execute a dismissal. Such is the nature of cricket that the smallest lapses in concentration and resulting errors can result in a loss by the smallest of margins [9].

Perceptual-cognitive skills are an important characteristic of elite sports performance, with research showing that experts outperform novices in anticipation and decision-making in a variety of sports [10]. Wicketkeepers must use the same visual cues as a batter to 'pick' the ball the bowler has bowled and assume an appropriate position to take the ball. They must also closely watch the batter and their position at the batting crease to execute any stumping opportunities. A small sample study of wicketkeepers (n = 12, sorted into expert and non-expert groups) found that expert wicketkeepers strategically select visual cues in order, with lateral information taking precedence over depth information [11].

Due to their position in the field, the wicketkeeper can make unique observations and assist team captains in setting field placements, bowling matchups and, in elite cricket, using Decision

Review System technology. By nature, wicketkeepers are often a 'busy' personality type, always wanting to be involved and contributing to the match. The wicketkeeper can lift the fielding side by camouflaging poor return throws from the field and encouraging their teammates.

6.3 Movement and Physiology

The wicketkeeper's position behind the stumps will change depending on the type of bowler; they will be standing back from the stumps for a fast bowler and will stand up to the stumps (directly behind the batter) for a spin, slow and occasionally medium-pace bowler. The movements and skills required of the wicketkeeper vary depending on these positions. Generally, a wicketkeeper is now required to wear a helmet when standing up to the stumps but will use a cap when standing back, meaning that a headwear change between overs is also a common requirement.

Typically, a wicketkeeper standing back from the stumps will either catch the ball directly or run towards the stumps to receive a throw from a fielder. Standing back from the stumps, a wicketkeeper has more time to react to the deviation of the ball but may have to cover a greater distance using lateral movements and dives. If they are standing up to the stumps for a spin bowler, the wicketkeeper has less reaction time but also generally less ground to cover, relying more on anticipatory movements, a strong base and quick reflexes. As previously mentioned, female wicketkeepers spend less time standing back from the stumps than their male counterparts and therefore will not be required to run up to the stumps as often.

A small handful of studies have attempted to evaluate the movements required of cricketers, which have found that movement requirements vary by both position and game format. Time-motion analysis has been considered important for coaches, trainers and other support staff to develop sport-specific conditioning programmes and tailor recovery periods based on quantified game demands [1, 9, 12, 13].

Petersen et al. [12] (as shown in Table 6.1) found that in T20 cricket, 7% of movements of wicketkeepers were spent in high-intensity efforts such as sprinting; despite this small percentage, these efforts are often in wicket-taking opportunities and are therefore important. The disadvantage of these time-motion analyses is that they do not consider the explosive movements of wicketkeepers such as diving and jumping.

Despite the relatively low-intensity level of the game, cricketers can be required to play for up to 6 hours a day over several days. A high level of aerobic fitness will help with recovery between days of play, heat stress and the ability to concentrate for long periods of time [14].

Very few studies investigating movement in cricket have investigated the wicketkeeper specifically [15–17]. Whilst wicketkeepers are found to spend a lesser amount of time in high-intensity sprints compared to fielders, they must perform highly repetitive explosive lateral movements from a squat position in order to get into position to catch the ball [9, 17]. A study by Rosen & Bower [15] identified numerous footwork patterns which varied according to personal preference and match situation. Furthermore, physical demands are dependent upon match format, with Petersen et al. [13] identifying that wicketkeepers covered a greater distance per hour in high-intensity efforts (running, striding and sprinting) in T20 matches (433 m) than in One Day matches (240 m) or multiday cricket (109 m).

To prepare themselves to be able to move appropriately to receive the ball, wicketkeepers typically adopt a variety of crouching positions: the full crouch, half crouch, and touch and move. The Australian wicketkeeper Sammy Carter (1878 to 1948) was the first player recorded to crouch down into a squatting position rather than simply bending at the waist [18].

The crouch position used by a wicketkeeper is usually influenced by their own personal choice and their physical ability. The most frequently reported choice of wicketkeeping stance is the full crouch, which is perhaps attributed to the fact that it has been used so successfully by players in the past [16]. Biomechanically, the full crouch is

Table 6.1 Percentage of time spent in each movement activity in T20 cricket [12]

% of time spent in activity	Fast bowling	Fielding	Batting	Wicketkeeping
Walking	51	54	68	73
Jogging	26	25	16	20
Running	7	6	3	3
Striding	9	8	6	3
Sprinting	9	7	7	1

Reproduced from Petersen et al. [12]. Percentage (%) of time spent at different speeds

deemed to be a resting position, taken up prior to moving into a 'power position' or loading phase. The half crouch and touch-and-move stances are loading phase stances. As per recommendations from a specialist wicketkeeping coach, a full crouch, or power position, should not be held for more than two seconds. This is to ensure that the power within the muscles is not lost prior to movement [9]. With the more dynamic touch-and-move stance, the wicketkeeper is moving from a counter-movement instead of a stationary position; therefore, the leg musculature is already activated when the movement starts [16].

Injuries.

Injury surveillance related to specific positions in cricket is a recent development, and few studies detail injuries specifically related to wicketkeeping [19, 20]. Due to the nature of their role, wicketkeepers could be considered at an increased risk of hand and finger injuries, head knocks, and lower body conditions associated with repetitive load. Most research into injuries in cricket positions combine wicketkeeping with fielders and does not specifically investigate injuries related to the position of wicketkeeper. A study published in 2002 [19] investigated cricket injuries in Australian cricket over a five-year period and recorded incidents of wicketkeepers sustaining hand and wrist, lumbar, knee and leg injuries. The same study also found that wicketkeepers had the lowest overall injury prevalence compared to other positions. It could be inferred that the reduced sprinting and throwing volume appears to be protective against common shoulder and other soft tissue injuries seen in their teammates.

It has also been suggested that due to the unique nature of the position, some wicketkeepers may under-report or under-investigate their injuries for fear of missing matches [19]. There may often be pressure to play injured due to a lack of available wicketkeeping replacements, or the player may be wary of being replaced in the team and losing a chance to cement their place in the side. For example, given the lack of sprinting required, keepers can often carry or hide low-grade hamstring, quadricep or calf strains behind the stumps more easily than outfielders. It is critically important that this practice is discouraged, especially in younger players, to prevent any lasting damage that could affect their future careers. Any decision to continue to play whilst injured should be well informed on the basis of available information and medical guidance.

Hand and finger injuries to wicketkeepers are common and may be sustained by direct impact from the ball, ground or even the bat. Despite being the only fielder permitted to wear gloves, a previous literature review [21] found that most hand injuries in cricket are sustained by wicketkeepers. This may be explained by the sheer volume of balls directed at them. An Australian study [22] reported that wicketkeepers have a higher risk of hand fractures (per player per 100,000 balls) compared to fielders for both males (1.59 > 0.48) and females (2.88 > 1.44). It should also be noted that female wicketkeepers have a higher rate of hand fractures than their male counterparts. The distribution of these fractures is generally focused on the palmar surface of exterior bones of the hand (generally fractures of the distal phalanx with fingers 1 and 5 more exposed than fingers 2, 3 and 4), as these are more vulnerable to direct impact [23]. The same study also found that, compared to fielders, wicketkeepers had a higher proportion of middle phalanx to distal phalanx fractures. Whether this is due to protection provided by wicketkeeping gloves to the distal phalanx or possible under-reporting of these injuries (generally more minor than middle phalanx injuries) is unclear. It is important to note that distal phalanx fractures are the most common and safest to continue playing with, as they are often non-articular and heal well, and even if they involve the distal interphalangeal joint, there doesn't tend to be a significant functional loss. Despite being less common, middle or proximal phalanx injuries involving the proximal interphalangeal joint should always be investigated and medically managed. These fractures heal poorly if they displace, and post-traumatic osteoarthritis can cause loss of ability to grip the bat and be career threatening. Depending on the location and articular involvement, hand fractures sustained whilst wicketkeeping may require referral to orthopaedic surgeons and occupational hand therapy for ongoing management. With regard to chronic and repetitive risk, it has been reported that repeated high-velocity impacts could lead to osteoarthritis of finger joints and recurrent collateral ligament damage [24].

Wicketkeepers are also at risk of head impacts, either from direct contact from a bowled delivery or throw, as well as deviation off the wickets, ground, bat or batter. This risk is especially present when keeping up to the stumps when reaction times are reduced. There is also an uncommon risk of a direct blow from the bat during the batter's bat swing or follow-through whilst the keeper is up to the stumps. To minimise concussion and other head injury risks, many governing bodies have enforced that wicketkeepers are required to wear a helmet when keeping up to the stumps, and it is strongly recommended that this is encouraged at all levels of cricket. Any head impacts should be taken seriously, and players should be screened for concussion symptoms before being allowed to continue.

Due to the nature of their repetitive crouching and power movements, wicketkeepers can be susceptible to chronic strains of the back, hips and lower limbs. Muscle groups under increased loading from these positions include hip flexors, quadriceps and gluteal muscles. Research has indicated that the full crouch position may trigger greater knee flexion and knee joint pressure compared to the half crouch and touch-and-move stances and suggests this technique be avoided by wicketkeepers with a history of knee injuries [25].

6.4 Coaching and Conditioning

As with other parts of the game, wicketkeeping coaching and conditioning practices are largely based on anecdotal experience rather than scientific evidence. An example being coaching advice such as '*when you're standing up, try and stand as close as you can, because the closer you are, the less deviation off the bat when the batsman nicks it, the more chance of it hitting your palm rather than the outside of your thumb*' as Harold Stephenson quoted in an interview [23], has dual benefits in terms of being able to better catch the ball and avoid injury to the thumbs.

However, the inclusion of sports scientists, performance analysts and data scientists into the coaching staff of professional teams means that practitioners are now able to collect scientific evidence to support their coaching practices. A professional cricket team's backroom staff can now include specialist bowling, batting and fielding coaches; physiotherapists; strength and conditioning coaches; nutritionists; mental skills coaches and sports scientists. These practitioners are now able to collect and use performance and health and conditioning data to monitor performance and fitness levels throughout the season. It is important that all parties work together to ensure the players they are working with have the skills, physical condition and mental capacity to play to the very best of their ability.

In recent years, a study was conducted by the science and medicine and coaching staff at the England & Wales Cricket Board, which investigated whether it was quicker for a wicketkeeper to remove the bails following an off target throw at the stumps from a fielder by standing in front of the stumps rather than the traditional method of remaining in their usual position behind the stumps [26]. The investigation found that the wicketkeeper was able to remove the bails more quickly if they stood in front of the stumps, allowing them to take the ball and remove the bails in one fluid motion. The key point made was that the wicketkeeper needed to know exactly where their stumps were to successfully save time by standing in front of the stumps. However, when the test was repeated with a bowler, it was determined that they were, in fact, slower at removing the bails from in front of the stumps, likely because they do not practice the skill of receiving the ball in from the fielders as wicketkeepers do.

Wong et al. [2] present a battery of tests to assess the physical fitness of wicketkeepers including anthropometry, movement screening, strength, power, aerobic capacity, speed and agility. Testing batteries such as these at regular intervals (for example, pre-, mid- and post-season) will assist practitioners in prescribing training and managing player workloads. For a wicketkeeper, building a solid aerobic base and then adding sprint work, agility and change of direction should form the basis of a conditioning programme. Based on the large volume of lateral activities performed by wicketkeepers, it would be beneficial to improve multidirectional reactive strength to enhance their diving ability [2] by including single-leg strength work. Wong et al. [2] present sample training plans specifically designed for wicketkeepers. Practitioners should be mindful of the different game demands and variances in the physiology of female wicketkeepers and tailor their practices accordingly.

Practitioners working with wicketkeepers can look to research in other sports with similar movements, such as football goalkeepers or baseball catchers, to gain insights which may benefit wicketkeepers.

6.5 Conclusion

Despite the recent evolution of the game of cricket, the wicketkeeper remains a specialist position within cricket fielding. The skills and movements required are unique to this position and must be considered and tailored to the specific individual when prescribing training practices. Coaches and medical practitioners working with wicketkeepers should be mindful of the need to rely on anecdotal evidence whilst there is a lack of scientific evidence in regard to physiological requirements and injuries.

References

1. MacDonald D, Cronin J, Mills J, McGuigan M, Stretch R. A review of cricket fielding requirements. S Afr J Sports Med. 2013;25(3):87–92. https://doi.org/10.7196/SAJSM.473.
2. Wong S, Lim J, McErlain-Naylor SA, Scanlan A, Goggins L, Ahmun R, et al. Strength and conditioning for cricket Wicketkeeping: a narrative review. Strength Condition J. 2024;47:1–12. https://doi.org/10.1519/SSC.0000000000000847.
3. cricinfo E: Netherlands vs England, 1st ODI at Amstelveen, NL v ENG, Jun 17 2022 – Full Scorecard. 2022. https://www.espncricinfo.com/series/england-in-netherlands-2022-1281442/netherlands-vs-england-1st-odi-1281444/full-scorecard. Accessed 21/07/2024.
4. cricinfo E: Team Records – Highest Innings Totals in IPL 2024. 2024. https://www.espncricinfo.com/records/tournament/team-highest-innings-totals/indian-premier-league-2024-15940. Accessed 21/07/2024.
5. Club MC. The laws of cricket. In: Club MC, editor. 2017 Code. 3rd ed. London, 2022.
6. MacDonald DC, Cronin JB, Macadam P. Key match activities of different fielding positions and categories in one-day international cricket. Int J Perform Anal Sport. 2018;18(4):609–21.
7. Shilbury D. An analysis of fielding patters of and 'A' grade cricket team. Sports Coach. 1990;13(4):41–4.
8. Lee TA, Novak AR, Rodriguez ECP. Position-specific fielding instances and utilisation in professional men's T20 cricket. Moore Park: Human Performance Research Centre, School of Sport, Exercise and Rehabilitation, Faculty of Health, University of Technology Sydney; 2024.
9. MacDonald DC. Performance analysis of fielding and wicket-keeping in cricket to inform strength and conditioning practice. Sports Performance Research Institute New Zealand. Auckland: Auckland University of Technology; 2015.
10. Hopwood M, Mann D, Farrow D, Nielsen T. Does visual-perceptual training augment the fielding performance of skilled cricketers. J Sports Sci Coach. 2011;6(4):1–15.
11. Houlston D, Lowes R. Anticipatory cues-utilization processes amongst expert and non-expert wicketkeepers in cricket. Int J Sports Psychol. 1993;24:59–73.

12. Petersen C, Portus M, Dawson B. Quantifying positional movement patterns in Twenty20 cricket. Int J Perform Anal Sport. 2009;9:165–70.
13. Petersen C, Pyne D, Dawson B, Kellett A. Movement patterns in cricket vary by both position and game format. J Sports Sci. 2010;28(1):45–52.
14. Johnstone J, Ford P. Physiologic profile of professional cricketers. J Strength Cond Res. 2010;24(11):2900–7.
15. Rosen B, Bower R. Analysis of the footwork patterns of elite wicket-keepers in cricket. J Hum Mov Stud. 2006;51:181–96.
16. Plunkett D, Salter C, Moore D. The difference in efficiency of movements to the ball between wicketkeeping stances Australian Sports Commission. 2005.
17. MacDonald DC, Cronin J, Mills J, Stretch R. Wicket-keeping in cricket: a literature review. Int J Sports Sci Coach. 2013;8(3):531–41.
18. Cashman R. The Oxford companion to Australian cricket. Oxford University Press; 1996.
19. Orchard J, James T, Alcott E, Carter S, Farhart P. Injuries in Australian cricket at first class level 1995/1996 to 2000/2001. Br J Sports Med. 2002;36:270–5.
20. Orchard JW, James T, Portus MR. Injuries to elite male cricketers in Australia over a 10-year period. J Sci Med Sport. 2006;9:459–67.
21. McGrath A, Finch C. Bowling cricket injuries over: a review of the literature. Critical review, 1985–1996. Monash University Accident Research Centre, Wellington Road, Clayton, Victoria, 3168, Australia.
22. Brooks K, ORchard J, Saw A, Kountouris A. Hand fractures and return to play in elite Australian cricketers. J Orthop. 2020;22(22):100–3.
23. Taylor B. Standing up to the wicket is what keeping is all about. In: Oliver S, editor. The cricket monthly. Online: ESPN Cricinfo; 2013.
24. Belleppa P, Barton N. Hand injuries in cricketers. J Hand Surg Br Vol. 1991;16(2):212–4.
25. Escamilla R, Fleisig G, Zheng N, Barrentine S, Wilk K, Andrews J. Biomechanics of the knee during closed kinetic chain and open kinetic chain exercises. Med Sci Sport Exerc. 1998;30(4):556–69.
26. Egan S. Analysis: should keepers stand in front of the stumps for run outs? 2018. https://crickether.com/2018/03/03/analysis-should-keepers-stand-in-front-of-the-stumps-for-run-outs/. Accessed 21/10/2024 2024.

Personal Protective Equipment in Cricket: The Past, Present and Future

7

Claire Bolton, Nick Peirce, Ifraah Naeem Naeem, and Andy Harland

7.1 Why Do Cricketers Need PPE?

Although not strictly a contact sport, cricket involves an extremely hard ball being delivered at high speeds (25–45 m/s) towards the batter [1]. A ball that leaves the hand at 90 mph still reaches the batter with a speed of approximately 75 mph. Therefore, batters, who stand approximately 20 m away from where the bowler delivers the ball, have 35–80 ms to react and make a judgement of what, if any, shot to play [2]. The ball also travels off the bat at high speeds, occasionally in unpredictable directions. The laws of cricket also allow a bowler to direct a ball at the batter when bowling, including towards their head (provided the ball bounces first). Therefore, batters and players standing in the immediate vicinity are at significant risk of being struck by the ball.

A ball strike can produce a force of greater than 600 g, exceeding thresholds for all human tissues including bones. This threatens multiple areas of the body, which require protection from contusions, fractures, head injuries and potentially uncommon but serious impact to the chest and resultant cardiac death (commotio cordis). There are no published studies specifically describing all ball strike injuries; however, Ranson et al. [3] showed areas of the skull struck by the ball and Deshmukh et al. [4] examined injuries to the hand. Player safety has attracted significant attention following several high-profile cases, primarily the death of Australian cricketer Phillip Hughes who was struck by a ball when batting in 2014, and other incidents of balls hitting batters, fielders, and support staff or umpires [2]. Some documented fatalities in modern cricket are outlined in Table 7.1.

Therefore, cricket has developed sport-specific personal protective equipment (PPE) to reduce the frequency and severity of injury. PPE

C. Bolton (✉)
The England and Wales Cricket Board, London, UK
e-mail: Claire.bolton@ecb.co.uk

N. Peirce
The England and Wales Cricket Board, London, UK

Loughborough University School of Sport, Exercise and Health Sciences, Loughborough, Leicestershire, UK
e-mail: Nick.peirce@ecb.co.uk

I. N. Naeem
Loughborough University School of Sport, Exercise and Health Sciences, Loughborough, Leicestershire, UK
e-mail: I.Naeem@lboro.ac.uk

A. Harland
Loughborough University School of Mechanical, Electrical and Manufacturing Engineering, Sports Technology Institute, Loughborough, Leicestershire, UK
e-mail: a.r.harland@lboro.ac.uk

B. Olivier, J. W. Orchard (eds.), *Cricket Sports Medicine*,
https://doi.org/10.1007/978-981-96-6321-7_7

Table 7.1 Summary of recorded fatalities due to ball strikes while playing cricket

Name	Level of cricket	Country	Age	Year	Activity	PPE	Cause of death	Summary
John Williams [6]	Amateur Club	Wales	80	2019	Umpiring	None	Head injury	Struck on the head by a ball which had been hit by a batter. Placed into an induced coma and died a month later in hospital
Bavalan Pathmanathan [7]	Amateur Club	England	24	2015	Batting	Unknown	Possible Commotio Cordis	Player hit on the chest by the ball when batting and collapsed on the pitch. Given CPR and taken to hospital but later died
Hillel Oscar [8]	Amateur Club	Israel	55	2014	Umpiring	None	Head injury	Struck in the jaw by a ball which had been hit by a batter, possibly after the ball ricochetted off the stumps. Taken to hospital but unable to be revived
Phillip Hughes [9]	State	Australia	25	2014	Batting	Helmet	Head injury	Struck on the back the neck by a bouncer during a match. The impact ruptured the vertebral artery. Hughes was resuscitated on the pitch but died of his injuries 2 days later
Darryn Randall [10]	Amateur Club (ex-first-class player)	South Africa	32	2013	Batting	Helmet	Head injury	Playing a domestic game and was struck on the side of the neck when attempting to play a pull shot. Was rushed to hospital after collapsing on the field
Zulfiqar Bhatti [11]	Club	Pakistan	22	2013	Fielding	None	Possible Commotio Cordis	While batting, the player was hit in the chest by the ball and collapsed. Unable to be resuscitated

(continued)

Table 7.1 (continued)

Name	Level of cricket	Country	Age	Year	Activity	PPE	Cause of death	Summary
Alcwyn Jenkins [12]	Club	England	72	2009	Umpire	None	Head injury	Suffered a head injury while fielding after being hit by a ball thrown by a fielder. Airlifted to hospital but didn't recover from injuries
Raman Lamba [13]	Club	India	38	1998	Fielding	None	Head injury	While fielding at short leg during a club match, the player was struck on the head by the ball. Suffered significant brain injuries and was pronounced dead after being placed in an induced coma

is now commonplace, with its use specified in the games' laws. Batters are permitted 'a helmet, external leg guards (batting pads), batting gloves and, if visible, forearm guards', fielders may wear a helmet, and wicketkeepers are permitted helmets, gloves and external leg guards [5]. Minimum standards for PPE are not explicitly outlined in the Laws of Cricket, but the British Standards Institution has published standards for various items of cricket PPE that are now generally accepted.

Some players are also at risk of being struck by objects other than the ball, most notably the bails. Bails are traditionally made of wood and sit on top of the stumps. After a ball hits the stumps or the bails, they can fly off potentially striking the wicketkeeper if they are close to the stumps. There are several documented incidents of serious, career-ending eye injuries after being struck by a bail. These have more commonly occurred in those not wearing a helmet but lead to calls for the bails to be tethered to the stumps. Since the introduction of mandatory helmets or facemasks for wicketkeepers standing up to the stumps, there have been no notable eye injuries. However, there is still a theoretical risk of the bails passing through the grill, meaning additional eyewear would improve protection.

7.2 History of PPE in Cricket

Cricket PPE has moulded, and been moulded by, the game itself. As bowlers began bowling overarm, batters found their lower legs were vulnerable to injury and sought options to protect them. The earliest leg pads comprised white-painted canvas with vertical strips of cane wood, heavy cotton stuffing and leather buckles. Unsurprisingly, these were heavy and restrictive, significantly limiting a batter's movement. Over time, batters took advantage of these large pads to deliberately block the ball from hitting the stumps. This resulted in a 1744 addition to the Laws of Cricket to prevent this, and leg before wicket (LBW) as a dismissal was born.

Interestingly, genital protectors (boxes) were introduced almost a century before helmets, with the first references in the early 1800s. Players wished to prevent themselves from pain, and resultant immobilisation, if they were struck in this area.

Helmet wearing was initially controversial, with boos and heckles from the crowd when Dennis Amiss first wore a helmet in the 1970s. Before long, Amiss' colleagues and teammates recognised the benefits of helmets. When a ball bowled by Andy Roberts broke David Hookes' jaw, Hookes asked if he could borrow Amiss' helmet the next time he played. On his return from injury, the first ball Hookes faced was another from Roberts, which he hit for six. Commentator Richie Benaud called this a 'defining moment for cricket' [14].

Batting gloves emerged to shield batters' hands from ball strikes and protect from the abrasive surface of the bat handle. Early gloves had leather palms and minimal finger protection before a cane was added to protect the back of batters' hands.

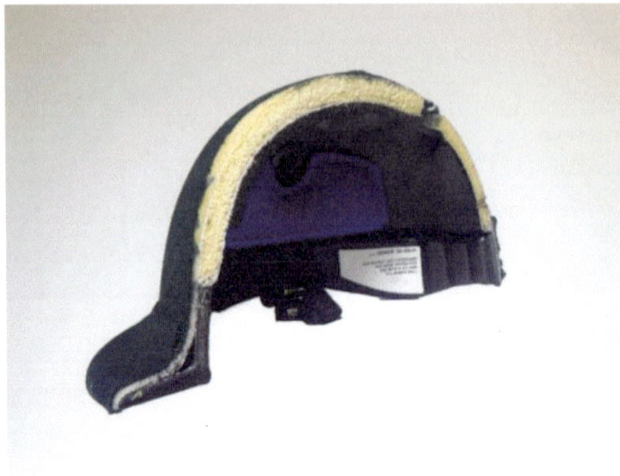

Fig. 7.1 Cross section of a batting helmet, showing the internal layers

7.3 What Forms of PPE Are There?

7.3.1 Helmets

Head injuries used to account for up to 23% of injuries [15]. As such, Helmets are now universally accepted and are incorporated into the cricketing laws to ensure the safety of the players [2].

Helmets are designed to protect the head by absorbing and distributing the energy generated on impact, dissipating energy into the inner protective padding to gradually transfer the impact load to the head and protect against penetration [16]. Helmets are made up of several elements. A stiff, generally fibreglass or acrylonitrile butadiene styrene, shell spreads the impact force, while a low-density polyethylene soft liner absorbs the impact energy [3]. A faceguard or grille attaches to the front of the helmet to protect the face from contact injuries. Helmets are held in place using an adjustable padded chin strap (Fig. 7.1).

Initial helmets had modifiable gaps between the peak and grill, which batters preferred large to maximise visibility. However, repeated career-ending eye socket injuries and academic findings [3], shown in Fig. 7.2, highlighted that a large gap left players vulnerable to injuries as the ball could pass through (as seen in Fig. 7.2). As such, grills and peaks were strengthened, and rigid attachments were designed to prevent batters from adapting the gap between the peak and grille. A new British Standard was introduced in 2014 (BS 7928:2013) and was mandated by the ECB across all professionals and under-18s. The ICC then adopted this as the international standard, and a list of helmets passing the standard is available on the ICC website.

7.3.2 Neck Protectors

The 2014 British Standard for helmets omitted protection for the lower occiput and neck, largely due to concerns around head movements being too restricted. However, research suggests that 17% of head injuries occurred at the back of the skull and 6% occurred at the neck with no contact with the helmet [3]. Combined with the tragic death of Phillip Hughes in 2014 due to a ball strike at the base of his skull, this leads to a new design and British Standard of neck protectors (BS 7928:2013+A1:2019). Neck protectors aim to reduce the frequency and severity of injuries to the base of the rear of the head (occiput) and upper neck (Fig. 7.3). *Neck protectors are now compulsory to wear when batting in English and Australian elite domestic cricket or playing for one of these two teams internationally. Most other countries have not yet made neck protectors compulsory, nor are they routinely used in amateur cricket.*

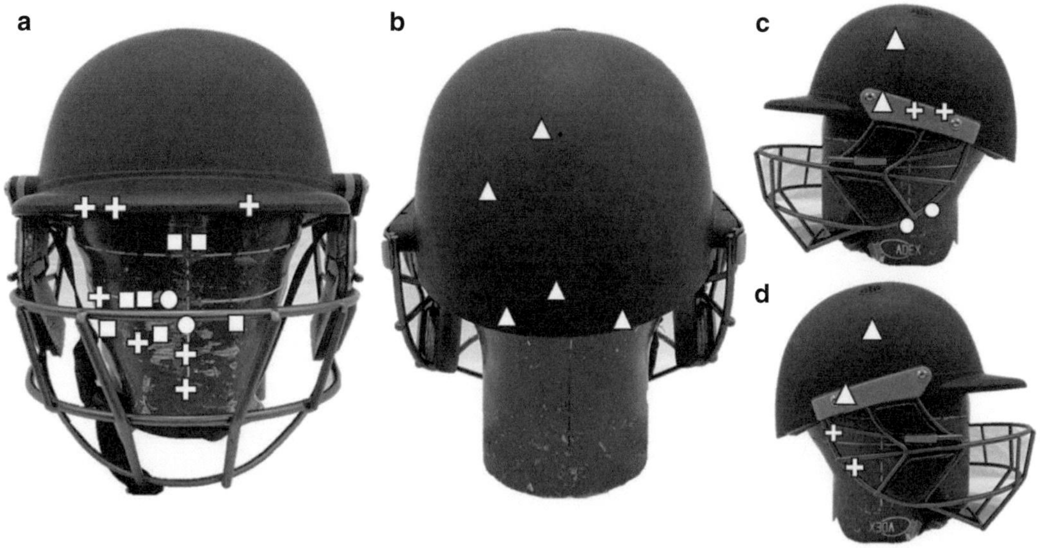

Fig. 7.2 Impact locations and primary injury types: (**a**) face, (**b**) back of the head, (**c**) non-dominant side of the head and (**d**) dominant side of the head. Injury symbols: triangle—concussion; cross—laceration; star—haematoma; circle—eye injury; square—fracture [3]

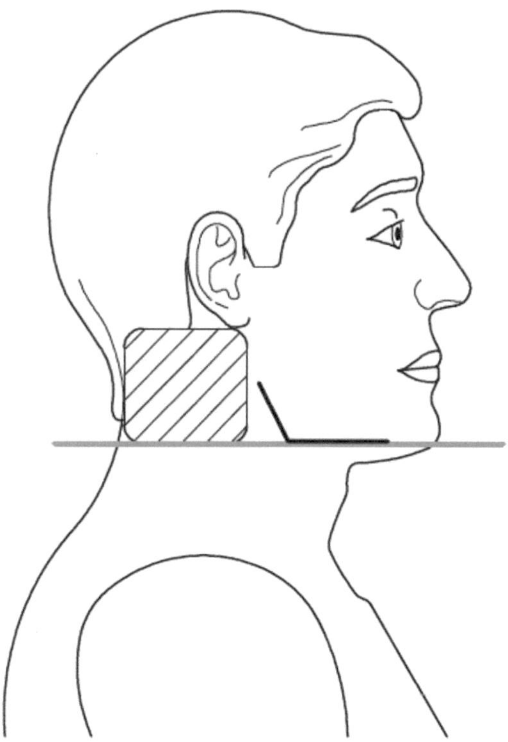

Fig. 7.3 Neck protector coverage. (Source: British Standard BS 7928:2013+A1:2019)

7.3.3 Gloves

Batters' hands are particularly vulnerable to ball strikes or being crushed against the bat handle. Figure 7.4 shows where the gloves appear to fail to protect fully during batting (a) or wicketkeeping (b) [4]. Glove designs have changed very little over the years, with minimal advancements in material and design to maintain affordable products.

7.3.4 Genital Protectors (Boxes)

Testicular injuries are relatively rare when compared to other sports injuries [17]. However, over half of all testicular injuries are sustained during sports, with blunt force trauma the cause of almost all sports-related male genital injuries [18]. In cricket, this trauma is somewhat preventable by wearing a box. The best performing genital protectors have a more rounded shape and greater internal depth, making them more difficult to distort by impact; boxes also offer the

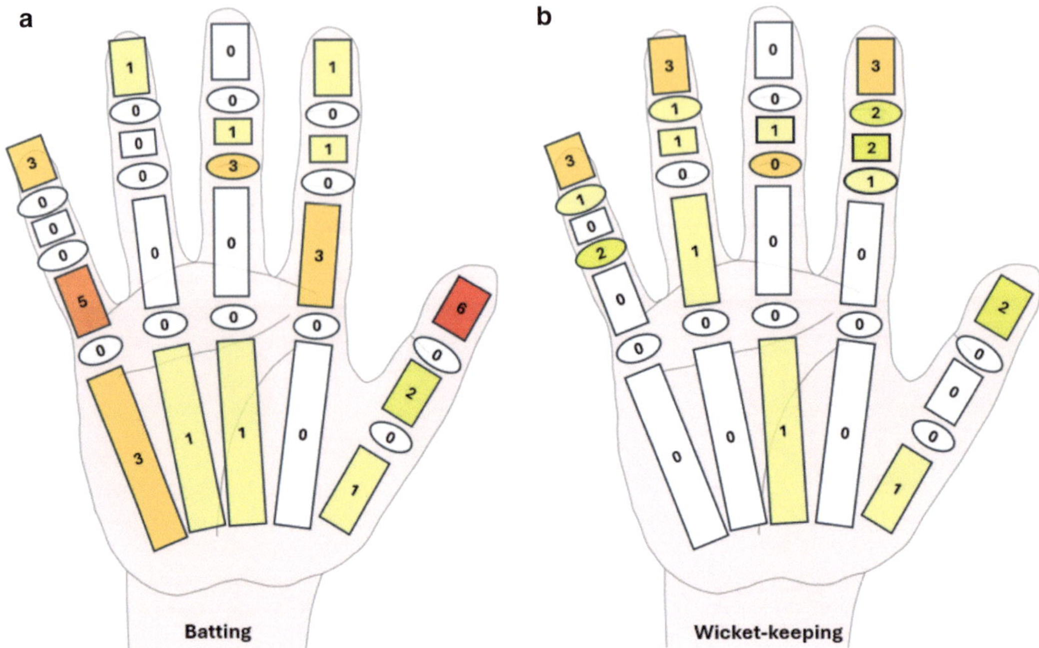

Fig. 7.4 Distribution of fracture and dislocation injuries occurring to areas of the hand during (**a**) batting (29 fractures, 0 dislocations) and (**b**) wicketkeeping (18 fractures, 7 dislocations) [4]

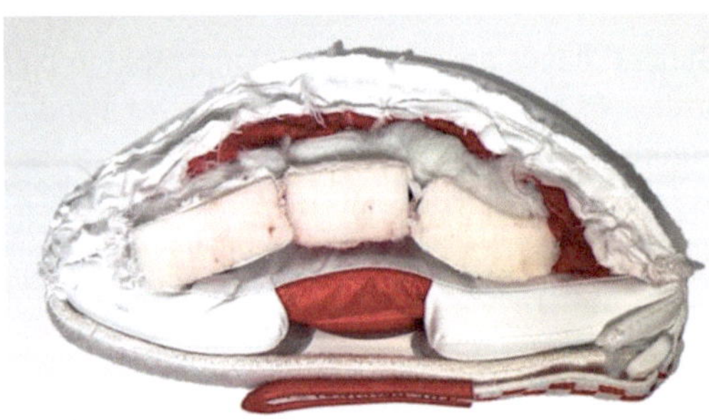

Fig. 7.5 Cross section of a cricket leg pad, taken from the top of the pad, showing the internal layers, vertical strips of padding, padded inners and strap

greatest protection when they are worn beneath any clothing. A British Standard (BS 6183-2:2000) was published in 2000 and outlines the structure and strength required for optimal safety. Since this standard was developed, little effort has been applied to research and the improvement of genital PPE, which has resulted in injuries occurring due to poor quality of boxes or boxes being worn incorrectly.

7.3.5 Leg Pads

Leg pads are designed to protect the anterior aspects of the lower leg and knee and are worn by batters, fielders in certain positions and wicketkeepers (Fig. 7.5).

The *face* of the pad protects the front of the lower leg and makes up the largest surface area. Vertical strips of padding are separated by rods, allowing the pad to wrap around the shin. The gap between each block of padding should not exceed 20 mm when the pad is strapped to the leg to ensure that the ball cannot contact the batter's leg.

Knee rolls offer extra flexibility around the knee by containing less stiff material than other areas of leg pads but with horizontal strips of protective padding. Knee rolls are less pronounced in wicketkeeping pads, offering greater flexibility and ease of movement. Knee rolls can assist umpires in determining the height of a ball in an LBW judgement. Although modern materials and designs mean traditional knee rolls are not necessarily required, players have reported being given out LBW more often when wearing pads without a knee roll, as the height of the ball was harder to judge.

The *top hat* sits above the knee roll to protect the lower thigh. Given that the lower thigh generally has greater muscle volume, there is less padding here than in other areas. In wicketkeeping pads where there is no knee roll, the top hat is less discernible from the rest of the pad.

The *wings* differ between batting pads and wicketkeeping pads, and asymmetric and symmetrically designed pads. Lighter asymmetric pads add protection only where it is needed (the inside of the rear leg and outside of the forward leg), while symmetrical pads are slightly heavier with even protection across each leg. Wicketkeeping pad wings are on the outside and provide wrap-around protection.

Several cushioned Velcro *straps* secure the pads to the legs.

The *instep* is an inverted U that fits over the player's shoe and protects the lower shin and ankle. This area of the pad contacts the bowlers' shoe, and occasionally the floor and therefore is typically reinforced to prevent against excessive wear.

Pad *inners* give extra support and comfort by providing a softer contact, and greater airflow behind the pad. Some inners are removable and washable, helping enhance hygiene.

7.3.6 Thigh Pads

Thigh protectors protect the thigh and hip that correspond to the batter's predominant thigh and may also cover their back leg. Thigh pads have several Velcro straps to allow for a close and comfortable fit.

7.3.7 Arm and Chest Guards

A ball strike to the ribs is not uncommon and can cause discomfort and occasionally rib fractures. Resultantly, some players wear chest guards around their leading rib cage (side-facing bowler). Chest guards are more common in those facing the extremes of fast bowling, in white ball cricket and in less skilled and confident batters in the lower order. Some chest guards now include modern shock-absorbing materials, and a British Standard (BS 6183-2:2000) is available. A direct strike to the chest wall can result in commotio cordis, which is a rare but potentially fatal condition. Commotio cordis occurs when an object (usually small and hard, like a cricket ball) strikes the chest directly over the heart during a critical time during a heartbeat. This immediately causes an abnormal heart rhythm (ventricular fibrillation) and cardiac arrest [18, 19]. Commotio cordis deaths have occurred in cricket, as indicated in Table 7.1. Coupled with the impact on performance and comfort, this may explain why full chest protectors across the sternum are not routinely worn despite the risk. Nevertheless, umpires are wearing chest protectors more commonly and are interested in improvements in their ergonomic qualities. It is worth noting, however, that research has reported that chest protectors may not be sufficient to substantially reduce the risk of commotio cordis in baseball [20]. Therefore, the effectiveness of chest protectors as PPE to prevent commotio cordis in cricket warrants further investigation.

Arm protectors speak for themselves in that they are worn on the leading arm against the fastest bowlers.

7.4 PPE for Coaches and Support Staff

Coaches and umpires have suffered severe and occasionally fatal injuries due to being struck by the ball. Subsequently, governing bodies are exploring strategies and policies to protect support staff. For example, the England and Wales Cricket Board and Cricket Australia have implemented policies that require support staff and coaches taking up certain positions during training sessions to wear helmets. Further, some umpires are seeking their own PPE solutions to the risk they are exposed to during matches. In many ways, cricket is a long way behind its

American cousin, baseball, on this matter, with baseball home plate umpires, who, albeit, are much closer to the path of the ball, wearing full PPE from helmets and chest guards right down to reinforced shoes.

7.5 The Impact of PPE on Cricket and Injuries

Much of the evidence on the effectiveness of PPE purports to helmets, as this most vital item of PPE to prevent severe or catastrophic injury. Helmets have been shown to be very successful in preventing specific head injury risks, especially moderate to severe head injuries, across several sports [3]. Wearing a helmet can lead to a reduction in the peak acceleration and the force applied to the skull, as well as a reduction in the skull's internal energy during a simulated ball strike [2]. This appears to have reduced head injuries, with a 16% reduction in the proportion of all head and neck injuries sustained by batters pre- and post-introduction of helmet regulations in July 2016 [21]. This effect is further displayed in unpublished ECB data for days lost to orbital facial injuries pre- and post-helmet standards and regulations shown in Fig. 7.6. Similarly, in recreational cricket in Australia the frequency of head, neck and facial injuries fell from 62% to just 4% when helmets were made compulsory [22].

It also appears that PPE has changed the way cricketers feel and how they play the game. England fast bowler Mark Wood sums this up 'To know you're not going to do any damage to anyone — that allows you to have that aggression in the game. Knowing that the other players are relatively safe gives you a lot of reassurance' [23]. Reassuringly, there is no evidence that wearing more effective PPE results in a greater number of injuries through abnormal risk-taking behaviour on the part of the batter or unsafe targeting by a bowler.

7.6 What Are the Challenges Associated with PPE in Cricket?

7.6.1 Cost

The manufacturing industry that underpins most cricket PPE has a tradition of using unsophisticated materials to support cost-effective equipment as part of a wider product range rather than bespoke and/or innovative designs. While more

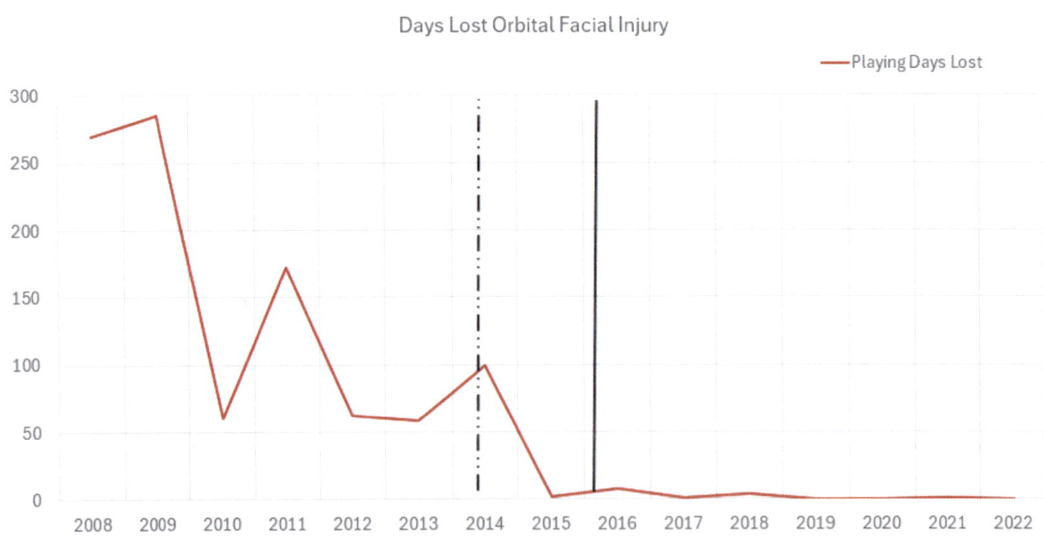

Fig. 7.6 Number of playing days lost due to orbital facial injury per year. Dashed line—introduction of helmet BSS; solid line—introduction of mandatory helmet wearing (Unpublished ECB data)

effective PPE could be produced with more expensive materials and designs, this would, for much of the game, be unaffordable. This, coupled with the desire to make cricket accessible to all, has stifled developments in some areas, as there is little incentive for manufacturers to explore more innovative designs.

7.6.2 Sustainability

As the sporting world seeks to reduce its environmental impact, the development of cricket PPE made with sustainable materials is becoming more necessary. However, the reluctance to invest in new developments and with each form of cricket PPE being multicomponent and multimaterial change in this area is challenging and has high costs associated. In the professional environment, repurposing is very difficult, and with teams changing kit providers and players moving between sponsors, PPE turnover can be high, which is largely unsustainable for a sport to encourage.

7.6.3 Mechanisms of Injury

Being struck by the ball is a common mechanism of injury across sports. However, the weight, hardness and size of a cricket ball are unique, as is the angle of release and the fact that the bowler is indirectly targeting the batter with the ball. This means that often, the outcomes of research in other sports cannot be directly applied to the development and provision of cricket PPE which must be specifically developed and tested, carrying financial ramifications.

PPE alone cannot prevent some injuries from occurring, particularly concussions which are caused by the linear and rotational acceleration of the brain, as well as direct impact [24]. While helmets prevent superficial or musculoskeletal injuries, they are less effective at preventing the movement of the brain inside the skull. While several new helmet designs are being postulated to reduce sports-related concussions, the effect of these helmets requires testing in the laboratory and on the field [25].

7.6.4 Player Opinions/Comfort

Most player complaints regarding PPE relate to the wearing of helmets, particularly neck protectors which are described as 'a distraction', making them 'feel claustrophobic' [26].

Furthermore, cricket PPE is ungainly and can impede a player's movement patterns. The comfort and fit of leg pads, and the subsequent impact on running performance, is an area of dissatisfaction among cricketers [27]. It is clear, and relatively obvious, that leg pads impede running performance when compared to running without PPE [28]. Running performance could be enhanced through the development of more ergonomic pads, potentially reducing the risk of being run out or allowing batters to complete more runs for a shot, which can both have significant impacts on games. Several wicketkeepers have moved away from traditional wicketkeeping pads in favour of smaller, more streamlined shin pads which allow greater agility behind the stumps.

7.6.5 Heat Stress

Wearing full PPE for a significant period has a large thermal effect, with core temperature increases of around 1 °C per two-hour session observed in batters [29]. Wearing a helmet can impede normal heat dissipation. This can result in heat stress, which has been mentioned by numerous players in reference to their discomfort when wearing helmets. Heat stress may reduce batting performance by hindering decision-making and focused attention. Subsequently, the development of a more 'breathable' helmet could improve player comfort and performance. The evolving challenges associated with climate change mean the issue of heat stress in sport is becoming more pertinent, demanding significant attention moving forward.

7.7 The Future of PPE

New materials and more flexible industry standards would allow for innovation and improvement of PPE, including lighter, more comfortable designs incorporating technologies from other industries such as Mips® Safety Systems. An example of this innovation is 3D-printed helmet inners, designed to maximise both comfort and protection for players. Scans of players' heads are used to produce latticed fillets which form helmet inners that are unique to each player's head. These create a closer fit, reducing helmet movement in the event of a ball strike, limiting the rattling of the head inside the helmet and preventing the grill from striking a player's face and causing injury.

There is an emerging concept of 'smart' helmets, fitted with sensors and accelerometers to provide real-time performance data on a player's movements, head position and impact forces and to detect medically relevant collisions. Impact sensors are popular in sports that require helmets (American Football) and those that don't (Football/Soccer, Rugby Union). While the use of these, and any accompanying research, is not commonplace in cricket currently, these could provide advantageous performance and medical data in cricket.

Women's specific PPE requires significant modernisation. Despite women's cricket being recorded as far back as 1745, women's hooped skirts famously resulting in the need for overarm bowling, and the first women's world cup predating the men's, cricket equipment has largely been developed to fit male anatomy and fulfil male needs. There are traditionally more male players, providing a more lucrative market for manufacturers to sell their products. However, recent increases in female participation and greater awareness around PPE have posed questions as to the suitability and effectiveness of existing PPE for females. This has highlighted the opportunity to research the specific needs of female players and for advancements to be made to the design and ergonomics of female PPE. These advancements should allow the comfort and the performance of the wearer to be improved. The British Standards for PPE use a full-sized cricket ball within its testing rather than the lighter and smaller women's ball. This makes it challenging to produce PPE for female players as the necessary requirements are not clear. As such, female-specific PPE is extremely limited, despite the obvious anatomical and physiological differences between the sexes.

References

1. Ahmad T, Jamshaid H, Mishra RK, Chandan V, Nazari S, Ivanova TA, Ahamad N, Ahmed S, Petru M, Kučera L. Development of lightweight cricket pads using knitted flexible thermoplastic composites with improved impact protection. Materials. 2022;15(23):8661. https://doi.org/10.3390/ma15238661.
2. Mohotti D, Fernando PL, Zaghloul A. Evaluation of possible head injuries ensuing a cricket ball impact. Comput Methods Prog Biomed. 2018;158:193–205.
3. Ranson C, Peirce N, Young M. Batting head injury in professional cricket: a systematic video analysis of helmet safety characteristics. Br J Sports Med. 2013;47(10):644–8. https://doi.org/10.1136/bjsports-2012-091898.
4. Deshmukh SR, Donnison E, Karantana A, Newman D, Peirce N. Epidemiology of hand fractures and dislocations in England and Wales professional cricketers. Int J Sports Med. 2021;43:381–6. https://doi.org/10.1055/a-1539-6955MCC.
5. Marylebone Cricket Club. Lord's Cricket Ground London | The Home of Cricket [Internet]. The Laws of Cricket Appendices | MCC | A.2 IMPLEMENTS AND EQUIPMENT. 2023 [cited 2024 Jul 31]. Available from: https://www.lords.org/mcc/the-laws-of-cricket/law-appendices#:~:text=For%20a%20batter,%20items%20permitted,and%20gloves%20are%20also%20permitted.
6. BBC News. BBC News [Internet]. Cricket umpire died after being hit by batsman's shot. 2019 [cited 2024 Oct 17]. Available from: https://www.bbc.co.uk/news/uk-wales-50585748#:~:text=Mr%20Williams%20was%20struck%20by,conclusion%20of%20accidental%20death%20recorded.
7. BBC Sport. BBC Sport [Internet]. Bavalan Pathmanathan dies after being struck in chest by ball. 2015 [cited 2024 Oct 17]. Available from: https://www.bbc.co.uk/sport/cricket/33425867.
8. BBC News. BBC News [Internet]. Israeli cricket umpire killed by ball. 2014 [cited 2024 Oct 17]. Available from: https://www.bbc.co.uk/news/world-middle-east-30260842.
9. BBC Sport. BBC Sport [Internet]. Phillip Hughes: Australian batsman dies, aged 25. 2014 [cited 2024 Oct 17]. Available from: https://www.bbc.co.uk/sport/cricket/30219440.

10. ESPNcricinfo [Internet]. Cricketer dies after blow to head. 2013 [cited 2024 Oct 17]. Available from: https://www.espncricinfo.com/story/cricketer-dies-after-blow-to-head-683131.
11. ESPNcricinfo [Internet]. Pakistan club cricketer dies while batting. 2013 [cited 2024 Oct 17]. Available from: https://www.espncricinfo.com/story/pakistan-club-cricketer-zulfiqar-bhatti-dies-while-batting-702269.
12. Home – BBC News [Internet]. BBC News – cricket ball throw killed umpire, Swansea inquest hears. 2010 [cited 2024 Oct 17]. Available from: http://news.bbc.co.uk/1/hi/wales/south_west/8634162.stm.
13. ESPNcricinfo [Internet]. The tragic death of Raman Lamba. [cited 2024 Oct 17]. Available from: https://www.espncricinfo.com/story/rewind-to-1998-the-tragic-death-of-raman-lamba-472228.
14. Amiss D with Graham-Brown J. Not out at close of play: a life in cricket. The History Press Limited; 2021.
15. Walker HL, Carr DJ, Chalmers DJ, Wilson CA. Injury to recreational and professional cricket players: circumstances, type and potential for intervention. Accid Anal Amp Prev. 2010;42(6):2094–8. https://doi.org/10.1016/j.aap.2010.06.022.
16. Curnow WJ. Bicycle helmets and public health in Australia. Health Promot J Austr. 2008;19(1):10–5. https://doi.org/10.1071/he08010.
17. Hunter SR, Lishnak TS, Powers AM, Lisle DK. Male genital trauma in sports. Clin Sports Med. 2013;32(2):247–54. https://doi.org/10.1016/j.csm.2012.12.012.
18. Eather S. 207 Cricket related Commotio Cordis. Heart Lung Circ. 2020 [cited 2024 Jul 31];29:S127. Available from: https://doi.org/10.1016/j.hlc.2020.09.214.
19. Spencer RJ, Sugumar H, Jones E, Farouque O. Commotio cordis: a case of ventricular fibrillation caused by a cricket ball strike to the chest. Lancet. 2014 [cited 2024 Jul 31];383(9925):1358. Available from: https://doi.org/10.1016/s0140-6736(14)60486-4.
20. Classie JA, Distel LM, Borchers JR. Safety baseballs and chest protectors: a systematic review on the prevention of Commotio Cordis. Phys Sportsmed [Internet]. 2010 [cited 2024 Oct 21];38(1):83–90. Available from: https://doi.org/10.3810/psm.2010.04.1765.
21. Eunson TH, Saw AE, Kountouris A, Orchard JW. Traumatic head and neck injuries in elite Australian cricket players: retrospective analysis from 12 seasons. Indian J Orthop. 2023;57:1584. https://doi.org/10.1007/s43465-023-00916-4.
22. Shaw L, Finch CF. Injuries to junior club cricketers: the effect of helmet regulations. Br J Sports Med. 2008;42(6):437–40. https://doi.org/10.1136/bjsm.2007.041947.
23. Spencer B. The Times & The Sunday Times [Internet]. How it works: the hi-tech cricket helmet to save batters. 2023 [cited 2024 Jul 30]. Available from: https://www.thetimes.com/sport/cricket/article/how-it-works-the-hi-tech-cricket-helmet-to-save-batters-8mxk6t3k0.
24. McIntosh AS. Evaluation of cricket helmet performance and comparison with baseball and ice hockey helmets. Br J Sports Med. 2003;37(4):325–30. https://doi.org/10.1136/bjsm.37.4.325.
25. Daneshvar DH, Nowinski CJ, McKee AC, Cantu RC. The epidemiology of sport-related concussion. Clin Sports Med. 2011;30(1):1–17. https://doi.org/10.1016/j.csm.2010.08.006.
26. Savage N. Fox Sports [Internet]. 'Stuck in an MRI scan machine': Australian cricketers facing dilemma as neck guards become mandatory. 2023 [cited 2024 Jul 30]. Available from: https://www.foxsports.com.au/cricket/stuck-in-an-mri-scan-machine-australian-cricketers-facing-dilemma-as-neck-guards-become-mandatory/news-story/65b8a1d2c60c4029187a9d6fdc66655d.
27. Webster JM, Roberts J. Incorporating subjective end-user perceptions in the design process: a study of leg guard comfort in cricket. Proc Inst Mech Eng Part P. 2009;223(2):49–62. https://doi.org/10.1243/17543371jset31.
28. Webster J, Roberts J. Determining the effect of cricket leg guards on running performance. J Sports Sci. 2011;29(7):749–60. https://doi.org/10.1080/02640414.2011.553962.
29. Stay S, Cort M, Ward D, Kountouris A, Orchard J, Holland J, Saw A. Core temperature responses in elite cricket players during Australian summer conditions. Sports. 2018;6(4):164. https://doi.org/10.3390/sports6040164.

8 Pre-Participatory Musculoskeletal Screening in Cricket

Jolandi Jacobs, Patrick Farhart, Ross Brosnan, and Steven Obst

8.1 Introduction

Cricket requires a combination of skill and physical fitness and can place significant demands on players' musculoskeletal and cardiovascular systems. Contrary to the perception of cricket being a low-intensity activity, contemporary research and expanding formats of the sport indicate that significant portions of many cricket matches are played at high physical intensities [1]. Seam bowlers are required to complete one-off and/or sustained episodes of very high-intensity efforts (e.g. bowling spells), increasing the likelihood of both traumatic and atraumatic overload injuries [2–4]. Between the 2015–16 and 2021–22 seasons, elite male cricket players in Australia experienced 136 injuries per 1000 match days, whilst elite female players sustained 101 injuries per 1000 match days [4]. Ensuring that players are adequately prepared to handle these demands is crucial for optimising their performance outcomes and reducing rates of injury [5]. Injury prevention in sports relies on understanding risk factors and injury mechanisms to create targeted programmes that effectively reduce injury risk [6, 7]. These injury prevention programmes can be individualised and tailored to address the specific needs of the player, although research on the effectiveness of injury prevention programmes is lacking [8]. Pre-participatory screening remains a recommended component of injury prevention in sports [6, 7] and aims to identify modifiable

Supplementary Information The online version contains supplementary material available at https://doi.org/10.1007/978-981-96-6321-7_8.

J. Jacobs (✉)
Wits Cricket Research Hub for Science, Medicine and Rehabilitation, Department of Physiotherapy, School of Therapeutic Sciences, Faculty of Health Sciences, University of the Witwatersrand, Johannesburg, South Africa

Physiotherapy Department, College of Health Sciences, School of Health Medical and Applied Sciences, Central Queensland University, Bundaberg, QLD, Australia

P. Farhart
School of Sport, Exercise and Rehabilitation, Faculty of Health, Human Performance Research Centre, University of Technology Sydney, Ultimo, NSW, Australia
e-mail: patrick.j.farhart@student.uts.edu.au

R. Brosnan
School of Health Sciences, University of Tasmania, Hobart, TAS, Australia

Sports and Performance Optimisation Research Team, University of Tasmania, Tasmania, Australia
e-mail: ross.brosnan@utas.edu.au

S. Obst
Physiotherapy Department, College of Health Sciences, School of Health Medical and Applied Sciences, Central Queensland University, Bundaberg, QLD, Australia
e-mail: s.obst@cqu.edu.au

B. Olivier, J. W. Orchard (eds.), *Cricket Sports Medicine*,
https://doi.org/10.1007/978-981-96-6321-7_8

physical factors that influence player readiness, injury risk [6, 9] and training interventions, including player load management and exercise prescription [10].

Most cricket injuries, particularly in fast bowlers, are non-contact events that are often linked (rightly or wrongly) to intrinsic physical factors such as faulty biomechanics, asymmetry, poor flexibility, neuromuscular strength and control, in addition to extrinsic factors such as training loads [11, 12]. Neuromuscular control is typically assessed using tests of movement quality and, in most sports, represents the first step of the pre-screening assessment process. Assessment of neuromuscular control is a recommended part of pre-participation screening for cricket [11] and many other sports with high rates of non-contact injuries (e.g. basketball [13, 14], netball [15], Australian football [16] and soccer [17]). The rationale for including assessments of movement quality is that 'suboptimal' movement patterns may contribute to a player's injury risk profile [11, 12, 18], provide insight into athletic performance and readiness to train/compete, can be used to guide further testing (e.g. strength and flexibility) and inform training load, match load and exercise prescription [11, 19, 20]. For example, injuries in fast bowlers are often linked to poor technique, poor physical preparation and/or overuse or overload, several of which may be underpinned by poor lumbopelvic-hip movement control, balance and/or proprioception [11, 12, 18, 21]. Importantly, because the link between movement quality and injury is tenuous, the purpose of assessing movement quality should not be to predict who is likely to be injured or to diagnose why a poor movement pattern exists but rather to highlight it and prompt the need for additional specific testing and/or to guide exercise prescription and player monitoring [22].

Based on the results of movement quality tests, additional specific testing might be indicated that quantifies aspects of muscular fitness, including strength, endurance and flexibility. Specific deficits in muscle strength and/or endurance (e.g. lateral trunk endurance) may contribute to suboptimal loading and increase a player's risk of sustaining an overuse/overload injury [11, 23]. Muscle strength screening could incorporate individual muscle or functional assessments of specific muscle groups, and results from these assessments may guide player monitoring and individual exercise prescriptions [22]. Another possible cause of suboptimal movement patterns observed in movement control testing could be reduced flexibility, which is assessed using a combination of muscle length, joint range of motion and/or neural mobility tests. Flexibility is essential for cricketers to optimise performance and prevent injuries related to the sport's dynamic demands [28, 29]. The key flexibility regions for cricketers include the shoulder, the hip and lumbar spine [18, 24] and the ankle [25]. Flexibility assessments are essential for identifying injury risk factors [25–27] and limitations that may hinder performance and the maintenance of muscle elasticity and joint health [28].

Aerobic and anaerobic fitness tests assess the capacity of a player to complete sustained low-intensity and repeated high-intensity physical efforts, which are important determinants of player performance and recovery. Aerobic tests such as time trials over set distances, maximal aerobic speed interval tests and intermittent recovery tests [29, 30] are frequently used in cricket settings worldwide to establish baseline measures of a player's aerobic power and capacity [10]. Anaerobic fitness tests measure the capacity for short bursts of high-intensity activity [31], and repeated sprint tests and cycle ergometry are commonly employed methods of assessment of anaerobic fitness [28]. Although cricket is an endurance sport that includes both aerobic and anaerobic demands, intermittent bursts of speed and power are essential to cricket-specific activities during batting, bowling and fielding that require acceleration, deceleration, change of direction, maximal velocity and agility [32, 33]. Speed and agility assessments are vital to determining a player's readiness to participate in these activities and are an objective tool that can inform individualised programmes to optimise speed development and monitor pre-season and through-season performance.

Whilst pre-participatory screening has limited predictive value for future injuries, it remains valuable for managing athlete health, establishing a baseline for monitoring fitness changes and fostering collaboration between medical practitioners, coaches and players. Injury prevention programmes for cricketers, such as those outlined by Forrest et al. [23], may address deficits identified by pre-participatory screening. Forrest et al. [23] present an exercise-based injury prevention programme with an exercise progression design through three phases: basic, intermediate and advanced. Cricketers should commence at an appropriate stage based on the results of neuromuscular screening, progressing individually as they master exercises with the correct technique. Whilst exercise progressions (basic, intermediate, or advanced) may be necessary for an entire team, individual advancement ensures players develop strength, endurance and balance effectively, reducing injury risk and optimising performance [23].

Screening tests typically measure modifiable variables [7]; however, the accuracy of commonly used screening tests is not certain, with several tests having either low-moderate or unknown reliability or validity estimates. Whilst cricket-specific pre-screening protocols have been developed, these are often implemented at elite and professional levels and may have limited validity in community-level players due to the lack of clinicians and resources [26, 27]. Whilst pre-screening has limited evidence-based support for predicting future injuries, its importance should not be overlooked [34]. During screenings, players can report any pre-existing injuries or concerns, which can be promptly addressed or flagged with a medical healthcare professional. Further, pre-screening tests provide a clinical and functional baseline for monitoring future changes in physical fitness [35]. To maximise the significance of pre-screening tests, the results should be used to tailor interventions based on a player's age, gender, injury history and the demands and requirements of their playing role. This includes personalised training areas for improvement and potential injury prevention strategies.

This chapter aims to provide an overview of user-friendly and scientifically sound screening tests that coaches and/or sports science and sports medicine practitioners could use across different levels of cricket participation. These tests aim to evaluate various aspects of physical ability, such as neuromuscular control, muscle strength, power and endurance, flexibility, speed and aerobic and anaerobic power.

8.2 Testing at Different Levels of Participation

Cricket is played at various levels of participation, which can be classified as community (non elite) [36], sub-elite [37] and elite [4]. Each level of participation requires unique pre-participatory screening and physical preparation. Screening is often seen at the sub-elite and elite levels [26, 27] and less common at the community level. Screening at the community level includes several limitations due to the lack of resources and qualified clinicians to implement the testing protocols. At the community level and school level, the focus is often on identifying and developing talent, which involves assessing essential physical fitness and growth-related factors [38, 39]. For semi-elite players, tests might concentrate on general fitness and injury prevention. Elite players, on the other hand, undergo comprehensive and detailed testing to ensure peak performance and minimisation of injury risks [11, 27]. Table 8.1 provides guidelines for details on how testing can be tailored for cricket programmes taking into account the level of programme, the goals of screening, available resources and desired outcomes of the screening process.

8.3 Limitations of Testing

Pre-participatory musculoskeletal screening is widely used in cricket to identify injury risk factors and inform player management strategies [1, 2]. Although designed to identify injury risk factors, screening may inadvertently pose a minor risk of injury or exacerbation of pre-existing conditions, specifically tests involving maximal effort or fatigue-based components. This risk is particularly relevant when testing is conducted at the sub-elite or community level, where sports science and medical support are limited.

Table 8.1 Levels of participation and testing focus

Level	Goals of screening	Limitations	Screening outcomes
Community/ youth	Assess basic functional fitness and readiness for participation	Screening would be done by teachers or coaches (as often no healthcare practitioners are available); lack of advanced testing equipment	Identifying and addressing limitations observed during fundamental movements necessary for participation
Semi-elite	Conduct specific screenings using basic equipment	Limited to basic equipment and testers	Personalised intervention for injury risk and performance, with tailored progression based on assessment
Elite	Specific screening using basic to advanced equipment for individualised outcomes	High cost and accessibility, requiring trained testers	Data-driven adjustments for performance and injury prevention, with tailored progression based on assessment

However, current research and findings on the reliability and validity of pre-participatory screening pose a challenge to accurately identifying risk factors for injury [3]. For screening to be accurate, it must be reproducible over time across different testers and the same individual [3, 4]. Poor reproducibility limits the accuracy and interpretation of the results, as significant errors can obscure the results [5, 6]. The reliability of tests used in cricket has been evaluated and included in this chapter [1, 2]. However, it has not been evaluated across different population groups or levels of participation.

Another evident limitation in pre-participatory testing is 'test creep', where several tests are included without robust evidence supporting their specific benefits in injury prevention. The sensitivity and specificity of commonly used tests remain variable, limiting their accuracy in identifying players genuinely at risk versus those unlikely to sustain injuries [3]. Given these constraints, it is essential to continue validating the reliability of musculoskeletal assessments and refining screening protocols to improve their clinical relevance and effectiveness in cricket.

8.4 Pre-Participatory Tests

The pre-participatory tests in this chapter include the following categories:

1. Neuromuscular control
   (a) Multi-component tests
   (b) Single-component tests
2. Muscle fitness
   (a) Strength
   (b) Power
   (c) Endurance
   (d) Flexibility
3. Cardiorespiratory fitness
   (a) Aerobic
   (b) Anaerobic
   (c) Speed

To help readers choose the most suitable test for their needs, Table 8.2 provides a matrix that details the unique tests for each category mentioned above. This table details the tests within each physical fitness domain and classifies them based on player experience, player role and rater experience.

Table 8.2 Matrix of pre-participatory tests in cricket

Test name	Player experience			Player role				Rater experience		
	Community/junior	Sub-elite	Elite	Bowler	Batter	Keeper	Allrounder	Novice	Intermediate	Expert
Multi-component movement assessments										
Functional Movement Scale™	Green	Green	Green	Green	Green	Green	Green		Green	Green
Athletic Ability Assessment		Green	Green	Green	Green	Green	Green		Orange	Green
16-PPM		Green	Green	Green	Green	Green	Green		Orange	Green
Motor Control Screen	Green	Green	Green	Green	Green	Green	Green	Green	Green	Green
AIMS-4	Green	Green	Green	Green	Green	Green	Green	Green	Green	Green
Single-component movement assessments										
Single leg squat and landing	Green	Green	Green	Green	Green	Green	Green		Orange	Green
Tests of lumbo-pelvic control		Green	Green	Green	Orange	Orange	Green		Orange	Green
Star Excursion Balance Test	Green	Green	Green	Green	Green	Green	Green	Orange	Green	Green
Lower quarter Y-balance test	Green	Green	Green	Green	Green	Green	Green	Orange	Green	Green
CKCUEST	Orange	Green	Green	Green	Orange	Orange	Green	Orange	Green	Green
Upper Quarter Y-balance test		Green	Green	Green	Orange	Orange	Green		Green	Green
Trunk mobility screen	Green	Green	Green	Green	Green	Green	Green	Orange	Orange	Green
Muscle strength assessments										
Isometric tests	Orange	Green	Green	Green	Green	Green	Green		Orange	Green
Upper/lower body RM (1-3-5) tests		Orange	Green	Green	Green	Green	Green		Orange	Green
Power and velocity-based tests			Green	Orange	Orange	Orange	Orange			Green
Flexibility assessments										
Active knee extension test	Green	Green	Green	Green	Green	Green	Green		Orange	Green
Modified Thomas test		Orange	Green	Green	Green	Green	Green		Orange	Green
Shoulder IR/ER	Green	Green	Green	Green	Orange	Orange	Green		Orange	Green
Knee to wall	Green	Green	Green	Green	Green	Green	Green	Orange	Orange	Green
Sit and reach test	Green	Green	Green	Green	Green	Green	Green	Orange	Orange	Green
Straight leg raise		Orange	Green	Green	Green	Green	Green		Orange	Green
Aerobic/anaerobic assessments										
Time Trials (1, 1.6, 2km)	Orange	Green	Green	Green	Green	Orange	Green	Orange	Green	Green
Interval Tests (MAS, YoYo IRT)	Orange	Orange	Green	Green	Green	Green	Green		Orange	Green
Distance Trials (e.g. 5- or 6-minute)	Orange	Green	Green	Green	Green	Orange	Green	Orange	Green	Green
Repeated Sprint Tests		Orange	Green	Green	Green	Green	Green		Green	Green
Speed assessments										
Change of direction tests		Orange	Green	Green	Green	Green	Green		Orange	Green
Max velocity tests		Orange	Green	Green	Green	Orange	Green		Orange	Green

Tool: *Green suggests the best option, orange suggests a potentially suitable choice, blank suggest a not-suitable option*

Footnote*: CKCUEST (Closed kinetic chain upper extremity stability test), ER (external rotation), IR (internal rotation), MAS (metabolic aerobic state), RM (repetition maximum), and YoYo IRT (YoYo intermittent recovery test).*

8.4.1 Neuromuscular Control and/or Movement Quality Assessments

8.4.1.1 Multi-Component Assessments

Multi-component movement assessments (MMAs) assess several aspects of neuromuscular control (e.g. strength, flexibility and balance) and offer a quick and effective solution to a pre-participation screening of athletes. Most MMAs include quantitative and qualitative assessments of 'fundamental' movements that encompass variations of squatting, lunging, pushing, pulling and abdominal bracing tasks. Most MMAs suitable for cricket pre-participation screening are quick and simple to administer, require very little equipment and/or training, and have acceptable reliability (Supplementary Table 8.1). Each MMA shares several fundamental movements relevant to cricket, and most include tasks that challenge unilateral-bilateral and static-dynamic control of lumbopelvic-hip movement in several planes of motion, making them particularly relevant to cricket-related injuries [11, 18, 21, 40].

The Movement Competency Screen (MCS) has acceptable content validity and reliability [41] and possesses the advantage of including several task progressions and guidance on subsequent exercise prescription, making it particularly useful for teams with expertise in strength and conditioning (e.g. strength and conditioning and physiotherapy professionals) [42]. Similarly, the Athlete Introductory Movement Screen (AIMS-4) includes several lower body movement tasks but, importantly, includes an abdominal bracing task, and hence may be more suitable for young sub-elite cricket players, particularly seam bowlers. Neither the MCS nor AIMS-4 includes a shoulder-specific test; hence, additional isolated tests of shoulder mobility or stability may be required. The Functional Movement Screen (FMS™), Athletic Ability Assessment (AAA) [43] and 16-PPM [44] each include specific tests of shoulder mobility or stability (e.g. CKCUEST). The FMS™ [45, 46] is the most widely used and researched MMA and includes seven fundamental movements suitable for all levels of participation but does require rater training to administer and, therefore, may be more suited to the sub-elite and elite level. Except for the 16-PPM, all MMAs listed in Supplementary Table 8.2 include fewer than nine items and can be completed within 15 minutes, reducing the influence of fatigue on test outcomes and making these tools suitable for pre-season team testing and/or individual player monitoring during the season. The AAA and 16-PPM are the most comprehensive MMAs and include a combination of qualitative and quantitative tests, with the added advantage of including a standardised test of standing balance (e.g. Y-balance and Star Excursion Balance Test (SEBT)); however, both require time and expertise to administer and may not be suited to the community level. The AAA and 16-PPM represent the most complete pre-screening assessment relevant to cricket, and each can be used as a standalone pre-screening tool for all levels of cricket, particularly if other isolated tests of strength, endurance, proprioception and balance are not readily available.

8.4.1.2 Single-Component Assessments

Single-component tests of neuromuscular control and/or movement quality are designed with a specific purpose (e.g. single-leg squat test assesses unilateral dynamic hip-knee control in the sagittal plane) and may be used in isolation or as part of, or in conjunction with, an existing MMA.

For cricket, several key focus points should guide the pre-screening assessment of movement control:

- Lower limb and lumbopelvic control during single-leg squatting, lunging and/or landing
- Lumbopelvic control during limb-trunk loading (i.e. anti-rotation/flexion/extension)
- Standing static and dynamic balance
- Shoulder stability/control

Although the evidence for an association between lower limb-trunk control and balance and low back pain in fast bowlers is inconsistent [12, 18], these tests should be considered for inclusion in the pre-participation screening of players, particularly seam bowlers at sub-elite and elite levels. Most tests use either realtime or video-assisted ratings using 3- and 4-point qualitative ordinal scales. Advanced evaluation of movement control using two-dimensional and three-dimensional motion analysis has traditionally only been available to elite teams. However, recent advances in computer vision analysis make this an option for sub-elite and even community-level participants.

Inadequate lower limb control during single-leg loading (e.g. dynamic knee valgus) is often cited as a risk factor for knee pain (e.g. PFPS [47]) and injury (e.g. ACL [48]) and has been shown to be predictive of low back pain in adolescent seam bowlers [18, 40]. Control of lumbopelvic and lower limb alignment during single-leg loading can be assessed whilst performing several different tasks (e.g. drop jump, tuck jump, lunge); however, the single-leg squat (SLS) test, with or without a decline, is the most common and well-developed variation [49, 50]. Inadequate lumbopelvic control during trunk loading is also considered a modifiable risk factor for non-contact injury in adolescent seam bowlers, as well as being linked to suboptimal bowling technique (e.g. knee collapse at BFC) and performance [18, 51]. Quantitative testing of lumbopelvic-hip control can be assessed using the 'lumbopelvic stability test' in crook-lying [40, 52, 53]; however, this test requires specialised equipment (pressure biofeedback unit) and training that is not readily available to most community or sub-elite players. Instead, lumbopelvic control may be assessed through other tests of abdominal bracing as part of some MMAs (e.g. active straight leg raise) or through other standardised test positions and tasks (e.g. waiter's bow, seated knee extension, bent knee fallouts [53]) (Table 8.3; Figs. 8.1, 8.2, and 8.3).

Lower limb control during single-leg loading is also influenced by ankle-knee-hip balance, which can be assessed using either the Star Excursion Balance Test (SEBT) [54, 55] or its variation, the Lower Quarter Y-balance test (LQ-YBT) [56]. The SEBT and the LQ-YBT features in the AAA (SEBT) and the 16-PPM (LQ-YBT) can be performed relatively quickly with minimal equipment and training. Each test involves the player standing on one leg and reaching in several directions with the opposing leg (8 directions for the SEBT and 3 directions for the LQ-YBT), with each reach distance being recorded and then summed as a composite score. Both tests possess acceptable reliability and validity and are commonly included in pre-participation sport screening [57–60]. Poor performance on the SEBT for the backfoot contact limb of seam bowlers (particularly in the posterior-medial direction) may assist the identification of those at higher risk of low back and/or lower limb injury during the season and the monitoring of adaptations through a season [53]. Alternatively, simple tests of single-leg standing balance time (up to 180 seconds) with eyes open or closed and/or standing on a stable or unstable surface may be used in younger populations and/or when time is limited.

Tests of neuromuscular control of the upper limb and shoulder are less developed. The closed kinetic chain upper extremity test (CKCUEST) [61] and the Upper Quarter Y-Balance test (UQ-YBT) [62] are the most popular tests, with the former included in the 16-PPM [44]. Both tests evaluate shoulder control in a weight-bearing push-up position. The CKCUEST assesses bilateral shoulder stability and speed of movement in a weight-bearing position and has established reference ranges for several different populations, including throwers [63], female athletes [64] and those with or at risk of shoulder pain [65]. The test is quick, easy to administer and suitable for all levels of cricket participation. Poor performance and/or pain during the CKCUEST may prompt additional testing of shoulder internal and external strength and/or trunk control, and in some cases, tests of shoulder integrity may be required. The UQ-YBT has the advantage of providing a left and right upper limb score and thus may be more suitable for monitoring unilateral throwing and/or bowling-related injuries and/or performance, and both tests have acceptable inter- and intra-rater reliability [44, 66]. Together with performance- and fitness-based assessments, tests of movement quality should form part of a comprehensive athlete screening in sport [37, 67, 68].

Table 8.3 Single-component movement assessments

Name of test(s)	Description	Equipment
Single-leg squat/landing (SLS)	The player performs a single-leg squat to ~45° of knee flexion. Observe the control of the lumbar spine, pelvis, hip, knee, ankle and foot from the side, front and rear.	Nil. Video analysis can improve reliability.
Tests of lumbopelvic control in standing [53]: Waiter's bow, dorsal pelvic tilt, single-leg weight shift	Waiter's bow: In standing maintain the spine in the neutral position during forward bending (flexion) to ±50° hip flexion. Dorsal pelvic tilt: In standing actively tilt the pelvis backwards to create lumbar flexion. Single-leg standing weight shift: Measure the lateral movement of the umbilicus during single-leg standing (position: Feet one-third of trochanter distance apart).	Goniometer to measure hip position. Tape measure to measure umbilicus movement. Qualitative rating requires some expertise in observational analysis of movement.
Tests of lumbopelvic control in 4-point kneel [53]: Forward and backward rocking	Forward and backward rocking: In a 4-point kneel player's weight shifts forward to 60° hip flexion.	Goniometer to measure hip position. Qualitative rating requires some expertise in observational analysis of movement.
Tests of lumbopelvic control in sitting and prone [53]: Active knee extension	Active knee extension: In upright sitting with lumbar lordosis player actively extend their knee without flexing the lumbar spine. Active knee flexion: In prone player actively flexes their knee without extending the lumbar spine.	Goniometer to measure hip position. Qualitative rating requires some expertise in observational analysis of movement.
Tests of lumbopelvic control in crook-lying using pressure biofeedback [52, 53, 69]	Assesses ability to maintain activation of deep abdominal muscles (e.g. transversus abdominis) and lumbar spine posture during controlled limb movements. A pressure biofeedback unit was placed under the lumbar spine and inflated to 40 mmHg. Participant contracts deep abdominal muscles to increase by 4–6 mmHg and maintain pressure whilst moving their lower limbs.	Pressure biofeedback unit or suitable sphygmomanometer cuff. Training required.
Star Excursion Balance Test (SEBT) [54, 55]	Standing on one leg, the player reaches as far as possible (along one of 8 directions) with the opposing foot and lightly touches each line without losing balance before reassuming the bilateral stance. Each direction is attempted, and distance is recorded. Up to 4 practice trials are provided. Reach distances can be normalised to either limb length or height (%) to allow comparison between players.	Marked lines on the floor (e.g. masking tape) arranged in a grid extending from a centre point at 45°. Reach directions are labelled as anterior, anteromedial, anterolateral, medial, lateral, posterior, posteromedial and posterolateral. Tape measure.
Lower quarter Y-balance test (LQ-YBT) [56]	As per the SEBT, it only includes 3 reach directions: Anterior, posteromedial and posterolateral.	Commercially available device testing kit (Y-Balance Test, Move2Perform, Danville, VA).

(continued)

Table 8.3 (continued)

Name of test(s)	Description	Equipment
Closed kinetic chain upper extremity stability test (CKCUEST) [61]	The player assumes a push-up position with the hands placed just inside athletic tape markers placed 36 inches apart (alternatively use 50% of height). Players then reach with alternating hands across their bodies to touch the athletic tape under the opposing hand. The number of cross-body touches performed in 15 seconds is recorded and averaged over 3 trials.	Masking tape and stopwatch. Stadiometer to measure player height.
Upper Quarter Y-balance test (UQ-YBT) [62]	The player assumes a push-up position with the feet no more than 12 inches apart and performs maximal effort reaches with the free hand in three directions (medial, superolateral and inferolateral) named in relation to the stationary hand. Record the average distance of 3 trials per direction and the sum for the total excursion score for left and right. Reach distances can be normalised to upper limb length or height (%) to allow players to compare.	Masking tape and tape measure. Stadiometer to measure player height.
Trunk mobility screen (seated rotation) [70]	The player sits on the floor with legs crossed and spine as straight as possible, holding a pole in front of the chest. A second pole, held by the tester >45° is positioned in front of the player. The player rotates their thorax, and the total range of rotation is measured.	Measurement tape, two poles.

8.4.2 Muscle Fitness Assessments

8.4.2.1 Strength, Power and Endurance Assessments

Muscle fitness assessments include tests for strength, power and endurance qualities. Functional testing further evaluates the performance of these traits in movements that replicate sport-specific activities [71] and gives practitioners and coaches an indication of a cricketer's ability to generate maximal external force in movements related to their sport [72]. Functional muscle strength testing, or power assessments, assess the rate with which force can be developed, and this can be considered as a triad of force, time and distance [73].

Muscle strength tests referred to in this chapter are based on current testing protocols used in

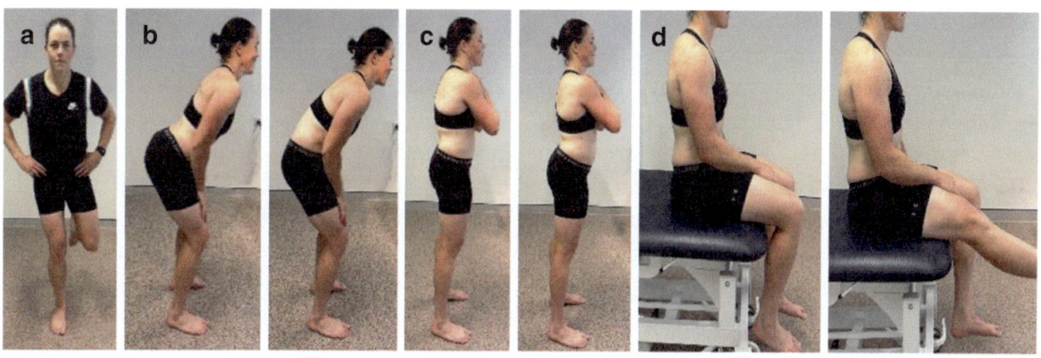

Fig. 8.1 Assessments of movement control—(**a**) single-leg squat, (**b**) waiter's bow, (**c**) dorsal pelvic tilt, (**d**) active knee extension in sitting

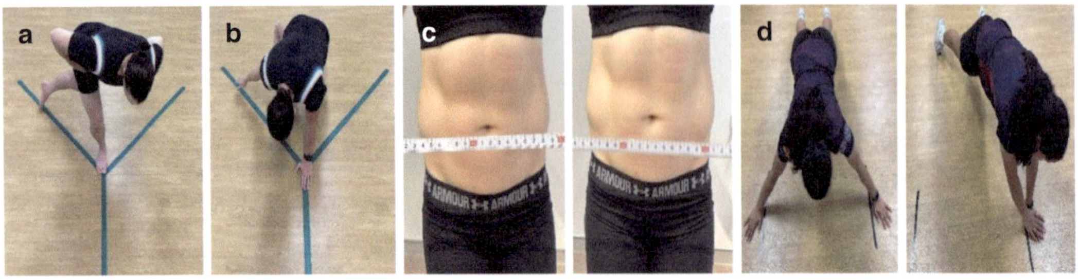

Fig. 8.2 Assessments of movement control—(**a**) lower quarter Y-balance test, (**b**) upper quarter Y-balance test, (**c**) single-leg weight shift, (**d**) closed kinetic chain upper extremity stability test

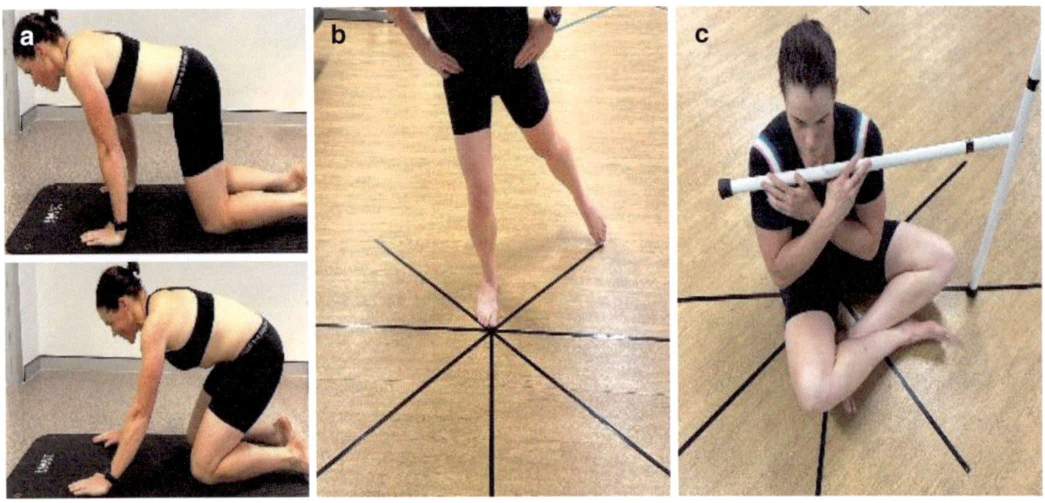

Fig. 8.3 Assessments of movement control—(**a**) forward and backward rocking, (**b**) star excursion balance test, (**c**) trunk mobility screen

cricket settings, published pre-screening tests used in cricket research [26, 27], and identified injury risk factors in male and female cricketers [23, 74–76]. For instance, studies have established an association between injury and a deficit in dominant shoulder internal rotation strength in both male and female cricketers [38, 75]. Additionally, asymmetries in strength between the dominant and non-dominant upper limbs are considered risk factors for throwing arm pain [77]. Reduced trunk endurance was identified as a risk factor for non-contact injury in adolescent pace bowlers [18]. Greater quadriceps strength in the non-dominant leg of fast bowlers was linked to an increased risk of lower back stress fractures [78]. Various strength tests are discussed and presented, including isometric tests, repetition maximum (RM) tests and functional strength tests (see Table 8.4 and Fig. 8.4). These tests measure the amount and rate of force development during tasks relevant to batting, bowling and fielding.

Strength testing may include isometric muscle tests to evaluate maximal strength of specific muscle groups, such as the calf or hamstring [79, 80], in addition to performance-based tests, such as the Isometric Mid-Thigh Pull (IMTP) [37]. Objective measurements for maximal strength can be obtained using dynamometry (e.g. handheld or instrumented) and/or force plates to enable accurate and reliable estimates of maximal strength and, where possible, maximal rates of force development and power. In the absence of dynamometry, functional muscle strength can be evaluated using either repetition maximal tests for the upper and lower body (e.g. 1RM, 3RM, 5RM), such as the bench pull, bench press, squat,

Table 8.4 Muscle strength, power and endurance assessments

Name of test(s)	Description	Equipment
Isometric tests		
Shoulder IR/ER [75]	The player lies supine with the shoulder abducted to 90° and performs isometric shoulder external and internal rotations. Record the maximum force exerted in each direction for comparison.	Handheld dynamometer (HHD), VALD ForceFrame™, or, regress, manual muscle testing (MMT) (compare to the other side).
Athletic Shoulder (ASH) Test [83]	The player lies in a prone position with elbow in full extension, forearm in pronation and heel of hand in contact with a force plate. Instruction is to push hand as hard and fast as possible into the force plate for 3 seconds in I (180° abduction), Y (135° abduction) and T (90° abduction) positions. Maximum force is recorded for each position and compared to the other side.	Force plate.
Hip abduction/ adduction [84]	The player lies supine with the hip at 0° of abduction and performs isometric hip abduction and adduction. Record the maximum force exerted in each direction for comparison.	Handheld dynamometer (HHD), VALD ForceFrame™, or, regress, manual muscle testing (MMT) (compare to the other side).
Hamstring [79]	The player lies prone with the knee flexed at 90° and performs isometric contractions of the hamstrings against a handheld dynamometer (HHD). Measure and record the peak force generated during these contractions.	HHD, VALD ForceFrame™ (or alternative hamstring testing equipment), MMT (compare to the other side).
Nordbord Isometric Hamstring Test [85]	The player is positioned on a NordBord at 30°, which is the angle between the trunk and the vertical line perpendicular to the floor. The player tries to hold this position until it succumbs to gravity, and the peak force (N) produced by dominant and non-dominant legs is recorded using wireless data acquisition.	VALD NordBord™.
Seated calf [80]	The player sits with the hip and knee flexed to 90° and performs isometric calf raises against a force plate. Record the maximum force exerted during the contraction for assessment.	HHD, force plate, MMT (compare to the other side).
Trunk side hold (alternative: Side bridge endurance test) [86]	The player performs a side plank hold on a glute-ham-raise bench (or legs held down on a mobile bed), with weight added for resistance. The hold duration is timed to assess the endurance and strength of the trunk stabilisers.	Timer, weight, glute-ham-raise bench.
Isometric Mid-Thigh Pull [37]	The player performs a maximal isometric pull from the mid-thigh position whilst standing on force plates and pulling against a barbell fixed in a rack. Record the peak force to evaluate lower body strength.	Barbell, fixed rack, force plate.
Eccentric tests		
NordBord Eccentric Hamstring test [87]	The player is positioned in a kneeling position on the NordBord device with knees at 90° and ankles secured by hooks superior to the lateral malleolus. The player then performs a Nordic hamstring exercise whilst decelerating forward, falling without hip flexion. The resultant force curve is registered on the NordBord application, and the highest achieved peak force is used for analysis.	VALD NordBord™.

(continued)

Table 8.4 (continued)

Name of test(s)	Description	Equipment
Upper/lower body RM tests		
1-3-5RM tests	The player performs a strength test with increasing weights to determine their one, three and five repetition maximums (1RM, 3RM and 5RM). Record the maximum weight lifted successfully for each repetition range. RM test could include bench pull, bench press, squat and/or deadlift.	Barbell, weights.
Single-leg calf raise [88]	The player balances barefoot on one leg with index fingers lightly touching a wall, keeping the knee straight, and performs maximum repetitions of maximum height vertical heel raises in time with a metronome set to 60 beats per minute. Count the maximum number of reps completed whilst aligning the middle of the ankle joint over the second toe, keeping the knee straight, without using excessive body movement and document the total if any cheating occurs.	Metronome device.
Single-leg hamstring bridge [89]	The player lies supine with one heel on a box measuring 60 cm high. The test leg is positioned in 20° of knee flexion and with arms crossed over the chest, the player pushes down through the heel to lift their bottom off the ground. The aim of the test is to do as many repetitions as possible until failure. The player needs to allow their bottom to touch the ground and then extend the hip to 0° without resting. The non-working leg is required to be held stationary in a vertical position to ensure that momentum is not gained by swinging this leg.	60 cm box.
Performance-based tests		
CMJ (or vertical jump alternative) [90]	The player performs a countermovement jump from a standing position by dropping into a self-selected countermovement depth, jumping as high as possible, and then landing back onto a force plate. Alternatively, a vertical distance measuring device can be used to record maximum jump height. In the presence of force plates, this test evaluates parameters of explosive lower body strength and vertical jump performance that are related to relative force and net impulse, jump height, rates of force development and reactive strength indices.	Distance measurement device, velocity-based technology (e.g. GymAware, force plates, vertec).
Repeated hopping [91]	The player performs multiple hops either on a single-leg or double legs, with force plates or a vertical distance measuring device used to record the height of each hop. This test assesses unilateral and bilateral vertical leg stiffness, lower limb strength, endurance and coordination through repeated jumping efforts.	Distance measurement device, velocity-based technology (e.g. GymAware, force plates, vertec).
Medicine ball throws [92]	The player performs throws with a medicine ball of varying weights, including vertical and horizontal throws. Record the distance of each throw. This test evaluates upper body strength, explosiveness and throwing capability.	Distance measurement device, velocity-based technology, medicine balls.

deadlift and their unilateral variations [81]. Performance-based tests of muscle power should also be considered, particularly for seam bowlers and power hitters, and these may include the countermovement jump (CMJ), squat jump (SJ) [82], drop jumps from various heights, repeated hopping tests, clean derivatives and bench press/pull [73] or medicine ball throw variations. Some of these tests require very little equipment and expertise to administer and provide a valid and reliable estimate of short-term muscular power suitable for all levels of cricket.

Table 8.4 provides basic details and descriptions for conducting commonly employed strength, power and endurance assessments, as well as the equipment required for each test. Most of these tests are easily administered throughout training blocks and can be integrated

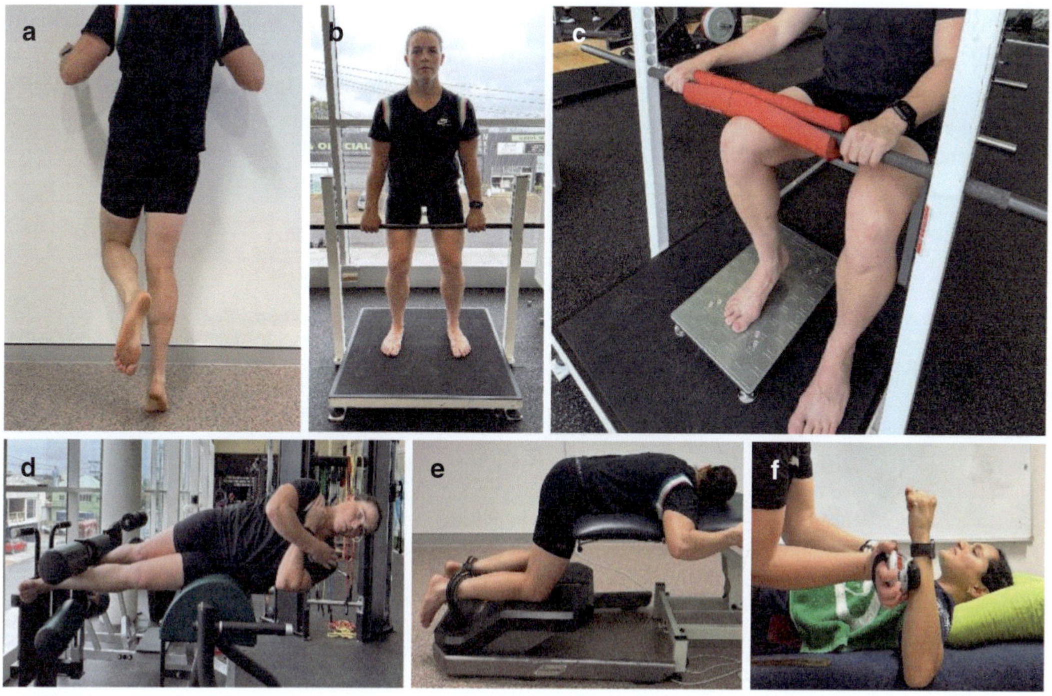

Fig. 8.4 Assessments of muscle strength, power and endurance—(**a**) single-leg calf raise, (**b**) isometric mid-thigh pull using force plates, (**c**) seated isometric calf strength test using force plates, (**d**) trunk side hold, (**e**) isometric hamstring strength test using an objective muscle testing device, (**f**) isometric shoulder internal rotation strength test using a handheld dynamometer

into training sessions through all phases of the season with the correct planning, communication, education and adaptability.

8.4.2.2 Flexibility Assessments

Flexibility assessments evaluate the range of motion (ROM) across joints, providing crucial insights into a cricketer's movement capabilities and potential injury risks. Unlike muscle strength testing, which focuses on force production and rate of force development, flexibility testing is the ability of joints and associated soft tissues (e.g. muscle, nerve, tendon) to move freely through a full ROM [93]. Deficits in neuromuscular and movement quality assessments can be underpinned by a lack of flexibility, highlighting the need for isolated muscle flexibility assessments. Flexibility is essential for cricketers to optimise performance and prevent injuries related to the sport's dynamic demands [26, 27]. For instance, limited shoulder internal rotation ROM has been associated with a higher risk of shoulder injuries [26]. Similarly, hip and lower back flexibility are essential for bowlers to maintain proper technique and avoid overuse injuries [18, 24]. Additionally, reduced ankle dorsiflexion is linked to increased injury risk in bowlers [25], whilst neural symptoms detected during screening are also identified as a risk factor for injury in cricketers [26]. Flexibility assessments are also essential for increasing recovery from physical activity by maintaining muscle elasticity and joint health [28].

Regular flexibility assessments are important for monitoring ROM changes during a season which might precede or be the result of a soft-tissue injury. As such, these tests need to be reproducible over time and by different observers [94]. Most flexibility measurements rely on either a goniometer or tape to measure the ROM of a specific joint(s). The muscle length tests included in the section are based on previous research on cricketers [26, 27], identifying injury risk factors in male and female cricketers [23, 74–76], and current clinical tests used in cricket settings. Joint-specific flexibility tests include the shoulder IR/ER ROM test [26], the trunk mobility screen test [70] and the knee to wall test for closed chain ankle dorsiflexion [27], and these are summarised in Table 8.5 and presented in Fig. 8.5. Most flexibility and tests can be adapted if specific equipment is unavailable. For example, basic tools like a measuring tape for ROM or visual assessment techniques with video analysis to evaluate movement quality and efficiency can be used.

Table 8.5 Flexibility assessments

Name of test(s)	Description	Equipment
Active knee extension [27]	The player lies supine with one leg extended and the other hip flexed to 90°. The player then extends the knee of the flexed hip as far as possible. The angle between the thigh and the leg is measured with a goniometer. Alternatively, the angle of the tibia relative to the vertical can be measured with an inclinometer. This test assesses hamstring flexibility and is recorded in degrees.	Goniometer, Range of Motion Inclinometer.
Modified Thomas [27, 95]	The player lies supine on the edge of a table, pulling one knee to the chest whilst allowing the other leg to hang off the table. The tester observes the angles of the hanging hip and knee with a goniometer or inclinometer to assess hip flexor, quadriceps and iliotibial band flexibility. Tightness in these muscles is indicated by an inability of the thigh to drop below the table level or knee extension.	Goniometer, Range of Motion Inclinometer.
Shoulder IR/ER [96]	The player lies supine with the shoulder and elbow flexed to 90°. The tester passively rotates the shoulder internally and externally, measuring the range of motion with a goniometer or inclinometer. This test assesses the flexibility and range of motion of the shoulder's rotator cuff muscles and is recorded in degrees.	Goniometer, Range of Motion Inclinometer.
Knee to wall [97]	The player stands facing a wall with 1 foot flat on the ground and the other knee bent, placing the toes of the bent leg against the wall. The player then attempts to touch the knee of the bent leg to the wall whilst keeping the heel on the ground. The distance from the wall to the big toe is measured, or alternatively, the angle of the tibia relative to the vertical can be measured with an inclinometer. This test assesses ankle dorsiflexion flexibility.	Measurement tape, Range of Motion Inclinometer.
Sit and reach [98]	The player sits on the floor with legs extended and feet against a box or wall. The player then reaches forward as far as possible, holding the position momentarily. The distance reached beyond the toes is measured. This test evaluates the flexibility of the lower back and hamstrings.	Measurement tape, Sit and Reach Box.
Passive straight leg raise [95]	The player lies supine with legs extended. The tester passively lifts one leg whilst keeping the knee straight, measuring the hip flexion angle at which the pelvis tilts or the opposite leg starts to lift. This test evaluates hamstring flexibility and is recorded in degrees.	Goniometer, Range of Motion Inclinometer.

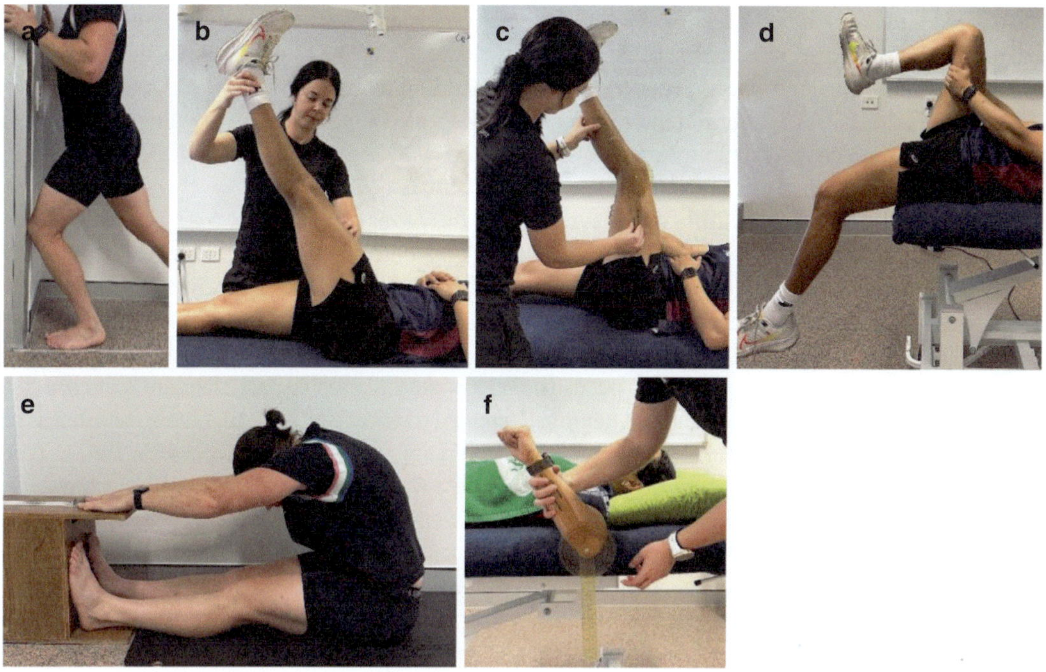

Fig. 8.5 Flexibility assessments—(**a**) knee to wall, (**b**) passive straight leg raise, (**c**) active knee extension, (**d**) Modified Thomas, (**e**) sit and reach, (**f**) shoulder range of motion

8.5 Cardiorespiratory Fitness Assessments

8.5.1 Aerobic and Anaerobic Assessments

Aerobic fitness refers to the body's ability to use oxygen efficiently during sustained physical activity and is linked to overall cardiovascular health and physical endurance. The gold standard measurement of maximal aerobic fitness uses a laboratory-based incremental exercise test (treadmill or cycle ergometer) to determine maximal oxygen consumption (i.e. VO_2 max test). Field-based alternatives are typically submaximal and provide relatively safe and cost-effective indirect estimates of maximal aerobic power and capacity [99]. Several standardised field-based tests are available, including multi-stage fitness, timed, or distance tests [29, 30, 100, 101].

Testing aerobic fitness is essential for cricketers to investigate how a player will:

- Recover between acute bouts of high-intensity events such as sprinting between wickets or to save a boundary
- Sustain prolonged physical activity, particularly during longer match formats, extended batting periods and prolonged bowling spells
- Recover from training games, matches, or events—this is highly relevant in cricket, in view of recent scheduling changes causing dense and sporadic playing seasons
- Perform cognitively at high intensities in relation to aspects of tactical awareness, technical ability, skill execution and decision-making

Aerobic tests, such as time trials over set distances (1, 1.6 or 2 km), maximal aerobic speed interval tests, YoYo intermittent recovery tests (YoYo IRT) [29], 30–15 intermittent recovery tests [30] and time-capped running tests, are all commonly used in applied cricket settings worldwide to establish a baseline measure of a player's aerobic fitness.

Anaerobic fitness is assessed by evaluating the ability to perform short bursts of high-intensity activity [31]. Anaerobic fitness, which includes qualities, such as strength, power and speed, is essential for batting, bowling and/or fielding activities [102]. There are numerous ways of assessing anaerobic fitness, such as the Wingate test and repeated sprint tests [28]. It has been suggested that if tests are to yield valid information relevant to competitive performance, they should include sport-specific movement patterns for relevant durations [28].

Anaerobic fitness testing is crucial for cricketers to investigate how an athlete will respond to:

- Repeat exposure to sprinting between wickets
- Repeat exposure to explosive movements in fielding
- Repeated high-intensity bowling actions during bowling spells in a variety of match formats

Anaerobic tests such as repeated Run a 2/3 tests, which are cricket-specific to batting scenarios, or repeated sprint ability tests, which display more fidelity to repeat exposures to explosive movement in fielding, are standard tests used in applied cricket settings to obtain baselines or time-point measures for a player's fitness (see Table 8.6).

8.5.2 Speed Assessments

Speed tests measure the rate at which an athlete can cover a specific distance [28]. Although cricket is an endurance sport that includes both

Table 8.6 Aerobic, anaerobic and speed assessments

Name of test(s)	Description	Equipment
Time Trials (1, 1.6, 2 km) [100]	Time trialled distance test that assesses the aerobic capacity of athletes. The result is the time taken to complete the required distance.	Timer, distance measurement device, GPS[a], heart rate monitors[a].
MAS Interval Tests [101]	Interval or shuttle test with work and rest periods that measures an athlete's maximal aerobic capacity. The shuttle/interval distances are marked out by cones.	Timer, distance measurement device, GPS[a], heart rate monitors[a].
YoYo IRT (level 1 or 2) [29]	Intermittent running test that focuses on the capacity to perform intermittent exercise (level 1) and the ability to recover from repeated higher intensity exercise (level 2).	Timer, distance measurement device, GPS[a], heart rate monitors[a].
Bronco [105]	This test consists of a total of 1200 m running a shuttle. Players are asked to run from a 0 to 20-m line and back to 0 m, then run to a 40-m line and back to 0 m, and then run to a 60-m line and back to 0 m. The execution of the 20–40–60 m shuttle is considered one repetition. Players have to complete 5 consecutive repetitions as fast as possible.	Timer, distance measurement device.
30:15 [30]	Intermittent running test that measures aerobic fitness whilst the athletes work at high intensities.	Timer, distance measurement device, GPS[a], heart rate monitors[a].
Distance Trials (e.g. 5- or 6-minute)	Distance trialled time tests that assess the aerobic capacity of athletes. The result is the distance covered in a particular time (e.g. 5- or 6 minutes)	Timer, distance measurement device, GPS[a], heart rate monitors[a].

(continued)

Table 8.6 (continued)

Name of test(s)	Description	Equipment
Repeated Run a 2/3 Tests	Assessing an athlete's ability to resist fatigue and/or increase power output correlated to explosive and repeated batting scenarios.	Timer, distance measurement device, camera and/or high-speed scrubbing app, timing gates[a].
Repeated Sprint Ability Tests	Assessing an athlete's ability to resist fatigue and/or increase power output correlated to explosive and repeated fielding or bowling scenarios.	Timer, distance measurement device, camera and/or high-speed scrubbing app, timing gates[a].
Run a 2 Test	Batter specific, testing the ability to accelerate, decelerate, and change direction whilst running between wickets with a bat in hand.	Timer, distance measurement device, camera and/or high-speed scrubbing app, timing gates[a].
505 Test [106]	Linked to the Run a 2, this test can assess an athlete's deceleration, change of direction and acceleration speed off both sides of the body.	Timer, distance measurement device, camera and/or high-speed scrubbing app, timing gates[a].
5, 10, 20, 40 m Max Velocity Test	Velocity tests covering both linear acceleration and max velocity qualities correlated to explosive fielding and batting scenarios.	Timer, distance measurement device, camera and/or high-speed scrubbing app, GPS, timing gates[a].

[a]This equipment may be readily available in a professional, international, or elite training facility. These aerobic, anaerobic, and speed tests can be completed without this equipment in a regressed model

aerobic and anaerobic demands, intermittent bursts of speed and power are integral to cricket-specific activities during batting, bowling and fielding that require acceleration, deceleration, change of direction, maximal velocity and agility [32, 33]. In line with the assessment of other fitness parameters previously discussed, there are numerous methods of assessing player speed that are relevant to cricket's outcome measures. For the convenience of this chapter, speed will encompass acceleration, deceleration, change of direction, maximal velocity and agility qualities.

Speed and agility testing benefits cricketers and provides information on:

- Tracking speed improvement, leading to improved batting, bowling and fielding performances
- Identifying movement pattern inefficiencies, allowing for targeted injury prevention
- Informing individualised programmes to optimise speed development
- Providing objective data for selection decisions and ensuring that the most athletic players are chosen for specific key roles in the field

Tests measuring a player's speed over a specific distance without addressing the reasons behind speed development are presented in Table 8.6. For insights into the 'why', readers should refer to work by Samozino, Nimphius and Morin, which is gaining attention in both research and applied settings [103, 104].

8.6 Conclusion

Pre-participatory screening tests are essential at all levels of participation, as they help identify deficiencies and guide targeted training interventions. Integrating various screening assessments (i.e. movement quality, strength, flexibility and cardiovascular fitness) ensures a thorough evaluation of a player's physical readiness to participate in cricket. Screening tests assist in identifying potential injury risks and optimising physical preparation. Although research on the effectiveness of these screening tests is still evolving, their practical application in cricket settings is promising and needs to translate into empirical studies. By adopting these screening protocols, cricket coaches and sports science and sports medicine practitioners can collaborate to ensure players are well-prepared to meet the physical demands of cricket. This proactive approach promotes a safer and more efficient training environment, enabling players to reach their full potential whilst reducing injury risk. As cricket continues to evolve, thorough and systematic screening to establish the aetiology of injuries will guide intervention programmes and remain a cornerstone of player development and well-being.

References

1. Vickery W, Duffield R, Crowther R, Beakley D, Blanch P, Dascombe BJ. Comparison of the physical and technical demands of cricket players during training and match-play. J Strength Cond Res. 2018;32(3):821–9. https://doi.org/10.1519/jsc.0000000000001528.
2. Vickery W, Dascombe BJ, Scanlan AT. A review of the physical and physiological demands associated with cricket fast and spin bowlers. Int J Sports Sci Coach. 2018;13(2):290–301. https://doi.org/10.1177/1747954117731051.
3. Jacobs J, Olivier B, Dawood M, Perera NKP. Prevalence and incidence of injuries among female cricket players: a systematic review and meta-analysis. JBI Evid Synth. 2022;20(7):1741–90. https://doi.org/10.11124/jbies-21-00120.
4. Orchard J, Inge P, Sims K, Kountouris A, et al. Comparison of injury profiles between elite Australian male and female cricket players. J Sci Med Sport. 2023;26:19.
5. Constable M, Wundersitz D, Bini R, Kingsley M. Quantification of the demands of cricket bowling and the relationship to injury risk: a systematic review. BMC Sports Sci Med Rehabil. 2021;13(1):109. https://doi.org/10.1186/s13102-021-00335-8.
6. Bahr R, Krosshaug T. Understanding injury mechanisms: a key component of preventing injuries in sport. Br J Sports Med. 2005;39(6):324–9. https://doi.org/10.1136/bjsm.2005.018341.
7. Finch C. A new framework for research leading to sports injury prevention. J Sci Med Sport. 2006;9(1–2):3–9; discussion 10. https://doi.org/10.1016/j.jsams.2006.02.009.
8. Bahr R. Why screening tests to predict injury do not work-and probably never will…: a critical review. Br J Sports Med. 2016;50(13):776–80. https://doi.org/10.1136/bjsports-2016-096256.
9. Finch CF, Bahr R, Drezner JA, Dvorak J, Engebretsen L, Hewett T, et al. Towards the reduction of injury and illness in athletes: defining our research priorities. Br J Sports Med. 2017;51(16):1178–82. https://doi.org/10.1136/bjsports-2016-097042.
10. Thompson PD, Arena R, Riebe D, Pescatello LS. ACSM's new preparticipation health screening recommendations from ACSM's guidelines for exercise testing and prescription, ninth edition. Curr Sports Med Rep. 2013;12(4):215–7. https://doi.org/10.1249/JSR.0b013e31829a68cf.
11. Olivier B, Taljaard T, Burger E, Brukner P, Orchard J, Gray J, et al. Which extrinsic and intrinsic factors are associated with non-contact injuries in adult cricket fast bowlers? Sports Med. 2016;46(1):79–101. https://doi.org/10.1007/s40279-015-0383-y.
12. Farhart P, Beakley D, Diwan A, Duffield R, Rodriguez EP, Chamoli U, et al. Intrinsic variables associated with low back pain and lumbar spine injury in fast bowlers in cricket: a systematic review. BMC Sports Sci Med Rehabil. 2023;15(1):114. https://doi.org/10.1186/s13102-023-00732-1.
13. Bird SP, Markwick WJ. Musculoskeletal screening and functional testing: considerations for basketball athletes. Int J Sports Phys Ther. 2016;11(5):784–802.
14. Legg J. Movement screen: minimum standards for AIS basketball scholarship. Canberra: Australian Institute of Sport and Basketball Australia; 2012.
15. Reid DA, Vanweerd RJ, Larmer PJ, Kingstone R. The inter and intra rater reliability of the Netball Movement Screening Tool. J Sci Med Sport. 2015;18(3):353–7. https://doi.org/10.1016/j.jsams.2014.05.008.
16. Haycraft JA, Kovalchik S, Pyne DB, Robertson S. Physical characteristics of players within the Australian Football League participation pathways: a systematic review. Sports Med Open. 2017;3:1–16.
17. McCunn R, Aus der Fünten K, Govus A, Julian R, Schimpchen J, Meyer T. The intra- and inter-rater reliability of the soccer injury movement screen (SIMS). Int J Sports Phys Ther. 2017;12(1):53–66.
18. Forrest MR, Hebert JJ, Scott BR, Brini S, Dempsey AR. Risk factors for non-contact injury in adolescent cricket pace bowlers: a systematic review. Sports Med. 2017;47:2603–19.
19. Kibler WB, Chandler TJ, Uhl T, Maddux RE. A musculoskeletal approach to the preparticipation physical examination: preventing injury and improving performance. Am J Sports Med. 1989;17(4):525–31. https://doi.org/10.1177/036354658901700413.
20. Nessler T, Mokha M. Using movement assessment to improve performance and reduce injury risk. Int J Athl Ther Train. 2013;18(2):8.
21. Olivier B, Stewart AV, McKinon W. Injury and lumbar reposition sense in cricket pace bowlers in neutral and pace bowling specific body positions. Spine J. 2014;14(8):1447–53. https://doi.org/10.1016/j.spinee.2013.08.036.
22. McCunn R, aus der Fünten K, Fullagar HHK, McKeown I, Meyer T. Reliability and association with injury of movement screens: a critical review. Sports Med. 2016;46(6):763–81. https://doi.org/10.1007/s40279-015-0453-1.
23. Forrest MRL, Scott BR, Hebert JJ, Dempsey AR. Injury prevention strategies for adolescent cricket

pace bowlers. Sports Med. 2018;48(11):2449–61. https://doi.org/10.1007/s40279-018-0981-6.
24. Orchard J, James T, Alcott E, Carter S, Farhart P. Injuries in Australian cricket at first class level 1995/1996 to 2000/2001. Br J Sports Med. 2002;36(4):270–4; discussion 5. https://doi.org/10.1136/bjsm.36.4.270.
25. Dennis RJ, Finch CF, McLntosh AS, Elliott BC. Use of field-based tests to identify risk factors for injury to fast bowlers in cricket. Br J Sports Med. 2008;42(6):477–82. https://doi.org/10.1136/bjsm.2008.046698.
26. Olivier B, Gray J. Musculoskeletal predictors of non-contact injury in cricketers – few and far between? A longitudinal cohort study. Phys Ther Sport. 2018;34:208–15. https://doi.org/10.1016/j.ptsp.2018.10.014.
27. Dennis RJ, Finch CF, Elliott BC, Farhart PJ. The reliability of musculoskeletal screening tests used in cricket. Phys Ther Sport. 2008;9(1):25–33. https://doi.org/10.1016/j.ptsp.2007.09.004.
28. Afonso J, Clemente FM, Nakamura FY, Morouço P, Sarmento H, Inman RA, et al. The effectiveness of post-exercise stretching in short-term and delayed recovery of strength, range of motion and delayed onset muscle soreness: a systematic review and meta-analysis of randomized controlled trials. Front Physiol. 2021;12:677581. https://doi.org/10.3389/fphys.2021.677581.
29. Dobbin N, Highton J, Moss SL, Hunwicks R, Twist C. Concurrent validity of a rugby-specific Yo-Yo intermittent recovery test (level 1) for assessing match-related running performance. J Strength Cond Res. 2021;35(1):176–82. https://doi.org/10.1519/jsc.0000000000002621.
30. Bruce LM, Moule SJ. Validity of the 30-15 intermittent fitness test in subelite female athletes. J Strength Cond Res. 2017;31(11):3077–82. https://doi.org/10.1519/jsc.0000000000001775.
31. Green S, Dawson B. Measurement of anaerobic capacities in humans. Definitions, limitations and unsolved problems. Sports Med. 1993;15(5):312–27. https://doi.org/10.2165/00007256-199315050-00003.
32. Lockie RG, Callaghan SJ, Jeffriess MD. Analysis of specific speed testing for cricketers. J Strength Cond Res. 2013;27(11):2981–8. https://doi.org/10.1519/JSC.0b013e31828a2c56.
33. Rudkin ST, O'Donoghue PG. Time-motion analysis of first-class cricket fielding. J Sci Med Sport. 2008;11(6):604–7. https://doi.org/10.1016/j.jsams.2007.08.004.
34. van Dyk N, Clarsen B. Prevention forecast: cloudy with a chance of injury. Br J Sports Med. 2017;51(23):1646–7. https://doi.org/10.1136/bjsports-2017-097861.
35. Cook G, Burton L, Hoogenboom BJ, Voight M. Functional movement screening: the use of fundamental movements as an assessment of function – part 1. Int J Sports Phys Ther. 2014;9(3):396–409.
36. McLeod G, O'Connor S, Morgan D, Kountouris A, Finch CF, Fortington LV. Prospective reporting of injury in community-level cricket: a systematic review to identify research priorities. J Sci Med Sport. 2020;23(11):1028–43. https://doi.org/10.1016/j.jsams.2020.04.023.
37. Jacobs J, Olivier B, Brandt C, Jafta G. Physical profiles of all-rounders, batters, and bowlers in sub-elite women's cricket. J Strength Cond Res. 2024;38(6):1095–102. https://doi.org/10.1519/jsc.0000000000004747.
38. Stretch R. Junior cricketers are not a smaller version of adult cricketers: a 5-year investigation of injuries in elite junior cricketers. S Afr J Sports Med. 2014;26(4):123–7. https://doi.org/10.7196/SAJSM.543.
39. Adirim TA, Cheng TL. Overview of injuries in the young athlete. Sports Med. 2003;33(1):75–81. https://doi.org/10.2165/00007256-200333010-00006.
40. Bayne H, Elliott B, Campbell A, Alderson J. Lumbar load in adolescent fast bowlers: a prospective injury study. J Sci Med Sport. 2016;19(2):117–22. https://doi.org/10.1016/j.jsams.2015.02.011.
41. Bennett H, Davison K, Arnold J, Slattery F, Martin M, Norton K. Multicomponent musculoskeletal movement assessment tools: a systematic review and critical appraisal of their development and applicability to professional practice. J Strength Cond Res. 2017;31(10):2903–19.
42. Kritz M. Development, reliability and effectiveness of the Movement Competency Screen (MCS). Auckland University of Technology; 2012.
43. McKeown I, Taylor-McKeown K, Woods C, Ball N. Athletic ability assessment: a movement assessment protocol for athletes. Int J Sports Phys Ther. 2014;9(7):862.
44. Barbosa GM, Calixtre LB, Fialho HRF, Locks F, Kamonseki DH. Measurement properties of upper extremity physical performance tests in athletes: a systematic review. Braz J Phys Ther. 2024;28(1):100575.
45. Cook G, Burton L, Hoogenboom B. Pre-participation screening: the use of fundamental movements as an assessment of function–part 1. N Am J Sports Phys Ther: NAJSPT. 2006;1(2):62.
46. Cook G, Burton L, Hoogenboom B. Pre-participation screening: the use of fundamental movements as an assessment of function–part 2. N Am J Sports Phys Ther: NAJSPT. 2006;1(3):132.
47. Herrington L. Knee valgus angle during single leg squat and landing in patellofemoral pain patients and controls. Knee. 2014;21(2):514–7. https://doi.org/10.1016/j.knee.2013.11.011.
48. Hewett TE, Myer GD, Ford KR, Paterno MV, Quatman CE. Mechanisms, prediction, and prevention of ACL injuries: cut risk with three sharpened and validated tools. J Orthop Res. 2016;34(11):1843–55. https://doi.org/10.1002/jor.23414.
49. Ressman J, Grooten WJA, Barr ER. Visual assessment of movement quality in the single leg squat

test: a review and meta-analysis of inter-rater and intrarater reliability. BMJ Open Sport Exerc Med. 2019;5(1):e000541.
50. Harris-Hayes M, Steger-May K, Koh C, Royer NK, Graci V, Salsich GB. Classification of lower extremity movement patterns based on visual assessment: reliability and correlation with 2-dimensional video analysis. J Athl Train. 2014;49(3):304–10. https://doi.org/10.4085/1062-6050-49.2.21.
51. Forrest M, Hecimovich M, Dempsey A. Lumbopelvic muscle activation patterns in adolescent fast bowlers. Eur J Sport Sci. 2016;16(6):677–84. https://doi.org/10.1080/17461391.2015.1135985.
52. Jull G, Richardson C, Toppenberg R, Comerford M, Bui B. Towards a measurement of active muscle control for lumbar stabilisation. Aust J Physiother. 1993;39(3):187–93.
53. Olivier B, Stewart AV, Olorunju SAS, McKinon W. Static and dynamic balance ability, lumbo-pelvic movement control and injury incidence in cricket pace bowlers. J Sci Med Sport. 2015;18(1):19–25. https://doi.org/10.1016/j.jsams.2013.10.245.
54. Hertel J, Braham RA, Hale SA, Olmsted-Kramer LC. Simplifying the star excursion balance test: analyses of subjects with and without chronic ankle instability. J Orthop Sports Phys Ther. 2006;36(3):131–7.
55. Gray GW. Lower extremity functional profile. Wynn Marketing, Incorporated; 1995.
56. Plisky PJ, Rauh MJ, Kaminski TW, Underwood FB. Star Excursion Balance Test as a predictor of lower extremity injury in high school basketball players. J Orthop Sports Phys Ther. 2006;36(12):911–9.
57. Batson G. Validating a dance-specific screening test for balance: preliminary results from multisite testing. Med Probl Perform Art. 2010;25(3):110–5.
58. Lisman P, Hildebrand E, Nadelen M, Leppert K. Association of functional movement screen and Y-balance test scores with injury in high school athletes. J Strength Cond Res. 2021;35(7):1930.
59. Gribble PA, Hertel J, Plisky P. Using the Star Excursion Balance Test to assess dynamic postural-control deficits and outcomes in lower extremity injury: a literature and systematic review. J Athl Train. 2012;47(3):339–57.
60. Plisky P, Schwartkopf-Phifer K, Huebner B, Garner MB, Bullock G. Systematic review and meta-analysis of the Y-balance test lower quarter: reliability, discriminant validity, and predictive validity. Int J Sports Phys Ther. 2021;16(5):1190. https://doi.org/10.26603/001c.27634.
61. Goldbeck TG, Davies GJ. Test-retest reliability of the closed kinetic chain upper extremity stability test: a clinical field test. J Sport Rehabil. 2000;9(1):35–45.
62. Gorman PP, Butler RJ, Plisky PJ, Kiesel KB. Upper Quarter Y Balance Test: reliability and performance comparison between genders in active adults. J Strength Cond Res. 2012;26(11):3043–8.
63. Roush JR, Kitamura J, Waits MC. Reference values for the Closed Kinetic Chain Upper Extremity Stability Test (CKCUEST) for collegiate baseball players. N Am J Sports Phys Ther. 2007;2(3):159–63.
64. Kardor S, Gorji Z, Ghotbi N, Attarbashi-Moghadam B, Shadmehr A, Gorji M. Upper extremity physical performance tests in female overhead athletes: a test–retest reliability study. J Orthop Surg Res. 2023;18(1):489.
65. Tucci HT, Martins J, Sposito GDC, Camarini PMF, De Oliveira AS. Closed Kinetic Chain Upper Extremity Stability test (CKCUES test): a reliability study in persons with and without shoulder impingement syndrome. BMC Musculoskelet Disord. 2014;15:1–9.
66. Westrick RB, Miller JM, Carow SD, Gerber JP. Exploration of the y-balance test for assessment of upper quarter closed kinetic chain performance. Int J Sports Phys Ther. 2012;7(2):139–47.
67. de la Motte SJ, Lisman P, Gribbin TC, Murphy K, Deuster PA. Systematic review of the association between physical fitness and musculoskeletal injury risk: part 3-flexibility, power, speed, balance, and agility. J Strength Cond Res. 2019;33(6):1723–35. https://doi.org/10.1519/jsc.0000000000002382.
68. Webster TM, Comfort P, Jones PA. Relationship between physical fitness and the physical demands of 50-over cricket in fast bowlers. J Strength Cond Res. 2022;36(3):e66–72. https://doi.org/10.1519/jsc.0000000000003542.
69. Mills JD, Taunton JE, Mills WA. The effect of a 10-week training regimen on lumbo-pelvic stability and athletic performance in female athletes: a randomized-controlled trial. Phys Ther Sport. 2005;6(2):60–6.
70. Frohm A, Heijne A, Kowalski J, Svensson P, Myklebust G. A nine-test screening battery for athletes: a reliability study. Scand J Med Sci Sports. 2012;22(3):306–15. https://doi.org/10.1111/j.1600-0838.2010.01267.x.
71. McGill SM, Andersen JT, Horne AD. Predicting performance and injury resilience from movement quality and fitness scores in a basketball team over 2 years. J Strength Cond Res. 2012;26(7):1731–9. https://doi.org/10.1519/JSC.0b013e3182576a76.
72. Reilly T, Morris T, Whyte G. The specificity of training prescription and physiological assessment: a review. J Sports Sci. 2009;27(6):575–89. https://doi.org/10.1080/02640410902729741.
73. McMaster DT, Gill N, Cronin J, McGuigan M. A brief review of strength and ballistic assessment methodologies in sport. Sports Med. 2014;44(5):603–23. https://doi.org/10.1007/s40279-014-0145-2.
74. Goggins L, Warren A, Osguthorpe D, Peirce N, Wedatilake T, McKay C, et al. Detecting injury risk factors with algorithmic models in elite women's pathway cricket. Int J Sports Med. 2022;43(4):344–9. https://doi.org/10.1055/a-1502-6824.
75. Murphy MC, Chivers P, Mahony K, Mosler AB. Risk factors for dominant-shoulder injury in elite female Australian cricket players: a prospective study. J Transl Sports Med. 2020;3(5):404–14.

76. Portus M, Mason BR, Elliott BC, Pfitzner MC, Done RP. Technique factors related to ball release speed and trunk injuries in high performance cricket fast bowlers. Sports Biomech. 2004;3(2):263–84. https://doi.org/10.1080/14763140408522845.
77. Clarsen B, Bahr R, Andersson SH, Munk R, Myklebust G. Reduced glenohumeral rotation, external rotation weakness and scapular dyskinesis are risk factors for shoulder injuries among elite male handball players: a prospective cohort study. Br J Sports Med. 2014;48(17):1327–33. https://doi.org/10.1136/bjsports-2014-093702.
78. Foster D, John D, Elliott B, Ackland T, Fitch K. Back injuries to fast bowlers in cricket: a prospective study. Br J Sports Med. 1989;23(3):150–4.
79. Kelln BM, McKeon PO, Gontkof LM, Hertel J. Handheld dynamometry: reliability of lower extremity muscle testing in healthy, physically active,young adults. J Sport Rehabil. 2008;17(2):160–70. https://doi.org/10.1123/jsr.17.2.160.
80. Warneke K, Keiner M, Lohmann LH, Hillebrecht M, Wirth K, Schiemann S. The influence of maximum strength performance in seated calf raises on counter movement jump and squat jump in elite junior basketball players. Sport Mont. 2022;20(2):191–9.
81. Kraemer WJ, Ratamess NA. Fundamentals of resistance training: progression and exercise prescription. Med Sci Sports Exerc. 2004;36(4):674–88. https://doi.org/10.1249/01.mss.0000121945.36635.61.
82. Cormie P, McGuigan MR, Newton RU. Developing maximal neuromuscular power: Part 1--biological basis of maximal power production. Sports Med 2011;41(1):17–38. doi: https://doi.org/10.2165/11537690-000000000-00000.
83. Ashworth B, Hogben P, Singh N, Tulloch L, Cohen DD. The Athletic Shoulder (ASH) test: reliability of a novel upper body isometric strength test in elite rugby players. BMJ Open Sport Exerc Med. 2018;4(1):e000365. https://doi.org/10.1136/bmjsem-2018-000365.
84. Thorborg K, Petersen J, Magnusson SP, Hölmich P. Clinical assessment of hip strength using a hand-held dynamometer is reliable. Scand J Med Sci Sports. 2010;20(3):493–501. https://doi.org/10.1111/j.1600-0838.2009.00958.x.
85. Akarçeşme C, Cengizel E, Alvurdu S, Bağcı E, Altundağ E, Cengizel ÇÖ, et al. Reliability and validity of the new portable Nordic hamstring test device (IVMES H-Bord). Proc Inst Mech Eng Part P: J Sports Eng Technol. 2024:17543371241239725. https://doi.org/10.1177/17543371241239725.
86. McGill SM, Childs A, Liebenson C. Endurance times for low back stabilization exercises: clinical targets for testing and training from a normal database. Arch Phys Med Rehabil. 1999;80(8):941–4. https://doi.org/10.1016/s0003-9993(99)90087-4.
87. Högberg J, Bergentoft E, Piussi R, Wernbom M, Beischer S, Simonson R, et al. Persistent knee flexor strength deficits identified through the NordBord eccentric test not seen with "gold standard" isokinetic concentric testing during the first year after anterior cruciate ligament reconstruction with a hamstring tendon autograft. Phys Ther Sport. 2022;55:119–24. https://doi.org/10.1016/j.ptsp.2022.03.004.
88. Green B, Coventry M, Pizzari T, Rio EK, Murphy MC. Form matters—technical cues in the single leg heel raise to failure test significantly change the outcome: a study of convergent validity in Australian football players. BioMed. 2024;4(2):89–99.
89. Freckleton G, Cook J, Pizzari T. The predictive validity of a single leg bridge test for hamstring injuries in Australian Rules Football Players. Br J Sports Med. 2014;48(8):713–7. https://doi.org/10.1136/bjsports-2013-092356.
90. Merrigan JJ, Strang A, Eckerle J, Mackowski N, Hierholzer K, Ray NT, et al. Countermovement jump force-time curve analyses: reliability and comparability across force plate systems. J Strength Cond Res. 2024;38(1):30–7. https://doi.org/10.1519/jsc.0000000000004586.
91. Maloney SJ, Fletcher IM, Richards J. Reliability of unilateral vertical leg stiffness measures assessed during bilateral hopping. J Appl Biomech. 2015;31(5):285–91. https://doi.org/10.1123/jab.2014-0254.
92. Stockbrugger BA, Haennel RG. Validity and reliability of a medicine ball explosive power test. J Strength Cond Res. 2001;15(4):431–8.
93. Behm DG, Chaouachi A. A review of the acute effects of static and dynamic stretching on performance. Eur J Appl Physiol. 2011;111(11):2633–51. https://doi.org/10.1007/s00421-011-1879-2.
94. Hayen A, Dennis RJ, Finch CF. Determining the intra- and inter-observer reliability of screening tools used in sports injury research. J Sci Med Sport. 2007;10(4):201–10. https://doi.org/10.1016/j.jsams.2006.09.002.
95. Gabbe B, Bennell K, Wajswelner H, Finch C. Reliability of common lower extremity musculoskeletal screening tests. Phys Ther Sport. 2004;5:90–7.
96. Cools AM, De Wilde L, Van Tongel A, Ceyssens C, Ryckewaert R, Cambier DC. Measuring shoulder external and internal rotation strength and range of motion: comprehensive intra-rater and inter-rater reliability study of several testing protocols. J Shoulder Elb Surg. 2014;23(10):1454–61. https://doi.org/10.1016/j.jse.2014.01.006.
97. Bennell KL, Talbot RC, Wajswelner H, Techovanich W, Kelly DH, Hall AJ. Intra-rater and inter-rater reliability of a weight-bearing lunge measure of ankle dorsiflexion. Aust J Physiother. 1998;44(3):175–80. https://doi.org/10.1016/s0004-9514(14)60377-9.
98. Wells KF, Dillon EK. The sit and reach—a test of back and leg flexibility. Res Q Am Assoc Health Phys Educ Recreat. 1952;23:115–8.
99. Sloth M, Sloth D, Overgaard K, Dalgas U. Effects of sprint interval training on VO2max and aerobic exercise performance: a systematic review

and meta-analysis. Scand J Med Sci Sports. 2013;23(6):e341–52. https://doi.org/10.1111/sms.12092.
100. Currell K, Jeukendrup AE. Validity, reliability and sensitivity of measures of sporting performance. Sports Med. 2008;38(4):297–316. https://doi.org/10.2165/00007256-200838040-00003.
101. Lacour JR, Padilla-Magunacelaya S, Chatard JC, Arsac L, Barthélémy JC. Assessment of running velocity at maximal oxygen uptake. Eur J Appl Physiol Occup Physiol. 1991;62(2):77–82. https://doi.org/10.1007/bf00626760.
102. Herridge R, Turner A, Bishop C. Monitoring changes in power, speed, agility, and endurance in elite cricketers during the off-season period. J Strength Cond Res. 2020;34(8):2285–93. https://doi.org/10.1519/jsc.0000000000002077.
103. Morin JB, Samozino P. Interpreting power-force-velocity profiles for individualized and specific training. Int J Sports Physiol Perform. 2016;11(2):267–72. https://doi.org/10.1123/ijspp.2015-0638.
104. Morin JB, Bourdin M, Edouard P, Peyrot N, Samozino P, Lacour JR. Mechanical determinants of 100-m sprint running performance. Eur J Appl Physiol. 2012;112(11):3921–30. https://doi.org/10.1007/s00421-012-2379-8.
105. Vachon A, Berryman N, Mujika I, Paquet JB, Bosquet L. Fitness determinants of repeated high-intensity effort ability in elite rugby union players. Int J Sports Physiol Perform. 2021;16(8):1103–10. https://doi.org/10.1123/ijspp.2020-0525.
106. Taylor JM, Cunningham L, Hood P, Thorne B, Irvin G, Weston M. The reliability of a modified 505 test and change-of-direction deficit time in elite youth football players. Sci Med Footb. 2019;3(2):157–62. https://doi.org/10.1080/24733938.2018.1526402.
107. Teyhen DS, Shaffer SW, Lorenson CL, Halfpap JP, Donofry DF, Walker MJ, et al. The functional movement screen: a reliability study. J Orthop Sports Phys Ther. 2012;42(6):530–40. https://doi.org/10.2519/jospt.2012.3838.
108. Mann K, O'Dwyer N, Bird S, Edwards S. Assuming rater reliability of a movement competency screen – is it true? J Sci Med Sport. 2017;20:22. https://doi.org/10.1016/j.jsams.2017.09.232.
109. Milbank E, Peterson DD, Henry S. The reliability and predictive ability of the movement competency screen in a military population. Sport J. 2016;2016:1.

Physical Performance, Psychological and Safety Considerations in Cricket Warm-Ups

9

Phil Scott

9.1 Introduction

'The act or process of "warming up" for a contest' [1] (Fig. 9.1) has been around since the late 1800s, according to sources. It precedes training or a match to give the athlete the best chance of entering the scenario as ready as possible, physically and psychologically, to perform at their best. All levels and age groups of sport will employ a warm-up, with varying reasons in mind. Fundamentally, alongside a collaborative approach to consistent training, nutrition and psychological preparation, the warm-up is there to acutely support improving the athlete's performance and reduce their chance of injuries. This chapter will focus on active warm-ups rather than the alternative options of a passive warm-up.

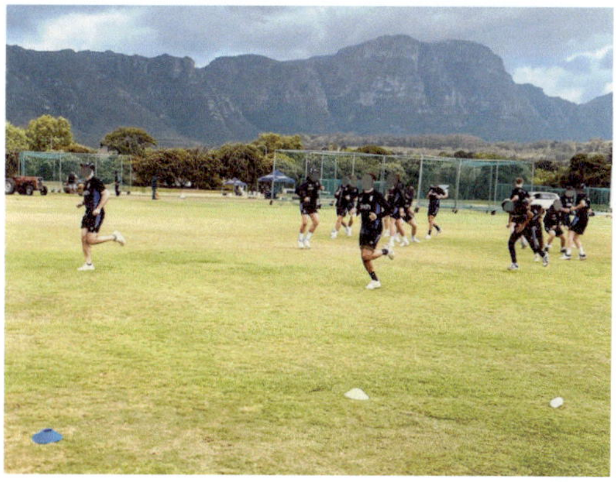

Fig. 9.1 A team warm-up on the field prior to a cricket training session

9.2 The Benefits and Mechanisms of the Warm-Up

Specifically, some of the most pertinent reasons relate to the physiological benefits, physical preparations and microdosing as well as the psychological preparations.

9.2.1 Physiological Benefits

The warm-up's most commonly understood benefit is the body temperature increase [2]. This increase, specifically in muscle temperature, has

P. Scott (✉)
England & Wales Cricket Board, London, UK
e-mail: phil.scott@ecb.co.uk

B. Olivier, J. W. Orchard (eds.), *Cricket Sports Medicine*,
https://doi.org/10.1007/978-981-96-6321-7_9

numerous positive effects on performance, including the following:

- Increases in muscle metabolism [3]: there is evidence of increased adenosine triphosphate (ATP) turnover as well as increases in anaerobic glycolysis and muscle glycogenolysis, which have been shown to improve subsequent exercise power production [4].
- Improvement in muscle fibre performance: with increased muscle temperature, there seems to be an increased performance of Type I fibres at lower contraction velocities and Type II fibres at higher velocities [5].
- Higher muscle fibre conduction velocities (MFCV): increases in temperature and higher MFCV and power outputs resulting from warm-up exercise may be a product of the increased Na^+/K^+ pump activity [6] and the ability to improve the speeds of muscle relaxation, which affect the athlete's ability to perform rapid cyclical movements, i.e. sprinting or fast bowling.

Another benefit of the warm-up is that it provides a period of time to alter our anaerobic and aerobic metabolism. Specifically, it has been shown that a bout of exercise prior to the main event can improve oxygen uptake kinetics [7]. By this, we mean there is an increase in the amplitude of the primary VO_2 response and a reduction in the VO_2 slow component, which will improve exercise tolerance and mean power outputs, leading to the sparing of an athlete's finite anaerobic energy stores [8]. We know that cricket demands a good level of aerobic capacity in order to recover between bouts of high-intensity efforts, i.e. bowling, sprinting and running between the wickets. Therefore, this would be a beneficial outcome if implemented correctly.

There are known neural benefits that can affect the power output of the athlete if performed at the right intensity with sufficient recovery before the activity. The effect of Post-Activation Potentiation (PAP) [9] has been shown to support acute improvements in jumping, sprinting and rotational power after performing an initial exercise. A lot of research has been exercise-focused within gym settings; however, there are practical parts to the research that can be applied to the on-field warm-up, such as the use of drop jumps for improved throwing [10]. The proposed mechanisms responsible for this improvement include an increased central drive to the motor neurons, increased reflex electrical activity in the spinal cord and phosphorylation of myosin regulatory light chains, which increase Ca^{2+} sensitivity of the myofilaments and increased concentration of sarcoplasmic Ca^{2+}, thus increasing actin-myosin cross-bridge cycling. The act of throwing commences from the ground up, which is the same as a drop jump. Therefore, it makes sense that there is an element of transfer between the two exercises alongside the proposed mechanisms.

9.2.2 Physical Benefits

The warm-up is a chance to acutely build the athlete up to the physical, psychological and skill level needed to perform at their maximum and best on the day. However, this is also an opportunity to top up and improve physical qualities whilst being another coaching opportunity. Another way of looking at it is by applying the concept of Microdosing [11]. In the world of cricket, if you take a 6-month season and you warm up every day you play or train, then you will arguably have 150 days of 10–15 minutes to utilise for 'micro-sessions'. If you convert that to hours, then you have around 37 hours of work time spread out throughout the season. If you reframe and deliberately plan this opportunity, then there is ample time not only to maintain but arguably improve some physical qualities throughout the season.

9.2.3 Psychological Benefits

Within the period of the warm-up, including the cricket-specific period, especially on match day, it is also a chance for the athlete to prepare psy-

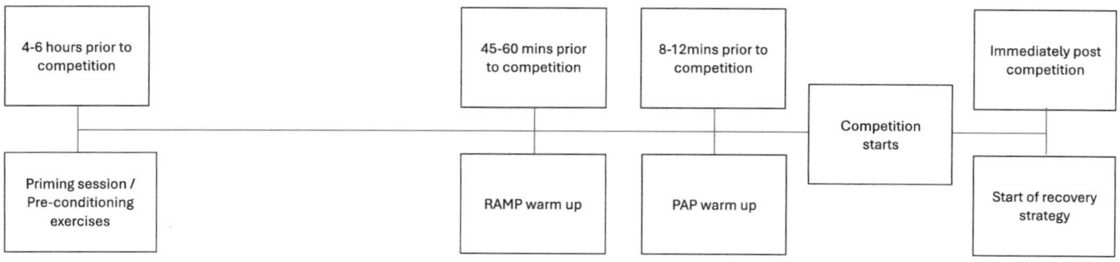

Fig. 9.2 Potential timeline of cricket warm-up strategies leading into competition. (Adapted from Kilduff et al. [22])

chologically for the upcoming demands [12]. Prior to competition, the athlete will have a mix of emotions, often underpinned by performance anxiety. The warm-up is an on-field chance for the athlete to start gathering their focus and control their emotions towards the performance. This is why, as much as we understand the underpinning mechanisms of physical preparation and the importance that it plays in their performance, we must always be cognisant and empathetic towards what they are going towards. This is a time to prepare the athlete physically but also support them in a fun, relaxed environment that allows them to get to their 'game state' as best as possible and not just tick off the boxes that we must have from a physical point of view. Getting this right is about finding the perfect blend of science and real-world practice. Finding the right games to stimulate the body and mind is key, considering that we are coaching cricket players who may or may not have extensive experience in other sports, i.e. football. Therefore, caution should be used when choosing the appropriate game for these cricket players.

9.3 Types of Warm-Up

As time and understanding have evolved, we have moved away from low-intensity and static stretching-based routines as we now understand that there may be impairments in both force [13] and repeated speed [14] outputs with performance. The use of more dynamic stretching [15] would be a preferred method, with static stretching being used in a targeted way if there are specific muscle length issues, and, ideally, dynamic stretching is the method that precedes any athletic movements [14]. Alongside this approach and armed with the knowledge of the improvements in physiology with temperature and muscle activation, there have been models and strategies put forward to optimise the pre-match preparation period both acutely (8–60 minutes prior to the match) and chronically (4–6 hours prior to the match), with Fig. 9.2 highlighting the potential time line of strategies to use.

9.3.1 Acute: RAMP Protocols: Up to 60 Minutes Prior to the Start of Play [14]

The 'RAMP' warm-up [16]: this model was proposed over 15 years ago around the principles of best practice within a warm-up. This framework (Table 9.1) allows practitioners freedom to deliver what is needed for their athlete and sport whilst having flexibility on exactly what is delivered. The acronym stands for:

R - Raise: we are looking to raise our body temperature, heart and respiration rate by working through a range of low to higher-intensity work. Utilising open or closed drills to engage the athletes in a fun but targeted manner is key in this first instance.

A - Activate & M - Mobilise: outside of moving the system globally, this is a chance to target key muscle groups and actively move through range with movements that are specific to the individual from a positional and an injury history point of view. For example, wicketkeepers will need good hip and thoracic mobility

Table 9.1 Examples of how coaches can utilise the RAMP [16] approach to a warm-up with cricket-specific examples

Warm-up method	Activity type	Cricket-specific examples
Raise	3–5 minutes of light jogging including multi-directional movements	Jog around the boundary, skipping, backwards jogging, cariocas, side shuffles, A-skips, B-skips, straight leg bounds, ground-based crawling movements
Activate	Core fundamental movements, i.e. overhead squats, lunges, RDL, press ups, rows, trunk bracing & rotations. Also, exercises for specific muscle groups for the position should be included.	*Bowlers:* SL hamstring bridges (Fig. 9.3), mini band targeting gluteus medius, SL squats, SL RDL, side plank bracing with rotation, resisted lateral flexion & rotation, resisted shoulder band work (throwing) *Batters:* Lateral lunges, mini band targeting gluteus medius, resisted rotations, resisted shoulder band work (throwing) *Wicket keepers:* Cossack squats, mini band targeting gluteus medius, SL squats, resisted rotations
Mobilise	Dynamic, though range, stretching	90/90 hip rotations, leg swings, long lunges with thoracic rotations, thoracic cat-camel, arm rotations and swings, dynamic upward and downward facing dog, deep squat with short holds
Potentiate	Increasing the intensity towards explosive and sport-specific exercises	*All players:* Running drills and skills working towards sprinting *Batters:* Explosive lateral work to simulate moving down the wicket, ISO batting rotations, explosive medball rotational work, plyometrics, change of directions with running between the wickets, clap press-ups *Bowlers:* Explosive medball slams, ISO holds specific to bowling positions, plyometrics *Wicket keepers:* Explosive medball throws for height and distance, ISO batting rotations, explosive medball rotational work, plyometrics, lateral hop & sticks

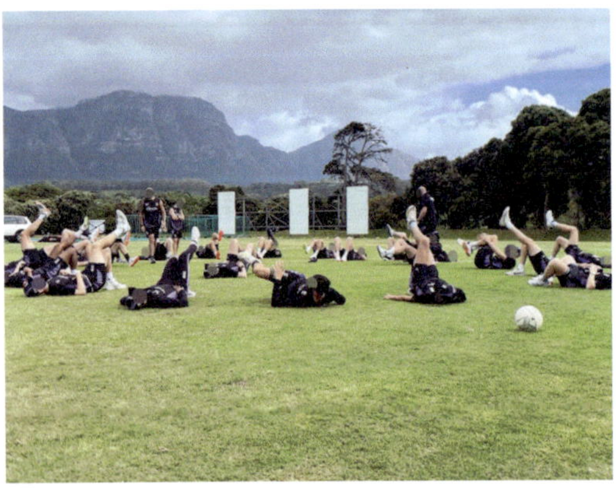

Fig. 9.3 A team performing activation exercises in the dynamic warm-up following the RAMP protocol

utilising a dynamic approach [17] and also be able to produce quality lateral movements. Therefore, targeting the 'cat-camel' stretch and the Gluteus Medius lateral band walks would be a strong option for this player. Understanding the key movement patterns used in the specific positions is key to the underpinning of programming in this phase.

P - Potentiate: the concept behind this term can be twofold. First, we are looking to take the players towards more specific movements and intensities, ensuring they are ready to perform their skill at full intensity. Second, as mentioned above, we will deliberately take advantage of the PAP effect [9]. There are various options for both gym-based and field-based PAP, which we will discuss later in the chapter.

9.3.2 Acute: PAP—Up to 8–12 Minutes Prior [19]

Acute methods relevant to cricket include the utilisation of PAP, which has been shown to improve performance and will peak between 8 and 12 minutes [18]. With the way cricket is set up and the traditional warm-up taking place up to 60 minutes prior to the start of play, this does not lend itself to being used. However, this is where we need to challenge tradition as to the best way forward. Understanding the effects and mechanisms will allow us to make informed decisions as to the best time to implement different 'warm-ups' or microdose training sessions for improved performance. For example, you can take advantage of isometrics whilst adopting a similar stance and position to batting for 5-second holds on both the 'top hand' and the 'bottom hand' to increase bat velocity [19]. Utilising this method, for example, would be simple to implement at the side of the pitch prior to players going out to bat.

9.3.3 Chronic: Priming/Pre-conditioning: Up to 6 Hours Prior [20, 21]

Priming or pre-conditioning is a useful strategy that combines the concept of microdosing a strength or power exercise between 4 and 6 hours prior to the competition. The proposed mechanisms include increased joint stiffness, high-frequency motor neuron activation, greater muscle fibre sensitivity to calcium ions as well as changes in hormonal status, specifically, increased levels of testosterone which have been linked to improvements in explosive performance [22].

9.3.4 Other Considerations

Aside from understanding the mechanisms that are in play with the warm-up, there are also some holistic and other angles to consider to be an effective coach in all circumstances presented.

9.3.4.1 The Individual Approach and Previous History

As alluded to, there are some general principles that can be applied to warm-ups and across the board for all players. However, understanding the individual within the team is essential to get the best out of that player as well as addressing their specific needs. For example, all players, bar the wicketkeeper, will consistently throw when fielding; therefore, there is a need to approach this area as a whole. However, there may be players within that group who have had a previous shoulder injury and need an extra volume of work or more targeted exercises. Understanding, prescribing and supporting the player to that degree will add up over the long term and also result in that player knowing they are being considered personally.

9.3.4.2 Group Versus Individual Warm-Ups and Multi-Day Versus One-Day

Generally, it is the custom to warm up the team as a whole all at the same time. However, the reality of cricket is that there are three formats and many roles within. For example, it may be prevalent in T20 cricket to warm up as a group 30–45 minutes prior to the start of play due to the short and intense nature of the whole match and the fact that the toss will take place 30 minutes prior to the start of play and the team will, therefore, know whether they are batting or bowling, whereas, in multi-day cricket, it may be more pertinent on day 2 when you know your side is batting all day and is yet to lose a wicket to warm up the batters as a group specifically for batting and even let the bowlers sleep in late and arrive for a mobility session closer to the start of play. There are obvious constraints to this, like coach preference, transport, team ethos, etc. However, it is worth considering all options for optimal preparation and recovery.

9.3.4.3 Environment

Although cricket is played in the summer months, there are still large variations in ambient temperatures from the height of a subcontinent summer at 35 °C+ to springtime in England, where snow can stop play. Therefore, it is worth asking how much warming up an athlete needs to do and whether they can have a shorter or minimal 'Raise' and move quicker to the 'AMP' since body temperature will clearly be less of a limiting factor to performance. There is no clear answer to this, but it is worth bearing in mind and utilising your coaching experience to judge what is best for the athlete.

9.3.4.4 Coach Integration

Although this has been alluded to, it is worth mentioning again, as we can end up working in silos and avoiding collaboration with the coaches. Clearly, there is a need for the initial parts of the warm-up to be led solely by the strength and conditioning coach; however, when and where appropriate, especially around the more sport-specific work, integrating and including the skills coaches is a great way for the players to see the relevance and also transition from general to more specific preparation. Being clear about what both yourself and the skills coach want and need from the session, alongside good communication, is essential for this process to work optimally; however, if it is executed to a high standard, then everyone will win.

9.3.5 Injury Prevention Considerations

Cricket warm-up is quite chaotic compared to other sports (such as track and field, the football codes, and court sports). As a result, warm-up injuries are probably more common than in other sports, with a challenge remaining for cricket to make the warm-up safer. In particular, a warm-up injury after the toss creates a major dilemma for the team, the umpires and the match referee and potentially an ethical choice for the opposition captain as to whether a player injured in the warm-up but prior to playing starting is allowed to be replaced in the starting team.

Convention dictates that the umpires and opposition captain will allow a replacement if a novel contact injury occurs inadvertently in the warm-up. However, pre-existing muscle soreness that has been slightly aggravated may not warrant a full replacement on the team sheet. Some injuries may be in a grey area between the two and present challenges. For this reason and also for the disruption itself, there is an incentive for teams to try to avoid warm-up injuries. Perhaps the most famous warm-up injury of all-time was Australian paceman Glenn McGrath in the 2005 Ashes, who rolled his ankle slipping on a stray ball on the field. This injury is particularly notable as it is said to have perhaps tipped the outcome of this series towards England, who subsequently won narrowly. Scenarios such as this are in play as risks for many cricket warm-ups because there will regularly be sections of the field where simultaneously one group of bowlers are warming up by bowling, others are doing running drills and another group might have coaches hitting balls to players who are practising catching. Because of a lack of definition of what part of the field is available to each group, stray balls can commonly impinge over to areas where others are running and bowling who might either get hit by a ball or trip over one.

A further injury mechanism that has emerged in recent years has been ankle sprains on the boundary rope when practising outfield catches. A surprisingly large percentage occurs in the warm-up, probably because of higher exposure (a player who attempts 1–2 boundary catches in a game may have been asked by a coach to practice ≥10 of these in a warm-up drill).

One of the traditions of cricket is for players to request other 'ball games' for some entertainment in the warm-up. Although there has been a trend away from actually playing variations of football games (such as soccer and touch/tag football), games can be much higher risk than the game of cricket itself. Knee anterior cruciate ligament injuries (a devastating injury more common in the football codes) have historically occurred in cricket warm-ups, as have concussions and head clashes. For the staff members in charge of warm-ups, there is a strong responsibility to balance the benefits of physical and psychological preparation with variant games and the additional injury risk they impose. In particular, wearing cricket spikes whilst participating in activities where close-range cutting manoeuvres are required (not normally a part of the sport of cricket) is likely to be a mismatch that adds to injury risk.

Finally, there is a small but non-zero risk of injury to staff and crowd members in cricket warm-ups. If catches are being practised near the boundary rope, there is a chance a stray ball might ricochet up into the grandstand area. Although this may not be at high speed, there is more potential for damage if the crowd and staff members are not watching the warm-up. Sometimes young children can be close to the fence. Stadiums may need to consider additional netting around the fence to make warm-ups safer for spectators.

References

1. Oxford English Dictionary, 2025. Available at: https://www.oed.com/. Accessed: 05/06/2025.
2. McGowan CJ, Pyne DB, Thompson KG, Rattray B. Warm-up strategies for sport and exercise: mechanisms and applications. Sports Med. 2015;45:1523–46.
3. Gray SR, Soderlund K, Watson M, et al. Skeletal muscle ATP turnover and single fibre ATP and PCr content during intense exercise at different muscle temperatures in humans. Pflugers Arch. 2011;462(6):885–93.
4. Gray SR, De Vito G, Nimmo MA, et al. Skeletal muscle ATP turnover and muscle fiber conduction velocity are elevated at higher muscle temperatures during maximal power output development in humans. Am J Physiol Regul Integr Comp Physiol. 2006;290(2):376–82.
5. Gray SR, Soderlund K, Ferguson RA. ATP and phosphocreatine utilization in single human muscle fibres during the development of maximal power output at elevated muscle temperatures. J Sports Sci. 2008;26(7):701–7.
6. Van der Hoeven JH, Van Weerden TW, Zwarts MJ. Long-lasting supernormal conduction velocity after sustained maximal isometric contraction in human muscle. Muscle Nerve. 1993;16(3):312–20.
7. Burnley M, Doust JH, Carter H, et al. Effects of prior exercise and recovery duration on oxygen uptake kinetics during heavy exercise in humans. Exp Physiol. 2001;86(3):417–25.
8. Jones AM, Wilkerson DP, Burnley M, et al. Prior heavy exercise enhances performance during subsequent perimaximal exercise. Med Sci Sports Exerc. 2003;35(12):2085–92.
9. Sale D. Postactivation potentiation: role in performance. Br J Sports Med. 2004;38(4):386–7.
10. Terzis G, Spengos K, Karampatsos G, Manta P, Georgiadis G. Acute effect of drop jumping on throwing performance. J Strength Cond Res. 2009;23(9):2592–7.
11. Cuthbert M, Haff GG, McMahon JJ, Evans M, Comfort P. Microdosing: a conceptual framework for use as programming strategy for resistance training in team sports. Strength Cond J. 2024;46(2):180–201.
12. Jose J, Joseph MM, Matha M. Imagery: it's effects and benefits on sports performance and psychological variables: a review study. Int J Physiol Nutr Phys Educ. 2018;3(2):190–3.
13. Power K, Behm D, Cahill FARRELL, Carroll M, Young WARREN. An acute bout of static stretching: effects on force and jumping performance. Med Sci Sports Exerc. 2004;36(8):1389–96.
14. Sim AY, Dawson BT, Guelfi KJ, Wallman KE, Young WB. Effects of static stretching in warm-up on repeated sprint performance. J Strength Cond Res. 2009;23(7):2155–62.
15. McMillian DJ, Moore JH, Hatler BS, Taylor DC. Dynamic vs. static-stretching warm-up: the effect on power and agility performance. J Strength Cond Res. 2006;20(3):492–9.
16. Jeffreys IBA. Warm-up revisited-the "ramp" method of optimising performance preparation. UK Strength Cond Assoc. 2007;6:15–9.
17. Nelson AG, Kokkonen J, Arnall DA. Acute muscle stretching inhibits muscle strength endurance performance. J Strength Cond Res. 2005;19(2):338–43.
18. Kilduff LP, Owen N, Bevan H, et al. Influence of recovery time on post-activation potentiation in professional rugby players. J Sports Sci. 2008;26(8):795–802.
19. Higuchi T, Nagami T, Mizuguchi N, Anderson T. The acute and chronic effects of isometric contraction conditioning on baseball bat velocity. J Strength Cond Res. 2013;27(1):216–22.
20. Nutt F, Hills SP, Russell M, Waldron M, Scott P, Norris J, Cook CJ, Mason B, Ball N, Kilduff LP. Morning resistance exercise and cricket-specific repeated sprinting each improve indices of afternoon physical and cognitive performance in professional male cricketers. J Sci Med Sport. 2022;25(2):162–6.
21. Cook CJ, Kilduff LP, Crewther BT, Beaven M, West DJ. Morning based strength training improves afternoon physical performance in rugby union players. J Sci Med Sport. 2014;17(3):317–21.
22. Kilduff LP, Finn CV, Baker JS, Cook CJ, West DJ. Preconditioning strategies to enhance physical performance on the day of competition. Int J Sports Physiol Perform. 2013;8(6):677–81.
23. Kellmann M. Enhancing recovery: preventing underperformance in athletes. Human Kinetics; 2002.

10 Strength and Conditioning for Injury Reduction and Rehabilitation

Anthony Weldon, Lee Pote, Jack Murfin, Helen Greenway-Shipman, and Rob Ahmun

10.1 Introduction

Strength and conditioning (S&C) aims to improve athletes' sporting performance and mitigate the risk of injury [1]. Although a traditional view of S&C may be the design and delivery of gym-based programmes, the roles and responsibilities of S&C coaches extend far beyond this in modern cricket [2, 3]. For example, S&C coaches play an integral role in injury reduction and the return to play process, which requires extensive integration and collaboration with the wider athlete support team [1–3]. Furthermore, with the growth of cricket (e.g. more extensive playing schedules), S&C coaches have various considerations (e.g. position-specific demands) and challenges (e.g. limited time) that need to be acknowledged when designing and delivering effective S&C provisions [3–6].

This chapter will explore the importance of S&C and how individualised training programmes can be informed and designed. Furthermore, we will discuss the practices employed and challenges faced by S&C coaches concerning implementing S&C for injury reduction and rehabilitation.

10.2 The Importance of Strength and Conditioning

In cricket, S&C plays an important role in the physical (e.g. strength, power, speed and mobility) and physiological (e.g. aerobic and anaerobic fitness) development of athletes [4, 7–10]. Superior physical and physiological attributes can differentiate athletes' playing and performance levels [7, 9, 11, 12]. Whilst more robust athletes can cope with the demands of modern cricket with an increased number and intensity of matches and the repetitive actions (e.g. running between the wickets, fast bowling and fielding) required in matches [13–15]. Accordingly, cricketers with superior physical and physiological abilities support the reduction of non-contact injuries and time loss due to injury [14], thus optimising an athlete's availability to train and

A. Weldon (✉)
Centre for Life and Sport Sciences, Birmingham City University, Birmingham, UK

Aston Villa Football Club, Aston Villa Foundation, Birmingham, UK
e-mail: Anthony.weldon@bcu.ac.uk

L. Pote
School of Sport and Exercise Science, University of Derby, Derby, UK
e-mail: l.pote@derby.ac.uk

J. Murfin
Warwickshire County Cricket Club, Birmingham, UK
e-mail: jackmurfin@edgbaston.com

H. Greenway-Shipman · R. Ahmun
England and Wales Cricket Board (ECB), ECB Performance Centre, Loughborough, UK
e-mail: Helen.Greenway-Shipman@ecb.co.uk; rob.ahmun@ecb.co.uk

B. Olivier, J. W. Orchard (eds.), *Cricket Sports Medicine*,
https://doi.org/10.1007/978-981-96-6321-7_10

compete. It is recognised that elite-level cricket leads to a much higher injury rate than community cricket due to the far greater intensity at the higher level (for example, pace bowling speeds are much higher at the elite level). If injuries do occur, S&C coaches can use their broad knowledge in sports science and sports medicine whilst working collaboratively with the wider athlete support team to rehabilitate an athlete and proactively put provisions in place (e.g. modified training programmes) to reduce the likelihood of reinjury [14, 16].

10.3 Considerations for the Design of Individualised Strength and Conditioning Training Programmes

Gone are the days when a single programme was sufficient to develop a team of cricketers. Nowadays, training programmes are designed to develop athletes based on their individual requirements [3]. Below are some areas that may be considered when individualising a training programme.

10.4 Match Format

The three main formats of the game include T20 (20 overs per team), One Day (up to 50 overs per team) and Multi-Day matches (played up to 5 days). The 'Hundred' format has also been introduced in the United Kingdom, where each team faces a maximum of 100 deliveries in five sets [17]. These formats differ in intensity and duration, and S&C programmes should be tailored to reflect these differences [6, 18–21]. Research has shown that as the match format becomes shorter, the intensity rises (i.e. T20 being the shortest and most intense), with fast bowlers subjected to the most demanding workloads [19, 21]. However, the long duration of multi-day matches produces a much larger overall physical load compared to shorter formats [19]. The movement category distances and variables for each format are shown in Tables 10.1 and 10.2.

More recent literature, using GPS monitoring, has compared the match demands of international fast bowlers between One Day and T20 formats. Greater match demands for all variables (relative to minutes played) were observed for T20 com-

Table 10.1 Movement variables for the three main formats of cricket (mean ± SD)

	Distance covered (metres/hour)				
Game format	Walking (0–2.00 m/s)	Jogging (2.01–3.50 m/s)	Running (3.51–4.00 m/s)	Striding (4.01–5.00 m/s)	Sprinting (≥5.01 m/s)
T20 (*n* = 83)	2083.6 ± 297.8	603.4 ± 194.8	132.6 ± 62.4	174.8 ± 84.4	170.0 ± 99.2
One Day (*n* = 126)	2121.8 ± 314.2	543.2 ± 157.4	117.4 ± 40.0	143.0 ± 60.4	127.6 ± 64.8
Multi-Day (*n* = 43)	2006.0 ± 296.5	454.3 ± 159.3	97.75 ± 42.0	114.5 ± 61.3	97.75 ± 60.0

Adapted from Petersen et al. [19]

Table 10.2 Movement category distances for the three main formats of cricket (mean ± SD)

Game format	Sprints per hour (n)	Mean sprint distance (m)	Maximum sprint distance (m)	Efforts per hour (n)	Recovery ratio (1:*x*)
T20 (*n* = 83)	11.2 ± 6.0	14.8 ± 3.4	24.6 ± 9.8	40.6 ± 18.2	44.0 ± 23.2
One Day (*n* = 126)	8.4 ± 3.8	15.0 ± 4.8	31.2 ± 12.2	34.4 ± 11.0	51 ± 20.6
Multi-Day (*n* = 43)	7.5 ± 5.0	10.6 ± 8.5	21.75 ± 9.0	28.75 ± 12.25	89.0 ± 41.5

Adapted from Petersen et al. [19]

Table 10.3 Physical demands (mean ± SD) of fast bowlers for One Day vs. T20 cricket matches

	One Day (*n* = 157)	T20 (*n* = 38)
Absolute physical performance		
Decelerations ≤4 m/s (n)	2.7 ± 2.3	3.0 ± 2.3
Decelerations −2–4 m/s (n)	25.9 ± 12.6	19.1 ± 7.8
Accelerations 2–4 m/s (n)	35.8 ± 18.9	29.1 ± 13.8
Accelerations >4 m/s (n)	4.2 ± 6.3	4.1 ± 3.1
Maximum velocity (km/h)	29.2 ± 2.5	30.0 ± 2.8
Total distance (m)	11927.0 ± 2726.1	6616.8 ± 962.2
Distance 0–7 km/h (m)	8317.5 ± 1919.5	4115.4 ± 970.5
Distance 7–15 km/h (m)	2147.4 ± 665.7	1545.2 ± 441.3
Distance 15–20 km/h (m)	563.0 ± 180.7	453.0 ± 160.4
Distance 20–25 km/h (m)	840.8 ± 298.2	354.5 ± 155.9
Overs	7.3 ± 2.2	2.4 ± 0.5
Duration (min)	208 ± 37	101 ± 15
Relative physical performance		
Decelerations ≤4 m/s (n/min)	0.01 ± 0.009	0.03 ± 0.03
Decelerations −2–4 m/s (n/min)	0.13 ± 0.06	0.19 ± 0.06
Accelerations 2–4 m/s (n/min)	0.18 ± 0.10	0.29 ± 0.12
Accelerations >4 m/s (n/min)	0.02 ± 0.03	0.04 ± 0.03
Metres per minute (m/min)	58.0 ± 10.3	66.0 ± 7.6
Distance 0–7 km/h (m/min)	40.3 ± 6.9	41.2 ± 8.9
Distance 7–15 km/h (m/min)	10.5 ± 3.0	15.4 ± 4.3
Distance 15–20 km/h (m/min)	2.7 ± 0.8	4.5 ± 1.3
Distance 20–25 km/h (m/min)	4.1 ± 1.5	3.5 ± 1.4
Distance 25+ km/h (m/min)	0.3 ± 0.2	0.6 ± 0.4

Adapted from Bliss et al. [22]

pared to One Day, besides for distance covered in the 20–25 km/h zone [22]. Specific movement category data for both formats are presented in Table 10.3.

To date, literature is scarce investigating the demands associated with female cricket, specifically the T20 format [23]. Results showed that international players cover 5250 ± 1664 m per match and 73 ± 62 m at speeds greater than 21 km/h [23].

10.5 Position-Specific Demands

Three main disciplines are associated with the game of cricket: batting, bowling and fielding (including wicketkeeping) [24]. Each discipline is associated with unique movement patterns and demands, which should be considered for S&C coaches when designing S&C, prehabilitation, or rehabilitation programmes (see Tables 10.4a, 10.4b, 10.4c, and 10.4d).

10.5.1 Bowling

Most research in cricket has been performed on bowlers (fast bowlers in particular) due to their high injury risk [25]. The bowling action requires an awkward combination of the run-up (at optimal speeds), extension, rotation and lateral flexion of the lumbar spine whilst attenuating high forces during the delivery stride [5, 26, 27].

10.5.2 Batting

Batters can score runs one of two ways. Firstly, they can sprint between the wickets, which requires accelerating, decelerating and changing direction. In particular, the deceleration and change of direction components place a significant eccentric demand on the lower limbs [28]. Secondly, batters can hit the ball towards or past the boundary. This requires considerable upper and lower body strength [10, 29].

Table 10.4a Position-specific considerations for programme design for fast bowlers

Quality	Importance	Exercises	Prescription
Strength (lower body)	Ability to cope with ground reaction forces (~6 times bodyweight). Develop the ability to produce high forces to increase ball release speed and bounce	Squat and deadlift variations (e.g. back squat, Romanian deadlift)	≥85% 1RM ≤6 repetitions 3–4 sets
Strength (upper body)	Correlation of upper body strength and delivery speed	Vertical and horizontal push/pull variations (e.g. bench press, shoulder press, bent over row, pull up)	≥85% 1RM ≤6 repetitions 3–4 sets
Power and reactive strength	Improves rate of force development during accelerative movements (i.e. ball release)	Weightlifting, jump and medicine ball variations (e.g. hang clean, drop jump, medicine ball chest pass)	
Speed, agility and quickness	Delivery speed ~95% maximal velocity	Acceleration, sprint, deceleration and change of direction drills	
Core	Optimise spinal function and control during the bowling action	Core movement and anti-movement variations (e.g. Turkish get up, medicine ball rotations, Pallof press)	
Conditioning	Develop repeated sprint ability	Repeated shuttles with associated work-to-rest ratios	80–100% maximum speed

Adapted from Mukandi et al. [35]

Table 10.4b Position-specific considerations for programme design for batters

Quality	Importance	Exercises	Prescription
Strength (lower body)	Force transferred via kinetic chain to distal joints to optimise ball impact	Squat, lunge, deadlift and hip extension variations (e.g. overhead squat, dumbbell lunge, hex bar deadlift, hip thrust)	≥85% 1RM ≤6 repetitions 3–4 sets
Strength (upper body)	Force generation associated with powerful hitting	Vertical and horizontal push/pull variations (e.g. bench press, shoulder press, bent over row, pull up)	≥85% 1RM ≤6 repetitions 3–4 sets
Power and reactive strength	Improves rate of force development during downswing and ball impact	Weightlifting, jump and medicine ball variations (e.g. hang snatch, depth jump and rotational medicine ball throw)	
Speed, agility and quickness	Develop ability to repeatedly run between the wickets	Acceleration, sprint, deceleration, change of direction and reactive drills	
Core	Explosive rotation of the torso leading to ball impact	Core movement and anti-movement variations (e.g. half-kneeling wood chop, isometric back extension)	
Conditioning	Improve match conditioning (i.e. ability to repeatedly bat and run between wickets)	Interval training with associated work-to-rest ratios	HRmean >75% HRmax

Adapted from Mathankar et al. [36]

Table 10.4c Position-specific considerations for programme design for fielders

Quality	Importance	Exercises	Prescription
Strength (lower body)	Improve force generation when performing accelerations, jumping, diving and various stops	Squat, lunge and deadlift variations (e.g. Bulgarian split squat, barbell deadlift, lateral lunge)	≥85% 1RM ≤6 repetitions 3–4 sets
Strength (upper body)	Increase throwing velocity and protect the glenohumeral joint.	Vertical and horizontal push/pull variations (e.g. bench press, shoulder press, bent over row, pull up)	≥85% 1RM ≤6 repetitions 3–4 sets
Power and reactive strength	Improves rate of force development during accelerative movements (e.g. jumping to catch a ball)	Weightlifting and jump variations (e.g. jump shrug, loaded squat jump)	
Speed, agility and quickness	Develops ability to run and decelerate over specified distances for ball retrieval	Acceleration, sprint, deceleration, change of direction and reactive drills	
Core	Develop trunk stiffness and momentum transfer to distal segments (i.e. during throwing)	Core movement and anti-movement variations (e.g. landmine rotations, dumbbell suitcase carry)	
Conditioning	Improve ability to repeatedly run various distances for ball retrieval	Interval sprints mimicking match pace and work-to-rest ratios	>75% HRmax

Adapted from Lim et al. [6]

Table 10.4d Position-specific considerations for programme design for wicketkeepers

Quality	Importance	Exercises	Prescription
Strength (lower body)	Improve force generation when performing short accelerations, jumping, diving and various stops from a ready position	Squat, lunge and deadlift variations (e.g. skater squat, unilateral deadlift, offset lunge)	≥85% 1RM ≤6 repetitions 3–4 sets
Power and reactive strength	Produce explosive multi-directional movements in reaction to the ball	Weightlifting and jump variations (e.g. clean, countermovement jump)	
Speed, agility and quickness	Recover the ball quickly and dismiss a batter by throwing or touching the stumps	Acceleration, sprint, deceleration, change of direction and reactive drills	
Conditioning	Maintain performance through extended innings	Aerobic training mimicking match speed and work-to-rest ratios	>75% HRmax
Flexibility, mobility and stability	To allow wicketkeepers to adopt an optimal ready position and perform diving and catching without restriction or increased injury risk	Assessment of imbalances or weaknesses, with appropriate exercises advised	

Adapted from Wong et al. [34]

10.5.3 Fielding

All players need to field and limit the runs scored by the opposition by covering varying distances at high speeds [24, 30]. This involves three phases: movement preparation, multi-directional movement and throwing [31, 32].

10.5.4 Wicketkeeping

Wicketkeepers are involved in every delivery, and the movement patterns associated with this position are highly unique [33, 34]. Various movements are required, such as jumping, shuffling, sprinting, rolling and diving at different speeds and distances [33, 34].

10.6 Sex

Males and females differ morphologically, physically (e.g. strength, power, speed) and physiologically (e.g. heart rate, oxygen consumption) [37, 38]. Typically, males are larger, have more muscle mass and have less body fat percentage than females [17, 39]. More specific to cricket, females have different force-velocity profiles, fielding characteristics and bowling speeds, which need to be considered when designing and delivering S&C and injury reduction programmes [40]. Research on fast bowlers has shown significant differences between males and females for ball release speeds, run-up speeds and kinematics at back foot contact, front foot contact and ball release [41]. This suggests that female bowlers generate less whole-body linear momentum during the run-up than their male counterparts [41]. Another important consideration when training female players is hormonal fluctuations due to the menstrual cycle, particularly for injury risk. Whilst this has not been investigated within a cricketing context, research in bat and stick sports has shown that female bone strength is compromised due to hormonal and menstrual irregularities prompted by high training loads [42]. Additionally, knee injuries are more prevalent in female athletes, perhaps due to hormonal fluctuations causing greater flexibility, laxity, range of motion and lack of strength [42]. Further research is needed about this, specifically in cricket.

10.7 Age

An increase in injury risk is a significant concern at younger levels; research has shown that injuries in adolescent cricket players are higher than in their adult counterparts [14, 43, 44]. Despite this, there needs to be more literature on S&C practices and injury prevention programmes for youth cricketers. Studies have suggested that for adolescent fast bowlers, S&C coaches should focus on improving the eccentric strength of the external shoulder rotators and hamstrings, increasing hip adductor strength, improving neuromuscular control of the lumbopelvic region, increasing trunk extensor endurance, managing bowling load and ensuring appropriate bowling technique [45, 46]. However, the prescription of programmes for adolescent athletes can be highly complex, with many individual factors to consider. For more information on training adolescent athletes, see the '*National Strength and Conditioning Association Position Statement on Long-Term Athletic Development*' and the ten pillars of long-term athletic development [47].

10.8 Contemporary Practices of Strength and Conditioning Coaches

A common phrase in high-performance sports is 'Evidence-Based Practice' [48–50]. This is when research in a particular area (e.g. injury reduction in cricket) is used to underpin, justify, or critique practices employed in a given discipline (e.g. S&C). Counterarguments to fully adopting this approach are that practitioners may use anecdotal practices (i.e. those that may work but lack evidence) [51] or that some evidence-based practices may lack ecological validity (i.e. the ability to generalise findings to real-life situations) [50]. To ascertain whether this is the case, various survey-based studies have been conducted across multiple sports, countries and levels to investigate the practices of S&C coaches [1, 2, 51–54]. More relevantly, several studies have specifically been conducted in cricket at professional, franchise and high-school levels [2, 3, 55]. Although these studies more generally investigated S&C practices, they provide some insight into certain practices used to reduce the risk of injuries, which are further described below.

10.9 Physical Testing

All S&C coaches across two survey-based studies implemented physical testing into their annual S&C programmes [2, 3]. Pre-season was the most common time for physical testing, although results indicated most S&C coaches conducted these all year round [2, 3]. Common assessments included muscular strength, endurance, power, speed and cardiovascular endurance [2, 3], which all underpin the various physical requirements for developing bowlers, batters and wicketkeepers. Furthermore, it helps inform S&C programme content and key areas for physical development. The most reported tests conducted were body composition and anthropometry [2, 3]. Measurements deriving from body composition assessments such as body fat percentage and muscle mass are often dictated by governing body guidelines or in-house data and targets of the cricket team. Such data may be important to establish whether S&C programmes achieve individual and team-based targets (e.g. decrease body fat and increase muscle mass). However, limited evidence suggests that body composition is related to performance or injury rates in cricketers. Still, it may provide normative data that an individual can target following an injury (e.g. the muscle mass of an injured limb).

10.10 Periodisation

According to survey-based research of S&C coaches in professional cricket, periodisation strategies are widely used [3]. For example, S&C coaches tend to conduct more training sessions, including more sets and reps for resistance training during the pre-season, which are then reduced during the in-season due to increased cricket training and competition [3]. During the in-season, S&C coaches tend to programme speed, strength and power sessions on the same day as cricket practice; however, they aim to provide ~36–48 h recovery before competitive matches [3]. This is likely because training is less intense and modifiable than competitive matches [3]. These approaches aim to provide an adequate training load and intensity whilst allowing appropriate recovery to optimise performance without increasing the risk of injury.

10.11 Types of Training

Survey-based research has revealed that in professional cricket, most S&C coaches include strength, speed, plyometrics and flexibility training within their programmes [2, 3]. The protective qualities of these training methods have been extensively highlighted in general and cricket-specific literature [14, 16, 56–59]. Interestingly, injury reduction was the second most common reason for using plyometrics beyond speed development in professional cricket [3]. Literature suggests when plyometric exercises are used in conjunction with other training modalities (e.g. strength and agility training), the occurrence of injuries (e.g. anterior cruciate ligament tear) is significantly reduced in different populations (sports, age and sex) [60]. The reasons for this may include increased muscle activation and proprioception, which supports a decrease in knee flexion, knee valgus and forces when landing [60]. In cricket, this may relate to fast bowlers improving their force attenuation qualities, thus reducing the risk of injury.

10.12 Workload Monitoring

Workload monitoring is also a key part of the role of the S&C coach and has been described elsewhere (Chap. 12).

10.13 Cricket-Specific Injury Reduction

Strength and conditioning coaches working in franchise-level cricket were explicitly asked in a survey study what they do for injury monitoring and prevention [2]. Participants disclosed that they recorded all injuries sustained, and the most common injuries were for fast bowlers to the hamstrings and lower back [2]. To mitigate these injuries, S&C coaches incorporated injury reduction programmes during the pre-season and in-season periods [2]. Furthermore, they prescribed prehabilitation exercises that focussed on strengthening the posterior chain and core whilst mobilising the hips [2].

10.14 Integration and Collaboration with the Wider Athlete Support Team

Strength and conditioning forms an integral part of an athlete's multidisciplinary support team. Accordingly, S&C coaches require broad knowledge and experience within their discipline and those worked with (e.g. data analysts, physiotherapists and sports coaches). Interestingly, research into the practices of S&C coaches in professional cricket showed that 40% held professional cricket coaching qualifications [3]. The perception of these S&C coaches was that the development of cricket-specific and broader knowledge of other disciplines in the wider athlete support team would become increasingly important in the future [3]. This may allow S&C coaches to become further integrated and involved in the implementation and decision-making processes of other disciplines, such as merging S&C and sports coaching in the form of integrated conditioning sessions or entering the rehabilitation/return to play process at an earlier stage. For example, an S&C coach and fielding coach co-designing fielding drills that expose athletes to repeated accelerations, sprints and decelerations whilst performing catches, ball retrievals and throws, with live GPS being used to ascertain when an athlete has met a designated workload.

10.15 Challenges to Implementing Effective Training Programmes

In an ideal world, the design and implementation of S&C programmes would be straightforward. However, as is commonplace in sports, particularly elite sports, many challenges make this difficult. A survey study of S&C coaches working in professional cricket found that the most common issues are associated with planning and periodising S&C programmes [3]. These issues were often associated with a condensed playing schedule, making it difficult to implement appropriate S&C and recovery strategies [3]. Other challenges included athlete adherence/buy-in to S&C and relationships with the wider athlete support team (i.e. opinion differences), which is likely more prominent for cricket players at club, franchise and international levels, whom S&C coaches may have intermittent contact with. These challenges can be reduced or overcome with the various mobile applications now available for communication, movement analysis, physical testing, programme design and programme monitoring.

References

1. Weldon A, Duncan MJ, Turner A, LaPlaca D, Sampaio J, Christie CJ. Practices of strength and conditioning coaches: a snapshot from different sports, countries, and expertise levels. J Strength Cond Res. 2020;36:1335.
2. Pote L, King G, Christie C. Strength and conditioning practices of franchise-level cricket trainers. South Afr J Sports Med. 2020;32(1):1–5.
3. Weldon A, Duncan MJ, Turner A, Christie CJ, Pang CM. Contemporary practices of strength and conditioning coaches in professional cricket. Int J Sports Sci Coach. 2020;16(3):585–600.
4. Bishop C, Weldon A, Hughes J, Brazier J, Loturco I, Turner A, et al. Seasonal variation of physical performance and inter-limb asymmetry in professional cricket athletes. J Strength Cond Res. 2021;35(4):941–8.
5. Christie CJ, McEwan K, Munro CE, King GA, Le Roux A, Olivier B, et al. Do South African international cricket pace bowlers have similar bowling volume and injury risk associates compared to other elite fast bowlers? Int J Sports Sci Coach. 2024;19(2):797–804.
6. Lim J, Wong S, McErlain-Naylor SA, Scanlan A, Goggins L, Ahmun R, et al. Strength and conditioning for cricket fielding: a narrative review. Strength Cond J. 2023;45(5):509.
7. Brazier TA, Tallent J, Patterson SD, Howe LP, Callaghan SJ. The physical profile of female cricketers: an investigation between playing standard and position. PLoS One. 2024;19(6):e0302647.
8. Jacobs J, Olivier B, Brandt C, Jafta G. Physical profiles of all-rounders, batters, and bowlers in sub-elite women's cricket. J Strength Cond Res. 2024;38(6):1095–102.

9. Noakes TD, Durandt JJ. Physiological requirements of cricket. J Sports Sci. 2000;18(12):919–29.
10. Weldon A, Clarke N, Pote L, Bishop C. Physical profiling of international cricket players: an investigation between bowlers and batters. Biol Sport. 2020;38(4):507–15.
11. Foden M, Astley S, Comfort P, McMahon JJ, Matthews MJ, Jones PA. Relationships between speed, change of direction and jump performance with cricket specific speed tests in male academy cricketers. J Trainol. 2015;4(2):37–42.
12. Stretch RA, Bartlett R, Davids K. A review of batting in men's cricket. J Sports Sci. 2000;18(12):931–49.
13. Dovbysh T, Reid D, Shackel D. Injury incidence within male elite New Zealand cricket from the early T20 era: 2009–2015. BMJ Open Sport Exerc Med. 2021;7(4):e001168.
14. Pote L, Christie CJ. Injury prevention strategies in cricket. Strength Cond J. 2018;40(5):34–43.
15. Stronach B, Cronin JB, Portus M. Part 1: biomechanics, injury surveillance, and predictors of injury for cricket fast bowlers. Strength Cond J. 2014;36(4):65–72.
16. Talpey S, Siesmaa E. Sports injury prevention: the role of the strength and conditioning coach. Strength Cond J. 2017;39(3):14–9.
17. Nicholls S, Keenan J, Cresswell AM, Pote L. An analysis of specific batting demands in the women's The Hundred competition. S Afr J Sports Med [Internet]. 2023 [cited 2024 Dec 10];35(1). Available from: https://journals.assaf.org.za/index.php/sajsm/article/view/15056.
18. Petersen C, Pyne DB, Portus MJ, Dawson B. Analysis of Twenty/20 cricket performance during the 2008 Indian Premier League. Int J Perform Anal Sport. 2008;8(3):63–9.
19. Petersen CJ, Pyne D, Dawson B, Portus M, Kellett A. Movement patterns in cricket vary by both position and game format. J Sports Sci. 2010;28(1):45–52.
20. Petersen CJ, Pyne DB, Dawson BT, Kellett AD, Portus MR. Comparison of training and game demands of national level cricketers. J Strength Cond Res. 2011;25(5):1306–11.
21. Petersen CJ, Pyne DB, Portus MR, Dawson BT. Comparison of player movement patterns between 1-day and test cricket. J Strength Cond Res. 2011;25(5):1368–73.
22. Bliss A, Ahmun R, Jowitt H, Scott P, Jones TW, Tallent J. Variability and physical demands of international seam bowlers in one-day and Twenty20 international matches across five years. J Sci Med Sport. 2021;24(5):505–10.
23. Garcia-Byrne F, Buckley JD, Bishop C, Schwerdt S, Porter J, Bailey D, et al. External and internal workload demands of women's twenty 20 cricket competition. J Sci Med Sport. 2020;23(1):89–93.
24. MacDonald Wells DC, Cronin JB, Macadam P. Key match activities of different fielding positions and categories in one-day international cricket. Int J Perform Anal Sport. 2018;18(4):609–21.
25. Orchard JW, James T, Portus MR. Injuries to elite male cricketers in Australia over a 10-year period. J Sci Med Sport. 2006;9(6):459–67.
26. Portus MR, Sinclair PJ, Burke ST, Moore DJ, Farhart PJ. Cricket fast bowling performance and technique and the influence of selected physical factors during an 8-over spell. J Sports Sci. 2000;18(12):999–1011.
27. Ranson C, Hurley R, Rugless L, Mansingh A, Cole J. International cricket injury surveillance: a report of five teams competing in the ICC Cricket World Cup 2011. Br J Sports Med. 2013;47(10):637–43.
28. Christie CJ, Elliot A, Pote L, Steenekamp T, Billaut F, Noakes TD. Effect of expertise on pacing strategies and sprint performance in batsmen. J Sci Med Sport. 2018;21(5):513–7.
29. Taliep MS, Prim SK, Gray J. Upper body muscle strength and batting performance in cricket batsmen. J Strength Cond Res. 2010;24(12):3484–7.
30. Sholto-Douglas R, Cook R, Wilkie M, Christie CJA. Movement demands of an elite cricket team during the Big Bash League in Australia. J Sports Sci Med. 2020;19(1):59–64.
31. Freeston J, Rooney K. Progressive velocity throwing training increases velocity without detriment to accuracy in sub-elite cricket players: a randomized controlled trial. Eur J Sport Sci. 2008;8(6):373–8.
32. MacDonald D, Cronin J, Mills J, McGuigan M, Stretch R. A review of cricket fielding requirements. S Afr J Sports Med. 2013;25:87.
33. MacDonald D, Cronin J, McGuigan M, Stretch R. A survey of the performance demands of cricket fielding and wicket-keeping. J Athl Enhanc [Internet]. 2014 [cited 2024 Dec 10];2013. Available from: https://www.scitechnol.com/a-survey-of-the-performance-demands-of-cricket-fielding-and-wicketkeeping-9Ffq.php?article_id=1667.
34. Wong S, Lim J, McErlain-Naylor SA, Scanlan A, Goggins L, Ahmun R, et al. Strength and conditioning for cricket wicketkeeping: a narrative review. Strength Cond J. 2024;47:8. https://doi.org/10.1519/SSC.0000000000000847.
35. Mukandi I, Turner A, Scott P, Johnstone JA. Strength and conditioning for cricket fast bowlers. Strength Cond J. 2014;36(6):96–106.
36. Mathankar A, Kirti S. Strength and conditioning for cricket spin bowlers. Strength Cond J [Internet]. 2021 [cited 2021 Nov 22]; Available from: https://journals.lww.com/nsca-scj/Abstract/9000/Strength_and_Conditioning_for_Cricket_Spin_Bowlers.99190.aspx.
37. Munro CE, Christie CJ. Research directions for the enhancement of women's cricket. Int J Sports Sci Coach. 2018;13(5):708–12.
38. Tahoor A, Koley S. Anthropometric variables and physical fitness characteristics in female cricket play-

ers of Maharashtra and Punjab: a comparative study. Int J Health Sci Res. 2019;9(3):1–6.
39. Rascon J, Trujillo E, Morales-Acuna F, Gurovich AN. Differences between males and females in determining exercise intensity. Int J Exerc Sci. 2020;13(4):1305–16.
40. McErlain-Naylor SA, Peploe C, Grimley J, Deshpande Y, Felton PJ, King MA. Comparing power hitting kinematics between skilled male and female cricket batters. J Sports Sci. 2021;39(21):2393–400.
41. Felton PJ, Lister SL, Worthington PJ, King MA. Comparison of biomechanical characteristics between male and female elite fast bowlers. J Sports Sci. 2019;37(6):665–70.
42. Perera NKP, Joseph C, Kemp JL, Finch CF. Epidemiology of injuries in women playing competitive team bat-or-stick sports: a systematic review and a meta-analysis. Sports Med. 2018;48(3):617–40.
43. Stretch R. Junior cricketers are not a smaller version of adult cricketers: a 5-year investigation of injuries in elite junior cricketers. S Afr J Sports Med. 2014;26(4):123–7.
44. Pote L, Christie CJ. Workloads placed on adolescent cricket players: a pilot study. [Internet]. [cited 2024 Dec 10]. Available from: https://journals.sagepub.com/doi/10.1177/1747954118810505.
45. Forrest MRL, Hebert JJ, Scott BR, Dempsey AR. Exercise-based injury prevention for community-level adolescent cricket pace bowlers: a cluster-randomised controlled trial. J Sci Med Sport. 2020;23(5):475–80.
46. Forrest MRL, Scott BR, Hebert JJ, Dempsey AR. Injury prevention strategies for adolescent cricket pace bowlers. Sports Med. 2018;48(11):2449–61.
47. Lloyd RS, Cronin JB, Faigenbaum AD, Haff GG, Howard R, Kraemer WJ, et al. National Strength and Conditioning Association position statement on long-term athletic development. J Strength Cond Res. 2016;30(6):1491–509.
48. Shurley JP, Todd JS, Todd TC. The science of strength: reflections on the National Strength and Conditioning Association and the emergence of research-based strength and conditioning. J Strength Cond Res. 2017;31(2):517.
49. Turner A. What is evidence-based practice in strength and conditioning? Strength Cond J. 2024:10-1519.
50. Waller G. Bridging the gap: the importance of evidence-based practice and collaboration within sports performance. Int J Strength Cond [Internet]. 2020 [cited 2024 Jun 20];1(1). Available from: https://journal.iusca.org/index.php/Journal/article/view/15.
51. Weldon A, Duncan MJ, Turner A, Lockie RG, Loturco I. Practices of strength and conditioning coaches in professional sports: a systematic review. Biol Sport. 2021;39(3):715–26.
52. Duehring MD, Feldmann CR, Ebben WP. Strength and conditioning practices of United States high school strength and conditioning coaches. J Strength Cond Res. 2009;23(8):2188–203.
53. Loturco I, Freitas TT, Alcaraz PE, Kobal R, Nunes RFH, Weldon A, et al. Practices of strength and conditioning coaches in Brazilian elite soccer. Biol Sport. 2021;39(3):779–91.
54. Weldon A, Cloak R, Kirk C, Ruddock A, Langan-Evans C, Detanico D, et al. Strength and conditioning (S&C) practices of judo athletes and S&C coaches: a survey-based investigation. J Strength Cond Res. 2024;38(4):e160–73.
55. Pote L, Christie CJ. Strength and conditioning practices of university and high school level cricket coaches: a South African context. J Strength Cond Res. 2016;30(12):3464–70.
56. Al Attar WSA, Soomro N, Sinclair PJ, Pappas E, Sanders RH. Effect of injury prevention programs that include the nordic hamstring exercise on hamstring injury rates in soccer players: a systematic review and meta-analysis. Sports Med Auckl NZ. 2017;47(5):907–16.
57. Barengo NC, Meneses-Echávez JF, Ramírez-Vélez R, Cohen DD, Tovar G, Correa Bautista JE. The impact of the FIFA 11+ training program on injury prevention in football players: a systematic review. Int J Environ Res Public Health. 2014;11(11):11986–2000.
58. Beato M, Maroto-Izquierdo S, Turner AN, Bishop C. Implementing strength training strategies for injury prevention in soccer: scientific rationale and methodological recommendations. Int J Sports Physiol Perform. 2021;16(3):456–61.
59. Kirkendall D, Dvorak J. Effective injury prevention in soccer. Phys Sportsmed. 2010;38:147–57.
60. Al Attar WSA, Bakhsh JM, Khaledi EH, Ghulam H, Sanders RH. Injury prevention programs that include plyometric exercises reduce the incidence of anterior cruciate ligament injury: a systematic review of cluster randomised trials. J Physiother. 2022;68(4):255–61.

11 A Comprehensive Guide to Fieldside Physiotherapy in Cricket

Cliffe Deacon, Benita Olivier, and Candice MacMillan

11.1 Introduction

Fieldside physiotherapy in cricket not only refers to the immediate, on-the-spot medical and therapeutic interventions provided to players during matches or practice sessions but also involves a series of preparatory activities that start long before the actual game and end a day after the game finishes. Cricket, a sport characterised by its diverse formats, Test, One Day International (ODI), and Twenty20 (T20), presents unique challenges for medical professionals. Each format represents a distinct physiological and psychological landscape, requiring tailored approaches to player preparation, injury prevention, and recovery.

This chapter comprehensively explores fieldside physiotherapy and a holistic view of the physiotherapist's responsibilities in a high-performance environment. It does not cover physiotherapy in a community, i.e. club or school, setting as this context has its own nuances to consider. However, much of the content of this chapter can be adapted to the community setting. From pre-game preparations and on-field interventions to post-match recovery strategies, the insights presented here illuminate the intricate decision-making processes behind the scenes of high-performance cricket.

It is acknowledged that numerous different perspectives exist, and many other physiotherapists may hold similar or opposing views, which is entirely acceptable. All approaches share the same fundamental principles; taking a preventative stance while preparing athletes for the highest level of workload, within safe parameters and for an appropriate duration, one can effectively manage the demands of a game, tour, or season [1].

Supplementary Information The online version contains supplementary material available at https://doi.org/10.1007/978-981-96-6321-7_11.

C. Deacon
Pakistan National Team, Pakistan Cricket Board, Lahore, Pakistan
e-mail: Cliffedeacon@cdphysio.co.za

B. Olivier (✉)
Centre for Healthy Living Research, Oxford Institute of Applied Health Research, Faculty of Health, Science and Technology, Oxford Brookes University, Oxford, UK

Wits Cricket Research Hub for Science, Medicine and Rehabilitation, Department of Physiotherapy, School of Therapeutic Sciences, Faculty of Health Sciences, University of the Witwatersrand, Johannesburg, South Africa
e-mail: Benita.Olivier@brookes.ac.uk

C. MacMillan
Faculty of Health Sciences, Department of Physiology, University of Pretoria, Pretoria, Gauteng, South Africa
e-mail: candice.macmillan@up.ac.za

B. Olivier, J. W. Orchard (eds.), *Cricket Sports Medicine*,
https://doi.org/10.1007/978-981-96-6321-7_11

Many contextual factors influence fieldside physiotherapy. Factors such as game format, player workload, cultural considerations, weather conditions, cricket rules related to on- and off-field medical care during a match, and logistical constraints are discussed. Through all this, the physiotherapist's role is a critical link between medical science, athletic performance, and team strategy.

11.2 Impact of Different Formats of the Game on Fieldside Physiotherapy

The format of the game impacts the timing and order of therapeutic interventions and player approaches, as well as critical decisions associated with these.

11.2.1 Twenty20 (T20)

T20 cricket is the shortest format of the game, played at high intensity and low volume. The time not utilised during the actual game is compensated for in the periods preceding and following the match, i.e. use the time at the hotel before/after the game. For a squad player to approach the physiotherapist on game day to discuss workload management, for example, would be incredibly difficult, as the time available to staff is extremely constrained.

The high intensity and brief duration of T20 cricket limit activities beyond those happening during the game itself, particularly regarding injuries. The primary challenge for the medical staff during a T20 game is that once a player is removed from the field for an off-field assessment, the rapid progression of the game may preclude the player's return and potentially have a significant impact on the match. It is crucial to ensure that the decision to remove a player from the game is based on sound medical reasoning. Unless dealing with an acute injury, generally a physiotherapist will be 'watching every ball from the dugout' because of the quick pace of the game.

11.2.2 Test Cricket

Test cricket is the longest format, played at lower intensity but high volume, and represents the opposite end of the spectrum. There is minimal time available outside of game time; however, the game itself provides sufficient time to accomplish necessary tasks, as one would not want players to lose out on sleep or recovery, or other important activities that can only be done outside game time. During the batting innings, one has considerable time to manage the other nine players' individual requirements (and even squad players) while simultaneously monitoring the two players currently engaged in the game.

11.2.3 One Day International (ODI)

One Day International (ODI) is the most taxing format, played at high intensity and high volume. This format presents the most significant challenge for any cricket player. It requires the same duration as a day in a Test match but maintains the intensity of the T20 format. The sole advantage is that it does not involve five consecutive days of play, and there is slightly more time available for players to return to the game if they must be removed from the field of play. Consequently, there is some time between games; however, unless a player is well-conditioned, they are at considerable risk when participating in a 5-game series, which is typically played over approximately 12 days. A crucial factor often overlooked in this scenario is that travel days do not constitute rest days, they physically impact the player.

11.2.4 Timings of the Start of Games

The time of day a game starts, i.e. whether it is a day, day-night or night game, primarily influences the quantity and type of supplementation (e.g. of fluids) planned; more intense and prolonged games necessitate increased supplementation. Additionally, to a lesser extent, it allows for the periodisation of sessions, as in some instances, there is an opportunity to conduct work on the morning of a game. From a logistical perspective, the time of day the game is played influences the scheduling and planning of each player's treatments, activations, taping, recovery, and conditioning.

11.2.5 Frequency of Games

An increased frequency of games necessitates greater efficiency in time management during gameplay.

11.2.6 Game Day Considerations

Knowing whether a game takes place the next day, the specific format of the game, and the anticipated requirements for the player in question significantly influence the treatment approach on the current game day. Additionally, this information affects the decision-making process regarding whether to allow the player to continue participation during a game or to remove the player from the current field of play.

Workload management typically determines the extent to which a player can or should engage in specific aspects of their training. It influences how the daily schedule is structured for each player in the squad participating in a particular match day. As the frequency of games increases, the significance of executing appropriate actions such as preventative treatment, taping, recovery, treatment periodisation, rehabilitation and adapting the intensity of rehabilitation/prehabilitation sessions at optimal times during each game day becomes paramount.

11.3 Other Factors Impacting Fieldside Physiotherapy

Numerous aspects, including gender, religion, country, security, host nation regulations, accommodation, transport, and weather, all influence the preparation and approach to game day.

11.3.1 Gender

Physiological requirements related to gender necessitate specific considerations. A notable issue is Relative Energy Deficiency in Sport (RED-S), with a large overlap of symptoms associated with the Female Athlete Triad [2], but also prevalent in males [3]. The similarities between the symptoms of RED-S and Overtraining Syndrome [2] and their different presentations in both male and female athletes warrant attention.

While acute low energy availability (LEA) can increase injury risk, its implications extend deeper into hormonal disruptions. RED-S seems to correlate with spontaneous ligament injuries, notably in high-force activities. Though cricket's biomechanical demands differ from Olympic lifting, the forceful movements in bowling create similar stresses on joints and ligaments. The compound effects of inadequate nutrition, especially during intensive tournaments, combined with sustained elevated cortisol levels, can create a complex interplay of physical and psychological vulnerabilities. This hormonal imbalance, while not immediately visible fieldside, requires physiotherapists to adopt a holistic approach that considers both the acute presentation and the underlying endocrine disruptions that may predispose athletes to injury.

11.3.2 Religion

Various religious traditions permit specific modalities and timelines, which others do not. Understanding how diverse cultures and religions approach the scheduling and periodisation of certain treatments, rehabilitation protocols, or recovery processes is essential.

In countries where the majority celebrate Ramadan, one tends to see games scheduled around religious timings. Games in countries with a predominantly non-Muslim population present greater nutritional challenges during Ramadan, as match schedules don't align with fasting times, requiring athletes to carefully optimise their pre-fast meals for sustained energy without compromising performance or comfort.

11.3.3 Country

Differences in weather and altitude associated with certain countries impose significantly greater physical demands on players. Australia serves as an example where both time zone differences and the large size of grounds impact players. Travelling to different countries impacts sleep and can result in travel fatigue and jet lag, depending on distance and time zones. The consensus statement on managing travel fatigue and jet lag in athletes by Janse van Rensburg et al. [4] contains valuable information in this regard. These factors influence the preparation of players, which subsequently has an indirect impact on their on-field treatment.

11.3.4 Security

Movement to and from cricket grounds and general movement outside hotels is restricted in some countries for security reasons. When security becomes an issue, it automatically requires a much more confined, controlled environment in which players must operate. The restrictions ultimately influence where, when and how players can train during or outside team training periods.

11.3.5 Host Nation Regulations

In certain nations, individuals are permitted to move to and from the venue in separate groups, whereas in others, a predetermined schedule is established for all activities. This organisational structure will determine the scheduling of activation sessions, taping procedures, treatments, recovery protocols, and other related activities before and after competitive events.

11.3.6 Accommodation and Transport

Accommodation near the game venue allows players more flexibility in their sleep schedule and personal time due to shorter travel times. As the distance increases, there is a greater inclination to conduct preparation and recovery activities at the game venue rather than having it delayed for 2 or 3 hours due to travelling. It is highly ineffective to postpone recovery activities until after an hour-long bus journey. Such a practice would be an inefficient use of the player's time, which could have been more productively allocated to rest.

11.3.7 Heat and Humidity

Certain countries adopt a rule where drink breaks are added in case the weather reaches a predetermined number on a given heat index under bilateral tour arrangements. On the other hand, some countries that incidentally have a lot worse or adverse weather conditions don't adopt these regulations. It then becomes the medical team's responsibility to make sure that players are prepared before a tour or game for what they are most likely to encounter. Heat and humidity play a major role in the amount of fluid a player loses for a set period and subsequently impact performance [5]. Adequate fluid replenishment is essential while avoiding overhydration, which has a delayed negative influence on fluid retention and sleep [6]. Strategies to deal with extreme heat include hydration monitoring, ice towels/vests/baths, and having bowlers come off the ground after a spell to have a quick cold shower and change into dry clothing.

11.3.8 Personal Well-Being

The physiotherapist is usually the first one up and the last one to go to bed. Strategies, such as taking personal time out and prioritising what is urgent, where possible, can help mitigate the risk of burnout. In addition, proper planning goes a long way to keep unforeseen circumstances at bay.

11.3.9 Treatment of Staff and Fans

Although this chapter mainly focuses on the approach to players, the physiotherapist is also sometimes responsible for the health of other medical and support staff members, such as the coaching staff. If travelling with a team doctor, the medical (illness) issues of the touring party are usually under the domain of the doctor; if not, the services of local general practitioners are often engaged. Also, on training or game days, the physiotherapist might be asked to occasionally treat injuries (other than cricket-related injuries), e.g. due to fans being 'over-excited' or protests or some other unexpected scenario in certain countries. In extremely rare situations, physiotherapy and medical staff might be the first responders for a cardiac arrest if it happens right next to the team room or dugout. For stadiums expecting large crowds or International Cricket Council (ICC) events like World Cups, there is usually a contract with the stadium for medical and paramedic services, meaning that the team staff are not required to manage injuries or illnesses in patrons.

11.4 A Physiotherapist's Approach Before, During and After the Game

This guide presents the approaches taken by Cliffe Deacon, the physiotherapist of Pakistan's National Cricket Team. The information provided in the rest of the chapter offers readers a comprehensive overview of the activities, tasks, and considerations pertinent to pre-game, in-game, and post-game scenarios.

11.5 Two Days Before the Game

11.5.1 Last Official Coaching Day

Two days before the match, commonly referred to as '2 days out', are typically designated as the last official training or coaching day. On this day, support staff, but primarily the technical staff, evaluate what they deem essential for the players to ensure adequate preparation.

11.5.2 Final Intensive Treatment Day

The final intensive treatment day occurs two days before the match. The playing 12 are typically announced 48 hours in advance of the game. This enables the alignment of treatment plans with the game plan.

The primary objective is to ensure that all players are prepared for the match. If any player is not ready, it is the responsibility of the staff to promptly inform the coaches, providing reasons, potential return-to-play timelines, and possible interventions for the following day to facilitate the player's return to play as expeditiously and responsibly as possible.

Players with the highest workloads, most frequently fast bowlers, receive their massages two days before the match, followed by a light bowling session the day after. In addition to the physiological benefits of massage [7], massage enhances the perception of recovery [8].

11.5.3 Adequate Rest

Adequate rest two nights before the match is crucial, particularly as many players are susceptible to pre-match anxiety the night before. An attempt is made to communicate with the players about the recommended bedtime based on periodisation principles.

11.6 The Day Before the Game

11.6.1 Optional Training Day

The day preceding the game, or '1 day out', is frequently utilised as an optional training day (with batters more likely than bowlers to take the training option). Ideally, on the day before the game, players should be allowed to focus on the upcoming match in their own way.

Occasionally, certain players request massage therapy on this day, particularly when they opt out of training. In some cases, the massage therapist typically remains at the hotel to attend to the players who are not participating in training.

11.6.2 Final Clearance and Assessment Sessions

Final clearance and assessment sessions are generally done for several reasons, primarily long-term maintenance. Another reason is a return-to-play scenario where a player requires specific interventions.

11.6.3 Soft Tissue Release

This day also presents an opportunity to implement indirect soft tissue release techniques that do not result in 'treatment pain' and align with the player's preparation needs for the following day.

11.6.4 On-Field and Next-to-Field Bags

Reviewing the bags' contents that will accompany the physiotherapist to the game is crucial. Treatment bags are duplicated, resulting in two identical bags containing consumables, electrotherapy equipment, taping materials, creams/oils, basic medication, splints, wound dressings, and other essentials. One of these bags is transported to the game venue, while the other remains at the hotel. Furthermore, the bag that gets transported to the venue consists of a next-to-field bag as well as an on-field bag (a smaller bag that gets taken onto the field when a player gets injured).

A comprehensive list of players requiring taping, including those with allergies to specific taping and specific types/purposes, is updated and used to prepare the necessary materials the evening before the game. This preparation facilitates efficient time management during the morning taping sessions, which may occur at the hotel or the venue, contingent upon logistical considerations and scheduling.

The physiotherapist may carry the medication but needs to consult with a physician dedicated to the team, whether during the game or in between games, as dispensing medication is outside of their scope of practice. A standardised inventory is regularly updated, and a similar approach is applied to medication management as it is used for treatment supplies.

Analysis of weather forecasts and periodisation allows for predicting supplement requirements on game day. A range of legal supplementation is employed to assist players in mitigating dehydration, cramping, and fatigue. All necessary items are prepared and packed on the eve of the game.

The contents of the on-field and next-to-field carry bags can be found as a downloadable checklist in the online supplementary material. It is important to, at any time, be aware of the World Anti-Doping Agency (WADA) regulations. Take, for example, tennis player Jannik Sinner, who tested positive for clostebol, an anabolic steroid, after this substance was transferred to him by his physiotherapist. His physiotherapist treated a cut on his own hand with Trofodermin, a dermatological cream containing clostebol as an active ingredient, and massaged Sinner without the use of gloves. The International Tennis Integrity Agency (ITIA) deemed this as a plausible explanation, and the ban was initially lifted, although at the time of writing this text, WADA was appealing the ban [9].

11.6.5 Reminders

In addition to reminding players about sleep hygiene, dietary guidance is provided. Particular emphasis is placed on maintaining a balanced proportion of all four macronutrients. Individual players' needs vary based on their workloads and body composition. In an ideal world, the specifics of nutritional requirements will be the role of the team's nutritionist or dietician.

The final task performed on the night preceding the game is the distribution of schedules for the following day. These schedules encompass taping sessions, specific activation exercises, and

Table 11.1 Match-day schedule

Date		
Match		
Team activities		
Time (00:00–00:00)	**Action**	**Specific notes/ comments**
	Breakfast	
	Pre-match meeting	
	Departure time	
	Arrival time	
Player prep (00:00–00:00)		
Time	**Player name**	**Specific notes comments**

other pertinent activities. Table 11.1 serves as an example.

11.7 The Morning of the Game

11.7.1 Breakfast

The importance of breakfast is widely recognised; however, many cricketers encounter difficulties with this meal. Several factors contribute to this issue, but the most prevalent appears to be sleep patterns, resulting in some players rising later in the morning.

11.7.2 Check-Ins

A status assessment is done during breakfast with the players present to inquire about their well-being. A 'check-in' is also performed during taping sessions before each training session or game.

11.8 Game Day: Pre-Game

11.8.1 Taping

The preferred location for taping varies depending on the venue, timing, and format of the sporting event. Several influential factors play a role, namely:

- Religious considerations: certain religious practices involve regular prayers that include ablutions, which cannot be performed with tape applied.
- Security protocols: some venues have stringent security measures beyond the team's control. If taping is to be conducted at the venue, it is necessary to ensure that transportation arrives with sufficient time to accommodate time for taping.
- Scheduling variations: particularly in Test cricket, the team entourage's early departure may allow taping to be performed in a more relaxed environment within the changing room, permitting athletes additional rest time.
- Gender considerations: privacy requirements may arise in an opposite-gender team environment, i.e. a male physiotherapist with a female team or vice versa, where taping can't be applied in the changing rooms between the other players.

11.8.2 Hydration Prep

One of the medical team members will be entrusted with the responsibility of managing hydration preparation. This process encompasses the preparation of water, electrolytes, and recovery beverages for transport to the game venue. The specific requirements vary based on the format of the game, the time of day, and the geographical region in which the event takes place.

11.8.3 Taping for Fingers and Hands

A supply of athletic tape is provided to players so they can perform their own general finger and hand taping. Most players are proficient in managing this task independently, except in specific injuries requiring specialised taping techniques.

11.8.4 Medical Meeting

The International Cricket Council (ICC) has implemented a mandatory medical meeting one hour before the commencement of any match or match day in tournaments [10], replicated in most bilateral series. Typically, this meeting is attended by the lead medical officer, stadium manager, lead paramedic, and match-day medical officer. The match-day medical officer also serves as the attending physician for teams with no medical doctor. These medical personnel are required to be present at the venue to attend to medical incidents from one hour before the match until one hour after the match concludes. While the doctor usually attends these meetings, the team physiotherapist will also find it beneficial, as a comprehensive understanding of the protocols is essential for navigating potential emergency situations and insulin dependence.

If it is not a professional match, it is unlikely that a medical meeting will take place. Here are some important considerations in terms of emergency care:

- Locate the nearest hospital beforehand. Get directions and an emergency response phone number.
- Be aware of whether the venue has a defibrillator and how it can be accessed in an emergency. If a cardiac arrest occurs, CPR needs to commence immediately and continue either until an ambulance crew arrives or it can be temporarily ceased to allow for defibrillator shock.
- Make sure the field is accessible to transport and ambulances and identify the easiest way on and off the field and out of the stadium.
- Collect the player's and staff's medical aid/insurance details or obtain a letter of guarantee from the club/union regarding coverage of the medical costs.

11.9 Game Day: Warm Up

11.9.1 General and Specific Activations

The Strength and Conditioning (S&C) typically conducts general activations. The physiotherapist assists individuals who may require specific activations, i.e. activating certain muscles or muscle groups by using specific movements to prepare these muscles for sport-specific movements. By this point, players have familiarised themselves with their own activation routines and can execute them efficiently. Many players use the gymnasium before departing for the grounds; however, time is still allocated for this activity at the venue, typically occurring before the general team warm-up.

11.9.2 Assisting S&C

During the general team warm-up, the physiotherapist takes on the role of assistant to the S&C and coaching staff until the game starts or if something goes wrong on the field.

11.10 Game Day: During Sessions

On game day, the physiotherapist will pay careful attention to players and rapidly respond. The most common concerns are discussed below.

11.10.1 When Batting

11.10.1.1 Concussion

Whether the team is batting or bowling, head impact and concussion are primary concerns that consistently warrant attention. The SCAT6 [11] represents the most current standard of concussion testing available, necessitating periodic baseline SCAT evaluations of players to establish a normative reference for comparative purposes.

11.10.1.2 Ball Strikes

Secondarily, ball strikes to areas other than the head include contusions and potential fractures, among other injuries.

11.10.1.3 Cramping/Hydration

Monitoring players who engage in prolonged batting or participate in sustained high-intensity situations is imperative.

11.10.2 When Bowling/Fielding

11.10.2.1 Hands/Finger Injuries

Although the chance of concussion still exists when bowling, the probability of it is significantly reduced. The most obvious injury to look out for here would be hand and finger injuries due to collecting, catching, stopping, bowling and throwing the ball.

11.10.2.2 Technique: Bowling and Diving/Sliding

Because bowling, throwing, and catching are repetitive actions, technical flaws or incorrect biomechanics may contribute to injury risk. Not all bowling, throwing and catching techniques work for all individuals, but there are some fundamentals to adhere to in order to minimise the probability of overuse injuries. Monitoring techniques while players perform under pressure may explain the mechanisms behind an overuse injury that may present itself later.

Careful observation of actions used in the throwing, catching, diving and/or stopping of the ball, especially when the player is under pressure, such as during a match, is imperative to identify 'risky' techniques before an injury is sustained.

11.10.2.3 Spatial Awareness

Spatial awareness is a proprioceptive aspect of the game and needs to be observed and noted down. Technically, it could be trained by teaching the correct diving techniques and interactive fielding sessions, where players need to be able to throw balls to the space where they believe another player should be by the time the ball reaches that specific area. Reduced spatial awareness would inherently increase the likelihood of players colliding with others, falling awkwardly, or placing themselves in compromised positions. This scenario presents a context where concussion becomes a highly probable outcome, as players collide, fall awkwardly, and potentially impact their heads. Proprioception training can be implemented if reduced spatial awareness is observed during a game.

11.10.3 On-Field Treatment Considerations

Medical personnel must be called on by the umpire in case of an injury, except in the case of a non-contact/medical collapse or a player or players collapsing due to head strikes (in which circumstances medical staff enter immediately without waiting to be called). This gets communicated during the pre-match meeting, and the match referee and the first aid responders get informed, especially when there is no team doctor and only a match-day medical officer at the game.

Players can leave the field to receive treatment, but there are some caveats to keep in mind [12]:

- If a batter sustains an external/impact injury, such as when a ball strike causes a laceration that requires stitching, they can leave and return at any position when a wicket falls.
- If a bowler/fielder sustains an external/impact injury, i.e. ball strike, they can leave and can immediately start bowling upon their return.
- If a batter is unable to continue batting due to an injury ('retired hurt'), no 'reserve' batter can replace them (with the exception of concussion). Therefore, the batter is deemed out and cannot return to bat later.
- Runners are no longer allowed in International cricket. Previously, a runner could run between the wickets on behalf of a batter if the batter sustained an injury and could not run as a consequence.

Be familiar with these rules as they appear in the ICC Playing Handbook [12] to ensure quick and confident decision-making, actions and reactions.

The physiotherapist or other medical staff member can only come onto the field to treat a specific injury sustained by a player twice during an innings. However, in the case of concussion monitoring, one can enter the field of play more than twice to monitor a player's symptoms. For every specific injury, one has 4 min initially; the second time one is allowed on the field for the same injury, only 2 min are granted. Thereafter, the physiotherapist or any other medical staff member is not allowed back onto the field of play for that specific injury. Related to this rule, cramping is a controversial point of discussion, as cramps are seen as the 'same injury', irrespective of which part of the body cramps. It's even gone as far as some match referees would deem supplementation sent to the players specifically for cramps (via the 12th player/reserves) as part of 'treatment received'.

If the 12th player comes onto the field, they are only allowed to field and not bowl or keep. If a keeper gets injured due to external injuries, a keeper may replace them as a keeper. However, once a player is deemed concussed, a like-for-like replacement can immediately replace the player in full. Both then get accredited for the runs they score, the wickets they take, etc., as part of their career stats.

Taping on the hands is allowed, but not while a player is bowling. Using cohesive taping instead of adhesive taping will allow the player to remove and reapply the taping during the game. For the fingers, the silicone sleeves/covers work well for this same reason.

The return-to-play decision is one of the most important decisions one needs to make under high-pressure conditions. The player may be experiencing a lot of pain, put the player at ease and respect pain. Ask the player: 'Where do you feel pain? Rate it out of 10'. Don't get frustrated if they don't answer immediately, it may take time if it is very painful. You don't have to make a decision/diagnosis in the first 3 seconds of arrival.

When making a decision as to whether the player can return to play or not, consider the following:

General considerations:

- What happened?
- How has the player responded to questions?
- Integrity tests and joint stability?

Red flags to consider in the decision-making process:

- Head injury—unconscious or diminished responsiveness.
- Uncontrolled bleeding.
- Fractures/serious dislocations.
- Inability to fully weight bear on limb.

In case you are dealing with a recurrent injury:

- Has the player just returned from injury?
- Treated or complained about the same injury during the week?
- Strapped joint/muscle before the game?

Also, consider the future risks in your decision:

- Risks vs benefits?
- If the player continues now, will the injury get worse?
- Which part of the season is it? (Beginning vs end).
- If the injury gets worse, how long will the recovery be?

Another consideration is the impact the player's injury will have on the team:

- When the player returns to the field, individual and team confidence in the player is key.
- When a player's injury affects his 'normal' ability, teammates might overcompensate, increasing their risk of injury.
- Is it worth giving the coach/team half a player?

11.10.4 Note-Taking

Medical and physiotherapy-related treatments take precedence; however, there is significant value in documenting observations about the game as it unfolds. Keeping notes helps one to identify factors that may influence technical, biomechanical, medical, or psychological outcomes.

Nevertheless, it is important to note that the security clearance process is completed before the commencement of the game. Often, only one person in the medical team (the most senior) is allowed access to a mobile device in case of a medical emergency. To be able to use a laptop for note-taking, one has to request permission from the anti-corruption officer, and it sometimes needs to be switched to flight mode with Wi-Fi and Bluetooth turned off.

11.10.5 Monitoring

Global Positioning System (GPS) devices provide functionality beyond mere distance measurement and are important in monitoring players. Additionally, records of the number of overs bowled by each player must be maintained while the Strength and Conditioning (S&C) trainers independently calculate and record workloads for each player, providing a basis for comparison with the GPS data.

11.10.6 Treatment if the Doctor Is Available

When a physician is available, conducting all maintenance procedures at the facility is preferable, allowing players to have unencumbered evenings.

11.11 Game Day: In Between Sessions

11.11.1 Periodisation

It is important to use this time to responsibly and progressively increase player workloads if they are not up to the required benchmarks for what they would face if they were to be selected for the next game. Periodisation is a combination of workloads and fixtures. It depends on the format of the game, the extent of participation thus far, the remaining duration, the timeframe within which one competes, and the subsequent events. In certain instances, it is necessary to augment the workload to mitigate abrupt increases, significantly elevating the probability of injury.

T20 cricket provides limited opportunities between sessions for substantial player development. Furthermore, due to the rapid pace of a T20 match, there is increased reluctance to engage reserve players during the game. However, if the team fields first, it is feasible to conduct some work during the break, albeit primarily technical in nature. Given that matches typically commence at approximately 18:00 or 19:00, the entire day is available for additional training, negating the need for on-site activities. Conversely, Test cricket essentially affords four intervals for developmental work: pre-game, post-game, lunch break, and tea break. The problematic format is ODIs, where the duration and intensity of the match are significantly high, resulting in minimal time for pre-game or in-game activities.

An additional factor that requires consideration is the squad status. This encompasses identifying resource requirements, their quantities, and associated timelines. The allocation of workloads and their specific details will inform the scheduling of these activities.

11.12 Game Day: Post-Game at the Ground

11.12.1 Immediate Recovery

Several factors warrant consideration in this context:

- What observations were made during the game?
- How do these correlate with each player's profile and pre-game status?
- Are there any emerging patterns that raise concerns?
- What is the periodisation?

The initial step typically involves consulting with the team doctor to swiftly assess individuals who have experienced injuries, while others proceed with cryotherapy, contrast therapy, and/or stretching. It is important to note that considerable conflicting scientific evidence exists regarding these practices. It would be inadvisable to inform a player immediately following a game that their chosen recovery method is scientifically ineffective. Instead, a more prudent approach involves finding a way to incorporate necessary interventions into methods that the player finds personally beneficial.

11.12.2 Severe Concerns

In the event that significant concerns or critical issues arise during the game, the doctor and physiotherapist allocate time to discuss and assess any specific observations or concerns communicated to them by the players.

11.12.3 Refuel First

It is important to refuel as soon as possible after a game. Various cultural norms dictate late dining and sleeping patterns, while individual preferences range from early to late meal and sleep schedules. Some individuals prefer frequent, smaller meals, while others adhere to intermittent fasting regimens.

11.12.4 Evening Scheduling

In the event of an urgent medical concern requiring immediate attention, the organisation of diagnostic scans necessitates a degree of administrative and logistical management. Subsequent scheduling is determined based on the severity of the condition and the anticipated activities for the following days.

11.13 Game Day: Post-Game at the Hotel

11.13.1 Less Severe Concerns

After a game, players will be categorised into groups: those requiring immediate medical intervention and those who will be consulting the following day for a range of potential actions, including a discussion, evaluation, maintenance, treatment, or a recovery session in the gymnasium or aquatic facility. Post-game treatments are determined based on the schedule established immediately following the conclusion of the game.

11.13.2 Post-Game Recovery

Players typically have their own personal preferences regarding post-game recovery [13]. Contingent upon the time of day and format, a pool session may be conducted upon return to the hotel. Some athletes prefer a light gymnasium session, and recommendations are typically provided based on their workload and physical condition.

11.13.3 Diet Reminders

Reminding the players to adhere to a healthy and balanced diet is important. The focus should be on ensuring the appropriate preparation of dishes rather than compelling players to consume unfamiliar food. This consideration is typically addressed, deliberated, and finalised during the signing of the tour Memorandum of Understanding (MOU).

11.13.4 Sleep Reminders

Achieving sleep after a competitive event presents significant challenges even under optimal conditions. This phenomenon varies due to factors such as adrenaline, emotional and mental states, and individual personality traits. Certain fundamental elements remain consistent when it comes to sleep hygiene. These are exposure to blue light, dietary habits, fluid consumption patterns, and a concept referred to as mental management. One factor that has become increasingly significant is the impact of social media on players. The effects are severe, necessitating psychological support as an essential requirement.

11.13.5 If Tomorrow Is another Game Day: 1 Day Out Again...

This represents an additional factor influencing post-game treatments. In certain instances, international teams participate in two matches within a 48-hour period, with a third match scheduled two days later, ensuring all fixtures adhere to a specific timeline.

11.13.6 Reporting Player Status to Coaches

This task requires immediate attention, albeit not before the completion of all treatments. Coaches require definitive information regarding players to facilitate planning and discussion of any borderline cases as necessary. A concise summary is to be disseminated immediately following the final treatment. The traffic light system is employed, wherein green indicates readiness, yellow denotes players under maintenance that do not impede their availability, orange signifies borderline players necessitating discussion, and red indicates complete unavailability.

References

1. Gabbett TJ. The training – injury prevention paradox: should athletes be training smarter *and* harder? Br J Sports Med. 2016;50(5):273–80. https://doi.org/10.1136/bjsports-2015-095788.
2. Stellingwerff T, Heikura IA, Meeusen R, Bermon S, Seiler S, Mountjoy ML, et al. Overtraining syndrome (OTS) and relative energy deficiency in sport (RED-S): shared pathways, symptoms and complexities. Sports Med. 2021;51(11):2251–80. https://doi.org/10.1007/s40279-021-01491-0.
3. Statuta SM, Asif IM, Drezner JA. Relative energy deficiency in sport (RED-S). Br J Sports Med. 2017;51(21):1570–1. https://doi.org/10.1136/bjsports-2017-097700.
4. Janse van Rensburg DC, Jansen van Rensburg A, Fowler PM, Bender AM, Stevens D, Sullivan KO, et al. Managing travel fatigue and jet lag in athletes: a review and consensus statement. Sports Med. 2021;51(10):2029–50. https://doi.org/10.1007/s40279-021-01502-0.
5. Gamage JP, De Silva AP, Nalliah AK, Galloway SD. Effects of dehydration on cricket specific skill performance in hot and humid conditions. Int J Sport Nutr Exerc Metab. 2016;26(6):531–41. https://doi.org/10.1123/ijsnem.2016-0015.
6. Li H, Early KS, Zhang G, Ma P, Wang H. Personalized hydration strategy to improve fluid balance and intermittent exercise performance in the heat. Nutrients. 2024;16(9) https://doi.org/10.3390/nu16091341.
7. Holly Louisa D, Samer A, Timothy James Ainsley C. Effect of sports massage on performance and recovery: a systematic review and meta-analysis. BMJ Open Sport Exerc Med. 2020;6(1):e000614. https://doi.org/10.1136/bmjsem-2019-000614.
8. Hemmings B, Smith M, Graydon J, Dyson R. Effects of massage on physiological restoration, perceived recovery, and repeated sports performance. Br J Sports Med. 2000;34(2):109–14; discussion 15. https://doi.org/10.1136/bjsm.34.2.109.
9. World Anti-Doping Agency: WADA appeals case of tennis player Jannik Sinner. https://www.wada-ama.org/en/news/wada-appeals-case-tennis-player-jannik-sinner; 2024.
10. International Cricket Council (ICC). Minimum medical standards for major ICC events 2020.
11. Echemendia RJ, Brett BL, Broglio S, Davis GA, Giza CC, Guskiewicz KM, et al. Introducing the sport concussion assessment tool 6 (SCAT6). Br J Sports Med. 2023;57(11):619–21. https://doi.org/10.1136/bjsports-2023-106849.
12. International Cricket Council (ICC): ICC Playing Handbook 2019–20 – The official handbook for international cricket players, officials and administrators. https://www.icc-cricket.com/news/playing-handbook (2019–20).
13. Venter R, Potgieter BJ. The use of recovery modalities by elite South African team athletes. S Afr J Res Sport Phys Educ Recreat. 2010;32:133–45.

Load Management in Cricket: Theory and Practicalities

12

John W. Orchard, Nico Grobler, Ross Herridge, and Dean McNamara

12.1 Introduction

When anyone talks about 'load management in cricket', there is a high likelihood that they are referring to fast bowlers. Before the turn of the twenty-first century, the term was hardly used or even mentioned. The first published studies were conducted in the early 2000s [1, 2]. It remains a relative afterthought with respect to batters, spin bowlers and wicketkeepers but is now a main-stream concept to manage pace bowlers, particularly in red ball (long format) cricket. It is worth starting with a discussion as to why pace bowling load monitoring is an important injury management and performance consideration that is unique in comparison to the other positional and competition-type demands across elite cricket.

J. W. Orchard (✉)
School of Public Health, University of Sydney, Sydney, NSW, Australia
e-mail: john.orchard@sydney.edu.au

N. Grobler
Wits Cricket Research Hub for Science, Medicine and Rehabilitation. School of Therapeutic Sciences, University of the Witwatersrand, Johannesburg, South Africa

R. Herridge
Cricket Australia, Melbourne, VIC, Australia
e-mail: Ross.herridge@cricket.com.au

D. McNamara
Sydney Sports & Exercise Physiology, Cricket New South Wales, Sydney, NSW, Australia
e-mail: dean@ssep.com.au; dean.mcnamara@cricketnsw.com.au

12.2 What Type of Sport Is Cricket?

Cricket is a sport which is a mix between a skill-based activity and a physical challenge, with a performance bias towards the task of skill proficiency. It is most analogous to its sister sport of baseball, as both sports are derivations of the original English sport of rounders [3].

Many sports at the other end of the spectrum are won by the fittest, fastest and strongest (albeit with a lesser dose of technique), such as track & field, swimming, cycling, weightlifting, rowing, etc. More extreme skill-based pursuits than cricket exist, and some have such a low degree of physical fitness that it is questionable whether they qualify as 'sports'. Golf, archery and lawn bowls are most definitely sports that retain some benefit from physical fitness. Further still, billiards and darts remove physical fitness requirements to such a degree that many taxonomists would classify them alongside chess and poker as 'games'.

The Mitchell classification of sports [4], used to determine thc risk of playing a certain sport with a cardiac disorder, was written by Americans unfamiliar with cricket. It mistakenly classifies cricket alongside golf and billiards as one with-

B. Olivier, J. W. Orchard (eds.), *Cricket Sports Medicine*,
https://doi.org/10.1007/978-981-96-6321-7_12

out any cardiac risk. Sadly, we know of rare examples of cardiovascular deaths in cricket [5]. Observational studies have further identified the high physical demands of cricket, particularly in pace bowlers [6].

The difference between the positions in cricket is that spin bowlers, batters and wicketkeepers are further along the skill-based spectrum (compared to pace bowlers). Physical fitness is still important for these positions but clearly less so than skill proficiency. Even at elite levels, we can discuss the occasional batters or wicketkeepers who have 'poor fitness levels', but there is no such thing as an elite batter with a poor skill base (of being able to hit the ball). Pace bowlers must have good skill acquisition but, at an elite level, must also be extremely physically fit in comparison [6].

Training and skill development for batters, wicketkeepers and spin bowlers has an 'old school' flavour to it. The best batsman who ever played cricket is considered to be Don Bradman, and attached to him is a famous story, which is that he grew up repetitively practising hitting the ball against a wall with a stump. This story is probably not the secret of his success. Still, if you asked him what the real secret was, his answer would have been very similar to Tendulkar's, Lara's or Heyhoe-Flint's: 'practice and then more practice' (meaning facing as many bowlers as possible in the nets and out on the ground). The best batters in the team are almost always said to 'train the hardest'. Facing more balls is likely to improve batting proficiency and is not particularly likely to result in injury.

Fast bowlers are somewhat different—they need to train 'efficiently'. Those fast bowlers who bowled the most balls in training, especially while young, didn't end up in the Hall of Fame. Many of them ended up in the casualty wards, with degenerative injuries of the lumbar spine in particular. Injury surveillance in cricket has consistently shown that fast bowlers (in the red ball format in particular) have higher rates of injury than the other positions [7–9]. More so than the different positions, fast bowlers need to be conscious of picking training loads that hit the sweet spot between skill development and refinement and diminished returns/avoiding injury.

12.3 How Much Is Too Much?

Load management in sports became a very popular topic in the 2010s, with an IOC expert consensus conference devoted to the subject [10]. 'How much is too much?' was the signature question, although 'how much is too little?' is an equally relevant consideration. The answer(s) are complicated but start with the concession that load tolerance can and should be developed. Fast bowlers, like runners, swimmers, cyclists and football players, can be trained to tolerate higher levels of load by gradual buildup of load. Although much consideration is given to the lumbar spine, fast bowlers can also get shoulder and leg injuries. Throwing and running loads (in the field and for fitness) can be relevant for these other injuries. Each injury represents micro- or macro-failure of a tissue in the appropriate body part and whether that tissue has coped with or failed to cope with the local repetitive and acute loads. Individual joint, bone, muscle and tendon loads are too complicated to measure. So, we measure the estimated total body load in fast bowlers by the number of balls bowled. This is either done for match balls bowled or total balls bowled (match and training) and is most commonly collated as weekly or seasonal (yearly) loads. In hindsight, too much can be defined retrospectively after injury. In terms of avoiding injury prospectively, we recommend that familiar loads generally be tolerated, but unfamiliar loads are likely to (but not always destined to) lead to injury.

12.4 Importance of Monitoring Training and Match Demand in Cricket

In recent years, there has been an increase in the demand for year-round player availability among elite-level cricketers [11]. This has resulted in more demanding schedules that involve multiple training sessions [11]. Monitoring training and match demand to optimise players' performance is important [12]. By tailoring training programmes (Fig. 12.1) to individual players and tracking volume patterns and associated perfor-

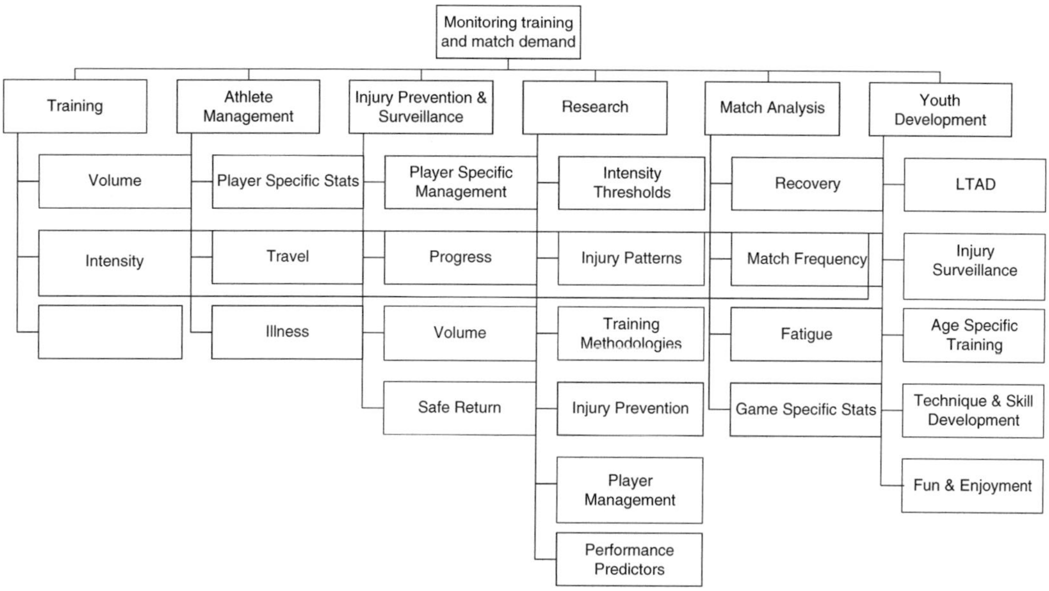

Fig. 12.1 There are a large number of interactions with match and training workloads

mance metrics and trends over time, coaches can identify optimal training volumes, intensities and recovery strategies for each player to maintain optimal performance levels throughout a season [12]. This personalised approach guides decisions on player selection, rest periods, or training and match demand adjustments, maximises performance potential and ensures players are adequately prepared for matches [12].

In today's dynamic cricketing landscape, with players being contracted to multiple teams across the globe and the ever-increasing demands of training and match schedules, ensuring the well-being and management of players has become a daunting task for cricketing institutions [13]. The complexities of managing player fatigue and injuries while ensuring that the players perform at their best highlight the need for a comprehensive and sustainable approach towards player welfare [13]. To mitigate these difficulties, coaches can benefit from utilising reliable, cricket-specific measures of fatigue and demand, particularly when players' access is limited [14]. The same can be said for returning players from an injury (Fig. 12.1) [15]. After an injury, gradually reintroducing a player and monitoring training demand during rehabilitation allows coaches and medical staff to track an injured player's progress, determine appropriate training volumes and ensure a safe return to play [6, 12, 14].

The impact of monitoring training and match demand extends beyond player performance and welfare. It plays a crucial role in talent identification and player progression (Fig. 12.1) [12]. By tracking training and match demand data from junior levels to elite cricket, coaches can spot promising players, monitor their development and make informed decisions about their progression to higher levels [16]. This approach also ensures that adolescent players are exposed to appropriate training and match demands, avoiding excessive physical demands that could impede their long-term development [16].

The data collected from monitoring cricket's training and match demand holds significant potential for cricket research and analysis (Fig. 12.1). Researchers can identify training and match demand thresholds, injury patterns and performance predictors by collecting and analysing training and match demand data from a large sample of players [12]. This knowledge can shape future training methodologies, injury prevention strategies and player management protocols [12].

12.5 The Acute:Chronic Workload Ratio (ACWR)

As it turns out, the most commonly used measure of workload in fast bowlers is also the most common in other sports. This is the ratio of the acute weekly workload in a given week (number of balls bowled) against the average workload of the previous weeks. The index (reference) week can alternatively be excluded or included in the calculation, bearing similar results [17]. The most common baseline is 4 weeks (the average weekly workload of the previous 4 weeks, Fig. 12.2), [18] but on occasions, 6-week, 8-week and 10-week baselines are used. It is also possible to look at 3-day, 2-week [19], 3-month and other loads and compare them to previous periods. The training and/or tissue adaptation residual should be considered when determining the chronic workload duration. Compared to previous seasons, seasonal (yearly) load is occasionally measured, particularly in young players. The 'ideal' ratio is 1.0 (this week's number of balls bowled is the same as the average number bowled in the previous four weeks). However, any range of 0.7–1.5 is considered 'low risk' for injury, whereas 'workload spikes' of greater than 1.5 are considered at increased risk for injury. Monitoring the ACWR is based on the assumption that a rapid increase or spike in acute training and match demand, relative to the chronic training and match demand, can increase the risk of injury [20–22]. When the ratio is too high, it suggests a rapid and significant increase in training and match demand for which the athlete may not be adequately prepared [20–22]. The sudden change in demand could lead to chronic fatigue, inadequate recovery and a heightened risk of overuse injuries [20–22]. Training below the ratio could lead to undertraining and injuries, as the player is underprepared for sudden spikes in the training and match demand [20–22]. There is a moderate amount of evidence that high workload spikes in cricket specifically are an injury risk in fast bowlers [1, 20, 23, 24], along with ample evidence in other sports [10, 25, 26]. Despite the published evidence, there remains some scepticism about workload management [27].

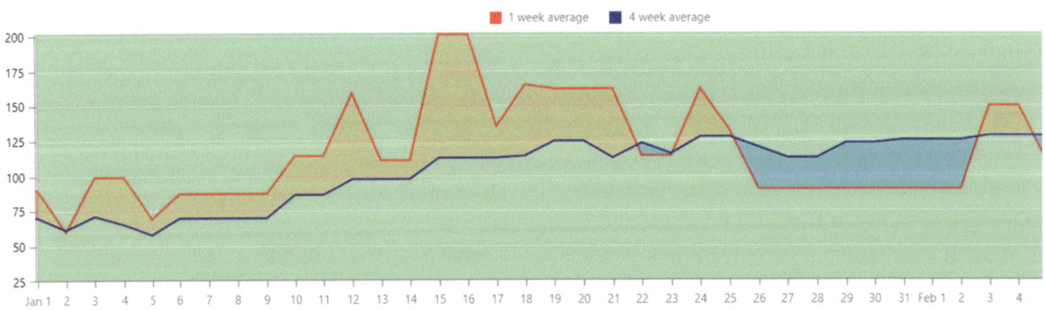

Fig. 12.2 Example plotting of Acute (Red) 1 week over Chronic (Blue) 4-week workload

12.6 Pace Bowlers Versus Baseball Pitchers

Notably, the position most similar to that of the fast bowler in cricket is that of the pitcher in baseball (Fig. 12.3), and they have many differences in approach to workload management. As an initial point of difference, baseball starting pitchers can generally only play every fourth or fifth day, as they will be too sore in the 2–3 days after a 'start' to be able to effectively pitch again. This has been the case for decades, and for this reason, load management has been much more part of the game of baseball for longer than it has been popular in cricket. Instead of 'weekly load', however, because baseball for starting pitchers works on a 4- or 5-day rotation, the key measurement is 'pitch count' (which is a match, not a combined training/match metric), and the baseline refers to previous 'starts' (which therefore is a pitches per 5 days measure, not pitches per week). A superb long review of the dilemmas of the baseball pitcher is the book 'The Arm' by Jeff Passan [28]. The title refers to the 'arm' generically but the ulnar collateral ligament of the elbow more specifically, as this is the pathognomonic injury of the baseball pitcher in the same way that the lumbar stress fracture is the pathognomonic injury of the cricket fast bowler. Passan [28] beautifully outlines that Major League Baseball franchises in the USA have a modern (and statistical) approach to workload management in starting pitchers, but this approach is not enough to solve the problem. He contrasts Japan as a comparison country that is still 'old school' and where coaches allow more latitude with pitch counts than in the USA. The first big problem in MLB is that the teams are extremely competitive (rather than cooperative) and see workload management as a competitive intellectual property. No franchise can get enough data, but the franchises do not share data, and there is very little data publication in the medical literature [29] (even though a lot of it exists at the franchise level). A second problem is that before being drafted/signed by an MLB franchise team, junior pitchers are free agents with the primary aim of putting themselves in the 'shop window'. Everyone is aware of the trade-off between skill acquisition and injury risk, but skill demonstration (to scouts) means that injury prevention is a secondary consideration for the vast majority of junior pitchers. Many of them have 'blown out their arm' (torn their UCL, requiring Tommy John reconstructive surgery) prior to even reaching MLB [28].

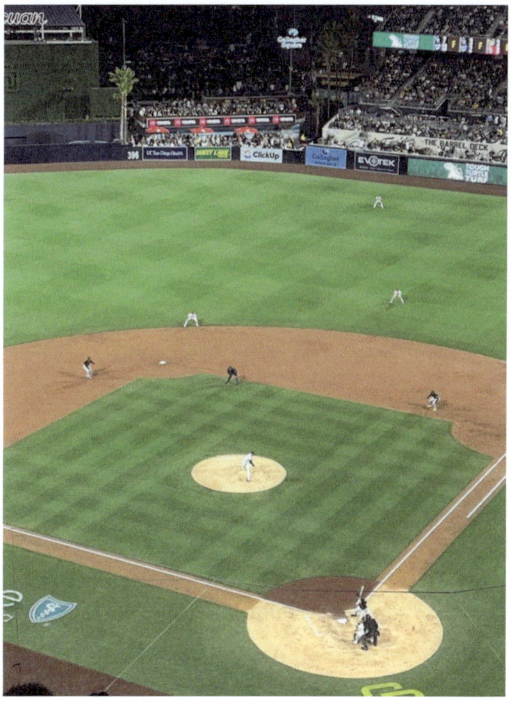

Fig. 12.3 Workload management (of pitchers/bowlers) is a common thread between baseball (pictured) and cricket

12.7 Fast Bowler Load Management in Different Countries

Load management is paid more attention in men's red ball cricket in Australia and England than anywhere else for reasons that are fairly straightforward. Along with India, England and Australia constitute a 'Big 3' of cricket that both have greater financial resources than other countries but also play more Test match (international red ball) cricket than other countries. Workload management of fast bowlers in India is less of a priority than in Australia and England because in India a far higher percentage of overs in red ball cricket are bowled by spin bowlers due to prevailing pitch conditions. Spin bowlers are able to bowl far more overs than pace bowlers without becoming injured due to lower bowling speeds (presumably imparting less force to the body) [9, 30].

The demands of first class domestic men's cricket vary from England to Australia. Pace bowlers in men's county cricket certainly bowl more overs in England than in any other country, due to the highest number of fixtures (and relative lack of conditions to suit spin bowling). However, the average delivery pace in England is slower than in other countries because of the specific conditions. All of the relative moisture of the pitch, the generous cover of ryegrass (which retains moisture more than warm-season grasses) and the use of the Dukes ball with a pronounced seam that retains the ability to swing the ball for longer mean that 'medium pace' bowling is particularly effective in England. No conversions have been published yet, but it may be the case that bowling 15 overs at 135–140 kph might be the equivalent of bowling, say, 25 overs at 125–130 kph.

12.8 Practicalities of Load Management

In any workload monitoring system, a clear definition of workload needs to be established. This needs to be established on two levels when using tools such as the ACWR. Firstly, the unit of workload and secondly, the duration of both the acute and chronic loads. The most common units of workload include distance, session RPE (AU), and in cricket, the number of balls bowled is defined as a workload. High-speed running (HSR) distance and efforts are usually captured in training and matches. Similarly to bowling workload, this allows practitioners to measure acute and chronic loads of high-intensity running so players aren't doing too little or too much high-intensity running, which is a risk factor for injury [6].

Simply counting balls bowled seems like a simple task, and if only match balls were counted, scorecards would provide all the relevant information to establish the bowling workload. However, both match and training bowling loads collectively contribute to determining bowling load. Therefore, a system is required to collect the bowling workload data. On a basic level and still practiced in elite cricket programmes are self-reported loads. The issue with self-reported load is the potential for false data due to miscounting or error in data input. Elite cricket programmes are now utilising wearable technology in training and matches. This technology is largely based around GPS outputs for the purposes of measuring running loads—both volume and intensity. Housed within these wearable technologies, however, exist accelerometers, gyroscopes and magnetometers in addition to GPS technology. Using all these technologies, sports scientists are able to extract with accuracy cricket-specific events automatically from a training session or match [31]. The outcome of this allows for the detection of bowling events, and therefore load reporting can exclude self-reported loads.

There are two major concerns in making inferences on athlete readiness when looking at bowling loads. Firstly, the accuracy of the bowling loads being reported; the second consideration is that by sampling using ball counts as the external load measure, the assumption exists that all balls are of equal loading. In practice, we know this to not be the case. Determining bowling intensity to build context in bowling load is required to further refine bowling load monitoring. Bowling velocity is one option to determine bowling intensity. There are some downfalls with using bowling velocity for intensity, however. Firstly, it is resource-heavy with no easy way to automate data collection in training settings. Secondly, with the changing tactical approaches in cricket, slower balls may wrongly be described as low intensity. Finally, it assumes that all fast bowlers are capable of being able to bowl with maximum velocity at any time. If a bowler can't reach their maximum velocity due to performance or fatigue, intensity could still be high. It could be argued that bowling velocity is a measure of fast bowling performance, not bowling intensity.

Since it has been established that bowling events can be detected with wearable technology, elite cricket programmes are able to further refine the intensity measures from the gyroscopes and accelerometers [32]. Practically, this enables support staff and coaches to more accurately prescribe and monitor fast bowlers in preparation for competition and return-to-play settings. This is more commonly done by reporting a relative score for the individual against a meaningful event or competition.

12.9 Load Management in Other Player Positions

The majority of injuries leading to missed playing time in batters and wicketkeepers are either contact injuries such as fractured hands, concussions, or acute muscle strains, which have not yet been associated with high workloads in batters [33, 34]. Spin bowlers do suffer from lumbar (and even cervical) stress fractures, on occasion, but generally have low injury prevalence. Spin bowlers will need return-to-play plans that involve a gradual increase in bowling loads after recovering from overuse injuries, using similar templates to pace bowlers. However, many uninjured spin bowlers pay little attention to load management plans and, despite this, enjoy low injury risk.

Occasionally, batters will develop overuse injuries such as tennis elbow (in the lead arm, so left elbow for a right-handed batter) [35]. Load management plans that limit daily and weekly batting practice time are important in the recovery from tennis elbow. It is very difficult to recover while still participating in red ball cricket, as batting times are relatively unlimited.

Throwing injuries (particularly to the shoulder, but sometimes affecting the elbow) are also relatively common in cricket, although many of them do not lead to much missed playing time. Throwing workloads (which relate more to training loads rather than match throwing loads) are related to the development of throwing injury symptoms [36].

References

1. Dennis R, Farhart R, Goumas C, Orchard J. Bowling workload and the risk of injury in elite cricket fast bowlers. J Sci Med Sport. 2003;6(3):359–67. https://doi.org/10.1016/s1440-2440(03)80031-2.
2. Dennis R, Finch C, Farhart P. Is bowling workload a risk factor for injury to Australian junior cricket fast bowlers? Br J Sports Med. 2005;39:843–6.
3. Hise B. Swinging away: how cricket and baseball connect. Scala Publishers Ltd; 2010.
4. Levine BD, Baggish AL, Kovacs RJ, Link MS, Maron MS, Mitchell JH. Eligibility and disqualification recommendations for competitive athletes with cardiovascular abnormalities: Task Force 1: classification of sports: dynamic, static, and impact: a scientific statement from the American Heart Association and American College of Cardiology. J Am Coll Cardiol. 2015;66(21):2350–5. https://doi.org/10.1016/j.jacc.2015.09.033.
5. List of Fatalities while playing cricket. https://en.wikipedia.org/wiki/List_of_fatalities_while_playing_cricket. Accessed 20/04/2024.
6. McNamara DJ, Gabbett TJ, Naughton G. Assessment of workload and its effects on performance and injury in elite cricket fast bowlers. Sports Med. 2017;47(3):503–15. https://doi.org/10.1007/s40279-016-0588-8.
7. Goggins L, Peirce N, Ranson C, McCaig S, Newman D, Langley B, et al. Injuries in England and Wales elite men's domestic cricket: a nine season review from 2010 to 2018. J Sci Med Sport. 2020;23(9):836–40. https://doi.org/10.1016/j.jsams.2020.03.009.
8. Orchard JW, Inge P, Sims K, Kountouris A, Saw AE, Saw R, et al. Comparison of injury profiles between elite Australian male and female cricket players. J Sci Med Sport. 2023;26(1):19–24. https://doi.org/10.1016/j.jsams.2022.12.002.
9. Orchard JW, Kountouris A, Sims K. Incidence and prevalence of elite male cricket injuries using updated consensus definitions. Open Access J Sports Med. 2016;7:187–94. https://doi.org/10.2147/OAJSM.S117497.

10. Soligard T, Schwellnus M, Alonso JM, Bahr R, Clarsen B, Dijkstra HP, et al. How much is too much? (Part 1) International Olympic Committee consensus statement on load in sport and risk of injury. Br J Sports Med. 2016;50(17):1030–41. https://doi.org/10.1136/bjsports-2016-096581.
11. Christie CJ, Barnard DV, Pote L, Munro CE. Workload monitoring in team sports: using elite cricket as an example. Indian J Orthop. 2020;54(3):271–4. https://doi.org/10.1007/s43465-020-00085-8.
12. French D, Torres RL. NSCA's essentials of sport science. Human Kinetics; 2022.
13. Halson SL. Monitoring training load to understand fatigue in athletes. Sports Med. 2014;44(Suppl 2):S139–47. https://doi.org/10.1007/s40279-014-0253-z.
14. Sholto-Douglas R, Cook R, Wilkie M, Christie CJ. Movement demands of an elite cricket team during the big bash league in Australia. J Sports Sci Med. 2020;19(1):59–64.
15. Noakes TD, Durandt JJ. Physiological requirements of cricket. J Sports Sci. 2000;18(12):919–29. https://doi.org/10.1080/026404100446739.
16. Pote L, Christie CJ. Strength and conditioning practices of university and high school level cricket coaches: a South African context. J Strength Cond Res. 2016;30(12):3464–70. https://doi.org/10.1519/jsc.0000000000001432.
17. Gabbett TJ, Hulin B, Blanch P, Chapman P, Bailey D. To couple or not to couple? For acute: chronic workload ratios and injury risk, does it really matter? Int J Sports Med. 2019;40(9):597–600. https://doi.org/10.1055/a-0955-5589.
18. Warren A, Williams S, McCaig S, Trewartha G. High acute: chronic workloads are associated with injury in England & Wales Cricket Board Development Programme fast bowlers. J Sci Med Sport. 2018;21(1):40–5. https://doi.org/10.1016/j.jsams.2017.07.009.
19. Ahmun R, McCaig S, Tallent J, Williams S, Gabbett T. Association of daily workload, wellness, and injury and illness during tours in international cricketers. Int J Sports Physiol Perform. 2019;14(3):369–77. https://doi.org/10.1123/ijspp.2018-0315.
20. Hulin BT, Gabbett TJ, Blanch P, Chapman P, Bailey D, Orchard JW. Spikes in acute workload are associated with increased injury risk in elite cricket fast bowlers. Br J Sports Med. 2014;48(8):708–12. https://doi.org/10.1136/bjsports-2013-092524.
21. Bourdon PC, Cardinale M, Murray A, Gastin P, Kellmann M, Varley MC, et al. Monitoring athlete training loads: consensus statement. Int J Sports Physiol Perform. 2017;12(Suppl 2):S2161–s70. https://doi.org/10.1123/ijspp.2017-0208.
22. Griffin A, Kenny IC, Comyns TM, Lyons M. The association between the acute: chronic workload ratio and injury and its application in team sports: a systematic review. Sports Med. 2020;50(3):561–80. https://doi.org/10.1007/s40279-019-01218-2.
23. Orchard J, Blanch P, Paoloni J, Kountouris A, Sims K, Orchard J, et al. Fast bowling match workloads over 5–26 days and risk of injury in the following month. J Sci Med Sport. 2015;18:26–30.
24. Orchard J, James T, Portus M, Kountouris A, Dennis R. Fast bowlers in cricket demonstrate up to 3- to 4-week delay between high workloads and increased risk of injury. Am J Sports Med. 2009;37:1186–92.
25. Hulin B, Gabbett T, Lawson D, Caputi P, Sampson J. The acute: chronic workload ratio predicts injury: high chronic workload may decrease injury risk in elite rugby league players. Br J Sports Med. 2015;50:231.
26. Blanch P, Gabbett TJ. Has the athlete trained enough to return to play safely? The acute: chronic workload ratio permits clinicians to quantify a player's risk of subsequent injury. Br J Sports Med. 2016;50(8):471–5. https://doi.org/10.1136/bjsports-2015-095445.
27. Carbone L, Sampietro M, Cicognini A, García-Sillero M, Vargas-Molina S. Is the relationship between acute and chronic workload a valid predictive injury tool? A Bayesian analysis. J Clin Med. 2022;11(19) https://doi.org/10.3390/jcm11195945.
28. Passan J. The arm: inside the billion-dollar mystery of the Most valuable commodity in sports. Harper Paperbacks; 2017.
29. Jazayerli R. Pitcher abuse points: a new way to measure pitcher abuse. Baseball Prospectus. https://www.baseballprospectus.com/news/article/148/pitcher-abuse-points-a-new-way-to-measure-pitcher-abuse/1998
30. Orchard J, James T, Kountouris A, Portus M. Changes to injury profile (and recommended cricket injury definitions) based on the increased frequency of Twenty20 cricket matches. Open Access J Sports Med. 2010;1:63–76. https://doi.org/10.2147/oajsm.s9671.
31. McNamara D, Gabbett T, Chapman P, Naughton G, Farhart P. The validity of microsensors to automatically detect bowling events and counts in cricket fast bowlers. Int J Sports Physiol Perform. 2015;10(1):71–5.
32. McNamara DJ, Gabbett TJ, Blanch P, Kelly L. The relationship between variables in wearable microtechnology devices and cricket fast-bowling intensity. Int J Sports Physiol Perform. 2018;13(2):135–9.
33. Orchard J, Blanch P, Paoloni J, Kountouris A, Sims K, Orchard J, et al. Cricket fast bowling workload patterns as risk factors for tendon, muscle, bone and joint injuries. Br J Sports Med. 2015;49(16):1064–8.
34. Orchard JW, Kountouris A, Sims K. Risk factors for hamstring injuries in Australian male professional cricket players. J Sport Health Sci. 2017;6(3):271–4. https://doi.org/10.1016/j.jshs.2017.05.004.
35. Orchard J, Kountouris A. The management of tennis elbow. BMJ. 2011;342:d2687.
36. Saw R, Dennis R, Bentley D, Farhart P. Throwing workload and injury risk in elite cricketers. Br J Sports Med. 2011;45(10):805–8.

13 Return to Play and Return to Performance in Cricket

Kevin Sims and David Beakley

13.1 Introduction

Injury is an inevitable part of professional sport, and therefore, so is returning to play following injury. While it is often not possible to prevent injury, a carefully managed return to play can reduce the chance of a reinjury and is something that the player and rehabilitation team can control. It is estimated that up to 21% of injuries are recurrent involving the same area [1]. The challenge in professional sports is to offset the risk of reinjury against the team performance, as it is known that team success is driven by player availability [2]. In cricket, hamstring and lumbar bone stress injuries (LBSI) are highly prevalent [3] and are prone to recurrence [4, 5] with lumbar bone stress injury having recurrence rates of up to one in four [5, 6]. Managing these common injuries, therefore, requires a robust process to safely and efficiently allow the athlete to return to optimal performance.

True high-performance management relies on the alignment and integration of all the disciplines impacting individual and team performance, including but not limited to coaching effectiveness, physical preparation, individual skill/talent, decision-making, team strategy and selection. Sports medicine practitioners are not able to influence or control all of these areas, and a collaborative, multi-disciplinary approach is therefore required to ultimately optimise performance. To this point, poor communication, a lack of consensus and inconsistency in expectations regarding return to play have the potential to lead to inadequate rehabilitation, premature return to play and increased risk of reinjury [7, 8].

This chapter will outline the principles of return to play, discuss the dichotomy of return to play versus return to performance and provide cricket-specific examples of return to play following a lumbar bone stress injury and shoulder tendinopathy.

K. Sims (✉)
Tennis Australia, University of Queensland, Queensland Sports Medicine Centre, Brisbane, QLD, Australia
e-mail: k.sims@qsmc.net.au

D. Beakley
PhysiPro Athletic, Melbourne, VIC, Australia
e-mail: david@physipro.com.au

13.2 Return to Play Principles

In the broadest sense, the return to play process can be considered a continuum of the following stages [9, 10]:

1. Injury management and rehabilitation.
2. Return to participation.
3. Return to sport.
4. Return to performance.

This section will outline some principles involved in planning this process.

B. Olivier, J. W. Orchard (eds.), *Cricket Sports Medicine*,
https://doi.org/10.1007/978-981-96-6321-7_13

13.3 Principle 1: Setting an Initial Timeline

Once the initial injury has been diagnosed, conversations on potential return to play timelines can begin. Our experience is that this step is crucial so all stakeholders (especially players/coaches/selectors) have a realistic understanding of the likely return date.

Firstly, the sports science and sports medicine (SSSM) team needs to be aligned in their projections to avoid confusion or mixed messaging. These conversations need to be based on an understanding of the pathology with input from a multi-disciplinary medical team (sports physician, physiotherapist, strength and conditioner and external radiologist, orthopaedic specialists when used). Having a realistic time frame reduces the risk of reinjury by allowing adequate time for tissue healing.

Next, there is a discussion with the player and coach/selectors in a shared decision-making process [11]. For example, there may be an important series or match where the risk of reinjury is offset by the potential benefit of having a key player available. We have found that a useful way of managing these conversations is to prepare 2–3 possible management options and, where possible, outline the risks and benefits (as objectively as possible) of each of them so an informed decision can be made. It is a pyrrhic victory if an overly conservative SSSM team succeeds in avoiding reinjury at the expense of team results when a player could have played [12].

Importantly, the shared decision-making should continue throughout the process as the athlete nears the final return to play date. Factors such as the athlete's confidence in their readiness and the coach's gauge of their level of performance are equally important as the SSSM team's more objective judgements. An added benefit of shared decision-making is that all stakeholders feel valued, making it much easier to modify, manage and progress training collaboratively.

13.4 Principle 2: Setting Milestones and Phases

Once a realistic return to play target has been agreed upon, the rehab team can map a timeline back from the projected return to play, which provides clarity on expected milestones on the pathway (e.g. return to run or return to bowl).

This can then allow more detail in planning as there may be several sub-phases within the major milestones as per Table 13.1. The phases are not mutually exclusive for example, a return to run and progressive gym loading will often occur simultaneously.

The control chaos continuum [13] (Table 13.2) provides a useful framework for progressing in the skill-specific loading phase of the process.

Table 13.1 An example of rehabilitation phases and transition criteria

Continuum	Description	Content	Transition criteria
Phase 1:	Acute injury management/ site protection	Focus on protecting injured tissue & gym-based rehab	Clinical measures e.g. pain/ swelling
Phase 2:	Load introduction	Gym-based rehab & gym-based preparation	Strength, function and endurance measures
Phase 3	Strength & Power Accumulation	Sport/injury-specific S&C rehabilitation	Strength, function and endurance measures
Phase 4:	Return to running, agility, jumping and landing	Progressive running, including volume and speed, agility, jumping and landing activities	Volume and high speed running and agility targets
Phase 5:	Training integration	Progressive sports-specific training incorporating control chaos continuum	Completed progressive exposure to uncontrolled training
Phase 6:	Full training	Need a defined time based on shared decision	All RTP criteria completed
Return to play			
Return to performance			
Maintenance			

Table 13.2 Control chaos framework with reference to cricket

Control	
Skill	Training content
Fielding	Planned training-player knows what is happening
	Low intensity
	Solo training with coach/rehab staff
	Stationary (2–3 steps) catching-mid range and boundary
	Stationary (2–3 steps) ground fielding
	Low-to-moderate intensity throwing to baseball mitt with partner
	Close monitoring of throwing volume
Bowling	Shadow bowling
	Avoid bowling to batsman (to keep intensity low)
	Walk through bowling using half net progressing to full net.
	Bowling off short run up (quarter to half run).
	Technical focus with low intensity.
	Closer monitoring of bowling volumes and intensity
Batting	Planned training-player knows what is happening
	Throw downs from coach
	Focus on specific shots (e.g. front foot only)
Control to chaos	
Skill	Training content
Fielding	Majority planned training -player mostly knows what is happening but progresses to some reactive work
	Progressive movement intensity
	Solo training but may join appropriate group drills
	Begin short catching
	Incorporate planned low-to-moderate intensity movement into catching drills -mid range and boundary
	Incorporate planned low-to-moderate intensity movement into ground fielding drills
	Throwing combined with low-to-moderate movement intensity
	Progress throwing volume and intensity
Bowling	Progress bowling to full run
	Progress intensity
	Begin bowling to batters once approaching moderate to full intensity
	Monitoring of bowling volumes
Batting	Majority planned training-player mostly knows what is happening
	Throw downs from coach but progress to reactive batting
	Batting against spin bowling
	Incorporating low-to-moderate intensity running between the wickets as appropriate
Chaos	
Skill	Training content
Fielding	Reactive training
	High movement intensity
	Training with rest of group
	Normal throwing volume and intensity
Bowling	Normal bowling intensity
	Bowling to batters
	Bowling centre wicket/battle zone scenarios
Batting	Facing all bowlers in nets
	Batting in centre wicket scenarios
	Incorporating high intensity running between the wickets

13.5 Principle 3: Setting Criteria

The next step in the shared decision-making process is to identify the key criteria that must be met before the athlete can be considered ready to play. These should not be solely time based. The criteria are ideally based on objective data; either from pre-season screening, in-season monitoring or from squad normative values. Example measures would include the following:

- Clinical (e.g. specific tests).
- Radiology (e.g. fracture healing).
- Strength (e.g. dynamometer).
- Rate of force development (e.g. force plates).
- Endurance measures (e.g. repeated calf raise).
- Function (e.g. an agreed number of high speed running sessions).
- Sports-specific measures (e.g. an agreed number of unrestricted bowling net sessions).
- Psychological readiness return to play (e.g. Injury Psychological Readiness to Return to Sport scale [14]).

Having clear criteria will assist in determining the content of the rehab in the phases. Once final return to play criteria have been established it is also helpful to establish criteria that determine when the athlete is ready to progress from one phase to the next. Expected time frames for healing and function are important considerations (for example, post-surgical protocols), but they should be underpinned with clinical testing, radiological status (e.g. fracture healing), strength, range and function measures which indicate a readiness to progress. Some examples would be clinical targets (e.g. resolution of swelling) that provide an indication of tissue healing and functional targets (e.g. painfree performance of consecutive single leg hops) that demonstrate the player's readiness to progress activity level (e.g. from walking to running).

It is usually relevant to ensure other members of the multi-disciplinary team, including a psychologist and dietitian, are involved in the process both in setting criteria and providing assistance to the player, particularly if the rehabilitation programme is likely to be prolonged.

13.6 Control Chaos Continuum

A return to play framework has been advocated in invasive sports (e.g. football and basketball) involving progressive exposure to increasingly complex sports-specific scenarios [9, 13]. The original framework proposes five phases:

- High control.
- Moderate control.
- Control to chaos.
- Moderate chaos.
- High chaos.

Cricket, by its relative lack of direct physical contact with other players and repetitive movements (e.g. bowling), is more controlled than football. Nonetheless, there is some potential to use this framework when an injured player returns to full fitness. Although the basic cricket skills are similar across all formats, shorter forms such as T20 cricket are high chaos environments from a movement perspective (e.g. more diving, higher throwing intensity, batting innovations and bowling variations) but far more predictable with respect to volume (e.g. bowlers are limited to 4 overs maximum). In contrast, test cricket is less chaotic from a movement perspective, but the loading of all skills, particularly bowling, is uncontrolled. Therefore, this continuum lends itself more to the movement demands and Table 13.2 provides some examples of how this may be done.

13.7 Return to Play for a Cricket Fast Bowler

Fast bowlers have the highest injury rates of cricketers and are, therefore, often the target of many of the long-term return to play plans. For this group, consideration must be given to several factors which will influence the effectiveness and success of a return to play programme, including the following:

- Resolution of symptoms and pathology.
- Physical competency.
  - Strength.
    - Capacity.
    - Endurance.

  - Movement.
    Control.
    Power.
- Gradual introduction of load.
  - Number of bowling days versus rest days.
  - Volume of balls bowled per session.
  - Intensity of balls bowled per session.
  - Increases in volume or intensity between sessions and across weeks.
- Functional competency.
- Skill requirements (e.g. test match consistency vs. T20 variations).
- Psychological competency.

The return to play for a fast bowler following a lumbar bone stress injury illustrates how the principles described above may be incorporated into a practical situation. In this case, allowing sufficient time for bony healing is an important aspect of the management [15]. Figure 13.1 summarises the phases of rehabilitation and transition/return to play criteria in this case.

The rehabilitation team must carefully manage the return to bowling after a lumbar bone stress injury. Long periods of not bowling, while important to facilitate bone healing, also lead to a loss of some of the specific bony adaptations to bowling in the lumbar vertebrae [16] leading to an increased risk of overload on the resumption of bowling. Planning a return to bowl programme should consider the following:

- The importance of rest days and breaks from bowling in relation to the risk of developing a lumbar bone stress injury. Evidence has suggested bowlers who had at least two rest days between bowling sessions and a 2-to-3-week rest period mid-season were up to 20% less likely to develop bone marrow oedema on MRI [17].
- A gradual progression of loading, avoiding large 'spikes' in acute (weekly) bowling load in relation to chronic (4-weekly) workload [18] which previous research has shown up to 4.5 times increased risk of sustaining an injury in the following week.

Taking into consideration the aforementioned factors, an example of a return to bowling plan following a long-term injury (e.g. lumbar bone stress injury) is shown in Fig. 13.2.

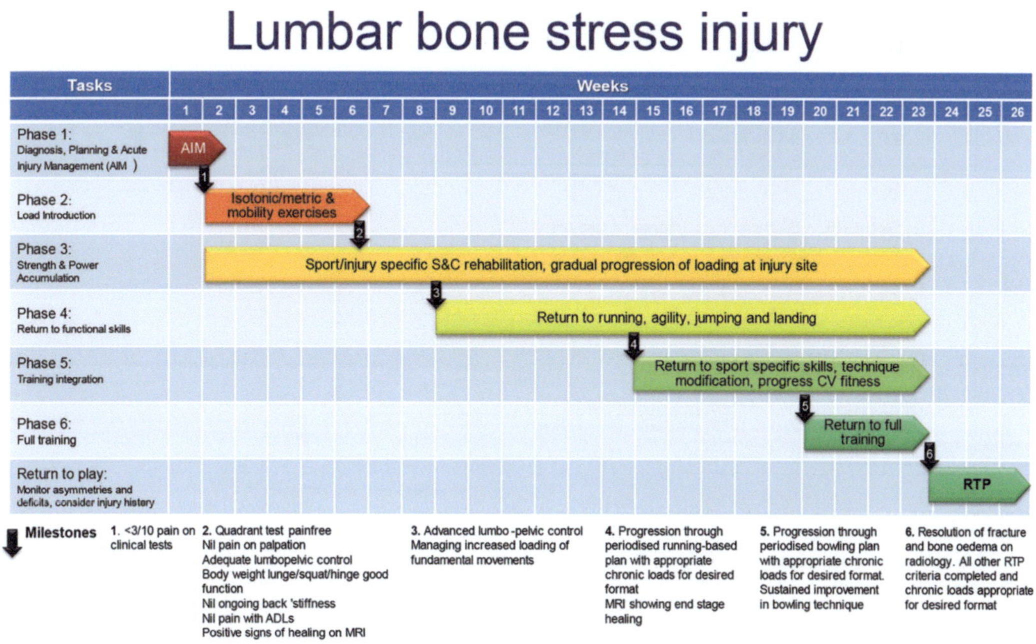

Fig. 13.1 Rehabilitation phases and transition criteria in a lumbar bone stress injury

Week	Session Number	Phase	Workload guidelines	Number of balls	Per wk	% increase from previous week
1	1	LOW Load, LOW Intensity	Walk through (4-5 steps) and bowl (max 100km/hr)	18	66	
	2		Walk through (4-5 steps) and bowl	12		
			Jog off ½ run and bowl (max 110km/hr)	12		
	3		Repeat previous session	24		
2	4		Walk through (4-5 steps) and bowl	6	72	9%
			Jog off ½ run and bowl (max 110km/hr)	18		
	5		Walk through (4-5 steps) and bowl	6		
			Jog off ½ run and bowl (max 110km/hr)	12		
		MEDIUM Load, MEDIUM Intensity	Jog full run and bowl (max 115km/hr)	6		
	6		Repeat previous session	24		
3	7		Jog ½ run and bowl	18	90	25%
			Full run (max 115km/hr)	12		
	8		Jog ½ run and bowl	12		
		MEDIUM Load, HIGH Intensity	Full run (max 120km/hr)	18		
	9		Repeat previous session	30		
4	10		Jog ½ run and bowl	12	108	20%
			Full run (max 120km/hr)	24		
	11		Jog ½ run and bowl	12		
			Full run (max 125km/hr)	24		
	12		Repeat previous session	36		
5	13		Full run (build up to max intensity)	36	114	6%
	14	HIGH Load, HIGH Intensity	Repeat previous session	36		
	15		Full run (build up to max intensity)	42		
6	16		Repeat previous session	42	138	21%
	17		Full run (build up to max intensity)	48		
	18		Repeat previous session	48		
7	19		Full run (build up to max intensity)	60	180	30%
	20		Repeat previous session	60		
	21		Repeat previous session	60		

Fig. 13.2 Example of a return to bowling plan. NB: This is a representative plan and will need to be adapted depending on the individual circumstances

Once the bowler has completed the seven weeks of return to bowl plan shown in Fig. 13.2, the focus then becomes ensuring the bowler is prepared for the volumes required in match situations. Finding the balance between ensuring the athlete is prepared to perform the demands of the sport, and limiting exposure and subsequent risk of injury, forms part of the skill required for successful workload management and performance. From our experience in managing elite Test cricket fast bowlers, cycling and periodising bowling workload between 150 and 180 balls per week seems to be the 'sweet spot', where balancing these competing factors is not only effective but sustainable.

Two examples of return to play programmes are detailed in Fig. 13.3 for Test cricket (Bowler 'X') and Fig. 13.4 for T20 cricket (Bowler 'Y'). While the time taken to build and periodise adequate workloads for the demands of Test cricket is the obvious difference, being able to execute the variety of different deliveries required for T20 cricket also requires some skill and consideration when planning a return to play programme. Collaborating with the athlete and coaching staff to ensure there are an adequate number of deliveries available to guarantee competent skill execution also needs to be taken into consideration.

An example of return to play following an upper limb (supraspinatus tendinopathy) provides an illustration around the planning involved in returning the shoulder to the demands of throwing. Figure 13.5 provides an example of the phases of recovery with transition criteria.

A controlled return to throwing is an essential part of returning an injured shoulder to the sport. Figure 13.6 is an example of a throwing programme that can be instituted from level 1 (in the case of a long-term injury, e.g. post-shoulder surgery) or at another appropriate point depending on the function of the player. In the example of the supraspinatus tendinopathy described above, level 4 may be suitable.

When returning to throwing, the following principles should be followed:

- No pain allowed.
- Alternate days throwing at the start of the programme.

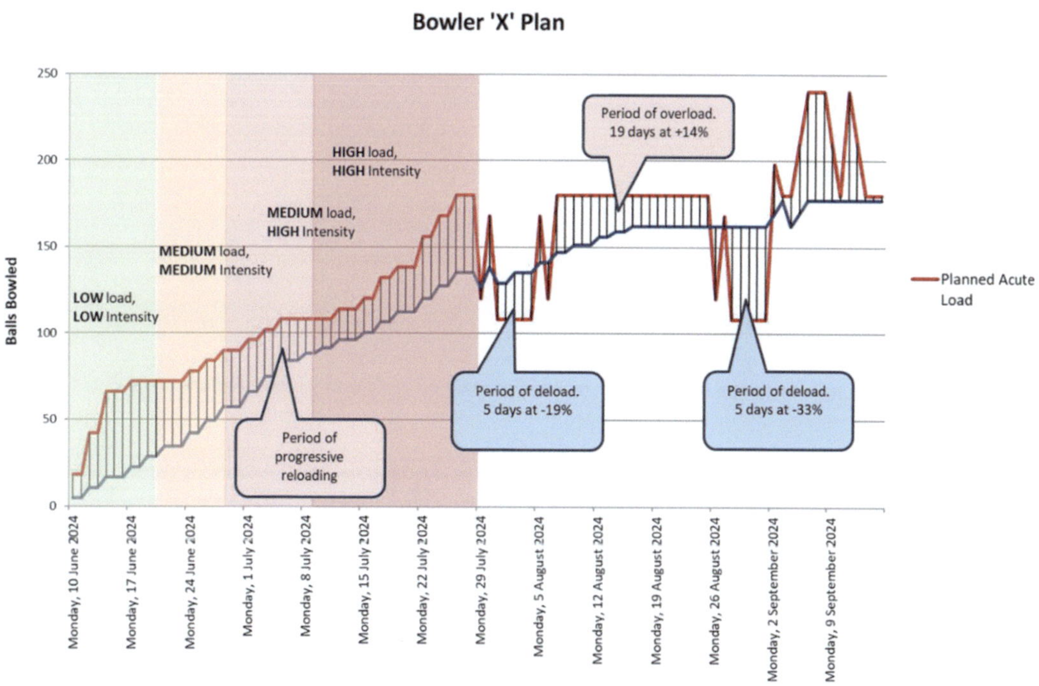

Fig. 13.3 Return to Test cricket bowling plan

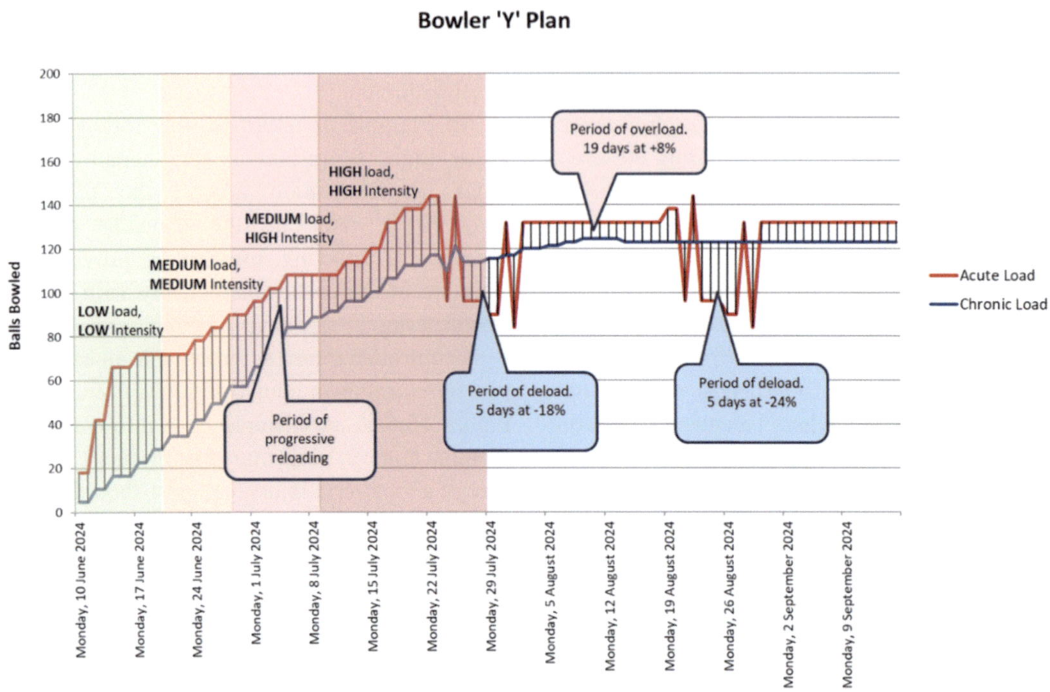

Fig. 13.4 Return to T20 bowling plan

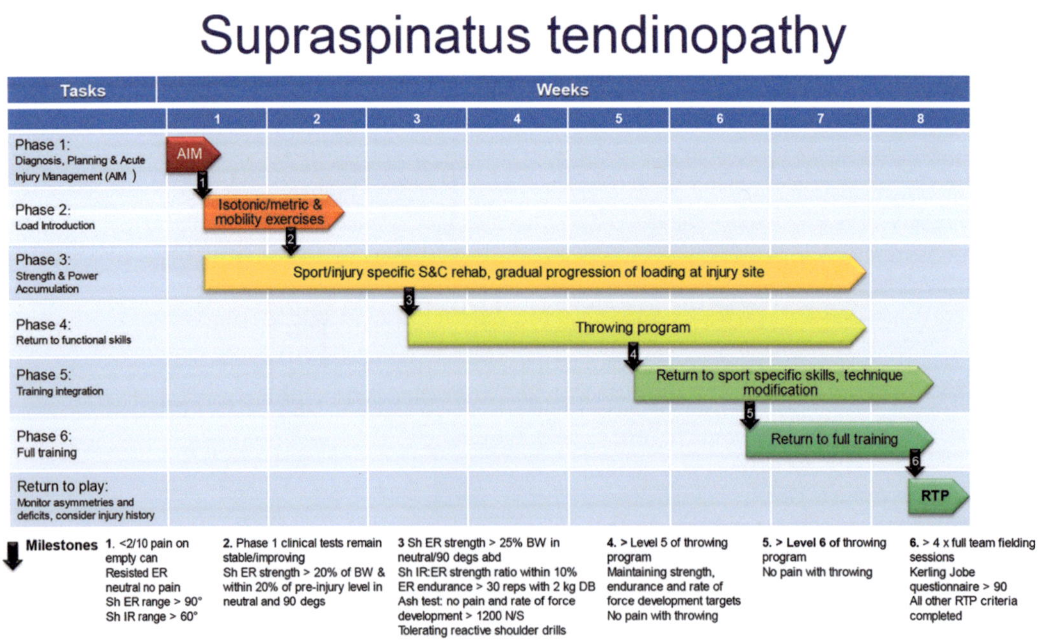

Fig. 13.5 Rehabilitation phases and transition criteria in a supraspinatus tendinopathy

Level	Session	Phase	Workload guidelines	Number of throws
1	1	Low ROM, Low Stress	Standing throw @ 50% (roll arm over) to glove @ 10m	2 x 6 throws
	2		Standing throw @ 50% (roll arm over) to glove @ 10m	2 x 8 throws
	3		Standing throw @ 50% (roll arm over) to glove @ 10m	2 x 10 throws
2	4		Standing throw @ 60% to glove @ 15m	2 x 6 throws
	5		Standing throw @ 60% to glove @ 15m	2 x 8 throws
	6		Standing throw @ 60% to glove @ 15m	2 x 10 throws
3	7		Standing throw @ 70% to glove @ 20m	2 x 6 throws
	8		Standing throw @ 70% to glove @ 20m	2 x 8 throws
	9		Standing throw @ 70% to glove @ 20m	2 x 10 throws
4	10	Medium ROM, Medium Stress	Warm-up throws: 1min, 15m to glove	-
			Crow step throw @ 80% to glove @ 30m	2 x 6 throws
	11		Warm-up throws: 1min, 15m to glove	-
			Crow step throw @ 80% to glove @ 30m	2 x 8 throws
	12		Warm-up throws: 1min, 15m to glove	-
			Crow step throw @ 80% to glove @ 30m	2 x 10 throws
5	13		Warm-up throws: 1min, 15m to glove	-
			1min, 20m at target on ground	-
			Crow step throw @ 80% to glove @ 40m	2 x 6 throws
	14		Warm-up throws: 1min, 15m to glove	-
			1min, 20m at target on ground	-
			Crow step throw @ 80% to glove @ 40m	2 x 8 throws
	15		Warm-up throws: 1min, 15m to glove	~10 throws
			1min, 20m at target on ground	~10 throws
			Crow step throw @ 80% to glove @ 40m	2 x 10 throws
6	16		Warm-up throws: 1min, 15m to glove	-
			1min, 20m at target on ground	-
			Crow step throw @ 80% to glove @ 50m	2 x 6 throws
	17		Warm-up throws: 1min, 15m to glove	-
			1min, 20m at target on ground	-
			Crow step throw @ 80% to glove @ 50m	2 x 8 throws
	18		Warm-up throws: 1min, 15m to glove	-
			1min, 20m at target on ground	-
			Crow step throw @ 80% to target @ 50m	2 x 10 throws
7	19	High ROM, Medium Stress	Warm-up throws: 1min, 15m to glove	-
			1min, 20m at target on ground	-
			Crow step throw to target @ 70m	2 x 6 throws
	20		Warm-up throws: 1min, 15m to glove	-
			1min, 20m at target on ground	-
			Crow step throw to target @ 70m	2 x 8 throws
	21		Warm-up throws: 1min, 15m to glove	-
			1min, 20m at target on ground	-
			Crow step throw to target @ 70m	2 x 10 throws
8	22	High ROM, High Stress	Warm-up throws: 1min, 15m to glove	-
			1min, 20m at target on ground	-
			Crow step throw to target @ 70m	6 throws
			Pick up and throw at target (stumps) @ 100% over 30m	6 throws
	23		Warm-up throws: 1min, 15m to glove	-
			1min, 20m at target on ground	-
			Crow step throw to target @ 70m	8 throws
			Pick up and throw at target (stumps) @ 100% over 30m	8 throws
	24		Warm-up throws: 1min, 15m to glove	-
			1min, 20m at target on ground	-
			Crow step throw to target @ 70m	10 throws
			Pick up and throw at target (stumps) @ 100% over 30m	10 throws

Fig. 13.6 Return to the throwing programme

- Do not increase volume and intensity in the same session.
- Consolidate for two to three sessions before progressing (either volume or intensity).
- Technique is important.

Level 6 in the throwing programme would be an appropriate level to be ready to follow some of the control chaos suggestions in Table 13.2. Once the player has reached level 7–8 full training can be incorporated (chaos in Table 13.2).

13.8 Return to Performance

Understanding the true impact of injury is challenging as the ability of an athlete to perform at their optimal level may be impaired by even small amounts of training loss [19]. It has been recommended that studies addressing return to sport adopt the consensus-based return to sport continuum [10] to capture the richness of the data illustrating that not all players will quickly return to their pre-injury level of performance. For example, studies of return to sport following hip arthroscopy have shown only 17–20% of subjects subjectively rate a return to the pre-injury level of sports performance [20, 21] with higher levels (55%) reported following ACL repair [22]. In basketball, there is a reduced performance level up to two seasons post Achilles tendon rupture [23].

To our knowledge, no cricket-specific study has reported a return to performance timeframes following a return to sport after injury. In the case of a cricket fast bowler, in addition to self-report, quantifying return to performance would require a combination of metrics including average and maximum ball speed, resilience to appropriate bowling volumes, accuracy, wickets and the ability to bowl variations as required. Ideally, this would be compared against pre-existing data on the same player or based on a comparison with their peers.

13.9 Summary

This chapter has described some cricket-specific considerations in the return to play process. The examples of the lumbar spine and shoulder injuries illustrate the use of time frames and transition criteria in assessing when a player is ready to progress and return to play. It is important to appreciate that a full return to play requires collaboration between multiple stakeholders to ensure that the player is exposed to adequate loading for the demands of the game (bowling and throwing in the examples provided) but in a progressive and controlled manner.

References

1. Bitchell CL, Varley-Campbell J, Robinson G, Stiles V, Mathema P, Moore IS. Recurrent and subsequent injuries in professional and elite sport: a systematic review. Sports Med Open. 2020;6(1):58. https://doi.org/10.1186/s40798-020-00286-3.
2. Goggins L, Peirce N, Stokes K, Williams S. Negative association between injuries and team success in professional cricket: a 9-year prospective cohort analysis. J Sci Med Sport. 2021;24(2):141–5. https://doi.org/10.1016/j.jsams.2020.07.007.
3. Orchard JW, Inge P, Sims K, Kountouris A, Saw AE, Saw R, et al. Comparison of injury profiles between elite Australian male and female cricket players. J Sci Med Sport. 2023;26(1):19–24. https://doi.org/10.1016/j.jsams.2022.12.002.
4. de Visser HM, Reijman M, Heijboer MP, Bos PK. Risk factors of recurrent hamstring injuries: a systematic review. Br J Sports Med. 2012;46(2):124–30. https://doi.org/10.1136/bjsports-2011-090317.
5. Singh SP, Rotstein AH, Saw AE, Saw R, Kountouris A, James T. Radiological healing of lumbar spine stress fractures in elite cricket fast bowlers. J Sci Med Sport. 2021;24(2):112–5. https://doi.org/10.1016/j.jsams.2020.06.018.
6. Sakai T, Tezuka F, Yamashita K, Takata Y, Higashino K, Nagamachi A, et al. Conservative treatment for bony healing in pediatric lumbar spondylolysis. Spine (Phila Pa 1976). 2017;42(12):E716–e20. https://doi.org/10.1097/brs.0000000000001931.
7. Ekstrand J, Lundqvist D, Davison M, D'Hooghe M, Pensgaard AM. Communication quality between the medical team and the head coach/manager is associated with injury burden and player availability in elite football clubs. Br J Sports Med. 2019;53(5):304–8. https://doi.org/10.1136/bjsports-2018-099411.
8. Grindem H, Snyder-Mackler L, Moksnes H, Engebretsen L, Risberg MA. Simple decision rules can reduce reinjury risk by 84% after ACL reconstruction: the Delaware-Oslo ACL cohort study. Br J Sports Med. 2016;50(13):804–8. https://doi.org/10.1136/bjsports-2016-096031.
9. Taberner M, Spencer N, Murphy B, Antflick J, Cohen DD. Progressing on-court rehabilitation after injury: the control-chaos continuum adapted to basketball. J Orthop Sports Phys Ther. 2023;53(9):498–509. https://doi.org/10.2519/jospt.2023.11981.
10. Ardern CL, Glasgow P, Schneiders A, Witvrouw E, Clarsen B, Cools A, et al. 2016 consensus statement on return to sport from the first world congress in sports physical therapy, Bern. Br J Sports Med. 2016;50(14):853–64. https://doi.org/10.1136/bjsports-2016-096278.
11. Dijkstra HP, Pollock N, Chakraverty R, Ardern CL. Return to play in elite sport: a shared decision-making process. Br J Sports Med. 2017;51(5):419–20. https://doi.org/10.1136/bjsports-2016-096209.

12. McCall A, Lewin C, O'Driscoll G, Witvrouw E, Ardern C. Return to play: the challenge of balancing research and practice. Br J Sports Med. 2017;51(9):702–3. https://doi.org/10.1136/bjsports-2016-096752.
13. Taberner M, Allen T, Cohen DD. Progressing rehabilitation after injury: consider the 'control-chaos continuum'. Br J Sports Med. 2019;53(18):1132–6. https://doi.org/10.1136/bjsports-2018-100157.
14. Glazer DD. Development and preliminary validation of the injury-psychological readiness to return to sport (I-PRRS) scale. J Athl Train. 2009;44(2):185–9. https://doi.org/10.4085/1062-6050-44.2.185.
15. Orchard JW, Saw R, Kountouris A, Redrup D, Farhart P, Sims K. Management of lumbar bone stress injury in cricket fast bowlers and other athletes. S Afr J Sports Med. 2023;35(1):1–6. https://doi.org/10.17159/2078-516x/2023/v35i1a15172.
16. Alway P, Peirce N, Johnson W, King M, Kerslake R, Brooke-Wavell K. Activity specific areal bone mineral density is reduced in athletes with stress fracture and requires profound recovery time: a study of lumbar stress fracture in elite cricket fast bowlers. J Sci Med Sport. 2022;25(10):828–33. https://doi.org/10.1016/j.jsams.2022.08.006.
17. Kountouris ASK, Beakley D, et al. MRI bone marrow oedema precedes lumbar bone stress injury diagnosis in junior elite cricket fast bowlers. Br J Sports Med. 2019:1236–9.
18. Hulin B, Gabbett T, Blanch P, Chapman P, Bailey D, Orchard J. Spikes in acute workload are associated with increased injury risk in elite cricket fast bowlers. Br J Sports Med. 2014;48:708–12.
19. Raysmith BP, Drew MK. Performance success or failure is influenced by weeks lost to injury and illness in elite Australian track and field athletes: a 5-year prospective study. J Sci Med Sport. 2016;19(10):778–83. https://doi.org/10.1016/j.jsams.2015.12.515.
20. Wörner T, Thorborg K, Stålman A, Webster KE, Momatz Olsson H, Eek F. High or low return to sport rates following hip arthroscopy is a matter of definition? Br J Sports Med. 2018;52(22):1475–6. https://doi.org/10.1136/bjsports-2018-099154.
21. Ishoi L, Thorborg K, Kraemer O, Holmich P. Return to sport and performance after hip arthroscopy for femoroacetabular impingement in 18-to 30-year-old athletes a cross-sectional cohort study of 189 athletes. Am J Sports Med. 2018;46(11):2578–87. https://doi.org/10.1177/0363546518789070.
22. Ardern CL, Taylor NF, Feller JA, Webster KE. Fifty-five per cent return to competitive sport following anterior cruciate ligament reconstruction surgery: an updated systematic review and meta-analysis including aspects of physical functioning and contextual factors. Br J Sports Med. 2014;48(21):1543–U46. https://doi.org/10.1136/bjsports-2013-093398.
23. Amin NH, Old AB, Tabb LP, Garg R, Toossi N, Cerynik DL. Performance outcomes after repair of complete achilles tendon ruptures in national basketball association players. Am J Sports Med. 2013;41(8):1864–8. https://doi.org/10.1177/0363546513490659.

14 Nutrition for Cricket Performance, Recovery and Injury/Illness Prevention

Michelle Cort, Ananya Somani Kanoria, Robert Naughton, and Bethanie Allanson

14.1 Introduction

Nutrition plays an integral role in the development, performance, injury risk, health and well-being of cricket players. Nutrition strategies should be individualised for each player and adjusted over time. A player's nutrition plan should vary based on numerous factors, including age and stage of development, training and match workload, physiological parameters, body composition goals, micronutrient status, injury status, role in the team, environmental conditions and match format.

M. Cort (✉)
Cricket Australia, National Cricket Centre, Brisbane, QLD, Australia
e-mail: Michelle.cort@cricket.com.au

A. S. Kanoria
Ananya Somani Nutrition, Mumbai, India

Indian Rugby Football Union, Mumbai, India

RxDX Healthcare, Bengaluru, India

R. Naughton
The England and Wales Cricket Board Lord's Cricket Ground London, London, UK
e-mail: Robert.Naughton@ecb.co.uk

B. Allanson
Western Australian Cricket Association, WACA Ground, East Perth, WA, Australia

Western Australian Institute of Sport, Perth, WA, Australia
e-mail: beth.allanson@wacricket.com.au

From a performance perspective, nutrition can impact the execution of cricket skills, a player's ability to effectively manage the physical load of extended periods of play and training, and the significant cognitive component of the sport. From an injury perspective, nutrition plays a role in both reducing risk and rehabilitation. It is important that sports nutrition research relevant to cricket is conveyed to players by an accredited sports dietitian/nutritionist in practical terms so that their performance, development and health are maximised. The role of the accredited sports dietitian/nutritionist is also important for preventing anti-doping outcomes that may occur due to inappropriate or high-risk supplement use.

14.2 Physiological Demands of Cricket

Cricket requires physical fitness, athleticism, technical skills and concentration. A player's nutrition strategies need to support all of these factors [1]. A player's workload will be unique to each training session and match. As such a player's nutrition plan should be adapted from day to day in order to meet these varying demands.

Workload data is commonly measured in training sessions and matches with elite and sub-elite cricket players (e.g. distance covered, time spent at different speeds, balls bowled). This data

B. Olivier, J. W. Orchard (eds.), *Cricket Sports Medicine*,
https://doi.org/10.1007/978-981-96-6321-7_14

provides valuable information to the sports nutrition professional when developing an individual player's nutrition plan.

In general, players cover more distance and undertake a greater number of repeated high-speed sprints during multi-day matches, whereas the shorter T20 formats demand more explosive power, speed, agility and a faster reaction time [2, 3].

Fast bowlers have the most physically challenging role, with repeated high-intensity bursts of acceleration and deceleration. They typically cover the most sprints per hour compared to other players across all formats of the game [4]. Nutritionally ensuring fast bowlers consume adequate fuel along with nutrients for recovery and muscle repair is a focus. Meanwhile, spin bowlers usually have less strenuous innings, covering lesser distances with fewer sprints [4].

Batters have a variable workload across matches based on the duration and intensity of their innings. Their nutrition requirements in matches will be dictated in part by these factors.

Wicketkeepers tend to have a higher workload in longer formats of the game, whilst in shorter formats, the intensity of their sprints can be increased [4]. An emphasis on fuelling and hydration especially during the longer formats is critical to performance.

Strength and power can benefit the performance of all players [2]. A player's nutrition can play a direct role in assisting strength gains and strength maintenance, when combined with an appropriate strength training program.

14.3 Physical Characteristics of Cricket Players

According to available literature, there is currently no optimal standard for the physical characteristics of a cricket player.

Anthropometric data indicates that male batters tend to be smaller and lighter than fast bowlers, who tend to be taller and heavier [4]. A similar trend has been reported amongst female cricket players [5]. However, one study found no difference in height between international male batters and bowlers, and the batters were actually heavier [2]. This highlights the earlier point that the 'optimal' physical characteristics of a player are difficult to define.

In terms of body fat, an average range of 12–14% of body fat has been reported among male batsmen and bowlers [2, 4]. Similarly, another study reported no significant difference in the sum of eight skinfold measurements in female cricket players across different roles in the team [5]. This data suggests that whilst the different roles can have varying physical demands in matches, body composition (in terms of body fat) may be similar across a team. There is currently no available data in the literature that reports on the lean muscle mass of cricket players.

Given a cricket team is made up of individuals with varying roles, physical demands, training status and injury history, it is dependent on high-performance staff working with individual players to identify what the most appropriate (modifiable) body composition is for their performance, health and (minimising) injury risk.

14.4 Training and Match Day Nutrition

As highlighted in the previous section, it is important to prescribe nutrition recommendations not just on format, but on player role within the game. Furthermore, even within the same format—nutrition, mainly carbohydrate, intake will be periodised in line with the day-to-day changes in physical load, i.e. match day vs rest day.

14.5 Macronutrients

Currently, there are no cricket-specific nutrition guidelines, so practitioners must look to the wider sport nutrition literature for guidance [6, 7].

14.5.1 Carbohydrate

Carbohydrates are the key to fuelling athletes, and this is no different in cricket. As previously

Table 14.1 Carbohydrate requirements in preparation for and during match play [9]

Format	Carbohydrate intake pre-play	Carbohydrate intake during play
Multi-day	6–10 g/kg BM	30–60 g/h
50 over/one day	4–8 g/kg BM	30–60 g/h
T20	3–6 g/kg BM	Small amounts (<30 g/h)
Training	3–8 g/kg BM	0–60 g/h

discussed, cricket is an intermittent sport, which involves actions of high-intensity with low-intensity movement—carbohydrates are necessary to support those high-intensity actions, such as bowling, running between wickets and chasing down a ball in the field. Carbohydrate (once digested into one of its components—glucose) is also the brain's primary energy source and is essential for optimal cognitive function.

For all formats, it is recommended that the consumption of carbohydrates be prioritised. How much and timings of carbohydrate intake are dependent on format, player role and workload during a match. For multi-day and one-day games, it is advisable to consume some carbohydrates in meals and snacks in the ~24 hours before the game. For T20, the shortest format of the game, carbohydrate requirements are reduced, and the focus on carbohydrate consumption can be on the ~12 hours before the game. There is no need for carbohydrate load for a cricket match.

Based on literature for other sports, estimated carbohydrate requirements are provided in Table 14.1 [9]. Fast bowlers, when undertaking a heavy workload, or batters when undertaking a long innings, should be at the higher end of the recommended ranges.

Some players with very high workloads (or those who have difficulty eating meals/snacks during matches) may need to utilise specially formulated sports foods (such as carbohydrate gels or carbohydrate sports drinks) to meet carbohydrate requirements. These products are easily digestible and, along with providing fuel for working muscles, can also provide a mouth-sensing benefit to the brain and central nervous system [8].

14.5.2 Protein

Protein plays a vital role in the maintenance and adaptation of skeletal muscle (lean muscle mass). Current recommendations advise a daily intake of 1.3–1.8 g/kg BM-1 [6]. Though, in cases of energy restriction (i.e. when losing body fat) or abrupt inactivity due to injury, an intake of 2 g/kg BM is advised to minimise any losses of muscle mass.

14.5.3 Fat

Dietary fat provides a valuable energy source and plays a vital role in general health. Unlike carbohydrate and protein, there is not a relative body mass recommendation for dietary fat intake. Rather, typical recommendations are provided as a percentage of total energy intake, with this value generally given at 20–30%. However, this may depend on individual training goals.

14.6 Vitamins and Minerals

When assessing micronutrient requirements, it is advisable to test players for current micronutrient status before making a specific intervention. Generally, single micronutrient supplementation is only required for the correction of a clinically specified medical reason, such as deficiency of a particular micronutrient [7]. Whilst all vitamins and minerals have an important role to play in the health of cricketers, there are three that require highlighting—iron, calcium, and vitamin D (Table 14.2).

Table 14.2 Selected micronutrient role and requirements [10]

Vitamin	Role	Daily required intake
Iron	Important for oxygen transport around the body	Male (19+)—8 mg
		Female (19–50)—18 mg
Calcium	Important for bone health, development and maintenance	Adults—1000 mg
		Adolescents—1200 mg
Vitamin D	Important to maintain serum calcium concentrations	5.0 μg/day

Table 14.3 Recovery recommendations [6–8]

	Carbohydrate	Protein	Fluid
Multi-day	1–1.2 g/kg/h for the first 4 hours	0.24–0.31 g/kg BM	1.5 x per kg lost with ~25 mmol/L sodium
50 over/one day	1–4 g/kg BM		
T20	1–4 g/kg BM		

14.7 Recovery

Whilst recovery is always important, the format of the match and specific player workload must be taken into consideration. For example, prioritised recovery in the multi-day format is extremely important as players must be ready to perform again the following day, and recovery nutrition strategies should start immediately following the close of play (or at the end of a batter's innings). Whereas the workload in T20 format is typically much lighter, and where back-to-back matches may not be played, recovery nutrition strategies can usually be incorporated into standard meals and snacks.

For recovery, a simple approach is to consider the three R's—Refuel, Repair and Rehydrate. Ensuring these are addressed in the first couple of hours after the end of the days, play/match will go a long way toward ensuring a player is ready to train or play as soon as possible.

Table 14.3 indicates the amount of carbohydrate, protein, fluid and sodium recommended for recovery purposes [6–8].

14.8 Hydration

Maintaining fluid balance can be challenging for players, especially when training or playing in the heat. If significant dehydration occurs, physical and mental performance, along with temperature regulation, is negatively impacted [9]. As dehydration progresses, especially in warm conditions, the risk of heat stress and serious health effects increases.

The opportunity to consume fluids during matches is governed by the ICC playing conditions. Drink intervals are prescribed at specific times for each of the three different match formats; however, an individual player may be given a drink at the fall of a wicket on the field, provided that no playing time is wasted.

14.8.1 Dehydration and Cricket Performance

Hydration has been researched extensively across a range of team sports and indicates that hypohydration impairs cognition, technical skill, and physical performance at around (3–4% body weight loss) [11, 12].

There have been several studies that have investigated hydration in cricket. One investigated the impact of dehydration on the performance of batters, bowlers and fielders [13] whilst playing in hot, humid conditions. Dehydration at levels of 3.7% (body mass loss) significantly impaired motor skill performance in all roles. The reduction in performance included the following:

- Fast bowlers—decreased bowling speed and line accuracy.
- Fielders—decreased overarm and sidearm throwing speed and accuracy.
- Batters—a reduction in speed when undertaking three runs.

Similarly, a study investigating motor skill performance of cricket bowling [14] found that bowling accuracy (line and distance) was impaired when subjects were dehydrated to 2.8% of body weight.

Whilst there are no cricket-specific studies assessing the impact of dehydration on concentration, decision making and reaction time, extrapolation of other sports research indicates that all of these parameters will be negatively impacted at levels of dehydration as low as 1% body weight loss [15].

14.8.2 Individualised Requirements

Sweat losses and fluid balance in cricket players are dependent on many factors, including environmental conditions, length of innings, workloads, duration of matches, rules regulating fluid intake, cricket uniforms and protective equipment, and the physiological characteristics of each player.

As shown in Table 14.4, player sweat rates vary considerably [13, 17–19], as do the fluid intake habits [16]. As such, the level of hypohydration (and, in turn, the impact on performance) that occurs in players can also vary substantially.

Given this, generalised fluid guidelines for cricket players are of little use. Individualised hydration plans should be developed for each player using a variety of information (e.g. individual player sweat rate, sweat sodium concentration, flavour preference and fuel requirements).

14.8.3 Practical Measures of Hydration Status

Before training or a match, on-waking urine specific gravity (USG) can provide a measure of a player's hydration status. If the equipment required for this isn't available, using a combination of urine colour, urinary volume and body weight (on waking) can assist in providing a more subjective assessment.

Body weight change in a training session, innings or match day can help to estimate the mismatch between fluid lost as sweat and fluid intake. This value can then be used to estimate rehydration volumes for players by replacing 1.5 litres of fluid for every litre/kilogram lost [20].

14.8.4 Fluid Options

Water can be a suitable choice for players in training and matches. However, a flavoured drink is often the preferred choice, given players are more likely to consume fluid if they enjoy the taste. When fluid needs are high, a player will often vary their drink throughout a match to avoid 'flavour fatigue'.

If a player has high fuel needs, a sports drink (containing 6–7% carbohydrate) can help to meet

Table 14.4 Sweat rates of cricket players [13, 17–19]

Author	Sweat rate	Environment	Subjects and setting
Gamage 2016	1208 ± 171 ml/h	30.8 ± 2.1 °C and 76 ± 9% RH	Elite male bowlers, batters, & fielders; outdoor field trials
	861 ± 148 ml/h	30.1 ± 2.1 °C; 77 ± 8% RH	
Soo 2007	300 ± 310 – 1440 ± 1250 ml/h	21.9–30.3 °C, 30–48% RH	Elite females; international competition
Bray 2007	0.73–0.93 kg/h	22.9 °C ± 1.1, 53.1% ± 7RH	Fast bowlers in match
	0.2 kg/h	20.6 °C ± 1.1, 39.5% ± 1.9 RH	Fast bowlers in training
Gore 1993	0.7 kg/h	22.2–27.1 WBGT	Fast bowlers match conditions

both fluid and fuel requirements. And when fast rehydration is required, a player should take advantage of high electrolyte-containing drinks or consume fluids when eating high-sodium foods/meals. The presence of sodium significantly improves post-exercise rehydration through its impact on fluid retention [21].

14.8.5 Cramping

Research supporting the theory that dehydration and electrolyte loss is a major cause of exercise-associated muscle cramps (EAMCs) is lacking [22]. The cause(s) of EAMCs remain unknown; however, it is likely that the cause is multifactorial and unique to each player [23]. Muscle fatigue is the one factor that nearly all studies in this area have identified as a contributing factor [22].

14.8.6 Overlap With Illness

Partially because substitutions for illness are not permitted in multi-day games, it is more likely in cricket than in some other sports that players might elect to continue to play if suffering from a gastrointestinal virus. This might tend to push them towards increasing dehydration in hot conditions. Additional emphasis on rehydration is required in these circumstances. It is important to note that the WADA code does not permit intravenous rehydration at either cricket grounds or hotel rooms. If a player is admitted to a hospital facility, intravenous rehydration can be used in the scenario of severe dehydration without breaching the WADA code.

14.9 Injury

Nutrition can play a significant role in both injury prevention and rehabilitation. Whilst injury can be inevitable at times, poor nutritional status can impede healing and recovery from injury.

14.9.1 Nutrition and Bone Health

Lumbar stress fractures are one of the most severe injury types in cricket, most commonly occurring in young fast bowlers

- *Maximising bone health and minimising fracture risk.*
  - Bone is a nutritionally modifiable, and dietary intake can have a significant influence on a player's bone health.
  - There are several nutrition considerations for optimising bone health, including ensuring adequate energy intake and meeting protein, calcium, magnesium, phosphorus, potassium and vitamin D requirements [24]. Meeting these nutrient requirements is especially important in young fast bowlers who are particularly susceptible to bone-related injuries such as lumbar stress fractures.
- *Calcium.*
  - Calcium is an essential element that is critical for skeletal mineralisation. It is the major component of bone and provides strength and structure. Dietary interventions relating to the amount and timing of calcium intake can be utilised to optimise bone health for players.
  - Whilst a daily calcium intake of 1000–1200 mg [10] is important, several research studies have shown that strategically consuming a calcium rich meal before exercise can lower markers of bone resorption during and after exercise. Integrating this practical strategy into a cricket player's individual nutrition plan can help to safeguard long-term bone health and reduce the risk of bone stress injuries [25–27].
- *Vitamin D.*
  - One of the key functions of vitamin D is to increase the absorption of calcium from the intestine, making it essential for skeletal health. It is almost impossible to obtain sufficient vitamin D from dietary sources alone.

- Cricket players at risk of vitamin D deficiency include those with naturally dark skin pigmentation and those with limited sun exposure (due to geography and season, weather conditions, indoor training environments, use of suncream/clothing that covers most of the body (i.e. cricket apparel)). It is recommended that these at-risk players should have their vitamin D status assessed via a blood test, and supplementation considered if levels are found to be low.

- *Energy Availability.*
  - Energy availability (EA) is the amount of dietary energy available to sustain physiological function after accounting for the energy cost of exercise. Maintaining energy availability can be challenging if energy output is increased (increased training or match workload), energy intake is reduced (e.g. reduced appetite, deliberate restriction) or both.
  - Low energy availability disrupts endocrine function and can negatively impact bone mineral density, increasing the risk of bone-related injuries [24]. Professional nutrition input should be sought for any player thought to be at risk of low EA.
- *Protein Intake.*
  - Bone mineral density is also positively associated with total protein intake. Several studies have shown that fracture risk may be lessened with a higher protein intake, providing calcium intake is also sufficient [28, 29].
- *Bone Fracture Healing.*
  - Sub-optimal calcium intake, low vitamin D levels and/or low energy availability will delay fracture healing.
  - It is essential that players are consistently consuming adequate energy during the bone healing period. Medical and sports nutrition professionals should also advise the player on whether supplementation with calcium and vitamin D is required [24, 30].

14.9.2 Soft Tissue Injuries

Most soft tissue injuries have two main stages—immobilisation and rehabilitation—both of which can be influenced by nutrition.

- *Immobilisation, Tissue Repair and Atrophy.*
  - *Protein and Energy:*
  - During the acute immobilisation period, energy requirements are often increased to assist with the healing process. It is important that players are not overly restricting energy intake at this time, as healing can be compromised. Any reduction in energy intake (with the goal of minimising body fat gain during this period of lower activity) should be well planned with the input of a nutrition professional.
  - Immobilisation (of any limb) reduces resting muscle protein synthesis and causes anabolic resistance to dietary protein intake. This, in turn, causes muscle tissue atrophy [29]. Players should ensure optimal protein intake (type, timing and amount) to minimise the loss of strength and lean muscle mass and to promote repair of the damaged tissue [31, 32]. Spreading dietary protein intake across the day provides a consistent stimulus for protein synthesis [32]. This is something many athletes, including cricket players, fail to do as the majority of protein tends to be consumed at the evening meal.
  - It is also important to note that sub-optimal protein and energy intake worsen the inflammatory response and slow down healing [32].
  - *Other Considerations:*
  - Creatine supplementation can assist in limiting muscle loss and/or helping to recover from the muscle atrophy caused by disuse and immobilisation [33, 34].
  - Omega-3 polyunsaturated fatty acids have the potential to enhance muscle regeneration by decreasing inflammation post-injury and limiting any reduction in muscle protein synthesis during periods of immobilisation. Consumption via food

sources (primarily oily fish) or supplementation should be considered [35].

- *Rehabilitation and Hypertrophy.*
- Following immobility, the primary nutrition goal will be to support muscle growth and increased strength.

  – *Protein & Energy:*
  – Muscle protein synthesis and remodelling require a significant amount of energy, and as such, energy requirements of the injured player will be increased during rehabilitation [31, 32].
  – The increase in energy should be met by ingestion of both carbohydrates and proteins. Carbohydrates will fuel any increased activity associated with the rehabilitation plan. When it is co-ingested with protein, carbohydrates will also stimulate insulin, improving net protein balance and muscle protein synthesis [36].
  – *Other Considerations:*
  – An increased intake of omega-3 fatty acids via consumption of oily fish or supplementation is also a consideration during the rehabilitation phase. These fatty acids are linked to enhanced rates of muscle protein synthesis and decreased expression of factors that regulate muscle protein breakdown [35].

14.10 Travel Considerations for Cricket

Most cricket players undertake travel for competition. Nutrition is one aspect of travel, which requires careful planning before leaving home to ensure performance and health aren't negatively impacted.

Nutrition considerations for travel include the following:

- Jet lag management.
- Training and match schedule.
- Accommodation—meal purchase, preparation and/or storage options.
- Food and drinks availability at the destination.
- Hygiene issues.
- Environmental conditions.
- Training and match venue facilities and food provision.

Minimising Jet Lag:

During travel, players should drink sufficient fluid to stay hydrated, and (where possible) eat meals at the mealtime of their destination. Once arrived (at the destination), caffeine should be avoided in the afternoon and evening and meals should be consumed at the usual time of the day.

Risk Minimisation:

Travel can increase the risk of a player being unable to meet their nutrition goals or developing an illness. One strategy that is useful for players and staff to undertake prior to departure is a travel nutrition 'risk management audit'. This will help to mitigate any nutrition-related issues that could impact performance or illness risk.

The audit lists down issues that could impact successful performance at the destination. Each 'risk' requires an associated risk management strategy. Table 14.5 shows an example of the audit process [37].

14.10.1 Illness Prevention

Gastrointestinal infections when travelling can often be food- and fluid-borne. Education of players, coaches and staff before travel is required to ensure high-risk items are avoided in high-risk locations (e.g. avoid local water, salads and peeled fruit). Probiotics and prebiotic consumption both before departure and during the travel period can assist in minimising the risk of specific infections [38].

Another important practical strategy to consider is monitoring the temperature (using a food thermometer) of meals served, especially where food is served as a buffet at training and match venues. It is necessary to avoid meals that are served between 6 and 60 °C, as food-poisoning bacteria can multiply to unsafe numbers in this temperature zone.

Table 14.5 Example of a travel nutrition risk management audit

Risk	Risk management strategy in place	Further strategy development required?	Level of risk	Level of risk with strategy in place
Example: Unknown food supply on long haul flight	Contact airline to discuss meal and snacks provided on flight	Plan to take own snacks on board if airline cannot provide special meal, or if unexpected changes occur to meal provision	Moderate	Low

The COVID-19 pandemic has provided additional education on the different types of spread of bacterial and viral disease and the subtle differences between mitigation of each transmission type, with the preference that preventive measures are taken against all types of infectious disease spread:

1. Food-borne transmission—cooking to high temperatures and/or refrigerating food until just prior to either eating or cooking mitigates against food poisoning.
2. Fomite spread—regular hand-washing and sanitising and the use of gloves when handling food mitigates against transmission.
3. Aerosol spread—masking in crowded indoor environments (such as during flights) and isolation of individuals with respiratory symptoms mitigates against transmission.

14.10.2 Additional Food Supplies

Packing a supply of food and sports foods from home will be useful if the food supply (type, quality, safety) is unknown, the player is a fussy eater, or if they rely on specific products around training sessions and matches.

14.11 Supplements in Cricket

Supplement use is widespread at all levels of sport, and cricket is no exception. Sports foods and supplements can play a small but important role when integrated into a player's individualised sports nutrition plan.

However, some supplements also have the potential to be harmful to a player's health and/or performance. Additionally, players need to be aware of the anti-doping risks of using supplements. Expert advice from an accredited sports dietitian/nutritionist and/or sports physician should be sought by players before consuming supplements. The following questions must be addressed to ensure an informed decision is made:

- Is the product effective?
- Is the product safe?
- Is the product permitted for use in the sport?
- Is the product appropriate to the players' age and development in cricket?

14.11.1 Anti-doping

A risk of using sports supplements is that they can contain prohibited substances that result in an anti-doping rule violation (ADRV). Issues that can increase the risk of anti-doping in a player include (but are not limited to): the false belief that supplements claiming to be 'natural' are fine to use, ingredients contained in the product not all being listed on the label (either by design or via contamination during manufacture), influence from those with questionable understanding of supplements, and confusing scientific names of ingredients on the product label.

It is difficult to know how many sports supplement products contain ingredients not listed on the product label. A 2016 survey conducted by the international doping laboratory LGC in Australia revealed that 19% of products tested contained substances banned in sport [39]. Another study found that ~15% of more than 600 products from around the world contained prohormone ingredients that were not declared on the label [40].

At least one professional cricket player has tested positive for a banned substance from this scenario. The player consumed a supplement that was proven to be contaminated (with a banned substance) during the manufacturing process. The player was subsequently banned from playing for a period of time.

The use of third-party batch analysis of supplements is one method that can be used by players to identify products that are at low risk of containing banned ingredients. However, this isn't an absolute guarantee.

Cricket players and support personnel should be familiar with the anti-doping codes that govern the sport. Players should also consult with their accredited sports dietitian/nutritionist and/or sports physician to help mitigate anti-doping risks associated with sports supplement use.

References

1. Noakes TD, Durandt J. Physiological requirements of cricket. J Sports Sci. 2000;18(12):919–29. https://doi.org/10.1080/026404100446739.
2. Weldon A, Clarke ND, Pote L, Bishop C. Physical profiling of international cricket players: an investigation between bowlers and batters. Biol Sport [Internet]. 2021;38(4):507–15. https://doi.org/10.5114/biolsport.2021.100148.
3. Biswas S, Bhattacharya R, Das A. Physical characteristics, movement pattern, and heart rate response of Indian cricketers during batting in Twenty20 (T20) matches. Int J Exerc Sci. 2023;16(6):1413–25.
4. Rosimus C. A review of the physical demands, physiological profile and the role of nutrition in cricket. EC Nutr. 2019;14(1):14–24.
5. Brazier TA, Tallent J, Patterson SD, Howe LP, Callaghan SJ. The physical profile of female cricketers: an investigation between playing standard and position. PLoS One [Internet]. 2024;19(6) https://doi.org/10.1371/journal.pone.0302647.
6. Phillips SM, Van Loon LJ. Dietary protein for athletes: from requirements to optimum adaptation. In: Nutrient reference values [Internet]; 2011. https://doi.org/10.1080/02640414.2011.619204.
7. Thomas DT, Erdman KA, Burke LM. Nutrition and athletic performance. Med Sci Sports Exerc. 2016;48(3):543–68. https://doi.org/10.1249/MSS.0000000000000852.
8. Burke LM, Maughan RJ. The governor has a sweet tooth – mouth sensing of nutrients to enhance sports performance. Eur J Sport Sci. 2015;15(1):29–40. https://doi.org/10.1080/17461391.2014.971880.
9. Burke LM, Hawley JA, Wong SH, Jeukendrup AE. Carbohydrates for training and competition. J Sports Sci. 2011;29(Suppl):1–27. https://doi.org/10.1080/02640414.2011.585473.
10. Eat for Health [Internet]. Available from: https://www.eatforhealth.gov.au/nutrient-reference-values
11. Burke LM, Hawley JA. Fluid balance in team sports. Guidelines for optimal practices. Sports Med. 1997;24(1):1–10. https://doi.org/10.2165/00007256-199724010-00004.
12. Nuccio RP, Barnes KA, Carter JM, Baker LB. Fluid balance in team sport athletes and the effect of hypohydration on cognitive, technical, and physical performance. Sports Med. 2017;47:1951–82. https://doi.org/10.1007/s40279-017-0738-7.
13. Gamage JP, De Silva AP, Nalliah AK, Galloway SD. Effects of dehydration on cricket specific skill performance in hot and humid conditions. Int J Sport Nutr Exerc Metab. 2016;26(6):531–41. https://doi.org/10.1123/ijsnem.2016-0015.
14. Devlin LH, Fraser SF, Barras NS, Hawley JA. Moderate levels of hypohydration impair bowling accuracy but not bowling velocity in skilled cricket players. J Sci Med Sport. 2001;4(2):179–87. https://doi.org/10.1016/s1440-2440(01)80028-1.
15. Lieberman HR. Hydration and cognition: a critical review and recommendations for future research. J Am Coll Nutr. 2007;26(5 Suppl):555S–61S. https://doi.org/10.1080/07315724.2007.10719658.
16. Garth AK, Burke LM. What do athletes drink during competitive sporting activities? Sports Med. 2013;43:539–64. https://doi.org/10.1007/s40279-013-0028-y.
17. Soo K, Naughton G. The hydration profile of female cricket players during competition. Int J Sport Nutr Exerc Metab. 2007;17(1):14–26. https://doi.org/10.1123/ijsnem.17.1.14.
18. Bray JW. The sweating response, body weight changes and voluntary fluid intakes during training and competition of fast bowlers: a case study [dissertation]. Chester: University of Chester; 2024. Available from: http://hdl.handle.net/10034/10915
19. Gore CJ, Bourdon PC, Woolford SM, Pederson DG. Involuntary dehydration during cricket. Int J Sports Med. 1993;14(7):387–95. https://doi.org/10.1055/s-2007-1021197.
20. Shirreffs SM, Maughan RJ. Volume repletion after exercise-induced volume depletion in humans: replacement of water and sodium losses. Am J Phys. 1998;274(5):75. https://doi.org/10.1152/ajprenal.1998.274.5.F868.
21. Shirreffs SM, Sawka MN. Fluid and electrolyte needs for training, competition, and recovery. J Sports Sci. 2011;29(Suppl):1–46. https://doi.org/10.1080/02640414.2011.614269.
22. Braulick KW, Miller KC, Albrecht JM, Tucker JM, Deal JE. Significant and serious dehydration does not affect skeletal muscle cramp threshold frequency. Br J Sports Med. 2013;47(11):710–4. https://doi.org/10.1136/bjsports-2012-091501.

23. Miller KC. Rethinking the cause of exercise-associated muscle cramping: moving beyond dehydration and electrolyte losses. Curr Sports Med Rep. 2015;14(5):353–4. https://doi.org/10.1249/JSR.0000000000000183.
24. Sale C, Elliott Sale KJ. Nutrition and athlete bone health. Sports Med. 2019;49(Suppl 2):51. https://doi.org/10.1007/s40279-019-01161-2.
25. Barry DW, Hansen KC, van Pelt RE, Witten M, Wolfe P, Kohrt WM. Acute calcium ingestion attenuates exercise-induced disruption of calcium homeostasis. Med Sci Sports Exerc. 2011;43(4):617–23. https://doi.org/10.1249/MSS.0b013e3181f79fa8.
26. Haakonssen EC, Ross ML, Knight EJ, Cato LE, Nana A, Wluka AE, et al. The effects of a calcium-rich pre-exercise meal on biomarkers of calcium homeostasis in competitive female cyclists: a randomized crossover trial. PLoS One. 2015;10(5):e0123302. https://doi.org/10.1371/journal.pone.0123302.
27. Lundy B, McKay AKA, Fensham NC, Tee N, Anderson B, Morabito A, et al. The impact of acute calcium intake on bone turnover markers during a training day in elite male rowers. Med Sci Sports Exerc. 2023;55(1):55–65. https://doi.org/10.1249/MSS.0000000000003022.
28. Mangano KM, Sahni S, Kerstetter JE. Dietary protein is beneficial to bone health under conditions of adequate calcium intake: an update on clinical research. Curr Opin Clin Nutr Metab Care. 2014;17(1):69–74. https://doi.org/10.1097/MCO.0000000000000013.
29. Wall BT, Snijders T, Senden JM, Ottenbros CL, Gijsen AP, Verdijk LB, van Loon LJ. Disuse impairs the muscle protein synthetic response to protein ingestion in healthy men. J Clin Endocrinol Metab. 2013;98(12):4872–81. https://doi.org/10.1210/jc.2013-2098.
30. Karpouzos A, Diamantis E, Farmaki P, Savvanis S, Troupis T. Nutritional aspects of bone health and fracture healing. J Osteoporos. 2017;2017:4218472. https://doi.org/10.1155/2017/4218472.
31. Close GL, Sale C, Baar K, Bermon S. Nutrition for the prevention and treatment of injuries in track and field athletes. Int J Sport Nutr Exerc Metab. 2019;29(2):189–97. https://doi.org/10.1123/ijsnem.2018-0290.
32. Tipton KD. Nutritional support for exercise-induced injuries. Sports Med. 2015;45(Suppl 1):93–104. https://doi.org/10.1007/s40279-015-0398-4.
33. Hespel P, Op't Eijnde B, Van Leemputte M, Urso B, Greenhaff PL, Labarque V, Richter EA. Oral creatine supplementation facilitates the rehabilitation of disuse atrophy and alters the expression of muscle myogenic factors in humans. J Physiol. 2001;536:625–33. https://doi.org/10.1111/j.1469-7793.2001.0625c.x.
34. Johnston AP, Burke DG, MacNeil LG, Candow DG. Effect of creatine supplementation during cast-induced immobilization on the preservation of muscle mass, strength, and endurance. J Strength Cond Res. 2009;23:116–20. https://doi.org/10.1519/JSC.0b013e31818efbcc.
35. Jannas-Vela S, Espinosa A, Candia AA, Flores-Opazo M, Peñailillo L, Valenzuela R. The role of omega-3 polyunsaturated fatty acids and their lipid mediators on skeletal muscle regeneration: a narrative review. Nutrients. 2023;15(4):871. https://doi.org/10.3390/nu15040871.
36. Morton RW, McGlory C, Phillips SM. Nutritional interventions to augment resistance training-induced skeletal muscle hypertrophy. Front Physiol. 2015;6:245. https://doi.org/10.3389/fphys.2015.00245.
37. Halson SL, Romyn G, Cort M, Driller M. Nutrition for sport exercise and performance. In: Travelling athletes. 2nd ed. Routledge; 2024. https://doi.org/10.4324/9781003321286-30.
38. Pyne DB, West NP, Cox AJ, Cripps AW. Probiotics supplementation for athletes – clinical and physiological effects. Eur J Sport Sci. 2014;15(1):63–72. https://doi.org/10.1080/17461391.2014.971879.
39. Limited LGC. Australian supplement survey 2016. LGC Limited; 2016.
40. Maughan RJ. Contamination of dietary supplements and positive drug tests in sport. J Sports Sci. 2005;23(9):883–9.

15 Recovery in Cricket: Practical Approaches for Optimising Performance and Preventing Injury

George Dunlop, Nimrat Grewal, and Simran Grewal

15.1 Introduction

In competitive cricket, where games might last several days and seasons are protracted and demanding, it is important to be fully recovered as quickly as possible to enable the athlete to perform at their highest possible level. Recovery techniques are regimes for restoring athlete's psychophysiological processes that occur in the body after a training load [1]. In cricket, recovery includes a wide range of exercises, intended to re-establish both physical and mental balance following the strenuous demands of practice and play. The process of recovering has several facets, including behavioural, psychological and physiological aspects. It is a multifaceted approach that incorporates restoration of structural, hormonal, neurological and psychological functions. The aim of prioritising recovery in cricket is essential for optimising performance and preventing injuries.

G. Dunlop (✉)
Department of Physiotherapy, Royal Dutch Cricket Association, Amstelveen, The Netherlands
e-mail: george@dunlop-fysio.nl

N. Grewal
Department of Cardiothoracic Surgery, Leiden University Medical Center, Leiden, The Netherlands

Department of Cardiothoracic Surgery, Amsterdam University Medical Center, Amsterdam, The Netherlands

Department of Anatomy and Embryology, Leiden University Medical Center, Leiden, The Netherlands
e-mail: n.grewal@amsterdamumc.nl

S. Grewal
Department of Orthopaedic Surgery, Shoulder and Elbow Unit, Onze Lieve Vrouwe Gasthuis (OLVG), Amsterdam, Netherlands
e-mail: s.k.grewal@olvg.nl

15.2 The Physiology of Recovery

Athletes subject their bodies to significant mechanical, metabolic and neural stress during cricket matches and training. This stress leads to acute changes in muscle tissue, energy stores and the nervous system. Exercise-induced tissue damage is characterised by breakdown of muscle fibres which causes an inflammatory response which consequently decreases an athlete's physical work capacity and sports performance [2]. Recovery after training and matches is therefore essential for the body's need to restore homeostasis, neuromuscular function, replenishing energy stores and promoting tissue repair [1].

15.2.1 The Autonomic Nervous System

The autonomic nervous system plays a crucial role in the recovery period, because it regulates respiration, metabolism and cardiovascular

B. Olivier, J. W. Orchard (eds.), *Cricket Sports Medicine*,
https://doi.org/10.1007/978-981-96-6321-7_15

function by balancing the sympathetic and parasympathetic nervous system. The sympathetic nervous system controls the 'fight or flight reaction', which is characterised by tachycardia, high adrenaline levels, increased cardiac output and bronchodilatation. However, after training, the parasympathetic nervous system needs to be activated to lower the heart rate, reduce blood pressure and enhance digestion and relaxation—all essential for an effective recovery [3]. The vagus nerve is a key player in promoting parasympathetic activity and can be activated by numerous interventions such as deep breathing exercises and cold water immersion.

15.2.2 Muscle Repair and Adaptation

Exercise-induced tissue damage is characterised by histopathological muscle tissue changes that originate from skeletal muscle damage. Following, the destruction of skeletal muscle fibres causes an inflammatory response that decreases the athlete's physical work capacity and sports performance [2]. Muscle recovery is a complex process involving the repair of microtears in muscle fibres, the replenishment of glycogen stores and the reduction of inflammation. The degree of muscle damage incurred during cricket depends on the intensity and duration of activity, as well as the specific actions performed (e.g. bowling, sprinting, throwing, batting). Effective muscle recovery not only alleviates soreness and stiffness but also promotes the adaptation process, where muscles become stronger and more resilient to future stress.

15.2.3 Energy System Replenishment

Nutrition aids recovery from training by refuelling the muscle and liver glycogen stores and replacing the fluid and electrolytes lost during sweat. Nutrition aids in manufacturing new muscle proteins and cellular components to aid in tissue repair.

15.3 Recovery Techniques in Cricket

Given the varied demands of cricket, a one-size-fits-all approach to recovery is insufficient. Instead, a comprehensive recovery programme should integrate multiple techniques tailored to the player's individual needs and the sport's specific demands. Recovery strategies can be classified into passive, active and proactive recovery [1, 4]. Passive recovery is the process in which the athlete is not actively participating, but recovers through external stimulations, active recovery involves participation through physical action, and proactive recovery involves self-initiated and social activities aimed at reducing psychological stress.

15.3.1 Passive Recovery

Passive recovery includes methods that do not require significant physical exertion and in which the body recovers through external stimulation. Important passive recovery strategies are sleep hygiene, massage and compression garments. Sleep has an adaptive and restorative function for both physiological processes and mental health [5, 6]. Several studies have shown a positive correlation between sleep and optimal performance, whereas compromised sleep quantity and quality have been shown to affect the neurologic-, immune- and endocrine systems adversely [7–10].

Massage therapy has shown positive results for reducing excessive post-exercise muscle tone, increasing muscle range of motion and increasing the circulation and nutrition to damaged tissues [11].

Compression garments work by applying graduated pressure to the limbs, which enhances venous return, reduces muscle oscillation and decreases the accumulation of metabolic waste products. Several studies have shown the positive effects of compression garments in post-match muscle soreness. Hydrotherapy and heat therapy help relax muscles and improve circulation.

The psychological demands of cricket can be as taxing as the physical ones. Mental recovery is essential for maintaining focus, motivation and overall well-being. Techniques such as mindfulness meditation, relaxation breathwork and visualisation can help players manage stress, reduce anxiety and improve sleep quality. Additionally, mental resilience training, which includes cognitive behavioural strategies and psychological skills training, can enhance a player's ability to cope with the pressures of high-level competition.

15.3.2 Active Recovery

Active recovery involves engaging in low-intensity exercise following a match or training session. Activities such as light jogging, swimming or yoga are ideal for increasing muscle length, reducing lactate concentrations, replenishing oxygen in the blood and supporting elevated circulation and ventilation [12]. Although the literature in this area remains inconclusive, several studies have shown positive effects of mobility exercises that focus on joint health, which is crucial for preventing overuse injuries common in cricket, such as tendonitis or stress fractures.

15.4 Measuring Recovery: Tools for Optimising Performance

An effective recovery strategy in sports, especially cricket, demands accurate monitoring of both workloads and recovery measures [13, 14]. To measure recovery, we often refer to measures of fatigue or neuromuscular fatigue (NMF). Managing fatigue is, therefore, key to ensuring athletes get the desired training adaptations, stay competition-ready and reduce the risk of injuries or illness [15].

Resources such as team budgets and skilled support staff play a significant role in analysing the data to make meaningful decisions about training and recovery. Below are a variety of options to measure recovery. Each needs to be combined with workload monitoring and assessed for team budget and practicality.

15.4.1 Subjective Recovery Measures

Subjective measures include self-reported assessments where players rate their perceived level of sleep, muscle soreness, stress, fatigue and readiness to train [16]. These measures can be used daily to monitor changes in recovery status, helping coaches and sports medicine professionals make informed decisions about training loads and recovery needs [16]. The greatest advantage of subjective measures is their cost-effectiveness. In order to be effective, player compliance needs to be high, driven by strong team culture as well as support staff and player feedback loops. There is an educational component of onboarding players and support staff, to understand wellness questions and scores, individual score variances (Z-scores) and forms of feedback that relate to meaningful performance related decisions.

15.4.2 Objective Recovery Measures

Continuous advances in technology are offering athletes, coaches and physicians deeper insights into recovery. However, with this wealth of information, we must determine which data holds real value (ie. reliable and consistent) and translate into meaningful performance related decisions in training and recovery. Metrics such as heart rate variability (HRV), velocity based training (VBT), force platform analysis, resting heart rate and sleep patterns provide valuable insights into an athlete's physiological state and readiness for training [17, 18].

15.4.3 Heart Rate Variability (HRV)

HRV refers to the variations in time between heartbeats, providing insights into the balance between the sympathetic and parasympathetic nervous systems [19]. HRV is a valuable metric for assessing an athlete's training status, adaptability and recovery, making it a helpful tool when evaluating readiness for training. The return of HRV to normal levels within 48 hours after an exercise bout is believed to indicate key bodily processes, such as temperature regulation, metabolism, blood flow and fluid balance, are recovering from the effects of physical activity [20].

15.4.4 CO_2 Tolerance Test

We can get an idea of how effectively we cope with stress by measuring our exhalation. The carbon dioxide tolerance test measures our bodies' ability to tolerate higher levels of arterial CO_2 (26). The depth and frequency of our breathing is a complex physiological process, which has been shown to be related to stress management, executive functions and cardiovascular functioning (27). Although breathwork has been practised for centuries to calm the mind and body, our research into understanding its effect on recovery is still in its infancy. A consistent practice of breathing exercises can positively influence our ability to tolerate arterial CO_2, which in turn helps regulate the nervous system, increase awareness and improve overall well-being.

15.5 Influencing Players' Recovery Habits

Player education is vital to create awareness around daily habits that influence recovery and for players to understand the influence of recovery or the lack thereof, having a direct effect on performance and injury prevention. Some simple examples to encourage recovery habits are to use recovery protocols, as seen in Fig. 15.1 using a recovery points system, or having a simple hydration chart (see Fig. 15.2) in the change room bathroom.

15.5.1 Building an Effective Recovery Routine

The cornerstone of a successful recovery routine focuses on building simple, consistent habits. Mastering the basics (hydration, nutrition and quality sleep) forms the foundation of optimal recovery. Once these core areas are in place, additional techniques can be incorporated to enhance and individualise recovery. There are increasingly more recovery protocols available, but at the end of the day, each player needs to individualise their recovery according to their desired adaptations and needs. Periodisation microcycles in-season help players recovery strategies between games and identify the right windows to effectively incorporate strength and conditioning sessions. Figures 15.2 and 15.3 illustrate two different recovery microcycles, based on either one or three games per week. Within a team environment, having a team recovery session is an important element of setting a team habit, and it becomes a part of the culture that allows for a group environment of relaxation, fun and connection (Fig. 15.4).

15.6 The Role of Sports Medicine Professionals

In high-performance cricket teams, recovery is managed through a coordinated system involving various specialists. This multidisciplinary approach ensures that all aspects of recovery—physical, nutritional, psychological and medical—are addressed comprehensively. Physiotherapists are an essential part of the cricket support team, overseeing recovery protocols and implementing injury prevention strategies through musculoskeletal screenings, wellness and workload monitoring, as well as working alongside, or in the absence of, a massage therapist, they provide hands-on treatments to support recovery between matches and after training sessions, helping to optimise players' readiness [22].

Strength and Conditioning (S&C) coaches play a vital role in the cricket support team by enhancing athletes' physical performance and reducing injury risk. They oversee post-match active recovery sessions, such as stretching, ice baths and pool sessions, and integrate recovery strategies such as workload management, biomechanical movement optimisation, into both short-term (micro) and long-term (macro) periodisation

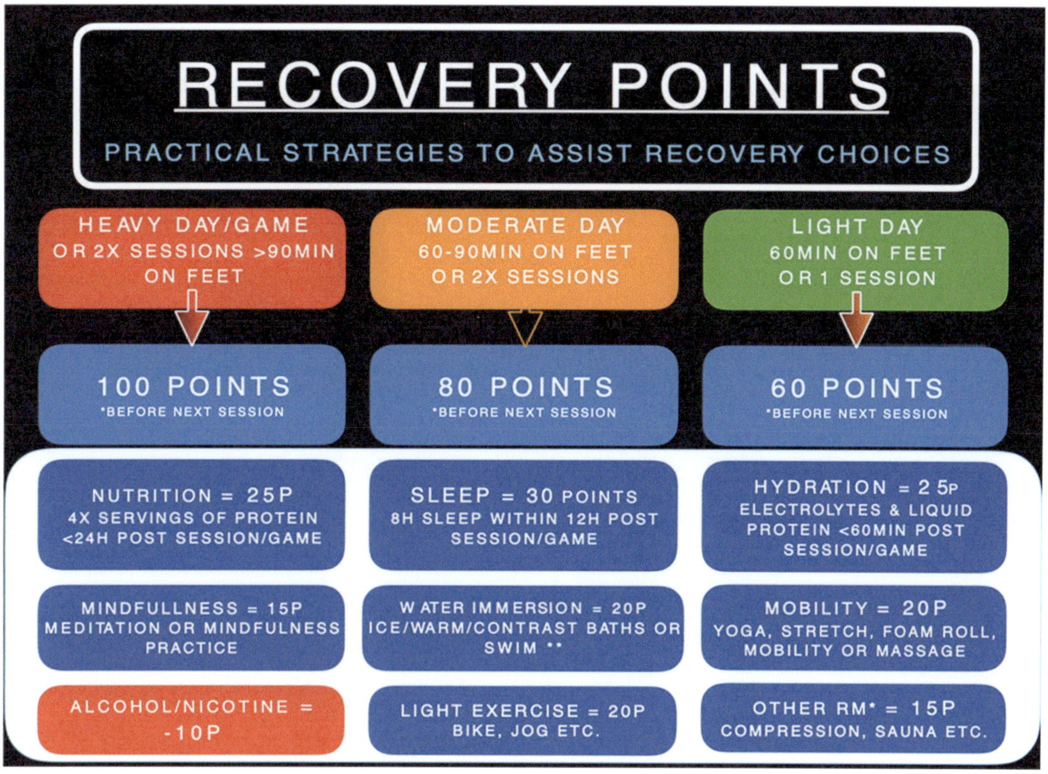

Fig. 15.1 Recovery points and strategies to assist recovery choices (modified from similar recovery point models) *RM = Recovery modalities ** Recovery swim with both swimming and active stretching or team beach/nature swim

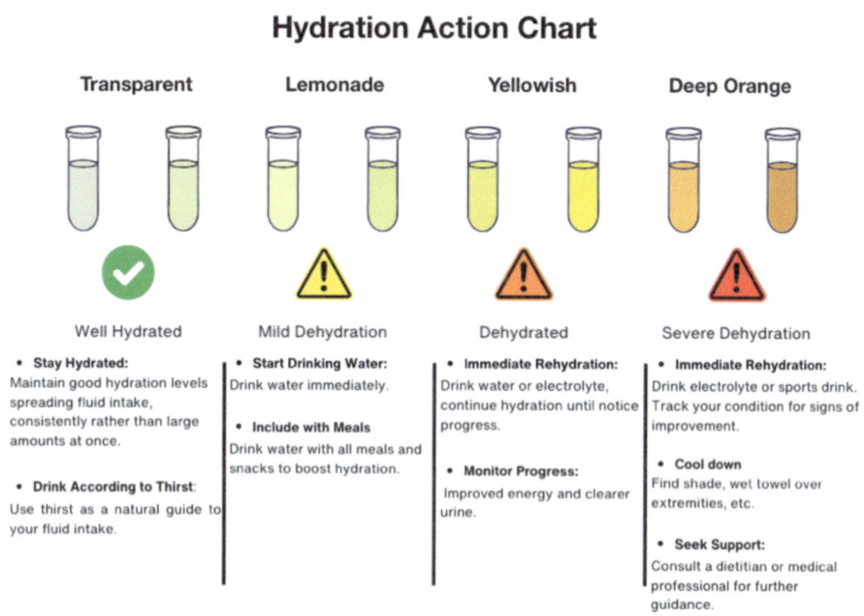

Fig. 15.2 Hydration Action Chart to determine hydration status

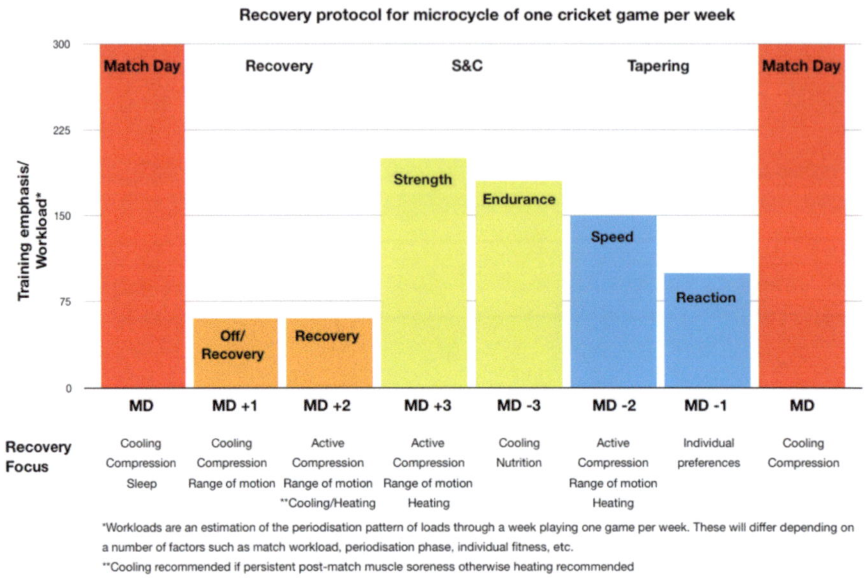

Fig. 15.3 Recovery protocol for microcycle of one game per week. (Modified from Aspetar Journal of Sports Medicine | Volume 11 | Targeted Topic—Sports Science in Football | 2022 [21])

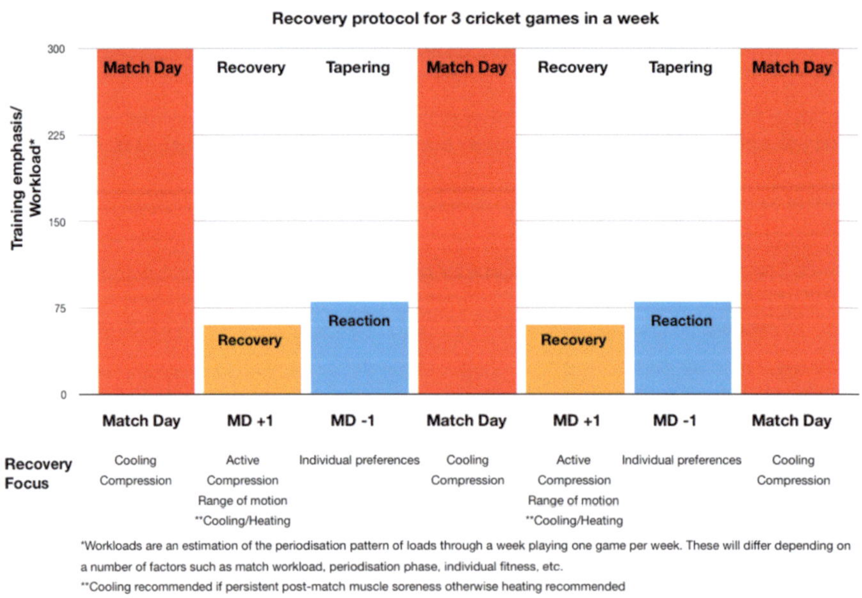

Fig. 15.4 Recovery protocol for microcycle of 3 games in a week. (Modified from Aspetar Journal of Sports Medicine | Volume 11 | Targeted Topic—Sports Science in Football | 2022 [21])

plans [23]. This approach ensures players are adequately rested and prepared to meet the physical demands of the season.

Sports psychologists play a role in recovery by providing mental support and strategies to help athletes manage the psychological demands of injury and the recovery process. They assist players in maintaining motivation, resilience and a positive outlook, which are essential for effective healing and a successful return to play.

Sports scientists contribute by analysing performance data and developing evidence-based recovery protocols that provide insights into optimising athletic performance. They look to monitor training progress and recovery to find patterns that ultimately may have an effect on performance.

Nutritionists tailor dietary guidance for players before, during and after training and matches to support individual adaptations and optimal recovery.

Team doctors oversee the medical aspects of recovery by managing injury rehabilitation, monitoring players' overall health and implementing illness prevention strategies. They play a crucial role in preventing respiratory illnesses through vaccinations and travel protocols, such as hand hygiene and mask use. When infectious diseases are identified, they act by isolating affected individuals to minimise illness, ultimately protecting players' recovery progress and maintaining their readiness for competition.

15.7 Psychological Aspects of Recovery

Psychological skills in high-level athletes are often overlooked yet are crucial for performance and health. A positive mindset is essential for maintaining focus, motivation and emotional balance [24]. Central fatigue and overtraining is a common pathology in professional athletes, particularly during training and competition seasons. Several studies show that factors influencing the central nervous system are key contributors to the development of chronic fatigue. When there is a disbalance in the sympathetic and parasympathetic nervous system, an athlete can remain sympathetically aroused, often characterised by disrupted sleep, changes in appetite and weight, decreased cognitive function and decreased motivation and depression, all of which can negatively impact performance [25].

Several psychological techniques are shown to lower this arousal level. As mentioned previously, adequate sleep and rest are important in calming this state and aid in the recovery process [7–10]. Techniques like mindfulness meditation, deep breathing exercises, and muscle relaxation can help players manage stress and reduce anxiety levels. Furthermore, mindfulness practices in which attention is paid to the present moment without judgment have been shown to enhance mental recovery and improve overall well-being [26].

15.8 Future Trends in Recovery

As the science of recovery continues to evolve, new trends and innovations are emerging that promise to revolutionise how cricketers approach recovery. There is a growing emphasis on integrating recovery into the overall training culture of teams, ensuring that players prioritise recovery just as much as they do training and performance. Furthermore, wearable technology that provides real-time feedback on recovery status, AI-driven recovery protocols that adapt to individual needs, and personalised recovery plans are promising developments to make recovery more effective, efficient and tailored to the specific needs of each professional cricketer.

15.9 Conclusion

Recovery in cricket is not merely a supplementary aspect of training; it is a critical component that underpins player performance, health and longevity in the sport. As the demands of cricket continue to grow, so does the need for effective recovery strategies. An approach based on the education of the importance of fundamentals such as sleep, nutrition and hydration along with multidisciplinary, evidence-based practice—one that involves measures of recovery integrating physiological, psychological and technological elements—cricket professionals can ensure that players are not only prepared for their next match but are also equipped to sustain long-term success in their careers. The ongoing evolution of recovery science promises to bring new innovations and insights, making recovery an ever more central focus in the world of cricket.

References

1. Kellmann M, Bertollo M, Bosquet L, Brink M, Coutts AJ, Duffield R, et al. Recovery and performance in sport: consensus statement. Int J Sports Physiol Perform. 2018;13:240–5.
2. Owens DJ, Twist C, Cobley JN, Howatson G, Close GL. Exercise-induced muscle damage: what is it, what causes it and what are the nutritional solutions? Eur J Sport Sci. 2019;19:71–85.
3. Alshak MN, Das J. Neuroanatomy, sympathetic nervous system. StatPearls; 2024.
4. Kellmann M. Preventing overtraining in athletes in high-intensity sports and stress/recovery monitoring. Scand J Med Sci Sports. 2010;20(Suppl 2):95–102.
5. Fullagar HH, Duffield R, Skorski S, Coutts AJ, Julian R, Meyer T. Sleep and recovery in team sport: current sleep-related issues facing professional team-sport athletes. Int J Sports Physiol Perform. 2015;10:950–7.
6. Ormsbee MJ, Gorman KA, Miller EA, Baur DA, Eckel LA, Contreras RJ, et al. Nighttime feeding likely alters morning metabolism but not exercise performance in female athletes. Appl Physiol Nutr Metab. 2016;41:719–27.
7. Kirschen GW, Jones JJ, Hale L. The impact of sleep duration on performance among competitive athletes: a systematic literature review. Clin J Sport Med. 2020;30:503–12.
8. Gupta L, Morgan K, Gilchrist S. Does elite sport degrade sleep quality? A systematic review. Sports Med (Auckland, NZ). 2017;47:1317–33.
9. Biggins M, Cahalan R, Comyns T, Purtill H, O'Sullivan K. Poor sleep is related to lower general health, increased stress and increased confusion in elite Gaelic athletes. Phys Sportsmed. 2018;46:14–20.
10. Grewal S, Theijse RT, Dunlop G, van Deurzen D, Van Den Bekerom M, Klautz R, et al. Exploring the impact of sleep on emotional and physical well-being in professional cricketers: a cohort study over an in-season training period. Front Sports Active Living. 2024;6:1389565.
11. Best TM, Hunter R, Wilcox A, Haq F. Effectiveness of sports massage for recovery of skeletal muscle from strenuous exercise. Clin J Sport Med. 2008;18:446–60.
12. Ortiz RO Jr, Sinclair Elder AJ, Elder CL, Dawes JJ. A systematic review on the effectiveness of active recovery interventions on athletic performance of professional-, collegiate-, and competitive-level adult athletes. J Strength Cond Res. 2019;33:2275–87.
13. Drew M, Vlahovich N, Hughes D, Appaneal R, Burke LM, Lundy B, et al. Prevalence of illness, poor mental health and sleep quality and low energy availability prior to the 2016 Summer Olympic Games. Br J Sports Med. 2018;52:47–53.
14. Brink MS, Visscher C, Arends S, Zwerver J, Post WJ, Lemmink KA. Monitoring stress and recovery: new insights for the prevention of injuries and illnesses in elite youth soccer players. Br J Sports Med. 2010;44:809–15.
15. Alba-Jiménez C, Moreno-Doutres D, Peña J. Trends assessing neuromuscular fatigue in team sports: a narrative review. Sports (Basel). 2022;10:33.
16. Duignan C, Doherty C, Caulfield B, Blake C. Single-item self-report measures of team-sport athlete well-being and their relationship with training load: a systematic review. J Athl Train. 2020;55:944–53.
17. Li RT, Kling SR, Salata MJ, Cupp SA, Sheehan J, Voos JE. Wearable performance devices in sports medicine. Sports Health. 2016;8:74–8.
18. Seshadri DR, Drummond C, Craker J, Rowbottom JR, Voos JE. Wearable devices for sports: new integrated technologies allow coaches, physicians, and trainers to better understand the physical demands of athletes in real time. IEEE Pulse. 2017;8:38–43.
19. Dong JG. The role of heart rate variability in sports physiology. Exp Ther Med. 2016;11:1531–6.
20. Manresa-Rocamora A, Sarabia JM, Javaloyes A, Flatt AA, Moya-Ramón M. Heart rate variability-guided training for enhancing cardiac-vagal modulation, aerobic fitness, and endurance performance: a methodological systematic review with meta-analysis. Int J Environ Res Public Health. 2021;18
21. Targeted topic—sports science in football. Aspetar J Sports Med 2022; 11.
22. Grant ME, Steffen K, Glasgow P, Phillips N, Booth L, Galligan M. The role of sports physiotherapy at the London 2012 Olympic games. Br J Sports Med. 2014;48:63–70.
23. Weldon A, Duncan MJ, Turner A, Lockie RG, Loturco I. Practices of strength and conditioning coaches in professional sports: a systematic review. Biol Sport. 2022;39:715–26.
24. Driediger M, Hall C, Callow N. Imagery use by injured athletes: a qualitative analysis. J Sports Sci. 2006;24:261–71.
25. Anish EJ. Exercise and its effects on the central nervous system. Curr Sports Med Rep. 2005;4:18–23.
26. Nuetzel B. Coping strategies for handling stress and providing mental health in elite athletes: a systematic review. Front Sports Act Living. 2023;5:1265783.

Communication in Cricket: The Roles and Responsibilities of Science and Medicine Staff

16

Thamindu Wedatilake, Raj Amarnani, Anna Warren, Pumi Senaratne, and Gurjit Bhogal

16.1 Introduction

Effective communication is crucial in sport to ensure good governance is maintained within structures. Communication in professional cricket is a multifaceted process that demands careful consideration of various ethical and practical aspects that are important to players. This chapter aims to provide a communication structure for sports science and medicine (SSM) staff working in professional cricket. Based on the authors' experiences, it first explores the needs and expectations of cricket players, methods for effectively conveying information to them and the intricacies of interactions with important stakeholders. Additionally, the chapter delves into the practical and ethical considerations whilst communicating within this unique environment.

T. Wedatilake (✉) · R. Amarnani · A. Warren
P. Senaratne · G. Bhogal
England and Wales Cricket Board, London, UK
e-mail: Thamindu.wedatilake@ecb.co.uk; Raj.amarnani@ecb.co.uk; Anna.warren@ecb.co.uk; Pumi.Senaratne@ecb.co.uk; Gurjit.bhogal@ecb.co.uk

16.1.1 Player Care: Players Best Interests

Cornerstone to player care is acting in a player's best interests. Clear and accurate communication is critical for good player care and should always be done with players' best interests in mind.

Defining a player's best interests is an important initial step before a discussion of communication processes is undertaken.

In the authors' experience, players' best interests are multifactorial, and they would suggest that SSM staff consider all aspects that affect them as a person and their career. These areas important to a player can be summarised by the acronym '*HAPPI*':

- *Health*—Being in good health.
- *Availability* to play cricket without injury/barriers.
- *Performance* in cricket.
- *Progress* as a person and their career.
- *Income* to have good quality of life.

Understanding these aspects is the initial step towards fostering a supportive and productive environment. When making decisions and subsequent communications about their care, players would expect all areas of HAPPI to be considered.

The SSM department should be structured in a way that ensures players' best interests are always

B. Olivier, J. W. Orchard (eds.), *Cricket Sports Medicine*,
https://doi.org/10.1007/978-981-96-6321-7_16

guarded. Figure 16.1 shows an example of how a professional sporting department could be organised, where there is a clear avenue to safeguard players' best interests.

16.1.2 Ethical Considerations of Communication

16.1.2.1 Player Confidentiality and Consent

Player confidentiality and consent are fundamental ethical principles in sports medicine. Safeguarding the player's privacy and ensuring informed consent are critical for maintaining trust and integrity in the player and SSM relationship.

Confidentiality refers to the obligation of medical professionals to keep a player's personal and medical information private [1]. This means that any information obtained during medical assessments, treatments, or discussions should not be disclosed to third parties without the player's explicit consent. In some environments, there may be an 'opt-out' or 'opt-in' process for sharing information amongst high-performance staff, but this should be carefully considered within the organisation. This principle is essential for protecting the player's dignity and autonomy.

In practice, maintaining confidentiality involves several key steps. During consultations, it is important to ensure a private setting where discussions cannot be overheard. Medical records should be securely stored and only accessible to authorised personnel. Digital records should be protected with passwords and encryption, whilst physical records should be kept in locked cabinets.

Informed consent is the process of providing the player with comprehensive information about their medical condition, treatment options and potential risks, allowing them to make knowledgeable decisions about their care. This involves a clear explanation of the proposed interventions, benefits, potential harms and side effects and timelines for recovery.

16.1.2.2 Communications with a Player

Each player has different thresholds for information, emotional responses and ways of processing news. Recognising and respecting these individual differences is crucial in establishing long-lasting and successful relationships. Players appreciate it when SSM staff take the time to tai-

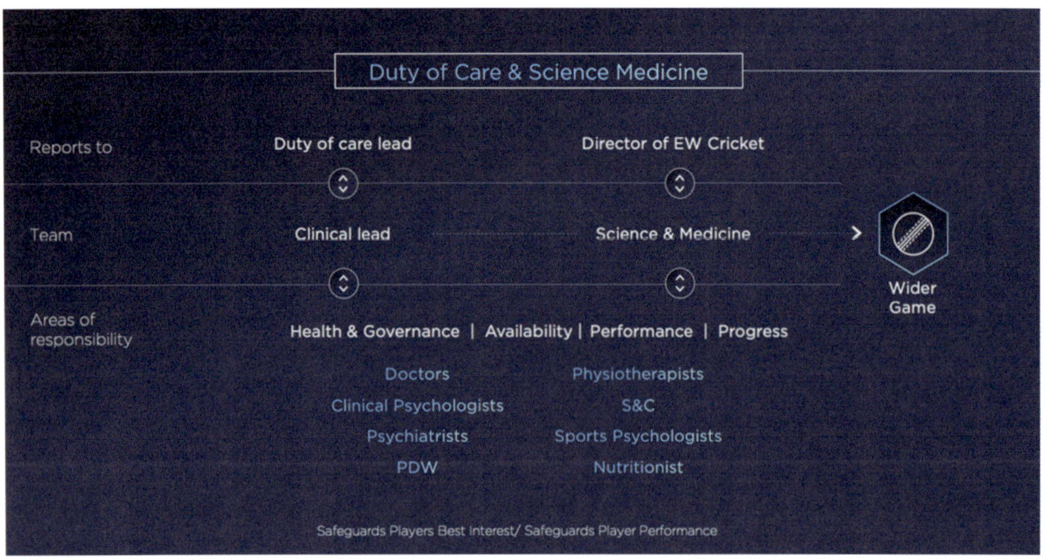

Fig. 16.1 Example of a Sport Science and Medicine team structure, outlining the various key roles and reporting pathways

lor their communication approach to fit the player's personality and preferences.

Furthermore, players want to be involved in decisions about their health and career. A collaborative dialogue openly explaining the options available, the pros and cons of each, and respecting the player's autonomy in making decisions about their health fosters a sense of control and partnership. A mutualistic consultation style where the player is actively involved and shares the decision-making process with the SSM team is important [2]. A paternalistic approach where SSM team members effectively make decisions for players should be avoided, as this often conflicts with player autonomy [3, 4].

Players also value ongoing communication, not just at the time of an acute injury or illness. Regular check-ins and updates, even when there is no immediate health concern, help maintain a continuous dialogue and a sense of involvement and trust.

16.1.2.3 Delivering Information to a Player

Delivering information to cricket players requires a strategic approach that considers both the content and the method of communication. First, it is important to ensure that the information is accurate and understandable. Using clear, non-technical language can help players understand the details of their health status and any recommended interventions. Visual aids, such as diagrams or videos, can also be effective in explaining complex medical conditions or procedures.

Timing and setting also play important roles in the delivery of information. Sensitive or potentially distressing information should be communicated in a private, comfortable setting where the player feels safe and supported. It is important to allocate sufficient time for these conversations, allowing the player to ask questions and express their concerns. Rushed and impersonal communication can lead to misunderstandings and anxiety.

Another key aspect is empathy and compassion. Delivering medical information, especially when it involves injuries or career-impacting news, requires a compassionate and sensitive style. Acknowledging the player's feelings and providing emotional support is just as important as conveying the facts. This empathy helps in building a trusting relationship and makes it easier for the player to accept and process the information. Some more challenging conversations are best done with another SSM practitioner, for example, a physiotherapist and a doctor together.

Follow-up and continuity are also important to address. It is beneficial to schedule follow-up meetings to address any further questions the player might have and to provide updates on their condition. This ongoing communication reinforces support and ensures that the player remains well-informed throughout their recovery process.

16.1.2.4 Further Considerations on Communication for SSM Staff

All SSM staff should sign a confidentiality agreement that has been produced and checked by the organisation's legal team so that the SSM staff clearly understand their role in communication and the medical governance that surrounds this. All players usually sign an agreement so that SSM staff can share information with other support staff, but if there is any doubt, the information should be checked with the player before any information is shared with a third party. When making communications regarding a player, there must be a clear appreciation of how such communication may lead to potentially even loss of earnings to the player and other third parties such as an agent. All SSM staff should abide by the standards of their respective healthcare professional governing body, such as the General Medical Council for doctors working in the United Kingdom. If there is any doubt or conflict regarding the ethics of communication, the individual healthcare professional should discuss the situation with appropriate peers and their own indemnity.

16.2 Communications Pathways

Cricket is a sport where players and staff are in tour/season or out of tour/season. Also, players play for multiple teams, including their international team, domestic team and a variety of franchises around the world. SSM communication pathways should cover all these aspects so there is always clear and concise communication about player care.

The key to good communication pathways is:

- Having a clearly documented process.
- Clear leadership.
- Clarity in roles and responsibilities of all staff.
- Effective multidisciplinary team working.
- Understanding medical governance in communication.

Whether on tour or not, in season or not, at defined time points, SSM staff should, as a minimum, have regular and structured SSM meetings, well-being meetings and workload planning meetings.

16.2.1 Communication on Tour

Touring with a cricket team presents unique challenges to the SSM team, arguably more so than other sports. This is due to a combination of factors, including the duration of the tours, often over a period of weeks to months, in locations that can have inadequate facilities to provide privacy, and the size of the travelling group which can often consist of 15–20 players and 15–20 staff members.

Whilst on a cricket tour, a clear communication structure and plan of action are vital to ensure staff cohesion and, importantly, protection of players interests. If the SSM team on the ground appears unorganised, this has the potential to create a difficult working environment for all relevant parties. Communicating with team management and coaching staff from the SSM team requires a nuanced and strategic approach. Each group has different interests and levels of involvement in the player's career and well-being.

SSM staff, including doctors, physiotherapists, nutritionists, strength and conditioning coaches, performance development and welfare officers and psychologists, require detailed and ongoing communication to provide coordinated care. This involves sharing comprehensive but appropriate medical information and updates about the player's condition, treatment plans and progress.

Importantly, there needs to be a clearly defined SSM lead 'on the ground', and this needs to be agreed upon well before the tour. This is usually a sports medicine doctor or a physiotherapist, depending on the environment and their familiarity with the players/coaching staff. A worked-through example of an on-tour communications structure can be seen in Fig. 16.2. Alongside this, having clear role allocations and job descriptions in a written format can be helpful (see Fig. 16.3).

Once this has been established, daily SSM meetings can facilitate effective communication within the SSM team, ensuring a holistic approach to the player's health. Again, having a structured approach to this can facilitate care, and we have outlined an example below that can be memorised with the mnemonic '*PIMMS*':

1. *Planning*

   This outlines what the events of the day are (e.g. training, matchday, timings, travel, media) to make sure everyone is aligned.
2. *Injury/Illness Status*

   This involves highlighting the current and suspected injuries and illnesses over the squad list, and updates are received from relevant members of SSM staff looking after them.
3. *Monitoring and Workload*

   Review of daily monitoring scores (e.g. sleep, mood, fatigue ratings) and workload monitoring (e.g. bowling, throwing loads, GPS) helps the SSM team make decisions around training or rehabilitation schedules for the team that day.
4. *Modifications*

   Once the above have been discussed, based on this information, training and match modification recommendations can then be agreed upon for individual players.

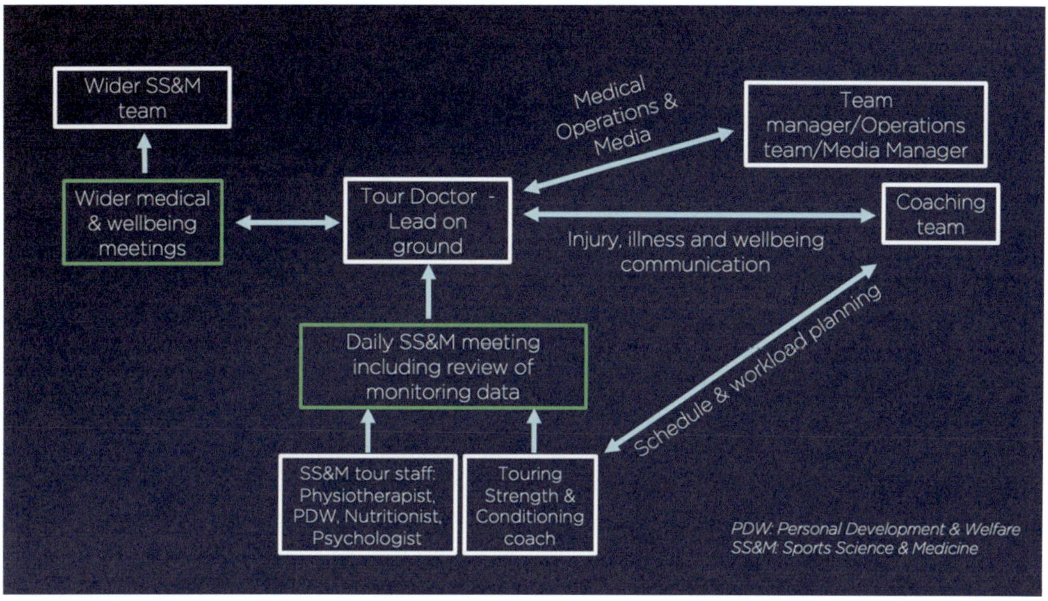

Fig. 16.2 Example of an on-tour communication structure

5. *Social*

   In the end, if there is time, highlighting a potential social opportunity for the SSM team to relax and take a break at the end of the day might be appropriate to ensure their well-being and prevent burnout, particularly on long and often rigorous tours.

Once the SSM meeting has concluded, the coaching, operational and media staff need to be informed in a coordinated manner. So that the same information is not relayed by multiple parties, which can clearly lead to confusion, the SSM lead has the responsibility to coordinate these communications. The SSM lead informs the relevant information initially to the head coach. Following this, other coaches (e.g. skills coaches), operations managers and media are informed of the relevant information. At times, due to the multitude of communications that are required simultaneously, the SSM lead may delegate certain communications to other SSM staff. For example, throwing modifications are to be discussed by the physiotherapist with the fielding coach. However, the ultimate control of all communication stays with the SSM lead to streamline this process and to avoid any confusion.

16.2.2 Communication Out of Tour

In a non-touring environment, managing player illness, injuries and concerns poses some challenges. It is very likely that players will be at a different location and possibly a different time zone from the SSM team. They could be under the care of another SSM team (e.g. domestic SSM team). Hence, it is imperative to maintain a clear structure of communication. Regular (at least weekly) and structured SSM meetings, well-being meetings and workload planning meetings become paramount to coordinate care, allocate appropriate resources and, importantly, streamline communication, avoiding any confusion for players and other stakeholders. This is illustrated in Fig. 16.4, which emphasises the importance of communication, a clear nominated lead and timely, accurate medical documentation.

Doctor	Strength& Conditioning Coach	Physiotherapist	Psychologist	Nutritionist	Personal Development &Welfare	Head of SS&M
Lead and organise daily medical meeting including setting up medical communication channels	Management and monitoring of player workload including using data monitoring platform	Coordinate all player reviews and logistics around this	Communicatio n of any performance psychology work of players to SS&M MDT	Ensure appropriate hydration and heat strategies in place	Safeguarding Lead for SS&M	Monitor SS&M staff wellbeing while on tour
Communicate injury, illness and wellbeing information to coaching team and contact point for coaching team	Liaise with coaching team regarding schedule/work load planning and inform SS&M team of these plans	Monitor any Injury and illness trends, red flags and lead on prevention strategies	Work with coaching staff on players performance psychology work-ons	Supplement lead role– ensuring all products used have no concerns	Monitor daily wellbeing on data monitoring platform	
Coordinate with non-touring SS&M team and lead medical & wellbeing meetings	Ensure players are completing daily monitoring and workloads on data monitoring platform	Line manages travelling soft tissue therapist	Wellbeing support	Attend and contribute to daily/wider medical meetings	Wellbeing support	
Communicate with team manager/opera tions team/ media	Attend and contribute to daily/wider medical meetings	Attend and contribute to daily/wider medical meetings	Monitor daily wellbeing data monitoring platform		Attend and contribute to daily/wider medical meetings	
Emergency care lead including organising pitch side emergency practice session			Attend and contribute to daily/wider medical meetings			

Fig. 16.3 Example of roles and responsibilities for each SSM staff member of the touring party

16.2.3 Communicating with the Players Regions/ Clubs/Counties/Franchises

Ensuring clear communication with players' clubs, counties, or franchises is paramount, as decisions made in isolation can be difficult and are often easy to criticise retrospectively. Clear communication before a camp or tour is essential, including reaching out to the respective teams for an SSM handover. Additionally, having a standardised format for an end-of-tour handover email compiled by the SSM staff on tour is important. Figure 16.5 provides an example of a pre-competition proforma, highlighting the usual necessary documents required by the SSM teams before the player attends their franchise or domestic competition. It is essential to have effective and secure IT systems in place to facili-

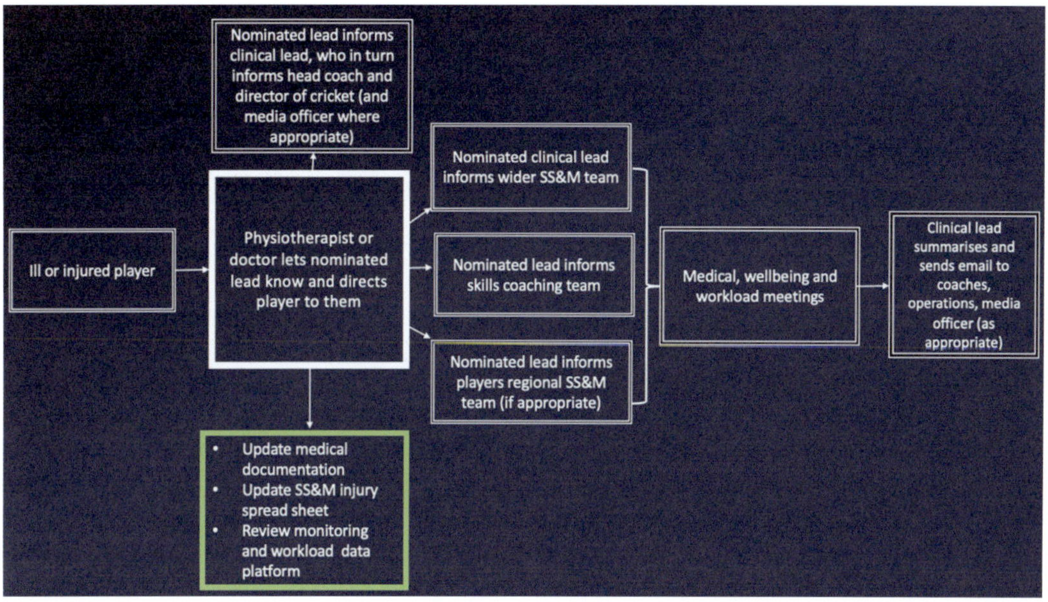

Fig. 16.4 Example of out-of-tour communication process

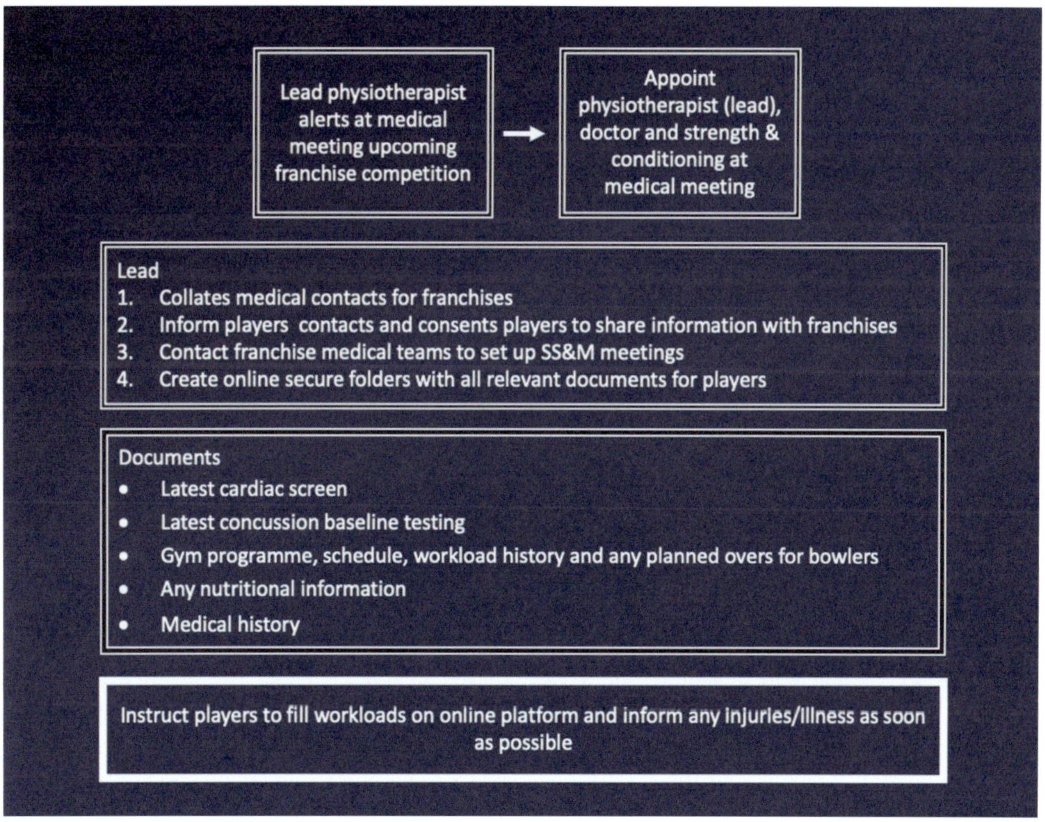

Fig. 16.5 Pre-competition communication example

tate the effective and secure sharing of player data.

Players who move between domestic teams, clubs, or leagues should have an SSM designated point of contact to guide injury and illness decisions. However, this setup will vary depending on the availability and provision of medical resources.

16.3 Considerations in Stakeholder Communications

16.3.1 Communicating with Coaching Staff

Team management, including the head coach, assistant coaches and skills coaches, need to be kept informed about players' health status to make informed decisions about team selection and training schedules. Communication with this group should be factual and timely, focusing on how medical conditions might impact a player's availability and performance.

However, it is important to balance transparency with confidentiality, ensuring that only relevant agreed information is shared without breaching the players' confidentiality. Informed consent from the player to share this information must be gained before this is communicated externally. Consent, depending on the problem, should be gained in every instance or written on to a pre-agreed document that the player has signed to give consent. If there is any doubt, the information should be checked with the player.

In some instances, the player may refuse to disclose certain information that may be important to the coaching staff and their day-to-day work. It is the duty of the SSM staff to carefully explain how sharing such information with coaching staff could help them achieve and 'push forward' 'HAPPI' objectives. Furthermore, players may need to be informed how this may impact the coaching staff's delivery of their work and their own well-being.

Continuous communication with the player must be maintained to ensure they are aware of the information that is being shared with the wider coaching staff. Importantly, the player should trust the SSM staff member that this is being done with the player's best interests in mind.

16.3.2 Communicating with the Media

Communicating with the media in the context of professional cricket is a delicate task that requires consideration of both the information conveyed and the manner of its delivery. The media plays a significant role in shaping public perception and can impact a player's career and personal life.

SSM staff should avoid communicating directly with media regarding a player health status. Instead, a media spokesperson, often the team's media manager, should be nominated to handle inquiries and make official statements. Only the appointed SSM lead should communicate with the media manager. A single point of contact helps in maintaining consistency and avoiding conflicting messages.

Transparency is important when communicating with the media manager, but a healthcare practitioner must ensure player confidentiality is maintained at all times and any information shared is with explicit player consent. Providing accurate and timely updates about a player's status can help manage public expectations and reduce speculation. However, it is essential to protect the player's privacy by sharing only necessary information and avoiding detailed medical disclosures unless the player has given explicit consent.

In instances where it may be beneficial or necessary for an SSM staff member to interact with the media, for example, to clarify a complex situation or as part of a media piece, the information that is shared should be discussed with players involved and guidance should be sought from the media manager. Before engaging with the media, it is also helpful to anticipate potential questions and prepare responses that align with the team's communication strategy. This preparation helps in delivering clear, concise and controlled messages, reducing the risk of miscommunication or misinterpretation.

Lastly, media training for SSM staff can be beneficial. Equipping SSM staff with the skills to handle interviews and public appearances can help them communicate effectively and confidently, reducing the likelihood of mishaps.

16.3.3 Communicating with Agents

With the growth of cricket over the last few decades, most professional players have agents or managers to look after their interests. They help players make decisions regarding their personal lives and careers and often hold very trusting relationships with the players. From an SSM staff perspective, communications with agents should be conducted with explicit player consent. Whilst agents are there to help their clients and have their best interests at heart, there are financial incentives to the agent, which has the risk of a potential conflict of interest. It is better to do these communications whilst the player is present so there is clear transparency to the player of what was discussed.

16.3.4 Communicating with Family Members

Family members often play a critical support role for players. Keeping them informed about the player's health and recovery can be beneficial for the player's ongoing development and emotional well-being. This is especially important if a player is considered a minor (usually under the age of 18, depending on the country of residence). Communication regarding minors has considerable ethical considerations that need to be discussed and considered on a 'case-by-case' basis.

Whilst communicating with family members, it is essential to respect the player's wishes regarding how much information is shared with family. Involving the player in these discussions and obtaining their consent ensures that their privacy is maintained whilst keeping the family informed and in a position to support the player appropriately. It is important that any communication with family is formal and not part of a social gathering or setting. It is better to do these communications whilst the player is present so there is clear transparency to the player of what was discussed.

16.4 Case Examples

16.4.1 Case 1

A skills coach asks the physiotherapist on tour about the status of one of the players who 'pulled up' with an injury during training that day. They ask this question during a social evening meal whilst on tour. The doctor, who is the nominated SSM lead on the ground, is in the process of reviewing radiology imaging for this injury and has not communicated anything yet or spoken to the player.

Things to consider:

- The doctor is waiting for radiology images to come back and does not have the necessary information to communicate effectively regarding the injury.
- The doctor has not yet spoken to the player to agree on communications and has not communicated anything to the head coach.
- The physiotherapist is not leading communication on the ground and, therefore, should not be communicating any injury information to the coaches.
- It is not uncommon for medical staff to be asked questions in social settings, which can compromise confidentiality and put staff in a challenging position.

16.4.2 Case 2

The Team's Performance Psychologist is asked in a wider staff meeting by the Head Coach to update the staff group on a player's mental health as they are trying to decide if it is appropriate for them to play franchise cricket.

Things to consider:

- A general staff meeting is not an appropriate forum to discuss sensitive medical information.
- Given this is a medical problem, any communications/questions should come through the SSM designated lead.
- It is important that any communication regarding mental health is first agreed upon with the player, as they may not want this information discussed with the coaching staff.
- Sharing mental health information pertaining to participation in franchise cricket without the player's consent breaches confidentiality and could impact their career prospects.

References

1. General Medical Council. Confidentiality: disclosing information for employment, insurance and similar purposes. 2017. Available from: https://www.gmc-uk.org/professional-standards/professional-standards-for-doctors/confidentiality%2D%2D-disclosing-information-for-employment-insurance-and-similar-purposes
2. General Medical Council. Good medical practice 2024. Available from: https://www.gmc-uk.org/professional-standards/good-medical-practice-2024
3. Gauthier-Mamaril É. Reframing patient-doctor relationships: relational autonomy and treating autonomy as a virtue. J Glob Ethics. 2022;18(1):32–47.
4. McKinstry B. Paternalism and the doctor-patient relationship in general practice. Br J Gen Pract. 1992;42(361):340–2. PMID: 1457157; PMCID: PMC1372178

17 A Psychological Perspective on Injury Rehabilitation in Cricket

Rasika Kalgutkar, Kiran Salunkhe, and Mugdha Bavare

17.1 Introduction

When we talk about injury prevention in sports, we're not just referring to proper warm-ups or good technique. Prevention also involves mental preparation, stress management, and a healthy balance between pushing limits and knowing when to rest. For instance, a cricket batter might use mindfulness techniques to stay focused during long innings, reducing the risk of a lapse in concentration that could lead to injury.

Rehabilitation, on the other hand, is the process of recovering from an injury and returning to play. It's not just about physical healing, it also involves overcoming mental hurdles like fear of re-injury or loss of confidence. Imagine a fast bowler coming back from a shoulder injury. Their rehabilitation might include not only physiotherapy but also visualisation exercises to rebuild confidence in their bowling action.

Throughout this chapter, we'll explore how the mind influences both the antecedents and responses to sport injury and intervention strategies used by psychologists to help athletes overcome their mental barriers. We'll look at real-world examples from cricket and other sports to illustrate key concepts. Whether you're an athlete dealing with an injury, a coach looking to support your team, a physiotherapist or support staff member providing essential care, or simply a sports enthusiast wanting to understand the full picture of athletic performance, this chapter will provide valuable insights into the crucial role psychology plays in sports injuries.

17.2 Antecedents and Responses to Sport Injury

Sport injuries jeopardise athletes' careers and achievement outcomes [1]. Injury rehabilitation in sports requires more than just healing the physical injury and returning to the levels of sports performance before injury. Despite this, injury prevention programmes seldom consider psychological elements [2]. Understanding the psychological effects of the injury on the athlete and the potential interactions between psychological variables and the recovery process is another essential component of optimising injury rehabilitation [3].

17.3 Psychological Antecedents to Sport Injury

Research suggests that sport injuries are influenced by both external elements (e.g. the nature of the sport and climate conditions) and internal elements (e.g. physiological and psychological aspects) [4]. Kleinert [5] put forth that an

R. Kalgutkar · K. Salunkhe · M. Bavare (✉)
Sports Psychologist, Mindsports, Mumbai, India

B. Olivier, J. W. Orchard (eds.), *Cricket Sports Medicine*,
https://doi.org/10.1007/978-981-96-6321-7_17

athlete's psychological condition may impact the occurrence of an injury. For instance, a batter who is emotionally frustrated for not being able to score against a bowler may run the risk of playing a hasty shot that leads to a muscle pull or a strain. Other examples include attention disruption, inadequate muscular coordination, and either high or low arousal.

This stream of research finds its origin in the cognitive appraisal models given by sports researchers as early as 1998. One of the most known models in this area is the "Stress and Injury Model" by Williams and Anderson (Fig. 17.1) [6]. It was developed with the intention of clarifying the antecedents that primarily lead to injury in sport. The model states that the probability of an athlete getting injured will be influenced by their perceptions of stress in any particular situation. According to the researchers, cognitive appraisal or in simple words, how one interprets a particular situation, bears much weightage in reaction to stress.

Cognitive evaluation of any circumstance presumes an equilibrium or disparity between two subjective views, namely, the primary and secondary appraisals [7]. Primary appraisal refers to the interpretation of a stressor or a situation as damaging or fearsome, and secondary appraisal refers to the degree to which one perceives that one has the resources to cope with this stressor.

To summarise the model, it states that the degree to which an athlete perceives stress in a certain environment will determine the chance of sustaining an injury and its recovery. It suggests that an athlete who has a personality prone to stress, incidence of past stressors, and an absence of perceived sufficient coping resources may have cognitive appraisals of the situation that may intensify their stress reaction and heighten their chance of acquiring an injury. For instance, an athlete who has a perfectionist personality and usually feels stressed if the training does not go the way he has planned may end up overtraining himself to failure, leading to an injury.

Stressful appraisals of a situation can cause detriments like increased muscle stiffness, loss of focus, and peripheral narrowing (missing out on task-relevant cues), which may lead to poor coor-

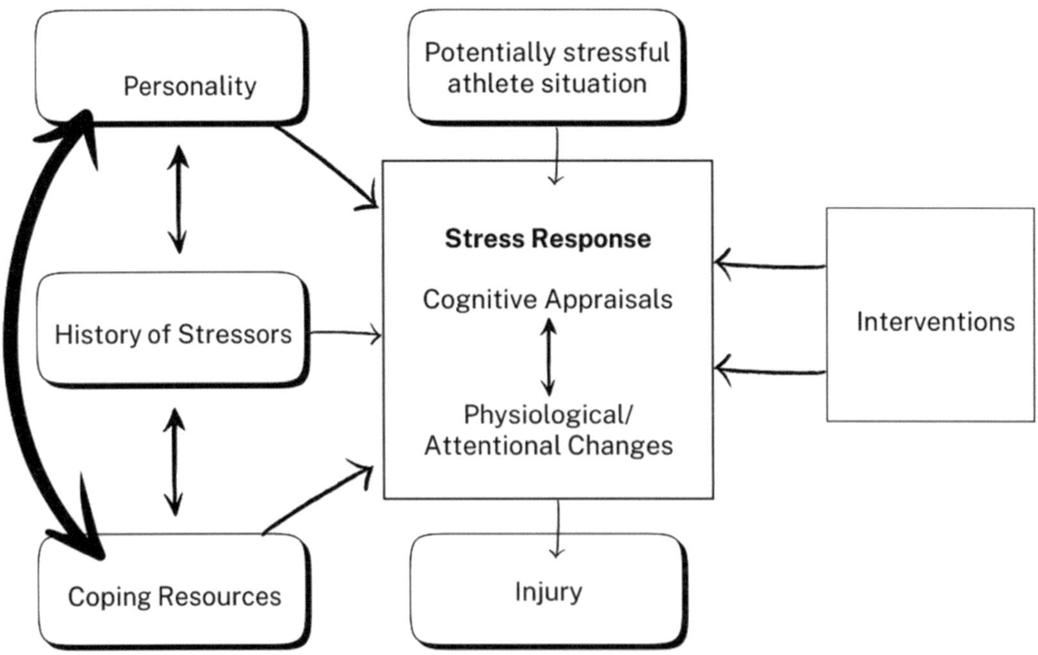

Fig. 17.1 The stress and injury model [6]

dination of muscles in athletes. Other determinants include problems in recognising situational cues, slowed decision-making, heightened reaction time, or other sensorimotor disturbances [8].

17.4 Psychological Responses to Sport Injury

Any major injury in any sport or otherwise requires good rest for recovery. However, sustaining an injury and taking a break from their sport can lead to significant emotional distress for athletes. Emotional disturbances range from sadness, isolation, loss of motivation, anger and frustration to anxiety, substance abuse, sleep loss, depression, or eating disorders. Understanding psychological responses to stress becomes crucial for the sport's medical professionals and the support staff as it impacts the athletes' rehabilitation process and its outcomes, and consequently on their return to the sport.

Various models have been used in relation to sports injuries to understand the athletes' responses. Adapting from the famous research by Kübler-Ross, the grief-response models presume that an injury is like a personal loss for any athlete, e.g. loss of the ability to play, loss of practice and daily routine), and it subsequently onsets a grieving process (Fig. 17.2). The individual goes through five stages of grief, namely denial, bargaining, anger, depression, and acceptance [9]. It is proposed that athletes react to an injury similarly to how they would react to the death of a loved one [10, 11]. On the other hand, as discussed in the previous section, cognitive appraisal models suggest that an athlete's emotional and behavioural responses to an injury would be determined by how they perceive and interpret the situation. According to the model, these appraisals are mediated by their personal and situational factors.

The biopsychosocial model of injury rehabilitation (Fig. 17.3) [12, 13] states that characteris-

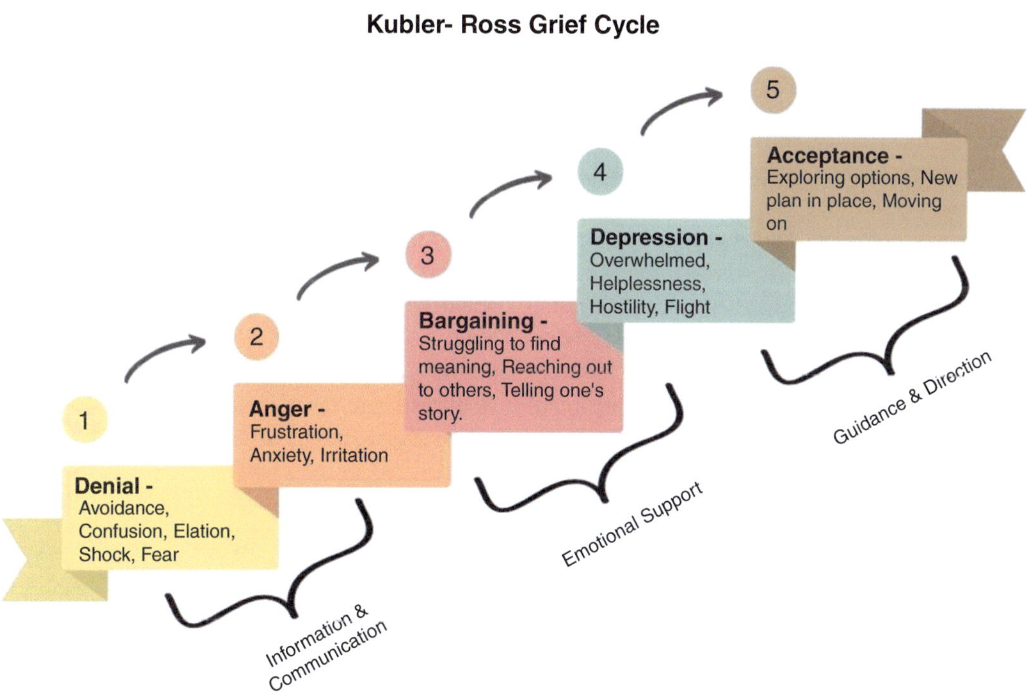

Fig. 17.2 Kubler-Ross grief cycle [9]

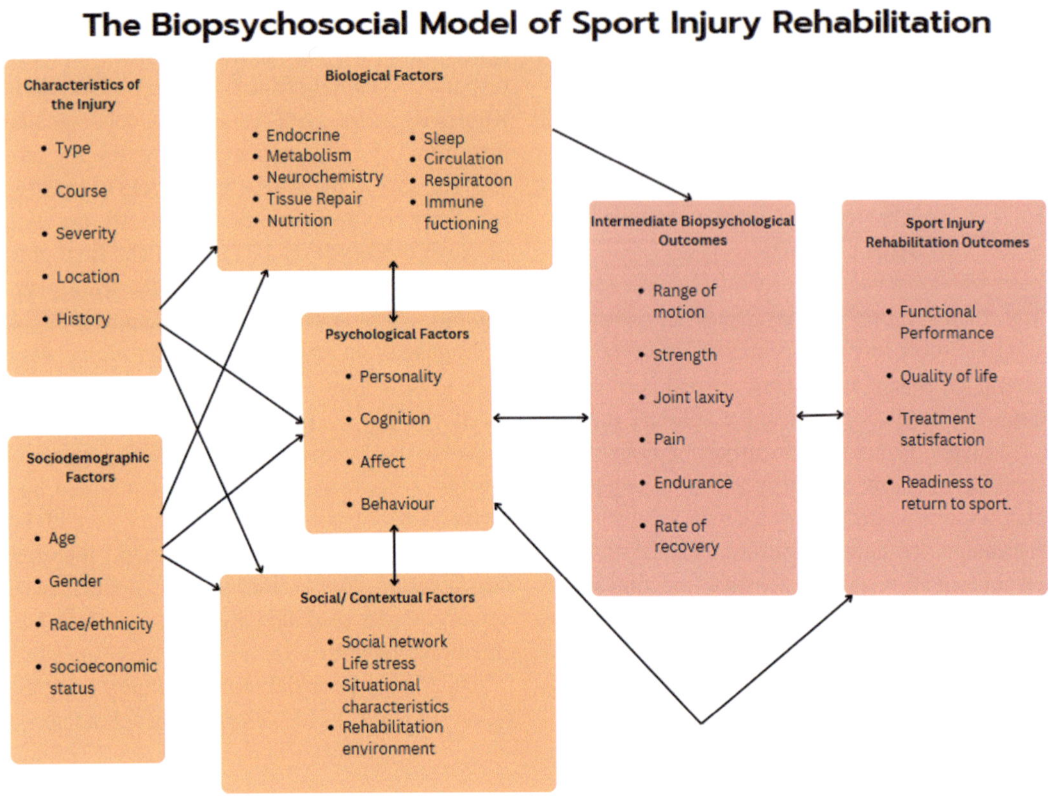

Fig. 17.3 The biopsychosocial model of sport injury rehabilitation [12, 13]

tics of the injury, the history of the athlete and their previous injuries, and the socio-demographic factors, such as athlete's age, gender, ethnicity, or socio-economic status, are factors that affect biological, psychological, and also social-contextual dimensions. Consequently, these three elements influence the intermediate results, including range of motion, muscular strength and endurance, joint laxity, pain perception, and recovery time. Functional performance, post-injury quality of life, treatment satisfaction, and readiness and willingness to return to sports are all examples of intermediate outcomes that ultimately affect rehabilitation outcomes. According to Santi and Pietrantoni, 2013 [14], psychological components are essential to this idea; in fact, they are reciprocally related to biological and socio-contextual factors and intermediate and ultimate rehabilitation results.

Nonetheless, Weise-Bjornstal et al. [15] proposed the most widely used and sophisticated model, the integrated model of response to sports injury, which included the mourning and cognitive appraisal models [16]. According to Weise-Bjornstal et al. [15], the idea explains the behavioural, emotional, and cognitive reactions to sports injuries and views injury as a dynamic process that considers both situational and personal factors in relation to rehabilitation adherence. Since recovery results are focused on the athlete's cognitive evaluation, emotional reactions, and behavioural reactions, it is inferred that all three can directly affect recovery outcomes.

17.5 Different Athlete Personalities and Their Varying Psychological Responses to Injury/Pain

Team medical staff are constantly having to assess how players are coping with injuries and, depending on their different personalities, whether they need encouragement to unload/rest more or whether they need encouragement to push through. Many athletes have a great ability to ignore pain and push through without missing any time. An athlete in this category needs to be watched carefully to ensure their performance isn't dropping if they are "ignoring pain". They might also need to have their use of pain-killing medications monitored, as it is a yellow flag if a player is starting to dose up on painkillers just to get through training sessions. For injury types that have a high risk of being serious in the longer term, such as low back pain in a fast bowler, medical staff will need to have a lower threshold to intervene and suggest that a player needs to get scanned if there are signs that the injury is serious. Another scenario where "non-presenting" players need to be carefully watched is the player who appears to have a nasty cough but is avoiding the medical staff. Not only might this mean being unable to access medication that might be helpful in managing this illness, in the modern era we understand that respiratory illnesses can easily spread throughout the team, so it becomes selfish to ignore symptoms and put other players and staff members at risk.

Despite the more common stereotype, there are certainly other players who have the opposite personality and are sometimes overly anxious about minor injuries and niggles. Some may present with highly anxious personalities. These players might have what objectively appear to be low or trivial grade injuries regularly which they present to physiotherapists and doctors regularly, often asking whether the condition might rule them out of the next match. It can become part of the player's coping routine that they always have something they need reassurance about, and decisive declarations can get them in the right mind-space to play, knowing that the medical team has reassured them. Obviously, this puts pressure on the medical team to make the right decisions, and these players might also need to have MRI scans regularly to "make sure".

These common variations between "regular presenters" and "routine non-presenters" to the medical team are an important part of understanding each individual player. Neither is the "right" or "wrong" personality; it is simply that these variations in psychology need to be understood, and injury management tailored with the personality of the player in mind.

17.6 Psychological Strategies

Over the last few years, psychological interventions have gained consideration and have been found to be playing a vital role in lowering the risk of sports injury [17, 18]. These interventions can deliver great benefits to athletes, both in the realms of prevention and rehabilitation [19–21].

As stated in the previous section, the stress-injury model proposes that athletes who experience high stress levels are more likely to fall under the risk of injury [6, 22, 23]. Thus, in relation to this, stress management strategies such as breathing exercises, seeking social support, cognitive restructuring, imagery, and practising mindfulness can work effectively to lower injury risks [17, 24, 25]. For example, a professional fast bowler who has been going through a tough season is under pressure to perform well, coupled with certain personal issues. His performance has been inconsistent, adding to his stress levels. Strategies like visualising successful deliveries and game scenarios and identifying and challenging negative thought patterns can not only help him reduce stress and stay in control but also reduce the risk of getting injured.

As per the cognitive-appraisal model, athletes' cognitive, emotional, and behavioural responses to injury are inter-connected [10]. An overall reaction to the injury is a dynamic process influenced by how an athlete appraises their situation cognitively (thoughts about injury severity and impact), which in turn shapes their emotional state (anxiety, fear, frustration) and behavioural actions (rehabilitation efforts, seeking information, social interactions). From an intervention point of view, it is important that athletes are educated about the cyclic nature of their thoughts, feelings, and actions [26]. Additionally, strategies such as cognitive restructuring and self-talk can be useful as they help athletes identify and reframe their negative thought patterns [27].

Using psychological interventions such as mental imagery, relaxation, and goal-setting often helps improve coping and reduce re-injury anxiety [28]. Athletes can use imagery during their rehabilitation phase with an integration of the emotions that they experience as well as during rehabilitation accomplishment, leading to a successful and safe return to sport. Relaxation techniques, such as abdominal breathing and progressive muscle relaxation (PMR), can support athletes in improving confidence levels by focusing on the right aspects and regulating their arousal levels in order to deliver optimum performance [28, 29]. Goal-setting is another strategy used in improving motivation levels by providing a direction towards recovery, ultimately resulting in a stronger return [30, 31].

While we have discussed the strategies briefly, it is important to ensure that their application is carried out by sports psychology professionals who adhere to ethical standards, as this can significantly impact the recovery of injured athletes. Sports psychologists are trained in tailoring interventions specific to athletes' needs and circumstances, thereby validating an effective use of the strategies.

References

1. O'Connor E, Heil J, Harmer P, Zimmerman I. Injury. In: Taylor J, Wilson G, editors. Applying sport psychology. Champaign: Human Kinetics; 2005. p. 187–206.
2. Engebretsen L, Bahr R. Why is injury prevention in sports important?. 2009. https://doi.org/10.1002/9781444303612.ch1.
3. Brewer BW, Cornelius AE, Raalte JL, Petitpas AJ, Sklar JH, Pohlman MH, Krushell RJ, Ditmar TD. Protection motivation theory and adherence to sport injury rehabilitation revisited. IEEE Trans Signal Process. 2003;17:95–103.
4. Williams JM, Andersen MB. Psychosocial antecedents of sport injury and interventions for risk reduction. In: Tenenbaum G, Eklund RC, editors. Handbook of sport psychology. 3rd ed. John Wiley & Sons, Inc.; 2007. p. 379–403. https://doi.org/10.1002/9781118270011.ch17.
5. Hackfort D, Kleinert J. Research on sport injury development: former and future approaches from an action theory perspective. Int J Sport Exerc Psychol. 2011;5 https://doi.org/10.1080/1612197X.2007.9671839.
6. Williams JM, Andersen MB. Psychosocial antecedents of sport injury: review and critique of the stress and injury model. J Appl Sport Psychol. 1998;10(1):5–25. https://doi.org/10.1080/10413209808406375.
7. Lazarus R, Folkman S. Stress, appraisal, and coping. New York: Springer; 1984.
8. Appaneal RN, Habif S. Psychological antecedents to sport injury. In: Arvinen-Barrow M, Walker NC, editors. The psychology of sport injury and rehabilitation. London: Routledge; 2013. p. 6–22.
9. Kübler-Ross E. On death and dying. London: Routledge; 1969.
10. Brewer BW. Review and critique of models of psychological adjustment to athletic injury. J Appl Sport Psychol. 1994;6:87–100.
11. Evans L, Hardy L. Sport injury and grief responses: a review. J Sport Exerc Psychol. 1995;17(3):227–45.
12. Brewer BW. Psychology of sport injury rehabilitation. In: Tenenbaum G, Eklund R, editors. Handbook of sport psychology. Hoboken: Wiley; 2007. p. 404–24.
13. Brewer BW. Injury prevention and rehabilitation. In: Brewer BW, editor. Sport psychology. Chichester: Wiley-Blackwell; 2009. p. 83–96.
14. Santi G, Pietrantoni L. Psychology of sport injury rehabilitation: a review of models and interventions. J Human Sport Exerc. 2013;8:1029–44. https://doi.org/10.4100/jhse.2013.84.13.
15. Wiese-Bjornstal DM, Smith AM, Shaffer SM, Morrey MA. An integrated model of response to sport injury: psychological and sociological dynamics. J Appl Sport Psychol. 1998;10(1):46–69.
16. Walker N, Thatcher J, Lavallee D. Psychological responses to injury in competitive sport: a critical review. J R Soc Promot Heal. 2007 Jul;127(4):174–80. https://doi.org/10.1177/1466424007079494.
17. Li S, Wu Q, Chen Z. Effects of psychological interventions on the prevention of sports injuries: a meta-analysis. Orthop J Sports Med. 2020;8(8) https://doi.org/10.1177/2325967120928325.
18. Tranaeus U, Ivarsson A, Johnson U. Stress and injuries in elite sport. In: Fuchs R, Gerber M, editors. Handbuch stressregulation und sport. Berlin/Heidelberg: Springer; 2018. p. 451–66.
19. Gennarelli SM, Brown SM, Mulcahey MK. Psychosocial interventions help facilitate recovery following musculoskeletal sports injuries: a systematic review. Phys Sportsmed. 2020;48:370–7. https://doi.org/10.1080/00913847.2020.1744486.
20. Gervis M, Pickford H, Hau T, Fruth M. A review of the psychological support mechanisms available for long-term injured footballers in the UK throughout their rehabilitation. Sci Med Footb. 2020;4:22–9. https://doi.org/10.1080/24733938.2019.1634832.
21. Heaney CA, Walker NC, Green AJK, Rostron CL. Sport psychology education for sport injury rehabilitation professionals: a systematic review. Phys Ther Sport. 2015;16:72–9. https://doi.org/10.1016/j.ptsp.2014.04.001.

22. Ivarsson A, Johnson U. Psychological factors as predictors of injuries among senior soccer players. A prospective study. J Sports Sci Med. 2010;99:347–52.
23. Rogers TM, Landers DM. Mediating effects of peripheral vision in the life event stress/athletic injury relationship. J Sport Exerc Psychol. 2005;27:271–88.
24. Ericksen S, Dover G, DeMont R. Psychological interventions can reduce injury risk in athletes: a critically appraised topic. J Sport Rehabil. 2022;31:224–9. https://doi.org/10.1123/jsr.2020-0315.
25. Simonsmeier BA, Andronie M, Buecker S, Frank C. The effects of imagery interventions in sports: a meta-analysis. Int Rev Sport Exerc Psychol. 2021;14:186–207. https://doi.org/10.1080/1750984X.2020.1780627.
26. Clement D, Arvinen-Barrow M, Fetty T. Psychosocial responses during different phases of sport-injury rehabilitation: a qualitative study. J Athl Train. 2015;50(1):95–104. https://doi.org/10.4085/1062-6050-49.3.52. Epub 2014 Oct 16. PMID: 25322346; PMCID: PMC4299742
27. Podlog L, Dimmock J, Miller J. A review of return to sport concerns following injury rehabilitation: practitioner strategies for enhancing recovery outcomes. Phys Ther Sport. 2011;12:36–42.
28. Schwab Reese LM, Pittsinger R, Yang J. Effectiveness of psychological intervention following sport injury. J Sport Health Sci. 2012;1(2):71–9, ISSN 2095-2546. https://doi.org/10.1016/j.jshs.2012.06.003.
29. Hooi LB, Wah TE. Injured athletes and a new invention of relaxation techniques. Int Res J Pharm Med Sci. 2018;1(4):78–81.
30. Vitale F. Recupero e prevenzione dell'infortunio sportivo: una ricerca sul contributo della pratica mentale (imagery). Giornale Italiano di Psicologia dello Sport. 2011;10:42–7.
31. Hamson-Utley JJ, Vazquez L. The comeback: rehabilitating the psychological injury. Athlet Ther Today. 2008;13(5):35–8.

Injury Prevention and Rehabilitation of Female Cricketers

18

Candice MacMillan, Licinda Pienaar, and Candice Christie

18.1 Introduction

This chapter provides an overview of both injury prevention and rehabilitation strategies specifically designed for female cricketers and also female-specific medical considerations. Over the past decade, the popularity of female cricket has surged, with increasing participation and viewership worldwide. Despite this growth, there remains a scarcity of research focused on the unique needs of female cricketers. Recognising the distinct physiological, biomechanical and psychological aspects of female athletes, this chapter emphasises the importance of customised approaches to reduce the risk of injuries and enhance rehabilitation outcomes. Tailoring these strategies to female cricketers is crucial, as imposing research and protocols designed for male cricketers can lead to suboptimal care and increased injury risk due to differences in anatomy, hormonal influences and the varied physical demands of the sport. By addressing these specific factors, we can improve player safety, performance and overall well-being, ensuring a more sustainable and successful athletic career for female cricketers.

18.2 Epidemiology of Injuries in Female Cricketers

Research on the epidemiology of injuries among female cricketers is essential to understand the incidence, prevalence and nature of injuries and inform evidence-based, targeted injury-prevention strategies. Elite female cricket players are more frequently injured than community cricket players [1]. The most prevalent body regions injured are the shoulder [1, 2] and knee, and fast bowlers sustain most. Injuries to the hand, wrist and fingers have the highest incidence and are most sustained by fielders [3]. Among Australian female cricketers, the most frequent match time-loss injuries for females over the seven seasons were hamstring and quadricep strains, concussion and shin/foot/ankle stress fractures [4]. Overuse injuries are common among community-level cricketers, with a significant number of injuries occurring in the shoulder [5].

C. MacMillan (✉) · L. Pienaar
Faculty of Health Sciences,
Department of Physiology, University of Pretoria,
Pretoria, Gauteng, South Africa
e-mail: candice.macmillan@up.ac.za;
Licinda.pienaar@up.ac.za

C. Christie
Department of Human Kinetics and Ergonomics,
Rhodes University, Grahamstown, South Africa
e-mail: c.christie@ru.ac.za

B. Olivier, J. W. Orchard (eds.), *Cricket Sports Medicine*,
https://doi.org/10.1007/978-981-96-6321-7_18

18.3 Factors Contributing to Injuries in Female Cricketers

Female cricketers face injury risks due to female-specific physiology, such as hormonal fluctuations; anatomical and biomechanical factors, including differences in hip structure and muscle strength; and the physical demands of the sport combined with challenges in training and workload management.

18.3.1 Female-Specific Physiology

Sex hormone fluctuations throughout the menstrual cycle are a distinct difference between male and female athletes. The menstrual cycle is typically separated into two main phases: the follicular phase, which spans from the first day of menstrual bleeding to ovulation, and the luteal phase, which occurs after ovulation. However, four distinct hormonal environments exist within a single normal cycle (Fig. 18.1). These include (1) the early-follicular phase, marked by low levels of both oestrogen and progesterone; (2) the late-follicular phase, characterised by high oestrogen and low progesterone levels; (3) the ovulatory phase, featuring medium oestrogen and low progesterone levels; and (4) the mid-luteal phase, distinguished by medium oestrogen and high progesterone levels.

Although studies on the impact of the menstrual cycle on female athletes' injury risk have yielded conflicting results, female cricketers, like all female athletes, may be particularly vulnerable to various sex-specific physiological risk factors for injury, influenced by hormonal fluctuations throughout the menstrual cycle [6, 7]. These fluctuations, e.g. rises in oestrogen during pre-ovulation and ovulation, can affect ligament laxity and joint stability, increasing their susceptibility to injuries, such as anterior cruciate ligament tears [6, 7]. Additionally, variations in bone density, particularly in relation to menstrual irregularities or conditions like the Relative Energy Deficiency Syndrome (RED-S) [8], can lead to a higher risk of stress fractures. Hormonal differences and menstruation symptoms can also impact recovery [9], potentially making female cricketers more prone to overuse injuries. For example, research has shown that a more effective recovery response, particularly regarding muscle damage and inflammation, is observed during the mid-follicular phase compared to the mid-luteal phase, when oestrogen and progesterone levels are lower [9]. Although research related to menstrual cycle phases, menstrual irregularities and hormonal contraceptives as contributing musculoskeletal injury risk factors

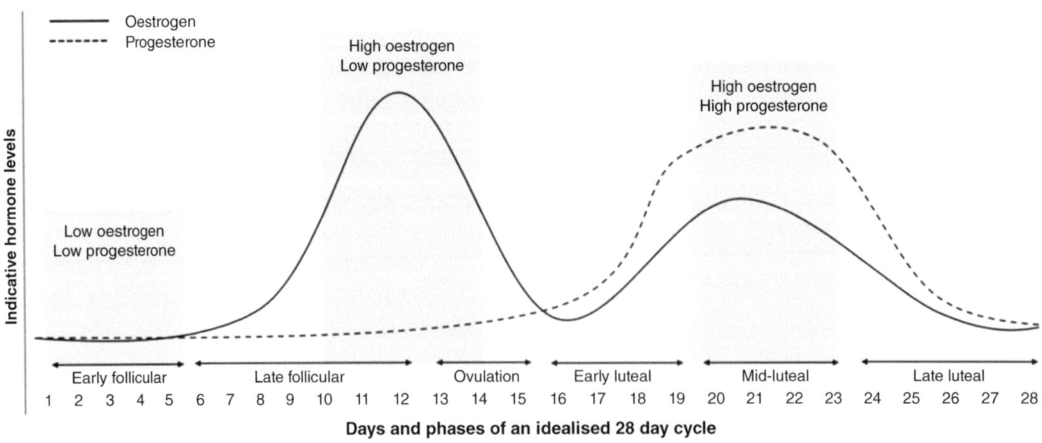

Fig. 18.1 Diagram illustrating hormone level changes throughout a normal menstrual cycle lasting 28 days, with the ovulation event occurring midway on day 14. While Fig. 18.1 demonstrates the hormonal fluctuations over a 28 day cycle, it should be noted that a normal menstrual cycle typically lasts 27–35 days

are increasing, several gaps have been identified [7]. These gaps include research from countries other than North America and Europe, athletes participating at levels other than elite level, athletes participating in team sports (including cricket), and the association between menstrual cycle phases and menstrual irregularities and muscle and tendon injuries [7]. Hormonal fluctuations should, therefore, not be considered as an isolated injury risk factor, but rather in combination with other factors as a possible contributing factor.

18.3.2 Anatomical and Biomechanical Factors

Sex differences in various sports, including soccer, handball and basketball, discuss biomechanical differences in general athletic performance, injury risk and specific movements like jumping and landing, also applicable to cricket. Research on cricket bowling mechanics among female cricketers, although less extensive than studies on their male cricketers, provides important insights into the unique biomechanical aspects and injury risks associated with the sport. Female cricket bowlers, like their male counterparts, are prone to injuries such as lower back pain and shoulder injuries. Research using inertial measurement units (IMUs) has highlighted that high peak accelerations at the back and front foot impacts during delivery can contribute to LBP [10].

The bowling mechanics in female cricketers also involve significant use of the shoulder joint. The shoulder undergoes complex motions, including external rotation during the backswing and internal rotation during the forward swing. While these movements are crucial for generating ball speed and maintaining accuracy, faulty bowling mechanics also predispose the shoulder to injury. Considering the high shoulder injury rates among female cricketers, research primarily focuses on the musculoskeletal aspects that contribute to shoulder injuries. The shoulder internal to external rotation (IR:ER) strength ratio greater than 1.00 is a significant risk factor for shoulder injuries in elite female cricketers [11]. Overuse injuries are a concern at the community level, pointing to the need for further research on biomechanical risk factors across different levels of play [5].

18.3.3 Physical and Nutritional Demands and Training and Workload Management

Workload management is crucial for female athletes' performance, injury risk reduction and overall health maintenance. Effective workload management involves balancing training intensity, volume and recovery to ensure athletes can perform at their best while minimising the risk of overtraining and injury.

Physical demands differ significantly across the four formats (T20, one-day, Test and Hundreds), with limited-overs matches involving more intense physical activity per unit of time and multi-day matches having higher overall demands. Bowling frequency, duration, intensity and volume—general measures of workload—are linked to injury risk, and research in this realm among female cricketers is expanding.

Athletes' recovery is essential because sufficient rest and sleep aid recovery and performance, and tailored recovery protocols should be designed for female athletes [12]. Furthermore, female athletes need adequate energy intake to support their training demands [13]. It is important to note that for normal menstruating female athletes, energy demands also differ across the menstrual cycle [14]. Overall, energy intake appears to be lower in the follicular phase than in the luteal phase, with a particular decrease in the days leading up to and including ovulation. The magnitude of these fluctuations is not yet clearly quantifiable and most likely varies between individuals and from cycle to cycle [14]. There is also a need for researchers and practitioners to consider anovulatory cycles and the potential effects of premenstrual disorders on dietary demands and intake.

Understanding the specific physical demands of female cricketers is crucial for developing effective training and workload management strategies. Available evidence provides insights into the physical and perceptual demands of female cricketers. External workload (i.e. distance covered at different intensities) of Australian women's T20 cricket matches is greater as the level of competition increases from Youth to National to International. However, youth athletes experience the intensity of match requirements as more demanding in comparison to players at the national and international levels [15]. In a simulated, Hundred's format match protocol, there were significant increases in heart rate and oxygen consumption [16]. From a practical perspective, findings from studies such as these should be used as guidelines for developing training programmes that mimic the demands of the women's format and focus on individualised exercise preparation.

18.4 Injury Prevention Strategies

Injury prevention for female cricketers involves a multifaceted approach that includes strength and conditioning programmes, technique optimisation and appropriate protective gear. Implementing these injury-prevention strategies can help female cricketers maintain peak performance while minimising the risk of injury, allowing for a more sustainable and successful sporting career.

18.4.1 Mitigating Menstrual Cycle-Related Injury Risks

Research related to interventions aimed to mitigate injury risk related to female hormonal fluctuations specifically is ongoing. It has been suggested that strength and conditioning programmes should be designed according to the different phases of the menstrual cycle. However, the efficacy and feasibility of such programmes are still under scrutiny [17]. Early detection and intervention of RED-S-related issues could prevent bone stress injuries. For example, structuring an individualised nutritional plan to restore energy availability can prevent more severe effects of RED-S. Therefore, educating female cricketers and team medical professionals about the signs and symptoms of RED-S is vital [18]. The Low Energy Availability in Females Questionnaire (LEAF-Q) is a screening tool to identify female athletes at risk of low energy availability and related health issues. It should be used to assess active females and female athletes who may be experiencing symptoms of energy deficiency and is utilised to help detect potential cases of Relative Energy Deficiency in Sport (RED-S) early on. A link to the tool is provided in the helpful resource table. Considering the injury risks related to ovarian hormone fluctuations, it was previously thought that the use of hormonal contraceptives to eliminate menstrual cycle-related hormonal fluctuations could decrease the risk of musculoskeletal injury. This notion has, however, been debunked [19].

18.4.2 Strength and Conditioning Programmes

Strength and conditioning programmes, including comprehensive warm-ups, enhance physical resilience and prevent injuries. These programmes should focus on developing core strength, flexibility and overall cardiorespiratory fitness to support the physical demands of cricket. More specifically, injury-prevention programmes that focus on maintaining a balanced shoulder strength ratio may be beneficial in reducing the burden of shoulder injuries among female cricketers.

Dynamic warm-ups that include stretching, agility drills and sport-specific movements can prepare the body for the stresses of training and competition, reducing the risk of muscle strains and joint injuries.

18.4.3 Technique Optimisation

Technique optimisation is crucial for safe batting, bowling and fielding performance. Coaches should emphasise proper techniques tailored to female cricketers, such as maintaining appropriate body alignment during bowling and using the correct grip and stance in batting. Safe fielding techniques, including proper catching and throwing mechanics, can prevent common injuries like shoulder strains and finger fractures. Optimal running or sprinting mechanics are also essential to prevent thigh strain injuries. Regular technical coaching sessions help players refine their skills and adopt safer, more efficient movement patterns.

18.4.4 Workload Monitoring

For female cricketers, monitoring workload is essential to prevent injuries and maximise performance, considering the specific physiological and biomechanical challenges they encounter. Cutting-edge wearable devices such as GPS trackers, accelerometers and heart rate monitors offer instantaneous data on physical activity strength, amount and regularity. These systems allow for accurate monitoring of specific workload patterns among female cricket players, enabling customised adjustments to training regimens based on each athlete's unique recovery needs and physical capabilities [20]. Furthermore, subjective data like session RPE and wellness surveys can provide a more comprehensive understanding of the stresses placed on athletes. Effective management of workload for female athletes necessitates a thorough, individualised strategy that considers physiological, psychological and social elements. By combining objective and subjective monitoring techniques, offering tailored assistance and prioritising recovery and mental well-being, coaching staff and support teams can enhance performance and minimise injury risk in female athletes.

18.4.5 Protective Gear

Protective gear and equipment recommendations should include sex-specific adaptations to ensure maximum safety and comfort. Female cricketers may benefit from protective equipment designed to fit their anatomical differences better, such as breast protection and well-fitted bras, helmets and pads. Ensuring that all protective gear is appropriately sized and worn correctly can significantly reduce the risk of impact injuries during play.

Protective sports gear, such as that worn in cricket, can hinder heat loss by trapping heat close to the body and limiting the evaporation of sweat, which is a key mechanism for cooling down. The heavy padding and helmets restrict airflow to the skin, reducing the body's ability to dissipate heat. This can lead to an increased risk of heat stress and dehydration as the body struggles to regulate its temperature under the added thermal load, especially during intense physical activity under hot and humid conditions. Continued research to improve the thermoregulatory properties of protective gear should remain a priority.

18.4.6 Recovery Strategies

Female athletes often have specific considerations regarding recovery due to physiological differences and potential hormonal influences. Proper nutrition is crucial for recovery. Female athletes should consume enough protein to support muscle repair and recovery. Adequate hydration is also essential, especially considering hormonal fluctuations affecting fluid balance. For example, blood plasma levels drop during the high hormonal phase (luteal phase) of the menstrual cycle. This impacts the hydrational strategies for short- and long-term recovery. Therefore, tracking the menstrual cycle can also help female athletes optimise training and recovery. Research suggests that during certain phases of the menstrual cycle (e.g. early-follicular phase), women may experience increased strength and endurance, while during others (e.g. luteal phase), recovery strategies might need adjustment.

18.5 Female-Specific Considerations During Injury Rehabilitation

Research on rehabilitation post-injury for female athletes indicates that a multifaceted approach that considers general and female-specific psychological, physiological and social factors is necessary. Psychosocial factors, including emotions, cognitions and behaviours, have been associated with rehabilitation outcomes, highlighting the need for practitioners to address these aspects during the rehabilitation process. Psychological factors, including self-efficacy, identity and fear of re-injury, may affect an athlete's ability to return to sports. Previous studies have reported that female athletes recovering from injury are often self-directed and exhibit greater levels of anxiety concerning an injury's impact on their lives and a loss of physical self-worth with injury when compared with male athletes [21]. Autonomous motivation, i.e. motivation that specifically aligns with players' intrinsic goals and outcomes, is particularly important for female athletes to adhere to rehabilitation programmes, as it plays a key role in ensuring their commitment to the process [22].

Sex-specific differences in injury profiles suggest that a tailored approach to rehabilitation and prevention may be beneficial. For example, sex-related differences in shoulder injuries among female athletes suggest the need for a comprehensive understanding of these injuries to enhance clinical decision-making and treatment.

18.5.1 Exercise During and After Pregnancy

While limited research exists regarding participation in bat and ball sports while pregnant, the general principles of safe exercise during pregnancy can be extrapolated to include sports such as cricket. For instance, moderate physical activity is recommended, and sports that pose a risk of abdominal trauma or balance loss are generally advised against [23]. Given the nature of cricket, which includes sudden movements and risk of impact from the ball, ground or another player, pregnant cricketers should be cautioned. As a general rule, when the uterus emerges from the pelvis to become abdominal (usually at the start of the second trimester or 12–13 weeks), the risk of trauma to the fetus should rule out participation in a sport with contact injury potential. Participation in general fitness activities, such as cardiorespiratory and strength training, included in cricketers' conditioning programmes, can still be considered individually for pregnant cricketers, beyond the first trimester.

Female athletes face a variety of challenges when resuming competition postpartum. These challenges include medical complications during and after pregnancy, societal pressures and a lack of evidence-based guidelines for their return to sport [24, 25]. A significant number of athletes experience perinatal complications such as anaemia and postpartum symptoms like low back pain and urinary incontinence, which can affect their physical function and return to competition [25]. Additionally, societal expectations and potential loss of sponsorships can further complicate the transition back to competitive sport [24]. Interestingly, while some athletes experience a decline in physical activity during pregnancy, others can maintain or even improve their performance postpartum [26]. The psychophysical aspects of returning to sport are also crucial, with both physical and psychological readiness being important for a successful return [27]. Moreover, cardiorespiratory fitness during pregnancy has been linked to a positive childbirth experience, potentially influencing postpartum recovery and return to sport [28].

Guidelines regarding the safe return to competition after pregnancy emphasise the importance of a safe and gradual return to exercise, taking into account each woman's unique circumstances, such as whether they had a vaginal or caesarean delivery and any postpartum complications like lower back and pelvic girdle pain, diastasis recti or pelvic floor issues [29]. The Australian Pelvic Floor Questionnaire (link provided in Table 18.1) is a screening tool for various pelvic concerns, including incontinence and prolapse. In the postnatal period, women can benefit from individualised assessment and guided pelvic floor rehabilitation for the prevention and management of urinary incontinence and pelvic organ prolapse and improved sexual function. The ePARmed-X+ questionnaire is a screening tool for returning to exercise postpartum. Links to the questionnaire, as well as helpful guidelines for return to participation postpartum,

Table 18.1 Quick links to helpful resources and tools

Tool	Description	Links
LEAF-Q Questionnaire/ REDs CAT2	The IOC REDs CAT2 is a clinical assessment tool for the evaluation of athletes/active individuals suspected of having problematic low energy availability (LEA) leading to REDs and for guiding the determination of the level of sport participation.	https://stillmed.olympics.com/media/Documents/Athletes/Medical-Scientific/Consensus-Statements/REDs/IOC-REDs-CAT-V2.pdf
ePARmed-X+	A screening tool for returning to exercise postpartum.	https://eparmedx.com
Australian Pelvic Floor Questionnaire	A screening tool for various pelvic concerns including incontinence and prolapse.	https://www.continence.org.au/resource/pelvic-floor-screening-tool-women?v=6373
Guidelines for return to exercise postpartum	Several authors have published guidelines that provide useful insights into returning to sport postpartum.	https://www1.racgp.org.au/getattachment/7c991ee7-3578-4e21-aa4c-a541bcb1787b/Exercise-after-pregnancy.aspx https://absolute.physio/wp-content/uploads/2019/09/returning-to-running-postnatal-guidelines.pdf
SMHAT-1	The International Olympic Committee Sport Mental Health Assessment Tool 1 (SMHAT-1) is a standardised assessment tool aiming to identify at an early stage elite athletes (defined as professional, Olympic, Paralympic and collegiate level; 16 and older) potentially at risk for or already experiencing mental health symptoms and disorders.	https://olympics.com/athlete365/app/uploads/2021/06/BJSM-SMHAT-1-Athlete365-2020-102411.pdf

are provided in Table 18.1. This tool is valuable for assessing a new mother's readiness to resume physical activity and sports participation. This comprehensive assessment helps identify postpartum-specific health concerns, provides individualised screening and aids in risk identification. Based on the results, healthcare providers can recommend appropriate activity levels and a gradual return to sport, ensuring the athlete's safety and optimal recovery postpartum. The questionnaire can prompt further medical evaluation if needed, guide the development of personalised exercise plans, and be used periodically to monitor progress and make necessary adjustments. By utilising the ePARmed-X+ questionnaire, healthcare providers and fitness professionals can ensure a safer, more individualised approach to postpartum return to sports. The guidelines stress the need for professional guidance, encouraging women to consult with healthcare providers or exercise professionals to develop an exercise programme tailored to their specific needs and health concerns. A supportive environment that encourages new mothers to engage in physical activity, ultimately promoting their long-term health and well-being, should be advocated.

Other important considerations include RED-S and mental health, specifically postpartum depression. New mothers often face sleep deprivation, altered eating patterns, irregular routines and increased nutritional needs for breastfeeding (around 600 kcal/day). These elements may lead to RED-S and related effects, making it essential to address these factors in their medical history and consider bone stress injuries if they report musculoskeletal pain when returning to exercise [29]. Postnatal depression (PND) affects around 20% of women, but up to 50% experience significant depressive symptoms without a formal PND diagnosis [30]. The Sport Mental Health Assessment Tool 1 (SMHAT-1) is a standardised assessment tool aiming to identify at an early stage athletes potentially at risk for or already experiencing mental health symptoms and disorders. In cases where practitioners recognise mental health symptoms or suspect mental health disorders, the SMHAT-1 tool can be used to screen athletes postpartum. Exercise is a recognised treatment for depressive symptoms and can sometimes be as effective as medication [31] and can enhance emotional well-being and alleviate anxiety and depression in the postpartum period.

A further consideration for national cricket boards is to develop pregnancy policies for female players. These probably need to be negotiated by players' associations but, at a minimum, need to provide for any maternity leave that is legislated in the specific country. It should be considered a right of female athletes in a team sport to have generous maternity leave provisions available to allow the choice of starting a family at a time which suits the individual. On return to play, childminding facilities and the ability for partners to travel with players are also critical for allowing players the choice to continue their careers (including touring) with young children.

18.6 Considerations for Long-Term Reproductive Health

Over the past decade and a half, women's cricket has experienced a substantial evolution, finally offering female athletes the chance to pursue full-time professional careers in the sport. Like their male counterparts, women cricketers now face considerable pressure to sustain high-performance levels and retain their contracts. As a result, elite female players often find themselves competing during their peak reproductive years, potentially forcing them to choose between starting a family and continuing their athletic pursuits. This dilemma, which affects both their professional and personal lives, can stem from various factors, including sport-specific issues, worries about pregnancy and post-birth recovery, insufficient maternity policies, or a lack of job security in their employment agreements [32, 33]. This, in turn, has potential implications for their reproductive health.

Research on retired female athletes has revealed several important findings regarding their long-term reproductive health. Although this research investigating long-term reproductive health among female cricketers is scarce, valuable insights can be gained from retired female athletes in other sports. Research conducted on former elite-level female athletes in rowing and rugby revealed high incidences of amenorrhea, later childbearing age and earlier menopause onset. These findings indicate a potentially reduced 'reproductive window' for women who participate in elite sports [32]. Among former female athletes who became pregnant after retirement, those with abnormal menstrual cycles during their active careers had significantly higher rates of infertility treatment compared to those with normal cycles [25]. This suggests that menstrual dysfunction persisting from active sports careers to post-retirement may be a factor in infertility when trying to conceive after retirement.

Implementing progressive pregnancy policies may facilitate the ability of some athletes to pursue childbearing during their professional years while retaining the option to resume their athletic careers. Fertility education is paramount for athletes who intend to continue their professional pursuits until their mid-30 s, with plans to start a family in their late 30 s. Although it may not be widely utilised or required, female professional athletes must be made aware of the availability of egg and embryo cryopreservation (i.e. freezing of eggs and embryos) as components of assisted reproductive technologies. The significance of early education lies in understanding that these techniques demonstrate high success rates when cryopreservation occurs before the early-to-mid 30 s, with success rates declining after that. Athletes can make informed decisions if they know about the reproductive techniques and associated success rates during their playing careers rather than only upon retirement.

18.7 Summary

In cricket, injury prevention and rehabilitation strategies are vital for sustaining peak performance and minimising downtime for both male and female players. However, it is crucial to acknowledge that male and female athletes may have unique physiological profiles and biomechanical patterns that influence injury risk and recovery. For female cricketers, research focusing on sex-specific aspects such as hormonal influences, menstrual cycle effects on injury susceptibility and recovery, and the impact of gender-specific training programmes is essential. Areas requiring further investigation include optimising nutrition and hydration strategies tailored to female physiology, understanding the role of menstrual cycle phases in injury occurrence and rehabilitation outcomes, and developing targeted strength and conditioning protocols that accommodate female biomechanics. By advancing our understanding in these areas, we can better tailor injury prevention and rehabilitation protocols to meet the specific needs of female cricketers, enhancing their performance and longevity in the sport.

References

1. Jacobs J, Olivier B, Dawood M, Panagodage Perera NK. Prevalence and incidence of injuries among female cricket players: a systematic review protocol. JBI Evid Synth. 2021;19:1977–83.
2. Pritchard G, Deshmukh P, Beerworth K, Saw A, Sims K. Incidence and management of shoulder injuries in female cricket. J Sci Med Sport. 2022;25:S57.
3. Jacobs J, Olivier B, Dawood M, Panagodage Perera NK. Prevalence and incidence of injuries among female cricket players: a systematic review and meta-analyses. JBI Evid Synth [Internet]. 2021 [cited 2022 May 27];Publish Ahead of Print. Available from: https://journals.lww.com/10.11124/JBIES-21-00120
4. Orchard JW, Inge P, Sims K, Kountouris A, Saw AE, Saw R, et al. Comparison of injury profiles between elite Australian male and female cricket players. J Sci Med Sport. 2023;26:19–24.
5. Zondo S, Abdullahi Y, Noorbhai H. Highlighting rural cricket: prevalence, Aetiology, and risk factors of injury among cricket players in a community setting. Open Sports Sci J. 2023;16:e1875399X2306050.
6. Hewett TE, Zazulak BT, Myer GD. Effects of the menstrual cycle on anterior cruciate ligament injury risk: a systematic review. Am J Sports Med. 2007;35:659–68.
7. MacMillan C, Olivier B, Viljoen C, Janse van Rensburg DC, Sewry N. The association between menstrual cycle phase, menstrual irregularities, contraceptive use and musculoskeletal injury among female athletes: a scoping review. Sports Med. 2024;54(10):2515–30.
8. Cabre H, Moore S, Smith-Ryan A, Hackney A. Relative Energy Deficiency in Sport (RED-S): scientific, clinical, and practical implications for the female athlete. Dtsch Z Sportmed. 2022;73:225–34.
9. Hackney AC, Kallman AL, Ağgön E. Female sex hormones and the recovery from exercise: menstrual cycle phase affects responses. Biomed Hum Kinet. 2019;11:87–9.
10. Senington B, Lee RY, Williams JM. Biomechanical risk factors of lower back pain in cricket fast bowlers using inertial measurement units: a prospective and retrospective investigation. BMJ Open Sport Exerc Med. 2020;6:e000818.
11. Murphy MC, Chivers P, Mahony K, Mosler AB. Risk factors for dominant-shoulder injury in elite female Australian cricket players: a prospective study. Transl Sports Med. 2020;3:404–14.
12. Fullagar H, Skorski S, Duffield R, Hammes D, Coutts A, Meyer T. Sleep and athletic performance: the effects of sleep loss on exercise performance, and physiological and cognitive responses to exercise. Sports Med. 2015;45:161–86.
13. Manore MM. Dietary recommendations and athletic menstrual dysfunction. Sports Med. 2002;32:887–901.
14. Rogan MM, Black KE. Dietary energy intake across the menstrual cycle: a narrative review. Nutr Rev. 2023;81:869–86.
15. Garcia-Byrne F, Buckley JD, Bishop C, Schwerdt S, Porter J, Bailey D, et al. External and internal workload demands of women's twenty 20 cricket competition. J Sci Med Sport. 2020;23:89–93.
16. Pote L, Nicholls S, Shaw A, Keenan J, Christie C. Physiological and perceptual demands during a simulated "the hundred" batting work-bout in female cricketers. J Sci Sport Exerc [Internet] 2024 [cited 2024 Jun 23]; Available from: https://link.springer.com/10.1007/s42978-024-00287-8
17. Elliott-Sale KJ, Ackerman KE, Lebrun CM, Minahan C, Sale C, Stellingwerff T, et al. Feminae: an international multisite innovative project for female athletes. BMJ Open Sport Exerc Med. 2023;9:e001675.
18. Mountjoy M, Junge A, Budgett R, Doerr D, Leglise M, Miller S, et al. Health promotion by International Olympic Sport Federations: priorities and barriers. Br J Sports Med. 2019;53:1117–25.
19. White L, Losciale JM, Squier K, Guy S, Scott A, Prior JC, et al. Combined hormonal contraceptive use is not protective against musculoskeletal conditions or injuries: a systematic review with data from 5 million females. Br J Sports Med. 2023;57:1195–202.
20. Ferraz A, Duarte-Mendes P, Sarmento H, Valente-Dos-Santos J, Travassos B. Tracking devices and physical performance analysis in team sports: a comprehensive framework for research—trends and future directions. Front Sports Act Living. 2023;5:1284086.
21. Sims M, Mulcahey MK. Sex-specific differences in psychological response to injury and return to sport following ACL reconstruction. JBJS Rev. 2018;6:e9.
22. Hildingsson M, Fitzgerald UT, Alricsson M. Perceived motivational factors for female football players during rehabilitation after sports injury—a qualitative interview study. J Exerc Rehabil. 2018;14:199–206.

23. Videmšek M, Bokal Vrtačnik E, Šćepanović D, Žgur L, Videmšek N, Meško M, et al. Priporočila za telesno dejavnost nosečnic. Slov Med J [Internet]. 2015 [cited 2024 Aug 12];84. Available from: http://vestnik.szd.si/index.php/ZdravVest/article/view/1220
24. Irani CR, Turner EHG, Rumps MV, Mulcahey MK. Recommendations for postpartum athletes returning to sport: the past, present, and future. Phys Sportsmed. 2024;52(6):533–40.
25. Nose-Ogura S, Yoshino O, Nakamura-Kamoto H, Kanatani M, Harada M, Hiraike O, et al. Medical issues for female athletes returning to competition after childbirth. Phys Sportsmed. 2024;52:147–53.
26. Pivarnik JM, Connolly CP, Marshall MR, Schlaff RA. Can pregnancy be an ergogenic aid to athletic performance?: a review. Women Sport Phys Act J. 2017;25:111–7.
27. Petruk I, Snizhko J. Psychophysical aspects of returning to active sports activities. Sci J Natl Pedagog Dragomanov Univ Ser 15 Sci Pedagog Probl Phys Cult Phys Cult Sports. 2023;127–31.
28. Jannah R, Utomo B, Abida LL, Kholifah B, Syafiq A, Wahyuddin W, et al. Adequate cardiorespiratory fitness during pregnancy for a better quality of childbirth. Healthc Low-Resour Settings [Internet]. 2024. [cited 2024 Aug 12]; Available from: https://www.pagepressjournals.org/hls/article/view/11967
29. Inge P, Orchard JJ, Purdue R, Orchard JW. Exercise after pregnancy. Aust J Gen Pract. 2022;5:117–21.
30. Dagher RK, Bruckheim HE, Colpe LJ, Edwards E, White DB. Perinatal depression: challenges and opportunities. J Women's Health. 2021;30:154–9.
31. Cooney GM, Dwan K, Greig CA, Lawlor DA, Rimer J, Waugh FR, et al. Exercise for depression. Cochrane Common Mental Disorders Group, editor. Cochrane Database Syst Rev [Internet]. 2013 [cited 2024 Aug 12];2013. Available from: http://doi.wiley.com/10.1002/14651858.CD004366.pub6
32. Thornton J, Rosen C, Davenport M, Mountjoy ML, Dorian P, Gouttebarge V, et al. Beyond the medals: a cross-sectional study exploring retired elite female athletes' health. BMJ Open Sport Exerc Med. 2023;9:e001479.
33. Carmody S, Den Hollander S, Elliott-Sale K, Mountjoy ML, Thornton JS, Massey A, et al. Self-reported reproductive health of retired elite women's footballers: a cross-sectional study. BMJ Open Sport Exerc Med. 2024;10:e002028.

19 The Youth Cricketer: Special Considerations for a Period Characterised by Rapid Growth and Maturation

Franso-Mari Olivier and Eirik Halvorsen Wik

19.1 Introduction

The years from early school-going age (8 years) up until approximately 20 years of age are a period in the youth cricketer's life characterised by rapid growth and maturation. This is also a phase where skill development and the fine-tuning thereof can be very exciting. On the flip side, it may involve a higher risk of injury. If not managed appropriately, these could lead to negative long-term health consequences, potentially ending an illustrious and lucrative sporting career.

In this chapter, we will be uncovering the topics of somatic growth and biological maturity status. We will also touch on non-invasive methods that can be used to estimate where an athlete is in their maturity process and whether they are maturing earlier or later compared to others their age [1]. Following this, we will touch on some important structural differences in the growing and maturing adolescent player's body, which will be discussed in the context of injury risk and clinical implications. Finally, we aim to provide actionable suggestions for anyone working with young players daily.

19.2 Growth and Maturation

Growth is the change in the size of the body as a whole or a body part [2]. Growth in height (i.e. getting taller) happens in a predictable distal-to-proximal pattern (bottom-to-top), meaning that bones in the lower extremities (e.g. the foot and lower leg) increase in length first, then the torso and upper limbs [3]. Maturation refers to changes in structures and organ systems, moving towards 'a mature state' (e.g. reaching your adult height); maturation therefore has a definite endpoint [4]. Although not discussed in this chapter, it is also important to acknowledge that many cognitive, behavioural, social and psychological developments take place during this time.

F.-M. Olivier (✉)
Wits Cricket Research Hub for Science, Medicine and Rehabilitation, Department of Physiotherapy, School of Therapeutic Sciences, Faculty of Health Sciences, University of the Witwatersrand, Johannesburg, South Africa
e-mail: fransomari@gmail.com

E. H. Wik
Institute of Sport and Exercise Medicine, Department of Exercise, Sport and Lifestyle Medicine, Faculty of Medicine and Health Sciences, Stellenbosch University, Tygerberg, South Africa
e-mail: ewik@sun.ac.za

B. Olivier, J. W. Orchard (eds.), *Cricket Sports Medicine*,
https://doi.org/10.1007/978-981-96-6321-7_19

Key Terminology

Growth: A change in the size (the entire body or body part).

Maturation: A process (progression to a mature biological endpoint).

Maturity status: How far in the maturity process someone has come at a given point.

Peak Height Velocity (PHV): The maximal growth rate in height, usually expressed in cm per year. Age at PHV is a common indicator of maturity timing.

19.3 Peak Height Velocity and the 'Adolescent Growth Spurt'

Many a coach would relate to the situation where a player returns after a long school holiday and 'everything has changed'. The long whites are no longer long enough, and the player standing in front of you looks, to say the least, extremely tall, scrawny and a little uncoordinated. You are witnessing the adolescent growth spurt. The maximal rate of growth in height during adolescence is known as peak height velocity (PHV). On average, a male athlete would be expected to reach PHV around the age of 14 years, and annual growth would be around 9–10 cm. Females usually reach PHV somewhat earlier, around 12 years of age and approximately 6–12 months prior to menarche (onset of menstruation), with slightly lower average growth rates compared to males (a maximum of around 8–9 cm increase in height per year) [3].

19.4 How Can We Estimate Growth and Maturity Status?

Awareness of where a player is in their growth and maturity process is important. For example, a club or team may end up selecting or giving more playing time to earlier maturing players at the expense of those maturing later. Although this is often misunderstood as a consequence of the relative age effect (i.e. where players born earlier in the year are favoured over those born later in the year), it is important to understand that these two selection biases are different. Relative age effects are a consequence of time and usually only differ up to one or two years, depending on the age band used (e.g. 12.0 to 12.9 years in a U13 group). Maturity, on the other hand, is driven primarily by genetic factors and can differ up to six years in a single age group (e.g. two players may have a skeletal age of 9.1 and 15.1 in an U13 group). Relative age is therefore more prominent pre-puberty, while maturity biases are stronger during and after puberty. As the onset of puberty is accompanied by increases in physical size and muscle mass, an earlier maturing player has a physical advantage (e.g. ability to bowl faster or hit the ball further) over a late maturing player, who might be lost to the game prematurely as a result of less exposure to good quality coaching and limited time on the field [5]. Another important application is to tailor training programmes to each individual to enhance performance or to reduce the chances of sustaining different injuries (refer to the section on injury patterns below). Although it is possible to get a general idea of maturity status within a team just by looking at players, objective methods are most often preferred.

The Khamis-Roche Method to Estimate Maturity Status

Requirements: Biological parent heights, age, height, body mass.

Outcome: Predicted adult height (PAH).

Use in practice: Bands of <85%, 85–96% and >96% have often been used to group athletes as "pre-PHV" (before the growth spurt), "circa-PHV" (during the growth spurt) and "post-PHV" (after the growth spurt), respectively.

Different methods are available, and the best choice depends on your specific context and resources (e.g. time, money, equipment, staff). The maturity of the skeletal system has been considered the best indicator, where X-rays of the hand and wrist are most often used to estimate skeletal age [6]. This approach is relatively expensive and requires both trained staff and specialised equipment. In a clinical setting, stages of maturity may be determined from secondary sex characteristics (e.g. pubic hair, breast development) as they are closely linked to hormones [6]. However, this is considered an invasive approach in non-clinical settings and is, therefore, not often used in sports.

To work around the challenges associated with the methods mentioned above, many youth sports programmes use estimates based on height and weight. One of the most popular equations is the 'Khamis-Roche method' [7]. This method includes parent heights to account for genetics, in addition to the players' current height, body mass and age. This calculates an estimation of how tall a player will be when they reach adulthood (predicted adult height; PAH), and you can see how far away they are from reaching this.

The percentage of predicted adult height (current height/predicted adult height * 100) is also commonly used to classify players in terms of their position to the adolescent growth spurt and estimate if they are likely before it ('pre-PHV': <85%), experiencing it ('circa-PHV': 85–96%) or after it ('post-PHV': >96%) [8, 9]. This way, you can get an indication of which players are more or less mature and which players are more likely to be going through a period of rapid growth.

19.5 Height and Weight Measurements—Important Considerations

When assessing height and weight in the youth cricketer, the rationale for doing so should be crystal clear and communicated to the players, for example, to estimate the player's position in relation to PHV. This assessment should not be performed more than four to six times per year, as players may experience an overemphasis on body composition, potentially leading to body dissatisfaction, body image disturbance, disordered eating and eventually resulting in Relative Energy Deficiency in Sport (REDs). The processes around this assessment should be executed in accordance with best practice guidelines. Consent and assent should be given by players and parents or guardians, measurements done privately and data captured, managed and reported confidentially [10].

19.6 Risk of Injury and Injury Patterns—Clinical Implication of the Adolescent Growth Spurt, Maturity Status and Timing

Most studies across sporting disciplines agree that athletes are at an increased risk of injury in the time around or right after PHV. Some adolescent athletes also experience something known as 'adolescent awkwardness', a temporary phase that can impact coordination and technique [11]. Although this topic has not been extensively investigated in cricket, we will use examples of studies from other sports to highlight how the adolescent growth spurt and maturity status and timing may affect injury risk.

Maturity Timing

Predicting at what age the athlete will reach PHV.

PHV earlier than the predicted age: early
PHV at the predicted age: on-time
PHV later than the predicted age: late.

Error of 1 year in 95% of the time [1]

19.7 Growth Spurt and Maturity Status

The skeletal attachment site (apophysis) is considered a 'weak link' in the muscle-tendon-skeletal chain in skeletally immature athletes [12]. It is, therefore, important in clinical practice to understand that the same mechanism of injury may result in vastly different diagnoses, depending on the maturity status of the player. For example, a 'simple' sprained ankle in the younger/less mature player may result in an avulsion fracture (a fragment of bone detaching from the insertion of the tendon on the bone), while a more mature player may be diagnosed with a ligament sprain or tear. Similarly, too much load over time may lead to irritations of the bony apophysis (apophysitis) in a skeletally immature player, while tendon problems (e.g. tendinopathy) are more likely in mature players [12]. Examples of these different diagnoses resulting from the same mechanism of injury are depicted in Fig. 19.1.

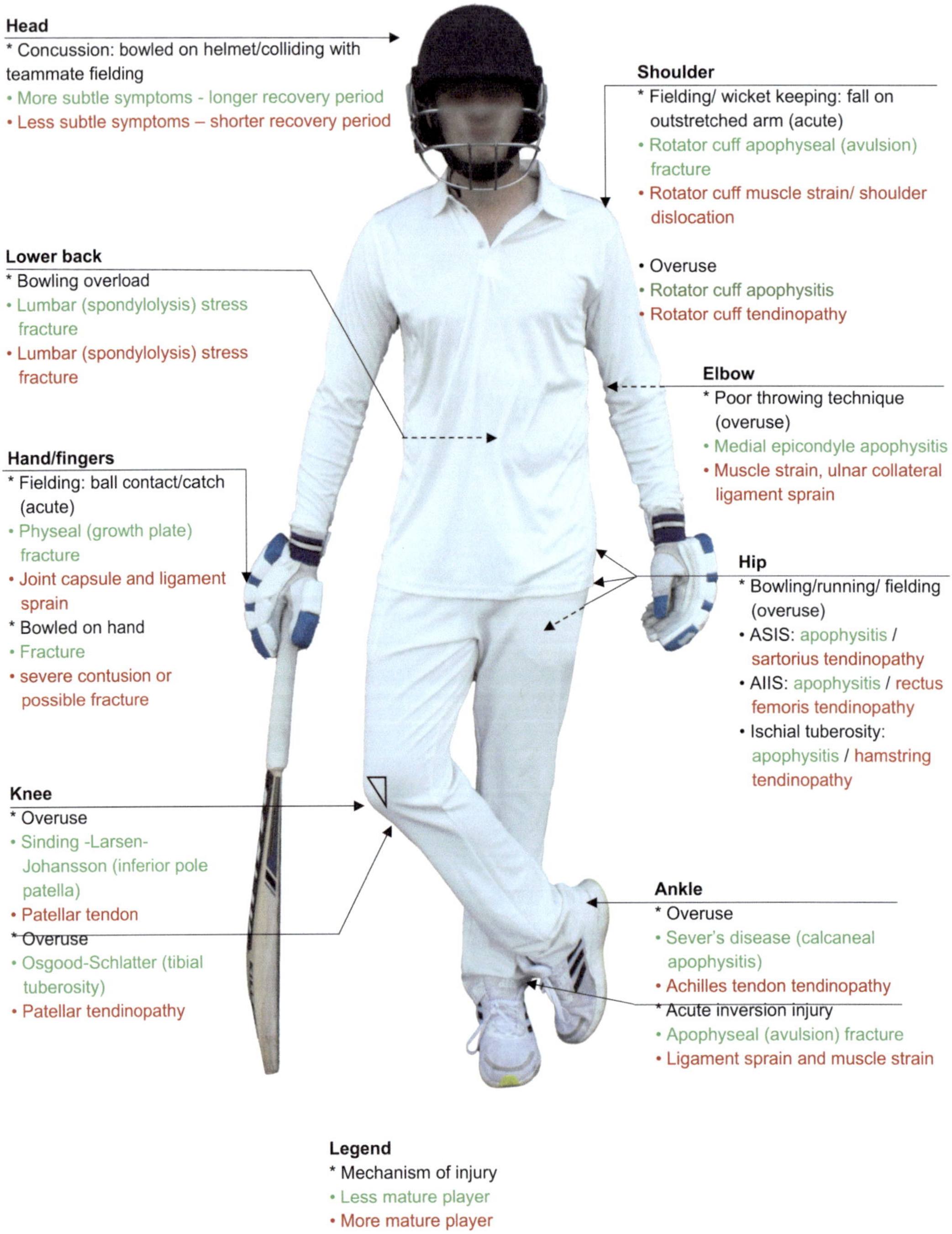

Fig. 19.1 The difference in cricket injuries between the less and more mature player

Injuries are more common in the circa-PHV period compared to the pre-PHV and post-PHV periods. For example, the highest injury risk was reported around 90% of PAH in competitive trampoline gymnasts [13] and elite youth soccer players [14, 15]. A distal-to-proximal injury pattern has also been confirmed, meaning that a less mature player is more likely to present with common growth-related injuries in the lower parts of the body (e.g. Sever's disease in the heel or Osgood-Schlatter disease in the knee), while more mature players are expected to be at greater risk of growth-related injuries higher up in the lower limbs (e.g. the hip/groin) and more muscle and joint or ligament injuries [16, 17].

Although it is less clear if athletes who mature earlier or later are at higher risk, there are some indications that it may affect injury patterns. For example, one study found that early maturing highly trained athletics, fencing and racquet sport athletes had a higher risk of injury compared to those maturing on time or late [18]. In a football study, early maturing players were shown to have the highest overall risk, although skeletally mature players had fewer lower limb apophyseal injuries compared to those who were not yet mature [19]. Similar trends were seen in another football study, where the overall risk was the same, but injury types were different depending on maturity status. Tendinopathies (overuse) and groin injuries were more common for early maturing players, while players maturing on time or late presented with more severe injuries and also osteochondral injuries [20].

19.8 Why the Youth Cricketer Gets Injured During the Growth Spurt

Athletes are at greater risk of injury around the adolescent growth spurt. The skeletally immature adolescent athlete's cartilage and growth plate are thicker around the age of PHV, making them more susceptible to injury. Just before this period, the bone-mineral density also decreases, potentially leading to an increase in acute fracture incidence during the growth spurt. Additionally, sudden skeletal growth has been suggested to increase moment arms (levers) and change the centre of mass in the limbs. Tendons and apophyses adapt slower to the lengthening skeleton than muscles; this disproportionate growth rate would result in reduced flexibility and strain on the weaker attachments (also referred to as 'soft tissue lag' [21–25]). The imbalance in growth and strength, accompanied by the loading of sports training and competition, may be why overuse injuries often occur in this phase. Teenagers will often play for multiple teams at one time (school plus club plus representative) and also often play multiple sports at one time. Because no central body is responsible for overall load management, some adolescents can find themselves playing sport multiple times per day and on all seven days of the week. Finally, the changes in bodily proportions and delay between muscle length and cross-sectional area caused by the adolescent growth spurt may result in compromised neuromuscular control and a higher risk of injury [26].

19.9 Youth Cricket Epidemiology

When describing the injury incidence rates for schoolboy-age cricketers, one should distinguish the level of play. Seasonal injury incidence rates for elite youth cricketers have been documented at 34% during elite level tournaments [27], whereas for the non-elite players this was higher at 49% during a retrospective study [28]. It can be expected that an elite male player will sustain approximately one injury per year [29]. Injuries are predominantly reported as sustained in the current competition season, and the literature reports a peak in the pre-season and again during periods when elite level tournaments take place [27]. More injuries are sustained during matches compared to practices, and bowling and fielding are the cricket activities leading to most injuries. The lower limb is usually the body region most affected, followed by the trunk and back and lastly the upper limb, but sometimes the differences between body regions are insignificant. Bone stress injuries are far more likely in adolescence compared to other injury types [30]. At the elite level, a very high percentage of junior male fast bowlers will develop lumbar stress fractures

[31]. In female elite juniors, lower limb stress fractures are more common than lumbar stress fractures, as running loads can be very high, although fast bowling loads are generally not as high as in males [32].

19.10 Differences Between Males and Females

Females experience PHV earlier than males, but that is not the only difference. Both sexes experience an increase in fat and fat-free (mainly muscle and bone) mass in early to middle adolescence. During puberty, fat-free mass continues to increase in males but plateaus in females. The opposite is the case for fat mass, where females continue to gain and more is distributed in the lower body compared to their male counterparts [2]. The differences in size and body composition are likely the reason why girls and boys perform relatively similarly in some sports before puberty, while boys outperform girls afterwards [33].

Flexibility and muscle strength seem to be other examples of sex differences. Females have greater musculoskeletal flexibility, reaching a plateau at around 14–15 years, while males experience a decrease at this point. The opposite is true of muscle strength, where male strength accelerates around 13 years, and females again reach a plateau around 14–15 years [3].

While the relationship between growth, maturity and injury is not well-researched among girls, one could hypothesise that many of the same patterns and mechanisms take place. For example, the same locations and structures might be prone to injuries, but perhaps at ages two years younger than what is observed for boys due to the earlier maturation process present in girls. On the other hand, the lower maximal growth rates seen for girls might mean that the growth spurt may pose less of an injury risk. With the earlier onset of the growth spurt, it could also be speculated that it happens for many players before training loads increase in the later adolescent years. One could also expect that the different changes in body composition (higher increase in fat and lower increase in muscle mass) impact injury risk differently.

19.11 Practical Tips for Managing the Adolescent Player

The first step in managing risk is to identify players who may be more susceptible to injury. As mentioned previously, some key risk factors have been identified in the literature, including maturity status, rate of growth in height and lower limb growth rate. But how can we manage these players? Some key factors to consider may be:

- Early detection of players at potential risk and players experiencing pain.
- Reducing aggravating mechanisms.
- Allowing adequate rest and recovery.
- Encourage adolescents and their families to take ownership of the total load from sport across the week, given that individual teams and sports may be completely unaware of training and match demands from alternate squads that the player is enrolled for.
- Regular height measurements during a season—2–3 times per season, to calculate predicted adult height and % of predicted adult height reached, thereby being informed about players' position in relationship to PHV. Other practical examples indicating growth—other than measuring height and weight—are rapid changes in shoe size and lower limbs suddenly appearing longer than the upper body.
- Modification and variation in the type of exercises: incorporate balance, coordination, landing skills and provide individual strength programmes.

One potential way to individualise training and competition based on growth and maturity—and counter selection biases—is to group athletes by biological characteristics ('bio-banding'), rather than calendar age [34]. Since it would be expected that some players mature later/earlier than others [35], the aim of this would be to 'even out' differences between players within the same-age group and to individualise training plans. For example, training groups, tournaments or matches could be organised, where biologically similar players are matched, using either measurements of size/body mass or maturity estimates. This can also be done within age groups, where the most mature players train or compete together (or in opposing roles) and similarly for the least mature players. In this instance, both groups compete against players of similar biological maturity and physicality. This may benefit both groups, whereby more mature players are encouraged to work harder against good competition, and less mature players get a chance to play without feelings of intimidation when playing against far more mature opponents [5]. This approach has been shown to benefit both early and later maturing athletes in soccer. Where later maturing players can better show their technical abilities when playing against biologically matched opponents, earlier maturing players may be more challenged physically than in their day-to-day training situation.

It is also possible to focus on different aspects of training before, during and after the growth spurt [36]. Taking steps to differentiate training during the growth spurt has also been effective in reducing injuries in academy soccer players [37]. For players who are in their growth spurt or symptomatic at growth-related injury locations (e.g. the heel or knee), reduced high-impact activities (e.g. those involving a lot of acceleration and deceleration or plyometric work) and more focus on motor skills, coordination, balance and technique is suggested. It would also be sensible to closely follow basic training principles, such as progressive overload and variation while considering a player's overall load (other sports, school, social life, etc.) and making sure they get enough recovery, sleep and nutrition throughout a training week [38].

19.12 Conclusion

This chapter highlights the perspective that the youth cricketer is not just a small version of the adult cricketer. This period of rapid growth and maturation is a sure telltale that these players are different and should be managed accordingly in clinical practice and in a team setup. Bodies of same-age players are not necessarily at the same level of maturation in relation to the period of fastest growth in height (PHV). Many youth programmes utilise methods to estimate adult height to inform coaching and medical staff, as players around their PHV may potentially be at higher risk of sustaining growth plate-related and overuse injuries. Monitoring load and modifying training for individuals could potentially result in improved management of players within the team.

References

1. Mirwald RL, Baxter-Jones AD, Bailey DA, Beunen GP. An assessment of maturity from anthropometric measurements. Med Sci Sports Exerc. 2002;34(4):689–94.
2. Malina RM, Bouchard C, Bar-Or O. Growth, maturation, and physical activity. Human Kinetics; 2004.
3. Brown KA, Patel DR, Darmawan D. Participation in sports in relation to adolescent growth and development. Trans Pediatr. 2017;6(3):150.
4. Cameron N. Chapter 13 - Assessment of Maturation: Bone Age and Pubertal Assessment. In: Glorieux FH, Pettifor JM, JÜPpner H, editors. Pediatric Bone. San Diego: Academic Press. 2003;325–38.
5. Walters SR, Renshaw I, Whatman C, Zoellner A, Harrison C, Millar S, Pithey R. Maturity status, relative age and bio-banding in youth cricket. N Z Cricket Rep. 2021;48:66–75.
6. Beunen GP, Rogol AD, Malina RM. Indicators of biological maturation and secular changes in biological maturation. Food Nutr Bull. 2006;27(4 Suppl Growth Standard):S244–56. https://doi.org/10.1177/1564826 5060274S508.
7. Khamis HJ, Roche AF. Predicting adult stature without using skeletal age: the Khamis-Roche method. Pediatrics. 1994;94(4 Pt 1):504–7.
8. Parr J, Winwood K, Hodson-Tole E, Deconinck FJ, Parry L, Hill JP, et al. Predicting the timing of the peak of the pubertal growth spurt in elite male youth soccer players: evaluation of methods. Ann Hum Biol. 2020;47(4):400–8.

9. Sanders JO, Qiu X, Lu X, Duren DL, Liu RW, Dang D, et al. The uniform pattern of growth and skeletal maturation during the human adolescent growth spurt. Sci Rep. 2017;7(1):1–9.
10. Mathisen TF, Ackland T, Burke LM, Constantini N, Haudum J, Macnaughton LS, et al. Best practice recommendations for body composition considerations in sport to reduce health and performance risks: a critical review, original survey and expert opinion by a subgroup of the IOC consensus on Relative Energy Deficiency in Sport (REDs). Br J Sports Med. 2023;57(17):1148–58.
11. Quatman-Yates CC, Quatman CE, Meszaros AJ, Paterno MV, Hewett TE. A systematic review of sensorimotor function during adolescence: a developmental stage of increased motor awkwardness? Br J Sports Med. 2012;46(9):649–55. https://doi.org/10.1136/bjsm.2010.079616.
12. Brukner P, Khan KM. Brukner & Khan's clinical sports medicine. 4th ed. New York: McGraw-Hill Medical; 2012.
13. Patel TS, McGregor A, Williams K, Cumming SP, Williams S. The influence of growth and training loads on injury risk in competitive trampoline gymnasts. J Sports Sci. 2021;39(23):2632–41.
14. Materne O, Farooq A, Johnson A, Greig M, McNaughton L. Relationship between injuries and somatic maturation in highly trained youth soccer players. International Research in Science and Soccer II. Routledge; 2015. p. 182–92.
15. Johnson D, Williams S, Bradley B, Sayer S, Murray Fisher J, Cumming S. Growing pains: maturity associated variation in injury risk in academy football. Eur J Sport Sci. 2020;20(4):544–52.
16. Monasterio X, Gil SM, Bidaurrazaga-Letona I, Lekue JA, Santisteban J, Diaz-Beitia G, et al. Injuries according to the percentage of adult height in an elite soccer academy. J Sci Med Sport. 2021;24(3):218–23. https://doi.org/10.1016/j.jsams.2020.08.004.
17. Materne O, Chamari K, Farooq A, Tabben M, Weir A, Holmich P, et al. Shedding light on incidence and burden of physeal injuries in a youth elite football academy: a 4-season prospective study. Scand J Med Sci Sports. 2022;32(1):165–76. https://doi.org/10.1111/sms.14059.
18. Rejeb A, Johnson A, Farooq A, Verrelst R, Pullinger S, Vaeyens R, Witvrouw E. Sports injuries aligned to predicted mature height in highly trained Middle-Eastern youth athletes: a cohort study. BMJ Open. 2019;9(3):e023284.
19. Materne O, Chamari K, Farooq A, Weir A, Holmich P, Bahr R, et al. Association of skeletal maturity and Injury risk in elite youth soccer players: a 4-season prospective study with survival analysis. Orthop J Sports Med. 2021;9(3):1–11. https://doi.org/10.1177/2325967121999113.
20. Le Gall F, Carling C, Reilly T. Injuries in young elite female soccer players: an 8-season prospective study. Am J Sports Med. 2008;36(2):276–84. https://doi.org/10.1177/0363546507307866.
21. Kucera KL, Marshall SW, Kirkendall DT, Marchak P, Garrett WE. Injury history as a risk factor for incident injury in youth soccer. Br J Sports Med. 2005;39(7):462.
22. Caine D, DiFiori J, Maffulli N. Physeal injuries in children's and youth sports: reasons for concern? Br J Sports Med. 2006;40(9):749–60.
23. Hawkins D, Metheny J. Overuse injuries in youth sports: biomechanical considerations. Med Sci Sports Exerc. 2001;33(10):1701–7. https://doi.org/10.1097/00005768-200110000-00014.
24. Faulkner RA, Davison KS, Bailey DA, Mirwald RL, Baxter-Jones AD. Size-corrected BMD decreases during peak linear growth: implications for fracture incidence during adolescence. J Bone Miner Res. 2006;21(12):1864–70.
25. Blimkie C, Lefevre J, Beunen GP, Renson R, Dequeker J, Van Damme P. Fractures, physical activity, and growth velocity in adolescent Belgian boys. Med Sci Sports Exerc. 1993;25(7):801–8.
26. Read PJ, Oliver J, De Ste CM, Myer GD, Lloyd DG. Assessment of injury risk factors in male youth soccer players. Strength Cond J. 2016;38(1):12–21.
27. Milsom N, Barnard JG, Stretch RA. Seasonal incidence and nature of cricket injuries among elite South African schoolboy cricketers. S Afr J Sports Med. 2007;19(3):80–4.
28. Stretch RA. The seasonal incidence and nature of injuries in schoolboy cricketers. S Afr Med J. 1995;85(11):1182.
29. Williams A, Peirce N, Griffin S, Langley B, McKay C, Stokes KA, Williams S. Annual incidence and prevalence of injuries in elite male academy cricketers: a 4-year prospective cohort study. J Sci Med Sport Plus. 2024;3:100050.
30. Blanch P, Orchard J, Kountouris A, Sims K, Beakley D. Different tissue type categories of overuse injuries to cricket fast bowlers have different severity and incidence which varies with age. S Afr J Sports Med. 2015;27(4):108–13.
31. Kountouris A, Sims K, Beakley D, Saw AE, Orchard J, Rotstein A, Cook JL. MRI bone marrow oedema precedes lumbar bone stress injury diagnosis in junior elite cricket fast bowlers. Br J Sports Med. 2019;53(19):1236–9.
32. Orchard JW, Inge P, Sims K, Kountouris A, Saw AE, Saw R, Beerworth K. Comparison of injury profiles between elite Australian male and female cricket players. J Sci Med Sport. 2023;26(1):19–24.
33. Tingelstad LM, Raastad T, Till K, Luteberget LS. The development of physical characteristics in adolescent team sport athletes: a systematic review. PLoS One. 2023;18(12):e0296181. https://doi.org/10.1371/journal.pone.0296181.
34. Cumming SP, Lloyd RS, Oliver JL, Eisenmann JC, Malina RM. Bio-banding in sport: applications to competition, talent identification, and strength and conditioning of youth athletes. Strength Cond J. 2017;39(2):34–47.

35. Radnor JM, Oliver JL, Dobbs I, Wong MG, Brown TW, Lloyd RS, Kelly AL. Selection into youth cricket academies: the influence of relative age and maturity status. J Sports Sci. 2023;41(3):272–9. https://doi.org/10.1080/02640414.2023.2208924.
36. Lloyd RS, Oliver JL. The youth physical development model: a new approach to long-term athletic development. Strength Cond J. 2012;34(3):61–72. https://doi.org/10.1519/SSC.0b013e31825760ea.
37. Johnson D, Williams S, Bradley B, Cumming SP. Can we reduce injury risk during the adolescent growth spurt? An iterative sequence of prevention in male academy footballers. Ann Hum Biol. 2023;50(1):452–60. https://doi.org/10.1080/03014460.2023.2261854.
38. Bergeron MF, Mountjoy M, Armstrong N, Chia M, Cote J, Emery CA, et al. International Olympic Committee consensus statement on youth athletic development. Br J Sports Med. 2015;49(13):843–51. https://doi.org/10.1136/bjsports-2015-094962.

Injury Prevention and Rehabilitation in Para-Cricketers

20

Candice MacMillan,
Dina C. Janse van Rensburg (Christa), Kirsty Elliott,
and Babette M. Pluim

20.1 Introduction

With its rich history and global appeal, cricket has become more inclusive, embracing athletes with diverse abilities. Para-cricket, a testament to this inclusivity, allows athletes with physical impairments to compete at high levels, showcasing their skills. This chapter explores the landscape of injury risk mitigation and rehabilitation specific to para-cricketers, underscoring the significance of tailored strategies to meet their unique needs. By understanding the types of physical impairments and common injuries prevalent among these athletes, we can develop strategies to maximise para-cricketers' short- and long-term performance and longevity in the sport. Additionally, it promotes a culture of safety and inclusivity within the sport, encouraging more individuals with disabilities to engage in cricket. Research on the epidemiology, prevention and management of injuries among para-cricketers is limited. However, extrapolating from the available studies on para-athletes and cricket players, one can infer that para-cricket players may experience a range of similar injuries. For instance, cricket's physical demands and repetitive motions are likely to pose similar demands and risks to para-cricketers, necessitating tailored injury prevention and management strategies. Also, some of the physical demands of wheelchair cricket are similar to those of wheelchair tennis, and therefore, the incidence and pathology of injuries among wheelchair cricketers could be comparable. This chapter discusses the injury rates, characteristics, risk factors and proposed injury prevention and management strategies per category of para-cricketers.

C. MacMillan (✉)
Faculty of Health Sciences,
Department of Physiology, University of Pretoria,
Pretoria, Gauteng, South Africa
e-mail: candice.macmillan@up.ac.za

D. C. Janse van Rensburg (Christa)
Section Sports Medicine, Faculty of Health Sciences,
University of Pretoria, Pretoria, South Africa

Medical Advisory Panel, World Netball,
Manchester, UK
e-mail: christa.jansevanrensburg@up.ac.za

K. Elliott
Sport, Exercise Medicine and Lifestyle Institute
(SEMLI), Faculty of Health Sciences, University of
Pretoria, Pretoria, South Africa
e-mail: kirsty.elliott@semli.co.za

B. M. Pluim
Section Sports Medicine, Faculty of Health Sciences,
University of Pretoria, Pretoria, South Africa

Medical Department, Royal Dutch Lawn Tennis
Association (KNLTB), Amstelveen, The Netherlands
e-mail: b.pluim@knltb.nl

B. Olivier, J. W. Orchard (eds.), *Cricket Sports Medicine*,
https://doi.org/10.1007/978-981-96-6321-7_20

20.2 Types of Physical Impairments Among Para-Cricketers

Para-cricketers are usually categorised into four groups: visual impairments (divided into three categories based on the degree of visual impairment), physical impairments (e.g. limb amputations, cerebral palsy, spinal cord injuries), intellectual impairments (e.g. learning disabilities) and hearing impairments. Various para-cricket tournaments have been established, showcasing the game's competitive spirit as well as the athletes' determination and skill. International tournaments where para-cricketers can compete include the Deaf Cricket World Cup, Deaf T20 World Cup, Blind Cricket World Cup and Physical Disability Cricket World Series.

Each type of impairment presents unique challenges and requires specialised approaches to injury prevention and rehabilitation. The diverse nature of these impairments means that a one-size-fits-all approach is ineffective, necessitating more individualised strategies.

20.3 Visually Impaired Cricketers

A review evaluating sport-related injuries, characteristics, risk factors and prevention opportunities reported that visually impaired athletes often experienced more injuries compared to other para-athletes [1]. Among the studies that identified injury mechanisms, overuse and collisions/contact were the most common causes.

20.3.1 Concussions

Sixty-two per cent of para-athlete concussions occur amongst athletes participating in visually impaired sports, including goalball, para-swimming and judo, with all sports-related concussions in visually impaired athletes resulting from collisions [2]. The management and diagnosis of concussions in visually impaired athletes present unique challenges. For instance, visually impaired athletes may have difficulty recognising and reporting concussive symptoms, like blurred vision, complicating timely and effective medical intervention [3].

Visually impaired cricketers are at risk of sustaining concussions from being struck by the ball or colliding with another player on the field. Considering the high concussion rates among visually impaired athletes, it is vital that medical and conditioning staff are familiar with and adhere to evidence-based pre- and post-concussion protocols, such as those proposed by the International Olympic Committee (IOC) [4].

20.3.2 Soft Tissue Injuries

Soft tissue injuries are common among visually impaired athletes, particularly in sports that involve a high level of physical contact or intense physical activity. For example, a study on goalball players found that soft tissue injuries were frequent, with upper limb injuries accounting for 92% of all reported injuries [1]. The most common soft tissue injuries among visually impaired athletes are muscle strains, ligament sprains and contusions. In goalball, the repetitive diving and blocking movements lead to a high incidence of shoulder and arm injuries, with the majority being epidermal abrasions, contusions and dislocations [1].

Similarly, visually impaired cricketers often run and dive on the field to restrict the number of runs the opposing team's batter can score or avoid a run-out by diving to reach the crease, leading to comparable injury patterns. While batting, players wear protective gear, but considering the potential for collision injuries, it may be advisable to use protective gear that does not hinder fielding performance. Coaching the correct driving and running technique could also mitigate the risk or severity of these injuries.

Additional risk factors for injuries among visually impaired athletes include para-sport type and visual classification, as they influence the specific physical demands, biomechanical stresses and potential hazards encountered during training and competition. Prevention strategies have rarely been evaluated, highlighting a gap in research and practice.

20.3.3 Injury Prevention Strategies

There is a notable gap in adapted injury prevention strategies for visually impaired athletes. Current mainstream approaches to injury prevention have not been sufficiently tailored to meet the specific needs of these athletes, resulting in a higher risk of injury [5]. However, valuable insights into strategies to mitigate injury risk among cricketers and para-athletes competing in bat-and-ball sports could also be relevant to visually impaired cricketers. For instance, the presence of certified athletic trainers for injury evaluation and management is beneficial. Understanding the mechanisms of injury, such as ball contact, could inform tailored prevention strategies for visually impaired athletes.

A national survey of visually impaired baseball players in Italy indicated that adapted versions of ball sports could improve the players' physical and psychological well-being [6]. This modified form of baseball, which includes safety modifications and assistance from sighted players, aims to mitigate injury risks while promoting the benefits of sports participation. Similarly, the rules of blind cricket are based on the standard laws of cricket with a few modifications to make participation possible and protect players from injury. The ball and stumps are, for example, bigger to allow partially blind cricketers to see the equipment, and the content of the ball (fitted with bells) allows completely blind players to hear the ball. Rules and modifications of this cricket format should be reviewed regularly to ensure continued player safety. Future research on the epidemiology, risk factors and prevention of injuries could guide governing bodies in amending the rules of the game if necessary.

20.4 Physically Impaired Cricketers

20.4.1 Wheelchair Cricket

Common injuries among wheelchair athletes include shoulder overuse injuries, wrist strains, carpal tunnel syndrome and hand lacerations. The repetitive motions required in wheelchair propulsion and the physical demands of sports contribute to these injuries. Pressure sores and skin abrasions are also prevalent due to prolonged periods of sitting and friction against the wheelchair. Improper wheelchair fit and poor technique can increase the risk of overuse injuries. Ensuring that athletes use well-fitted wheelchairs and receive proper training in propulsion techniques can mitigate some of these risks. Protective equipment, such as gloves and padded seating, can also help reduce injury incidence.

20.4.1.1 Shoulder Injuries Among Wheelchair Cricket Players

Wheelchair tennis players are prone to shoulder injuries due to the combination of wheelchair propulsion, overhead activities and daily wheelchair activities [7]. Common shoulder issues are acromioclavicular pathology, osteoarthritic changes, joint effusion and rotator cuff tears [7]. Some of the physical demands of wheelchair cricket, such as quick wheelchair propulsion and overhead throwing, are similar, suggesting that the injury rates, pathologies and risk factors for shoulder injuries may be comparable between the two sports. Risk factors for shoulder injuries in both wheelchair tennis and cricket include overhead movements, repetitive activation of the anterior muscle chain and internal rotators, as well as a higher spinal cord injury level. Muscular imbalance with stronger internal rotators, increased external range of motion, decreased internal range of motion and reduced total arc of motion are commonly observed musculoskeletal adaptations due to an unbalanced load [7]. Effective prevention strategies include strength and conditioning programmes designed to improve upper body resilience and flexibility, with a focus on shoulder and core strengthening to reduce the risk of overuse injuries.

20.4.1.2 Biomechanical Considerations for Wheelchair Cricket Players

The broader context of adaptive sports and the unique biomechanics and injuries in wheelchair athletes compared to non-disabled athletes underscore the need for medical providers to be aware of these differences. Research into the scapular kinematics of wheelchair tennis players reveals significant bilateral asymmetries in scapular kinematics, with greater scapular posterior tilt and upward rotation on the dominant side [8]. These findings are significant as they differ from non-disabled individuals with shoulder impingement and may inform the development of preventative and treatment exercise programmes for wheelchair users at risk of shoulder injury and pain. Interestingly, while scapular asymmetries are present, they are not exacerbated by increased speed during wheelchair propulsion and have limited associations with shoulder pain [9]. These findings suggest that the propulsion kinematics of highly trained athletes may not be the primary cause of pain. Additionally, wheelchair tennis players demonstrate significant biomechanical adaptations, such as larger forward trunk rotation and higher trunk angular velocity/acceleration, which may serve as compensatory mechanisms for the lack of lower limb and trunk function [10].

20.4.1.3 Other Injury Risk Considerations

In contrast to wheelchair tennis, where players are securely strapped to their chairs, wheelchair cricketers are not. While fielding, wheelchair cricketers, therefore, often fall forward out of their chairs to catch or stop the ball, increasing the risk of fractures and dislocations in the shoulder and clavicle. Wheelchair cricket, like other grass-surface sports, poses risks to athletes. However, it demands more from cricketers due to the nature of the grass surface. Wheelchair tennis, played briefly during the grass-court season on specially maintained surfaces on smaller courts, contrasts sharply with wheelchair cricket, which takes place on larger, uneven cricket fields with thick grass outfields. To enhance the sport, a surface more conducive to wheelchair movement or adjusting wheelchair tyre sizes for better grass terrain handling should be considered. Although similar research on wheelchair cricketers is needed, these findings could provide valuable insights for developing conditioning and skill training programmes for this population.

20.4.2 Amputee Cricketers

Amputee athletes participating in bat-and-ball sports face unique challenges, primarily involving injuries related to their residual limbs and prosthetic use. For instance, amputee baseball players often experience overuse injuries in their intact limbs and stump-related issues due to the demands of swinging a bat and running bases. The repetitive nature of these sports can also lead to soft tissue injuries such as muscle strains and joint sprains in the shoulders and arms, especially on the side opposite the amputation. As cricket also involves batting and running between wickets, amputee cricketers may face comparable injury risks. Effective injury prevention strategies for amputee athletes include tailored strength and conditioning programmes, proper fitting and maintenance of prosthetics and sport-specific training to improve technique and reduce stress in vulnerable areas. The importance of multidisciplinary support, including medical, psychological and technical assistance, to enhance the athletes' performance and mitigate injury risks cannot be overstated.

20.5 Intellectually Impaired Cricketers

Research on injury risk among athletes with intellectual impairments indicates that these athletes face specific challenges and injury patterns. Intellectually impaired athletes frequently have conditions such as ocular and visual defects, congenital cardiac anomalies and atlantoaxial instability that predispose them to injuries [11]. Injury profiles among intellectually impaired athletes may also be influenced by factors specific to their impairment, such as coordination challenges, communication difficulties and differences in cognitive processing. Considering the nature of cricket, where hand-eye coordination and quick decision-making are essential, these coordination and cognitive challenges may heighten these cricketers' injury risk. The effective communication skills of sports recreation specialists play a vital role in enhancing the experience and satisfaction of athletes with intellectual impairments, indirectly contributing to better injury risk management [12].

20.6 Hearing-Impaired Cricketers

Hearing-impaired athletes participating in bat-and-ball sports, such as baseball or cricket, may present unique challenges due to their specific communication and sensory needs when injured. While comprehensive data specifically targeting hearing-impaired bat-and-ball athletes is limited, there are broader insights into injury patterns and prevention strategies for hearing-impaired athletes. Hearing-impaired athletes in bat-and-ball sports may experience similar types of injuries as their hearing counterparts, such as muscle strains, ligament injuries and concussions. However, the communication barriers might contribute to a higher risk of misunderstandings during play, leading to collisions or missed cues, increasing the likelihood of injuries.

Effective injury prevention strategies for hearing-impaired athletes must be tailored to address their specific needs, including the following:

- Enhanced Communication: Utilising visual signals and ensuring clear, visible cues during games and practices to reduce the risk of misunderstandings and subsequent injuries.
- Education and Training: Training programmes for coachcs and players to understand the specific needs of hearing-impaired athletes, including using sign language or other communication aids.
- Modified Equipment and Environments: Ensuring that equipment and playing environments are adapted to enhance safety, such as ensuring visual cues supplement auditory signals.

20.7 Injury Rehabilitation for Para-Cricketers

Research on the rehabilitation of injuries in para-athletes indicates that while their injuries are often specific to their impairment and sports, the rehabilitation methods and outcomes can be similar to athletes without impairments. However, para-athletes also sustain a variety of injuries with unique patterns and risk factors related to their sport and disability [13]. Para-athletes' rehabilitation encompasses a variety of considerations, including the development of assistive devices, psychological factors and the enhancement of other sensory abilities to compensate for para-athletes' specific impairment. In addition to sport-specific injury rehabilitation, para-cricketer rehabilitation strategies must be tailored to address the unique challenges faced by these athletes. Specific considerations for visually, physically, intellectually and hearing-impaired athletes are summarised in Table 20.1.

Table 20.1 Considerations for injury rehabilitation of para-cricketers with specific impairments

Visually impaired cricketers	Unique challenges
	1. Navigation and mobility: Visually impaired individuals often rely on tactile and auditory cues for navigation, which can be disrupted during injury rehabilitation
	2. Proprioception: Visual impairments can affect proprioception, the sense of body position, which is crucial during rehabilitation exercises
	3. Communication: Clear verbal instructions and hands-on guidance are essential for effective rehabilitation
	Rehabilitation strategies
	1. Adapted physical therapy: Utilising tactile, auditory and proprioceptive feedback to guide exercises
	2. Assistive technology: Developing innovative devices has become part of injury prevention and rehabilitation practices in visually impaired athletes. These devices and applications provide audio feedback and simulate real-life scenarios. Lately, these technologies include the development of assistive devices for running, trajectory correction systems in sprinting and enhancing audio spatial cognitive abilities [17–19]. These technological advancements are crucial for the rehabilitation process as they provide alternative means for orientation and mobility during athletic performance
	3. Collaborative approach: Involving a team of specialists, including physiotherapists, occupational therapists and trainers familiar with visual impairments
	General comments
	Among the Para-athlete population, visually impaired athletes are particularly prone to sustaining concussions. While the current literature on concussion rehabilitation provides a foundation for understanding potential interventions, there is a clear need for research specifically focused on visually impaired Para-athletes, as their experience and reporting of symptoms throughout the recovery process differ from those of athletes without visual impairments. The IOC provides evidence-based guidelines for a safe return-to-play post-concussion [4]
Wheelchair cricketers	Unique challenges
	1. High rates of shoulder injuries, due to composite sport-specific and daily activity load
	2. Postural issues: Maintaining proper posture in a wheelchair is crucial to prevent primary and secondary complications related to the athlete's disability and injury sustained
	3. Thermoregulation: Spinal cord injuries can affect the body's ability to regulate temperature, making athletes more susceptible to heatstroke or hypothermia that can occur especially during the later phases of rehabilitation when more vigorous exercises are done in preparation for return-to-play
	Rehabilitation strategies
	1. Shoulder injuries necessitate specific rehabilitation strategies that often focus on core and trunk stabilisation. Exercises that simulate daily activities and sports-specific movements to ensure a smooth transition back to sport. Despite the high incidence of shoulder injuries among wheelchair athletes, there is a lack of sports-specific injury data, which hampers the development of targeted rehabilitation and prevention strategies
	2. Emphasising correct posture and alignment throughout the rehabilitation process reduces the risk of secondary musculoskeletal issues and optimises performance
	3. Cardiovascular function is an important consideration in the rehabilitation of Para-athletes with spinal cord injury (SCI), although current classification systems may not accurately reflect the degree of autonomic cardiovascular control [20]. Cricketers with SCI face unique challenges, such as differences in thermoregulatory responses that should be considered during the rehabilitation process

(continued)

Table 20.1 (continued)

Amputee cricketers	Unique challenges
	1. Prosthetic integration: Proper fitting and training with prosthetic devices are crucial for the performance and rehabilitation of injury. Prosthetic fit and type can also be reconsidered if deemed a contributing factor to injury
	2. Biomechanics of adapted movement patterns due to amputation and accommodation prosthesis
	Rehabilitation strategies
	1. Prosthetic training: Tailored prosthetic training programmes significantly improve rehabilitation outcomes post-injury as well as subsequent athletic performance
	2. Biomechanics**:** Biomechanical analysis has led to improvements in prosthetic design and training and rehabilitation protocols, contributing to better performance and reduced risk of recurring injury. Practitioners' knowledge of the biomechanics of the different activities in Para-cricket and athletes' activities of daily living is therefore crucial
Intellectually impaired	Rehabilitation of intellectually impaired athletes involves unique considerations that address both cognitive and physical aspects
	Unique challenges
	1. Cognitive function: Understanding the athlete's cognitive abilities to tailor rehabilitation programmes appropriately
	2. Communication: Adapting communication methods to ensure clear instructions and feedback
	3. Motivation and engagement: Employing strategies to maintain motivation and engagement throughout the rehabilitation process
	4. Safety and supervision: Ensuring a safe environment and adequate supervision during exercises and activities
	Rehabilitation strategies
	1. Simplified instructions: Using clear, concise and straightforward instructions to facilitate understanding and execution of exercises
	2. Visual and tactile aids: Incorporating visual cues and tactile feedback to enhance learning and performance
	3. Routine and structure: Establishing a consistent routine to provide stability and predictability can be particularly beneficial for intellectually impaired athletes
	4. Holistic approach: Combining physical rehabilitation with cognitive training and psychological support
Hearing-impaired cricketers	Rehabilitation of hearing-impaired athletes involves unique considerations that address their specific needs in communication, balance and sensory integration
	Unique challenges
	1. Communication: Adapting communication methods to ensure clear and effective instructions
	2. Balance and vestibular function: Addressing potential balance issues related to inner ear dysfunction
	3. Sensory integration: Enhancing the use of other senses to compensate for hearing impairment
	4. Psychosocial support: Providing support to address any psychological and social challenges related to hearing impairment
	Rehabilitation strategies
	1. Visual and tactile cues: Using visual aids, hand signals and tactile feedback to enhance communication during rehabilitation exercises
	2. Balance training: Incorporating exercises that specifically target balance and coordination
	3. Environmental modifications: Ensuring the training environment is conducive to the needs of hearing-impaired athletes, such as reducing background noise and providing clear visual cues
	4. Holistic approach: Combining physical rehabilitation with social and psychological support

20.8 Psychosocial and Environmental Factors That Influence Injury Risk and Rehabilitation

Research on psychosocial factors indicates that emotions, cognitions and behaviours are associated with sports injury rehabilitation outcomes [14]. While psychosocial interventions such as relaxation, positive self-talk, and goal setting have been found to facilitate recovery in athletes, their specific impact on para-athletes remains unexplored [15]. Although psychosocial factors are recognised as important in the rehabilitation of athletes, there is a lack of research specifically addressing the rehabilitation of para-athletes in bat-and-ball sports. Environmental factors, including equipment design and field conditions, have been shown to affect injury risk in bat-and-ball sports. Additionally, para-athletes face unique challenges due to the nature of their disabilities and the adaptations required for participation in sports, which may influence rehabilitation [16]. Practitioners working with para-athletes should be aware that injuries can present a greater challenge for these athletes than for those without impairments, as they may impede their ability to perform daily activities such as transferring from one location to another. This can have significant consequences for the psychosocial well-being of these athletes.

20.9 Conclusion

The benefits of sports practice for daily living are well established in individuals with impairments. However, for safety reasons, more research is warranted to investigate the nature, aetiology, mechanisms, severity and risk factors of sports injuries and their possible association with specific sports and types of impairments. Research on para-cricketers, particularly regarding their injuries, is extremely limited. Developing studies in this realm could lead to the creation of tailored therapeutic and preventative training programmes, enhancing players' functional independence, sports performance and overall health. Advancing research will ultimately reduce the incidence of sports injuries and improve the quality of life for impaired athletes.

References

1. Jewell C, Rockliff C, Black A. 892 BO38 – Spotlight on visually impaired (VI) athletes: a review of sport-related injuries, characteristics, risk factors, and opportunities for prevention. Brief Oral Abstr [Internet]. BMJ Publishing Group Ltd and British Association of Sport and Exercise Medicine; 2024. p. A66.1–A66. Available from: https://bjsm.bmj.com/lookup/doi/10.1136/bjsports-2024-IOC.114
2. Patatoukas D, Farmakides A, Aggeli V, Fotaki S, Tsibidakis H, Mavrogenis A, et al. Disability-related injuries in athletes with disabilities. Folia Med (Plovdiv) [Internet]; 2011. p. 53. Available from: http://content.sciendo.com/view/journals/folmed/53/1/article-p40.xml
3. Weiler R, Ahmed OH, Mechelen WV, Verhagen E, Bolling C. Concussion through my eyes: a qualitative study exploring concussion experiences and perceptions of male English blind footballers. Br J Sports Med. 2023;57:578–89.
4. Patricios JS, Schneider KJ, Dvorak J, Ahmed OH, Blauwet C, Cantu RC, et al. Consensus statement on concussion in sport: the 6th international conference on concussion in sport, Amsterdam, October 2022. Br J Sports Med. 2023;57:695–711.
5. Ahmed OH, Hussain AW, Beasley I, Dvorak J, Weiler R. Enhancing performance and sport injury prevention in disability sport: moving forwards in the field of football. Br J Sports Med. 2015;49:566–7.
6. Mirandola D, Monaci M, Miccinesi G, Vannuzzi A, Sgambati E, Manetti M, et al. Psychological well-being and quality of life in visually impaired baseball players: An Italian national survey. Federici S, editor. PLoS One. 2019;14:e0218124.
7. Mayrhuber L, Rietveld T, De Vries W, Van Der Woude LHV, De Groot S, Vegter RJK. A scoping review on shoulder injuries of wheelchair tennis players: potential risk-factors and musculoskeletal adaptations. Front Rehabil Sci. 2022;3:862233.
8. Warner MB, Wilson D, Heller MO, Wood D, Worsley P, Mottram S, et al. Scapular kinematics in professional wheelchair tennis players. Clin Biomech. 2018;53:7–13.
9. Mason BS, Vegter RJK, Paulson TAW, Morrissey D, Van Der Scheer JW, Goosey-Tolfrey VL. Bilateral scapular kinematics, asymmetries and shoulder pain in wheelchair athletes. Gait Posture. 2018;65:151–6.
10. Ju Y-Y, Chu W-T, Shieh W-Y, Cheng H-YK. Sensors for wheelchair tennis: measuring trunk and shoulder biomechanics and upper extremity vibration during backhand stroke. Sensors. 2021;21:6576.

11. Klenck C, Gebke K. Practical management: common medical problems in disabled athletes. Clin J Sport Med. 2007;17:55–60.
12. Tohamy B. Towards effective communication between sports recreation specialists and intellectually disabled athletes: an exploratory study. Int Sci J Phys Educ Sport Sci. 2018;6:33–43.
13. ChangSheng Z, Shin H-K, Kim YS. Study on the injury and rehabilitation of racket athletes with disabilities. J Korean Phys Ther. 2019;31:228–35.
14. Forsdyke D, Smith A, Jones M, Gledhill A. Psychosocial factors associated with outcomes of sports injury rehabilitation in competitive athletes: a mixed studies systematic review. Br J Sports Med. 2016;50:537–44.
15. Gennarelli SM, Brown SM, Mulcahey MK. Psychosocial interventions help facilitate recovery following musculoskeletal sports injuries: a systematic review. Phys Sportsmed. 2020;48:370–7.
16. Webborn N. The disabled athlete in ball sports. In: Chick G, editor. Acute chronic finger Inj ball sports [internet]. Paris: Springer; 2013. p. 817–30. Available from: http://link.springer.com/10.1007/978-2-8178-0382-1_12.
17. Júnior LAQC, Oka GTR, Bastos MP, Baima RL, Ferst NC, Lima ACO, et al. Trajectory correction for visually impaired athletes on 100 m Paralympic races. In: Antipova T, editor. Comprehensible Sci [internet]. Cham: Springer; 2022. p. 393–401. Available from: https://link.springer.com/10.1007/978-3-030-85799-8_33.
18. Shiota K, Tokui A. Audiospatial cognitive ability of visually impaired athletes in static and dynamic spatial cognitive tasks. J Phys Ther Sci. 2017;29:1981–6.
19. Afghani A. Android shape independent of aerobic fitness: a risk factor for low bone mineral content in overweight and obese Latina women. Clin Med Insights Womens Health. 2013;6:25–30.
20. West CR, Krassioukov AV. Autonomic cardiovascular control and sports classification in Paralympic athletes with spinal cord injury. Disabil Rehabil. 2017;39:127–34.

21 The Lived Experience of Injury in Cricket

Subhan Jay

21.1 I Am Subhan

My name is Subhan Jay, and I am 21 years old. I am studying Sports, Coaching and Physical Education at Oxford Brookes University. I am a semi-professional cricketer chasing my dream to be a professional cricketer. I showed interest in cricket early in my life (Fig. 21.1), and I was 9 years old when I decided to pursue my career as a cricketer. It is quite an early age to decide, but I believe there are a few things which you do not decide; rather, you are born with it. Coming from a very underdeveloped region and starting on the streets of Rawalpindi, Pakistan, it is never easy to make it big when a lot of talent is competing against you.

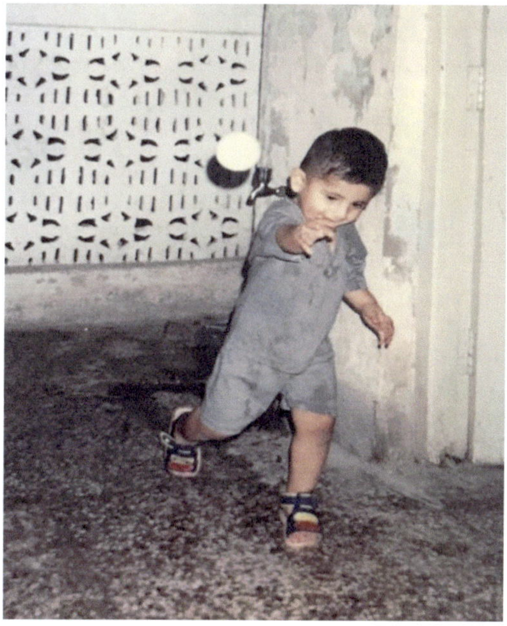

Fig. 21.1 Me, practising my bowling skills at a young age

21.2 Early Cricket Journey in Pakistan

I played my first senior team cricket game at the age of 9, and it is quite sad to say that I just fielded in that game. At that time, I felt incredibly happy to be involved because I just wanted to be on the field, and running around the entire day was extremely joyful. Naturally, I was never very good at cricket compared to other kids of my age,

S. Jay (✉)
Cricket Player, Oxford, UK

B. Olivier, J. W. Orchard (eds.), *Cricket Sports Medicine*,
https://doi.org/10.1007/978-981-96-6321-7_21

but what set me apart from the rest was my confidence, hard work, desire to improve, and never-give-up mentality, all of which I am happy to have maintained to this day.

At the age of 13, I enrolled in Pakistan's top cricket academy, and a year later, I was named senior team captain. I captained the senior team for the first time when I was 14 years old, and the amount of jealousy I received that day was unbelievable. Many older players were dissatisfied with my appointment as captain and left the club. They also thought that my average cricket skills did not make me a suitable leader. The academy coaches promoted me to captain because they saw my potential, influence and on-field demeanour, and we won the All Academy competition held in the UAE against academy teams like ICC and MS Dhoni. I was declared as the player of the tour (Figs. 21.2 and 21.3). This tour was a turning point in my journey and made me determined that against all the odds, I would stand tall and keep proving everyone wrong.

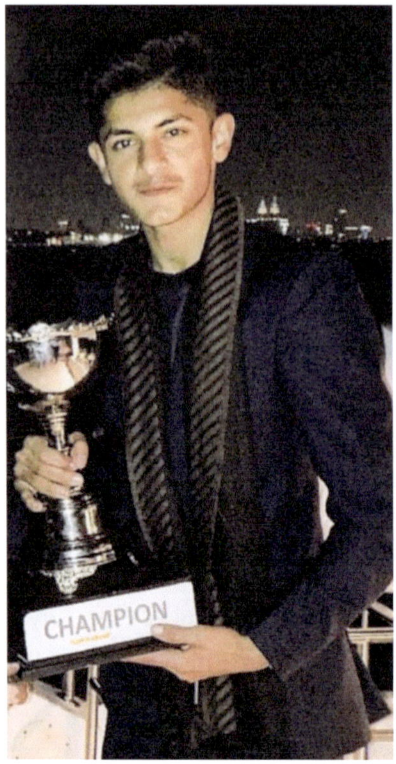

Fig. 21.3 Cruise dinner after winning the trophy

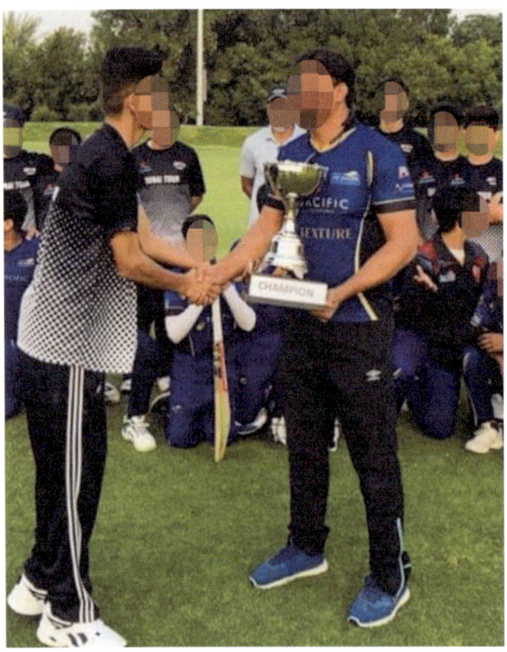

Fig. 21.2 Receiving the trophy as a winning skipper

21.3 Moving to England: A New Chapter

At the age of 15, I decided to leave my family, friends, school, and country and move to the UK (Fig. 21.4). This decision was extremely hard because I was very close to my mother since childhood and never thought of living a day without her, but to succeed, one must make a sacrifice, and I chose to leave my family, friends, and relatives behind to follow my ambition. I went to a cricket school in Sussex which gave me a tremendous opportunity to grow academically as well as a cricketer. The fitness standards and the skill level were top-notch. We had strength and conditioning sessions, where I had never heard of this term before. As weeks passed, I had never felt that insecure and underconfident before in my life.

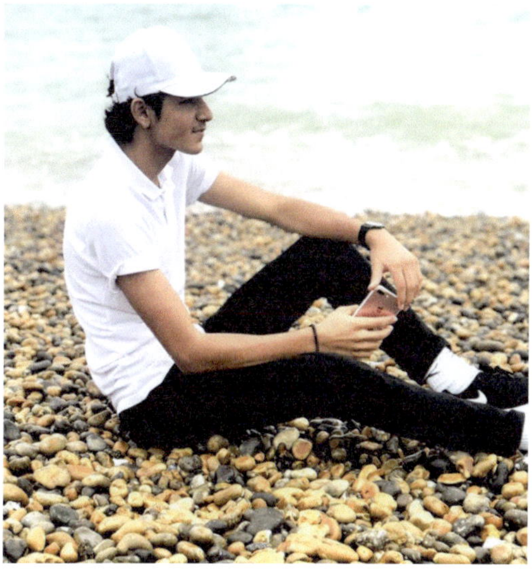

Fig. 21.4 First week in England in the city of Brighton

Before going to this academy, my view towards the cricketing world was entirely different, but the reality check brought me to my knees; I weighed about 43 kilos, which kept me underconfident.

I was dealing with some family issues, too, and in combination this affected me mentally, and at the time I just wanted to run away from all of it. I felt like quitting because the atmosphere around me was mentally exhausting. The added academic pressure made it even worse.

In my head, I clearly thought that I would disappear without telling anybody, but at the same time, there were some positive thoughts which were battling against these negative thoughts because I sacrificed a lot just to come to this stage, and what would I tell everyone back home about why I came back? Because it was hard and tough? I could not just screw up the expectations people had for me, especially my mother. So, that was the only motivation I had, and I decided to fight back.

I joined a nearby gym, and after college, I would head straight there daily (Figs. 21.5 and 21.6). The challenge was to be in the first team against all the odds. As a cricket player himself, my father's statements really influenced my work ethic. My father never gave me praise because he did not want me to develop a delusional mindset

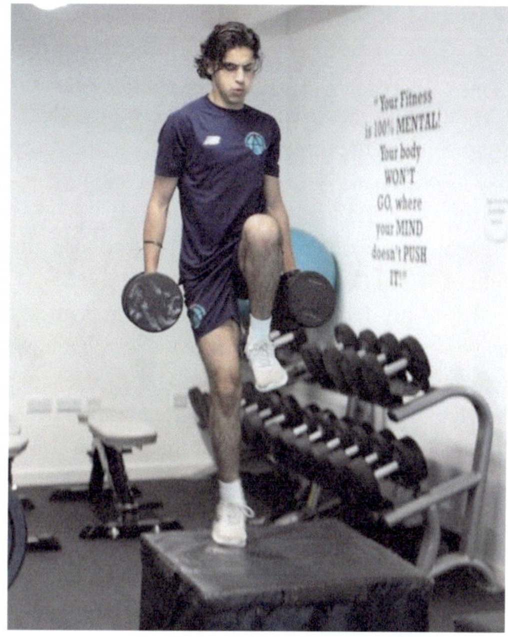
"Your Fitness
is 100% MENTAL!
Your body
WON'T
GO, where
your MIND
doesn't PUSH
IT!"

Fig. 21.5 Strength and conditioning at the academy

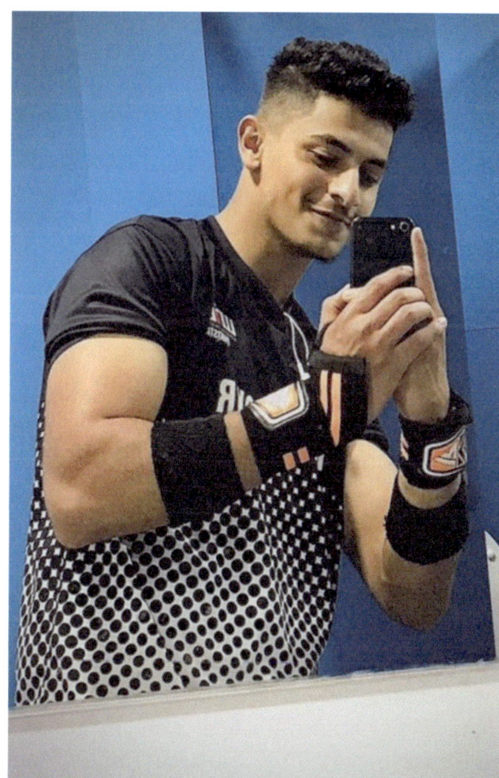

Fig. 21.6 A local gym in the city

in which I began to believe that I was too excellent. 'You are not good enough to be in the first team', 'Leave fast bowling, you are too weak for it', and 'Join cheerleading academy in college' were some of the things he would say to me every day as criticism. With determination and remembering ALLAH daily, I made it into the first eleven. The coaches and trainers produced the title of 'Hard Grafted One' for me.

I told my father about the selection with joy and my dad was already prepared to challenge me again, asking, 'Would you be the leading bowler?' And after taking a big breath upon hearing it, I decided to move on to the next task. My ambition to prove myself was tragically dashed by the COVID-19 pandemic. I continued to work and got stronger for my second year during the lockdown, but fate had other ideas. I damaged my shoulder, which affected my second year. I returned to my academy with the injury, which led to my dismissal from the team. Due to the injury, I did not perform up to par.

21.4 Battling Injuries and Setbacks

My performance suffered greatly when the bowling speed dropped. I lost my natural spark, flexibility and power somewhere, and the shoulder issue persisted even after receiving the necessary care. My injuries caused me a lot of pain, and it was emotionally draining to lose the speed I had developed.

I lost the muscles I had built after having to miss four months in the gym due to the shoulder problem. After recovering from the shoulder injury, I played my first season for a Sussex club alongside some incredible current Sussex star players and ex-England players. Being a member of the first eleven and competing against the top players in the league was an incredible experience. Since club performance was a requirement for selection, this was also my opportunity to return to my academy's first team. However, I had fewer opportunities to express myself and showcase my skills because I was the only youngster on the team and part of the squad. To regain my match fitness, I needed to bowl a lot of overs, but I only bowled four or five overs every game, which was obviously not helping me at all.

It was devastating; despite being the most diligent and wanting to wear the badge, I only had the opportunity to play one game for my academy. I bowled a fair number of overs in a few games before the season finished, but not enough to regain my pace, fitness, or confidence. In one of my academy's games, I took three wickets in three overs, scored in the 20s, and was dismissed. Since it was not a major squad game, I did not care that I was my team's best player. However, scoring runs and taking wickets is always fantastic, no matter where you play.

I left the academy after the completion of my A-levels and left Sussex with a heavy heart, as this place played a massive role in shaping my character and gave me the worst as well as best moments of my life. I thanked the players, coaches, and trainers for the support they provided me. Although it did not end the way I wanted due to the COVID-19 pandemic and my injury, I still wanted to leave with a smile on my face and get ready for the new challenges in life.

21.5 University Cricket and County Dreams

My primary motivation for applying to Oxford Brookes University was to play for the Oxford University Centre of Cricketing Excellence (UCCE). Before I joined, UCCE was regarded as first-class, and it was a fantastic quality where you play against county teams, establish yourself, and perhaps land a contract. Going into it, I knew I would not be able to get in straight away since it was a performance squad, and my club performance was not great because of the limited opportunities. The coach really liked my attitude and love for the game and gave me the chance to be a net bowler for the entire year. I felt good playing along with some great cricketers, but at times, I felt a bit unhappy, too, because I knew regardless of how well I bowled, there would not be any reward for me. I bowled for continuous 6 months selflessly and expected a reward in the future.

I joined a new club in Oxford and preferred continuing my cricket career in Oxfordshire.

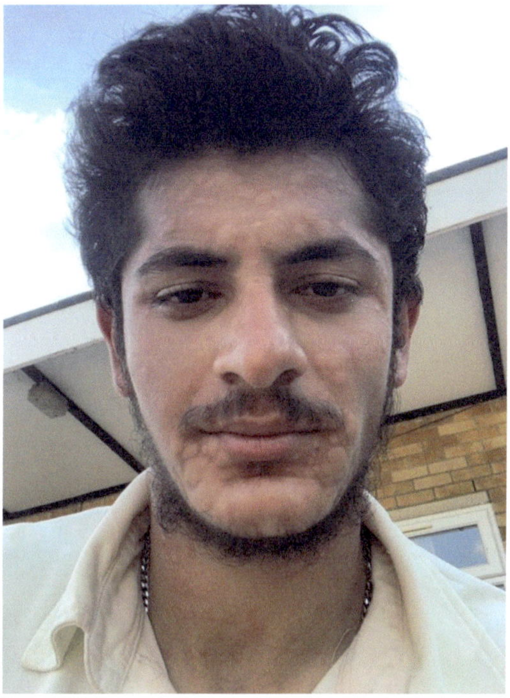

Fig. 21.7 Skin allergic attack during the game

Prior to the season, the objective was to take the most wickets and get unhindered entry into the UCCE main squad. I trained with a 'no mercy' mentality and pushed myself absurdly hard. I participated in 15 Red Ball matches, 6 Twenty20 matches, and 8 Under-19 matches for my team. I took over 50 wickets during the season, finishing as the league's second-highest wicket-taker and the club's top. In addition to being the top fielder for my team, I also picked up the most catches and run-outs. I had an excellent season overall and played some helpful knocks with the bat.

I experienced a medical crisis during the season due to shoulder pain and skin allergy (Fig. 21.7) attacks on the pitch, but I had a clear aim and refused to allow these things to affect how I was operating. I played the entire season despite these problems.

I was devastated with myself for not winning the match for my team while I was competing in the under-19 finals, as it was the last game of the season. Sitting on the side by myself, heated up, disappointed, and thinking negatively, I held a medal in my hand. What had I won after such a brilliant season? I had allergic reactions and would not leave the field. I attempted bowling quickly despite the pain, but what did I get for my constant effort?

But we plan and then ALLAH plans too. I saw an Oxfordshire chairperson walking up to me and approached me to be in the senior squad for the next season. I was completely unaware of who he was until he mentioned it himself. He observed me throughout the game and loved the passion I showed even though I lost the game. I did not collect many wickets or score any runs; it was just the confidence and hunger that everyone could witness. He invited me to winter nets with the county, and I felt a lot more relieved after hearing it because I told myself that, okay, I had achieved something.

The cricket season ended, and UCCE cricket started, and this time, my numbers were good enough to be in the squad. The team sheet came out, and I was in a provisional squad alongside 35 others. Now, the goal was to be in the main squad; now, I have to maximise my hard work. I created a very disciplined routine alongside an extremely strict diet plan and was excited to follow it.

21.6 Personal Struggles and Mental Health

Then came the most tragic chapter in my life. Back in Pakistan, I had fallen in love with a girl in my class when I was still at school. I always wanted a daughter like her. She was a walking art with unmatched grace and class. She was there for me through thick and thin, constantly convincing me that I was good enough to make it at the professional level. When everyone used to label me 'skinny' and make me feel horrible about myself physically, she was the one who constantly pulled me up and reminded me that everything would be worth it in the end.

The day came when she, the person I loved with my whole soul, decided to break-up with me. I was in the UK, and she was in Pakistan. I meant to go to Australia for a cricket season, but I promised her that I would come to Pakistan on her birthday. I burned the boats, left cricket, university, and my job and went to Pakistan on her birth-

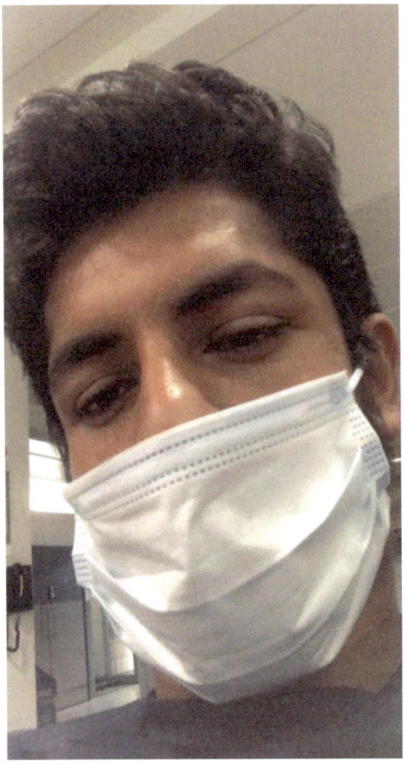

Fig. 21.8 Depression and anxiety attacks

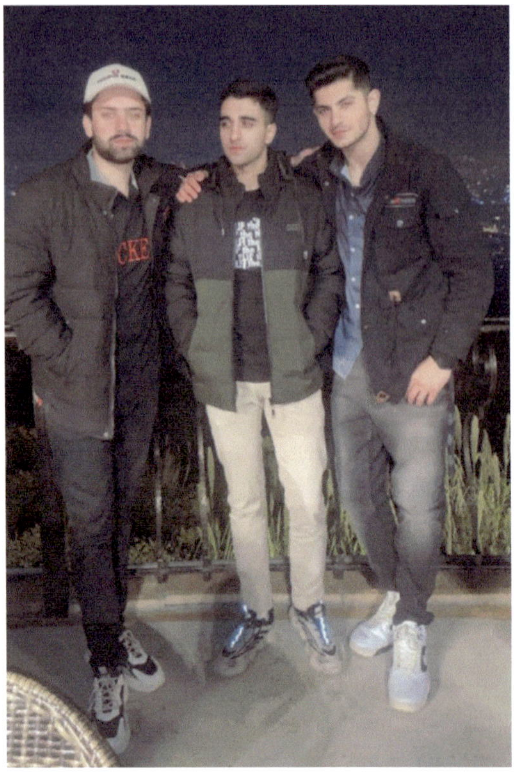

Fig. 21.9 My best friends back in Pakistan

day with the hope that she would come back to me. She denied seeing me and asked me to leave respectfully. She once told me that whenever she has a son, she wants him to be exactly like me. Seeing the same person turning cold made the world seem blurry, and I always wanted to be a cricketer for her, and even cricket seemed very irrelevant, too. Then, I went into depression and started experiencing anxiety attacks (Fig. 21.8).

I had two friends named Abu Bakar and Daniyal who were with me for 17 years (Fig. 21.9). They encouraged me and told me that I cannot give up. I should use this as motivation and become an even better person and athlete. I kept a smile on my face but came back to the UK with a broken heart. I dealt bravely with my illness and fought through it and told myself that I could not screw up the expectations people had for me.

I used to train in Ramadan while fasting, utilising an absolutely devastating routine. I used to leave my bed at 5 am daily and train for seven continuous hours for UCCE, including the nets and gym sessions daily. Then, I used to go to my lectures and was doing a part-time job alongside it, and I did it for the whole month. By the time of breaking the fast, I would be exhausted, but my passion did not let me stop. There were days when I could not do it anymore, but I said to myself that before, it was for her, and now I have to do it for myself.

My coach made it clear that no fast bowler would be a part of a 3-day game against Northampton County whose Yo-Yo score would be below 19. I took my fitness to the next level and promised myself that I would not stop running until I was dragged off the pitch. I scored 19.3, which was the fourth-highest score on the squad. I scored 18.1 previously, and seeing this improvement was satisfactory for me. I ticked all the boxes of selection criteria, but on the selection day, I was not selected. I had no hard feelings towards the coach, but I felt very hurt as all the hard work I did to achieve my dream did not pay off. I ignored the fact that I was not selected and worked even harder.

I was included as a 12th man for the following games due to my patience and hard work. I was on the bench for five consecutive games. Finally, a day came when I was in the playing 11, but fate was against me; the game got called off due to rain. I managed to play just one T20 game and bowled four overs with figures of 2–21. I got dropped without any explanation and never got a callback.

The cricket season started, and I went to play for the same club. I can say that I was bowling absolute wheels, and everyone at the club witnessed the massive gain in my pace and power. I changed my bowling action a bit and used my lower back a lot more than I was doing before. The concerning bit was that I was not picking up the wickets despite bowling quick.

During training sessions, I could feel that my lower back and hip region were continuously hurting, but I did not pay attention. As weeks passed, I never felt that insecure and underconfident. During a league game, I bowled three overs, and I could feel something was not right in my hip region. I came to bowl the fourth over, and on the second ball of my fourth over, I fell so badly and could not even move. I felt like someone was chopping a knife into my back. I could not comprehend what had just happened. I went to see a doctor, and they advised me to rest for 4–6 weeks.

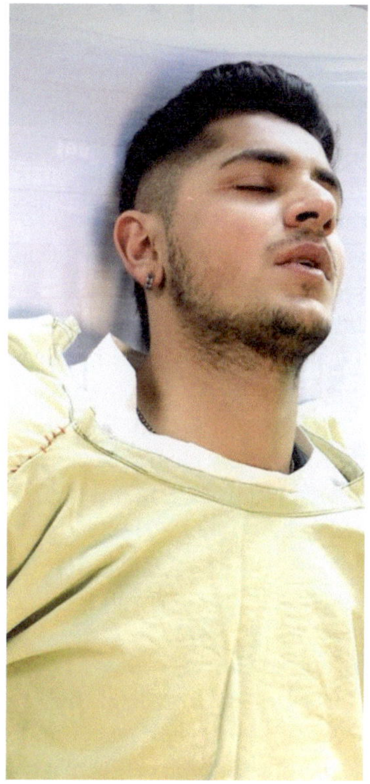

Fig. 21.10 After treatment of spinal injury

21.7 The Road to Recovery

After hearing that, I thought, how am I going to survive without cricket? But I had no option other than to give myself a chance to recover and be patient about it. With each day, my pain got worse, and I could not even move without support. My cricket season ended that year, and with it, the chance to represent UCCE and Oxfordshire. All these thoughts piled up and pushed me towards the same condition I was in during my break-up. But, as I learned a lot during those months, I again decided to fight with a smile on my face and be grateful to ALLAH regardless of my condition.

Seeing everyone play was hurtful, and that is the worst sight for any cricketer. I kept telling myself that it is for good, and ALLAH gives hard battles to strong soldiers, so fight through it and stand tall. After being in bed for four months with no improvement, I went back home for proper treatment (Fig. 21.10). I got steroid injections, hours of physiotherapy and exercises. I had L2, L3 and L4 disc bulges which impacted my groin, quadriceps, and tensor fasciae latae muscle. After the treatment, I went through rehabilitation, and I just kept saying to doctors, 'Please make me better; I want to play cricket again'. My mother was constantly there with me, encouraging me that I would play again and a lot better than before. But obviously, she could not see me in the painful state and showed her concern for me to opt for some other profession. I just kept telling her that I could not leave. I had left everything for the game, and if the game decided to leave me, then it was fine, but there was no way I was leaving it.

I cried on stretchers, with both negative and positive thoughts that will I be ever able to stand again and bowl fast? Would my childhood dream stay a dream? But the dream only ends when you stop dreaming, so I trusted ALLAH, stopped worrying about external factors, and decided to focus on what is under my control because if you focus on what is controllable, uncontrollable will automatically be in your control.

During my recovery, there were times when I was so sick and tired of doing the same thing repeatedly with no impact, but I used to watch my bowling videos, and I desperately wanted to fly the same way. You need to be mad and crazy if you want to be a fast bowler, and I had that madness. People love hitting sixes, I loved preventing them from hitting those sixes.

Finally, after one long year, I recovered, and my old club got relegated from the premier league, so I joined a new club. This year's season was also mentally very challenging, as the fear of getting injured again stuck in my head and every time I tried to bowl quickly, I would hold myself back. I played with body straps and painkillers just to give myself the chance to play for UCCE.

Whatever I have been through, ALLAH was always by my side, along with the prayers of my parents (Figs. 21.11 and 21.12). I consider myself an unsuccessful successful person. I have not made it to a professional level yet, but the respect and lifelong lessons I have received are unmatched. I am unlucky in love and in my cricketing life, but still grateful for every moment they have given me. Cricket has made me a better man, and so did the girl I was with. I believe in myself and still think that I will be a professional cricketer one day.

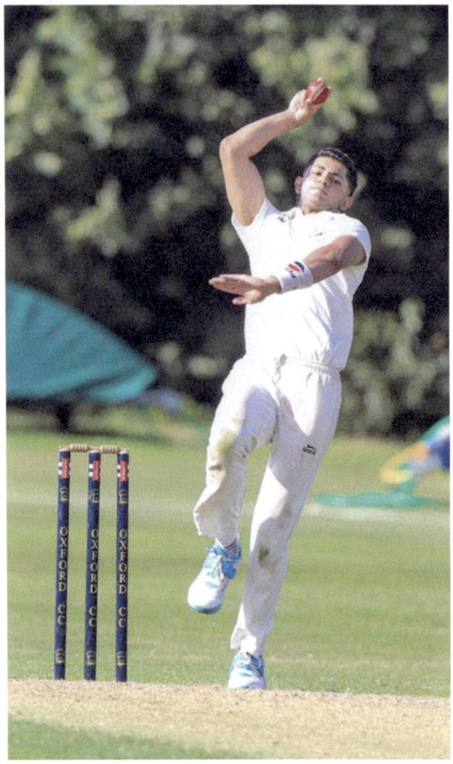

Fig. 21.12 Bowling after the injury of 1 year

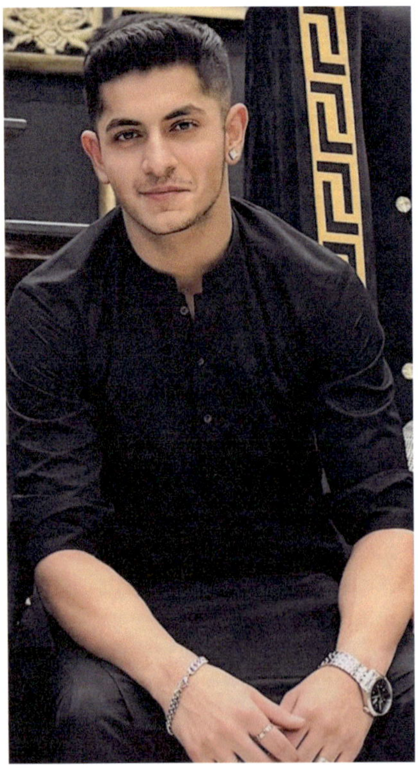

Fig. 21.11 Present day

People think I am arrogant and do not consider anyone better than me, which is not true. In my head, I am always the best without pushing anyone down. I do not get bothered by what people think of me; my fight and competition started with myself, and I will be the only barrier in my life that stops me from achieving what I want to achieve. My wicket-taking celebration is also based on self-belief, a positive mindset, believing in yourself and believing in ALLAH because he is always there. For my love life, I would leave the last page blank, just in case… and for my cricketing life, I would turn my dream into reality and bring a smile to my mother's face.

I want to be different from the rest of the guys, and I strive to be the best. I believe that 'I am not the one in the crowd, I am a crowd in one man'.

Part II

Specific Medical Considerations in Cricket

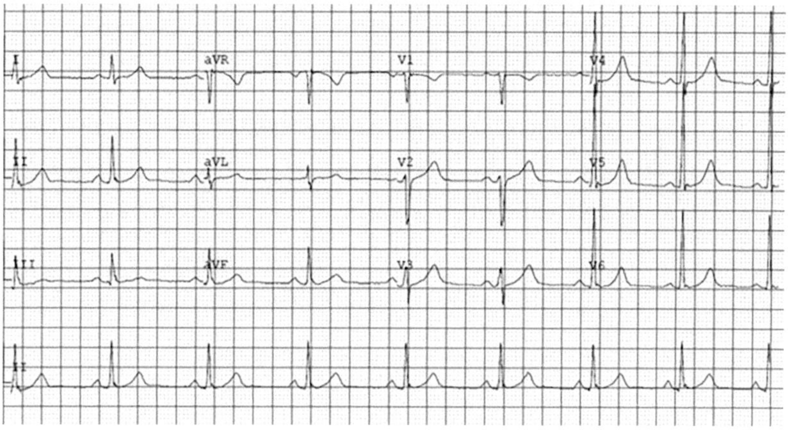

A normal athlete ECG

Pre-participation Cardiac Screening in Professional Cricket

22

Jessica J. Orchard, Hamish MacLachlan, Asela J. B. Ratnayake, and Nicholas Peirce

22.1 Introduction

The sudden unexpected death of young adults and children creates significant distress for families, friends, team environments and society and can be extreme when a collapse and sudden death occurs on the public stage, notably on the sporting field. With the spotlight on these tragedies now increasing exponentially through television and social media, a single event can have a profound impact. Cricket is no different and society now has an expectation that these events should be prevented. Consequently, sports have increasingly sought to implement measures for primary and secondary prevention and fulfil an expected duty of care.

This imperative has led to a strong desire to identify athletes at risk of young sudden cardiac death (SCD). We have moved past the arguments that considered the pre-participation evaluation (PPE) screening programme to likely produce too many false positives, end careers unnecessarily and be especially costly. The evidence now is clear that many of the conditions associated with SCD can be detected through pre-participation cardiac screening (PPCS) with an electrocardiogram (ECG)-based protocol. Furthermore, following screening and identification, there are evidence-based, disease-specific interventions such as lifestyle changes, drug therapy, surgical interventions and insertion of implantable cardioverter defibrillators to reduce the risk of SCD in affected athletes, many of whom can choose to continue. Sport now uses PPCS to meet the primary objectives: to identify underlying cardiovascular disorders predisposing to SCD, with the intent to reduce morbidity and mortality in its environment and on the field, whilst providing individualised, patient-centred, and disease-specific medical management [1].

There is widespread agreement that SCD in young individuals is an important public health issue, although national screening programmes for whole populations are not routine. Nevertheless, the European Society of Cardiology (ESC) and the American Heart Association (AHA) advocate PPCS for young athletes on legal, medical and ethical grounds [2, 3]. Since these recommendations were published, PPCS programmes have been established within various sporting organisations around the world,

J. J. Orchard (✉)
Sydney School of Public Health, The University of Sydney, Sydney, NSW, Australia
e-mail: Jessica.orchard@sydney.edu.au

H. MacLachlan
St George's University of London, London, UK
e-mail: Hamish.maclachlan@nhs.net

A. J. B. Ratnayake
Sport & Exercise Medicine Centre, Khoo Teck Puat Hospital, Singapore, Singapore

N. Peirce
England and Wales Cricket Board, London, UK
e-mail: Nick.peirce@ecb.co.uk

B. Olivier, J. W. Orchard (eds.), *Cricket Sports Medicine*,
https://doi.org/10.1007/978-981-96-6321-7_22

including the International Olympic Committee [4].

The global governing body for cricket, the International Cricket Council (ICC), provides a minimum medical standard to its 108 member nations for all ICC-organised events [5]. From a cardiac perspective, these standards focus on effective secondary prevention measures such as the requirement for a protocol and chain of command in the case of a cardiac arrest, including an ambulance on match day stationed close to the playing area, which is supported by appropriately trained staff. The minimum standard also requires the event chief medical officers to submit a detailed post-event medical report to the ICC. Whilst information on PPCS is requested in the medical report, this practice is not mandated by the ICC. As such, the nation members have autonomy over their decision to implement PPCS programmes for their registered athletes.

22.2 Magnitude of SCD in Athletes

SCD is widely accepted as the leading cause of medical death in young athletes [6].

However, there remains significant variation in the reported incidence of SCD (0.09 to 13.09 per 100,000 PY) [7]. This variation is explained by significant heterogeneity in study populations, definitions of SCD and methods of case ascertainment, including an accurate numerator (number of deaths per year) and an exact denominator (number of athlete participants per year) in the population studied. In the absence of established registries for young SCD, epidemiological studies have historically employed data identification methods which are hindered by ascertainment and selection biases. Examples include retrospective analyses of media reports and insurance claims which will underestimate the incidence of SCD. The only systematic review of SCD incidence in the young (12–39 years) general population was undertaken by Couper et al. [8]. There was no restriction of language or date in their review of 38 studies which also reported on subgroups of incidence according to sex, age and athletic status. Once again, significant heterogeneity in study populations, definitions of SCD and methods of case ascertainment precluded a meta-analysis. A notable limitation of the review was that survivors of SCA were not included. The main analysis included 26 studies and reported a median incidence of SCD in the general population as 1.7 per 100,000 person-years (PY) (IQR 1.3–2.6, range 0.75–11.9) [8]. After subgroup analysis, the investigators concluded that the majority of studies reported an incidence in the range of 1–2 cases per 100,000 PY.

Evolving epidemiological data supports a differential risk profile for SCD among specific population of athletes. The risk appears to be determined by: (1) Increasing age—athletes aged over 35 years are at 5 to 10 times greater risk than younger counterparts [9], (2) Sex—male athletes at 3 to 10 times greater risk than female counterparts [8], (3) Ethnicity—Black athletes at 3 to 5 times greater risk than white counterparts [6, 10] and (4) Sporting discipline and standard of competition—elite basketball, American football and soccer [6, 11].

These high-risk groups challenge the uniform approach to PPCS set out by the AHA and ESC. A risk-based approach may provide sporting organisations with a more cost-effective strategy for PPCS, particularly in the setting of limited resources, although this approach is not without important ethical considerations.

There are a number of relevant ethical issues that arise in the design and implementation of cardiac screening programmes [12]. One important consideration is whether the programme is mandatory (with or without enforcement, meaning 'no screen, no play'), opt-out (with or without a written waiver) or opt-in. In a survey of Australian elite sporting organisations' cardiac screening policies, about half were mandatory without enforcement and about a quarter were opt-out [13]. If using an opt-out programme, it is ideal to provide information about screening to athletes in advance to ensure they have sufficient time to make an informed decision about whether to participate. However, whichever model is used, the most important things are that the screening programme is well-run and that all

ECGs (and echocardiograms, if included) are interpreted by a physician with relevant expertise and that results are communicated and followed up (if needed) [12].

22.3 Cricket and the Risk of SCD

Cricket is a sport that has different disciplines within it that have different physiological demands. It is routinely played in the summer months internationally and often in hot conditions. It is played outdoors and often requires the individuals to spend prolonged periods undertaking repeated sprints of 20–50 metres. A bowler, for instance, will cover up to 45 km in a test match (5 days) through fielding and bowling. Approximately 7 km will be covered with repeated running at 18–20 km/h. In a one day international (typically 7–8 hours), players cover up to 15 km in the field, and if you include batting and perhaps scoring 100 runs, an all-rounder could cover 20–25 km. Cricket players could cover 1.5 km of that distance over the speed of 20 kph and players have been recorded reaching maximum speeds of around 34 kph in the field whilst chasing the ball to the boundary and players can do up to 200 high intensity/explosive accelerations off the mark. For comparison, an average elite midfield soccer player covers 10 km in one game.

However, the reality is that the incidence of SCD and SCA in professional cricket players is unknown. There are limited cases identified from media reports as detailed in Table 22.1. A complete review of media reports describing all traumatic cricket-related (cardiac and non-cardiac) fatalities in Australia was published in 2018 [14].

It is widely recognised that sport per se is not the direct cause of mortality in athletes; rather, it acts as a trigger for sudden cardiac arrest in predisposed individuals with underlying cardiovascular disease. Exercise may provide an arrhythmogenic setting due to a higher probability of hyperthermia, circulating catecholamines, and shifts in cardiac electrolytes and the acid-base balance. Sustained physical activity also holds the potential to accelerate the phenotype of arrhythmogenic cardiomyopathy which is one of the target conditions of PPCS [15, 16]. These factors are determined by the exercise intensity of the sporting discipline, which includes the static and dynamic demands of the physical activity.

These components are considered in the Mitchell classification of sports, which is referenced in the AHA and American College of Cardiology guidelines for eligibility and disqualification for competitive athletes with cardiovascular abnormalities [17]. It has been argued that cricket has been misclassified as a sport with 'low' static and dynamic cardiovascular demands and where 'impact is not expected' [18]. This may have important clinical implications in terms of recommendations for players with a cardiovascular diagnosis or who are taking anticoagulants. Consequently, cricket is likely to be reclassified in the next version of the Mitchell classification. Of note, cricket is not referenced in the equivalent classification system adopted in the 2020 ESC guidelines on sports cardiology and exercise in patients with cardiovascular disease [19].

Table 22.1 The incidence of SCD and SCA in professional cricket players from media reports

Name	Age at death (years)	Year of death	Team	SCA or SCD	Aetiology
Wilf Slack	34	1989	Middlesex, UK	SCD	Unknown
Parvaz Shirma	25	1996	Worcestershire, UK	SCD	Unknown
Joshua Baker	20	2024	Worcestershire, UK	SCD	Sudden arrhythmic death syndrome
Scott Mason	28	2005	Tasmania, Australia	SCD	Previous surgery for aortic valve replacement

Neither classification considers the sport-specific environmental factors, which are clearly relevant to cricketers who are typically exposed to long days in the sun. These conditions heighten the risk of hyperthermia and acidaemia, which serve as triggers for sudden cardiac arrest, as outlined above.

Cricketers who have a substrate for sinister ventricular arrhythmia and are deemed high-risk for sudden cardiac arrest may be considered for implantation of a primary (or secondary) prevention implantable cardioverter defibrillator (ICD). The AHA guidelines on athletes with ICDs seemingly apply a blanket recommendation against sports participation besides 'low-intensity' IA-level activities, including cricket, provided they are free of ventricular arrhythmia and device therapy for 3 months [17]. The notion that cricketers implanted with an ICD are safe to resume competitive sport should be approached with caution. The physical and environmental demands placed on cricketers, mistakenly considered safe in the return to low-intensity IA sport, may induce shifts in metabolic and electrolyte states may affect the device's detection and therapy algorithms and reduce the efficacy of shock therapy [20]. Another consideration for athletes with ICDs participating in sports such as cricket with pronounced, repetitive arm movements, is the increase in the risk of lead damage due to subclavian crush [21]. An understanding of this risk is particularly relevant to the device operator who may wish to consider implantation on the contralateral side of the dominant throwing arm, or submuscular placement which may promote device durability. An accurate understanding of the athlete's expected heart rate profile during their sport is warranted to ensure appropriate detection cut-off rates are programmed. The athlete should be aware of and avoid these heart rates throughout their physical activity. Conversely, detection zones need to be high enough for the athlete to meet the physical demands required and reduce the occurrence of inappropriate shocks [22]. Finally, device function may be compromised because of blunt trauma, which is relevant to a batter who may be hit in the chest by a hard cricket ball travelling at high speed from the bowler's arm. It is worth noting that force from a cricket ball to the chest is significant enough to cause SCD by commotio cordis.

There are several examples of cricketers experiencing commotio cordis. Commotio cordis occurs when a person receives a sharp blow to the chest, which causes a disruption to the heart rhythm (ventricular fibrillation) and sudden cardiac arrest [23]. These include the following (fatal) cases:

- Ankit Keshri, age 20, who bumped into the bowler whilst taking a catch in Bengal, 2015. [24]
- Martin Bedkober, age 22, who was batting was hit in the chest by the ball in Brisbane, 1975. [25]
- Abdul Aziz, age 18, who was struck in the chest by the ball whilst batting in Karachi, 1959 [25].

Another non-fatal case has been described of a 25-year-old at training, who was struck by the ball over the precordium whilst batting (without a chest protector) [26]. He was found unconscious, given CPR by coaching staff and successfully defibrillated by paramedics 9 minutes after the injury.

For the reasons described above, clinicians should avoid the one-size fits approach to athletes who are being considered for return to play following the diagnosis of a condition associated with ICD, and/or implantation of an ICD. Clearly, the athlete's risk of SCD associated with a return to yoga (IA) and riflery (IA) may differ significantly from cricket (IA). Contemporary guidelines have shifted towards a more individualised disease and sport-specific approach to risk assessment, and shared decision making which involves the athlete patient [27].

22.4 Existing Policies for Primary Prevention of SCD in Elite Cricketers

The landscape of cardiac screening in professional sports worldwide has evolved significantly, with increased awareness of the risk of SCD among athletes driving more comprehensive screening protocols. The screening protocols adopted by sporting organisations are influenced by differences in healthcare infrastructure, resource availability and differing interpretations of the cost-effectiveness and sensitivity of screening methods. As the debate over the best practices continues, the overarching goal remains the early detection of potentially life-threatening cardiac conditions to ensure athlete safety.

22.5 Cricket Australia

In 2016, Cricket Australia implemented a policy recommending players at the elite level are screened with personal/family history and physical examination (H&P) and resting 12-lead electrocardiogram (ECG). Players are screened on entry to the elite system and then every 2 years (up to age 21) or every 5 years (for those aged 21+ years) [28]. This protocol is similar to most other elite sports in Australia [13]. It is an opt-out policy and those who choose not to be screened are able to sign a waiver.

A detailed audit of the Cricket Australia programme was published in 2020 [28]. This paper reviewed cardiac screening results of all current players at the time (n = 710). The cohort comprised 62% male players/38% female (a reflection of the relative size of the elite and pathway programmes) and the mean age was 20.4 ± 4.9 years (range 14–37 years). Compliance with the programme was excellent at 98%, meaning that 98% had an up-to-date screening or waiver.

Importantly, no players were diagnosed with a condition associated with sudden cardiac death (SCD), no one was excluded from the sport for a cardiac reason and there were no major cardiac incidents reported in the previous 5 years. Almost 7% of players required follow up of some kind (most commonly an echocardiogram) and a small number of other diagnoses were made. These include bicuspid aortic valve (0.8%) and <0.7% for each of pulmonary valve lesion, Wenckebach heart block, supraventricular tachycardia, atrial fibrillation and mitral regurgitation (without mitral valve prolapse).

A detailed review of the ECGs showed that the rate of abnormal ECGs was low at 2.0% when interpreted using the International Criteria for Athlete ECG Interpretation [29]. Several benign athlete heart changes were common, e.g. sinus bradycardia (33.5%) and left ventricular hypertrophy by voltage criteria (LVH) (16.3%). LVH was 15 times more prevalent in male cricketers compared to females and most common in junior male pace bowlers. T-wave inversion was more common in female cricketers compared to males, both overall (8.0% vs. 1.2%, $p < 0.0001$) and in the anterior leads (V3–V4: 1.3% vs. 0.2%, $p = 0.049$).

Importantly, the programme is supported by a system of other measures to prevent cardiac emergencies [30]. This includes regular audits and reviews for ongoing quality improvement, an expert sports cardiology panel that provides 'sports cardiology infrastructure' and detailed match/training emergency planning procedures including CPR training for staff and access to automated external defibrillators (AEDs) [31].

22.6 England and Wales Cricket Board (ECB)

The PPCS programme in cricket was introduced by the England and Wales Cricket Board (ECB) in 2008. Initially reserved for the national squads, the programme soon expanded to include all national age group squads, disability squads and all first class counties.

The ECB's initial protocol included a health questionnaire (HQ), a 12-lead ECG and a clinical consultation with a sports cardiologist. Transthoracic echocardiography (TTE) was initially adopted as a second line screening tool, reserved for those with abnormal findings on their HQ or ECG. The ECB's screening protocol was updated in 2018, and required all cricketers to undergo an assessment with a 'one-off' TTE, preferably at their index screening. The frequency of screening using the standard ECG-based protocol was determined by the athletes' age (repeated every 2 years during adolescence and then 5 yearly after 21 years of age).

Outcomes from the ECB's nationwide screening programme were published in 2022. The screening protocol which evolved over the data collection period provided MacLachlan et al. with a unique opportunity to additionally report on the impact of repeat cardiac evaluations and first-line, one-off echocardiography, on top of ECG-based screening [32].

The study included 1208 cricketers who were screened between 2008 and 2019. After initial evaluation with the standard ECG-based protocol, 47 (3.9%) athletes underwent additional on-site assessment with TTE. TTE cleared 12 individuals, leaving 35 (2.8%) who were recommended follow-up (Fig. 22.1). After comprehensive secondary evaluation, 4 athletes (0.3%) were diagnosed with cardiac conditions associated with SCD, including 1 athlete with hypertrophic cardiomyopathy, 1 with arrhythmogenic cardiomyopathy and 2 with a Wolff–Parkinson–White pattern.

No additional conditions or adverse cardiac events were reported over a mean follow up of 5.8 ± 2.9 years. The overall prevalence of conditions associated with SCD in this study was 0.6%, which is similar to that reported in similar studies of athletic populations [5, 26].

The study highlighted the value of the on-site clinical consultation when one considers that 12% of athletes reported a symptom on their HQ but only a fraction (1.3%) of these prompted referral for further evaluation. Indeed, an experienced on-site physician is required to interpret symptoms and family history of heart disease in order to reduce the number of false-positive referrals [27, 28].

The cost of the standard ECG-based protocol was £106 per athlete and £25,569 per cardiac condition associated with SCD. These findings suggest that a sport-specific, nationwide, ECG-based cardiac screening programme for elite athletes can be cost-efficient, with 80% of costs attributed to first-line investigations.

22.7 Additional Value of Periodic Screening

Despite normal initial evaluation with the ECG-based protocol, 493 athletes underwent repeat screening at a cost of £50,151. Repeat evaluation demonstrated new ECG findings (Fig. 22.2) in 3 athletes, 1 of whom was referred for secondary evaluation and was diagnosed with hypertrophic cardiomyopathy. These findings support the ESC's recommendation to periodically screen athletes every 2 years [2].

22.8 Additional Value of Routine Screening with TTE

Despite normal findings with an ECG-based protocol, 342 athletes underwent first line assessment with TTE. This £200 test identified 2 athletes with cardiac conditions associated with SCD, including 1 with a bicuspid aortic valve with severe aortopathy and aortic regurgitation and 1 with a haemodynamically significant atrial septal defect. An additional 10 athletes were identified with minor valvular and congenital abnormalities. These findings demonstrate that TTE has the potential to identify structural heart diseases not detected by the ECG [33]. The enhanced sensitivity must be carefully balanced against cost. In this study, the cost of first-line TTE averaged £238 per athlete and £40,761 per cardiac condition associated with SCD. These findings suggest that an ECG-based protocol (with second line TTE) is a more cost-efficient screening protocol if the target conditions are those only associated with SCD. This may explain why TTE is typically adopted by financially endowed sporting organisations. A recent survey of 603 physicians who regularly screen athletes revealed that up to 65% use TTE as a first-line screening tool [34].

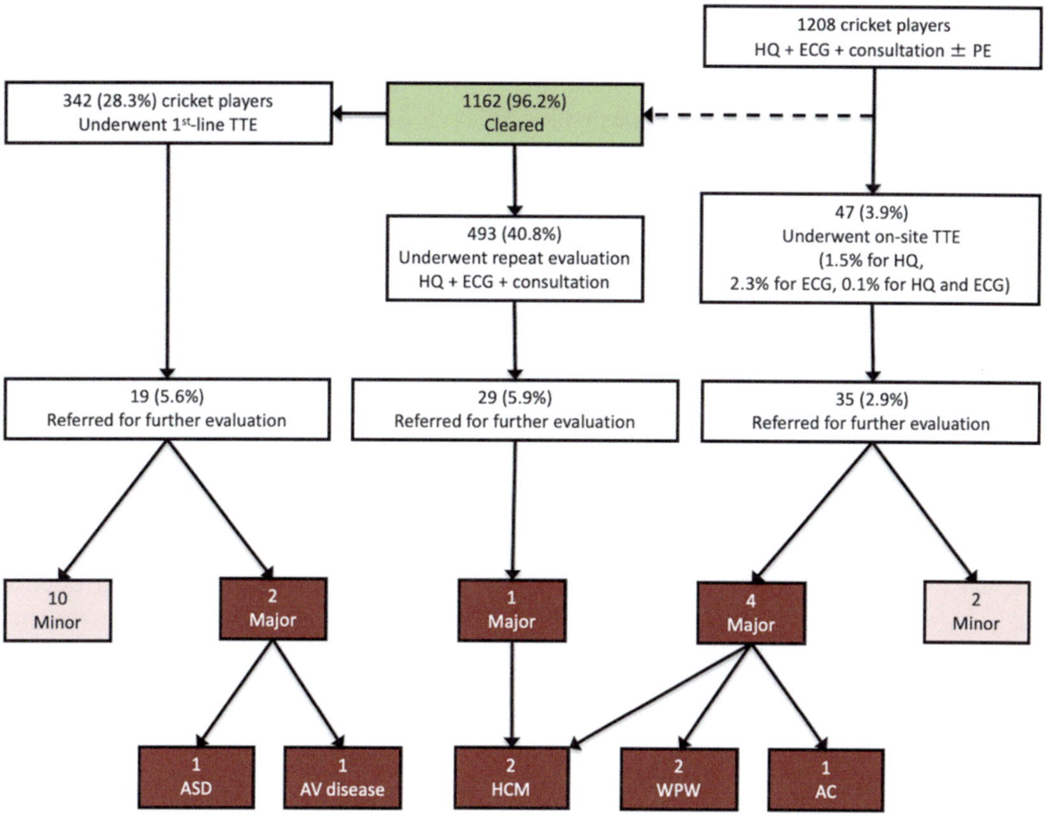

Fig. 22.1 Flow chart of cardiac screening programme in young, elite cricketers. *AC* arrhythmogenic cardiomyopathy, *ASD* atrial septal defect, *AV* aortic valve, *ECG* electrocardiogram, *HCM* hypertrophic cardiomyopathy, *HQ* health questionnaire, *TTE* transthoracic echocardiogram, *WPW* Wolff–Parkinson–White ECG phenotype [32]

The limitations of available resources, time and cost associated with TTE have been challenged by recent studies, which have evaluated the performance of focused protocols and novel hand-held devices [35, 36].

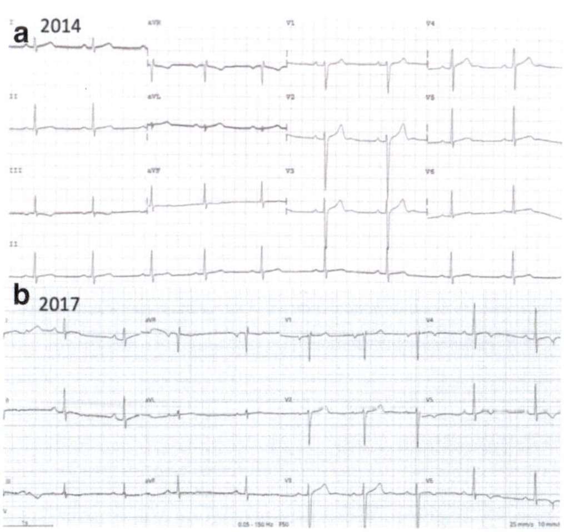

Fig. 22.2 Initial (**a**) and routine follow-up ECG (**b**) demonstrating new T-wave inversion in lateral leads

Regardless of the device or protocol being used, TTE interpretation can be challenging in athletic individuals when one considers cardiac adaptations to exercise may mimic mild phenotypes of cardiomyopathies. Incorrect interpretation of the athlete's heart by inexperienced clinicians may result in a significant number of unnecessary and costly secondary evaluations. Despite this, the majority of abnormalities identified with first-line TTE are congenital or valvular. If left untreated, these conditions may be associated with increased morbidity later in the athletes' life and should therefore be considered as target conditions.

22.9 Sri Lanka

Sri Lanka has a universal national programme of screening, which was introduced through the Ministry of Health in 2015 by the sports medicine development committee. This national pre-participation medical examination (PPE) programme is recommended for competitive athletes/sports and is compulsory for certain sports in all age groups [37]. In Sri Lanka, cricket is one of the sports that draws special consideration for a recommendation of PPE with its modern high-rated activity level and continuous exposure.

The cardiac screening section of the PPE includes a detailed examination of the cardiovascular system examination with a mandatory 12-lead ECG. The positive cases are further referred to either cardiology or electro-cardiophysiology for a specialised opinion before clearance for sports participation. Clearance for sports is conducted through the sport and exercise medicine centres in the main hospitals, through the trained medical doctors in the peripheral hospitals and private medical centres with authorised medical doctors. The PPE should be obtained at least 3 months before the sports event and pre-event examination (PEE) should be taken at least 2 weeks before the event. The validity period for the PPE is 12 months.

22.10 Secondary Prevention Strategies for SCD in Athletes

No cardiac screening programme will be able to offer absolute prevention of SCA. As such there have been great efforts to improve education and resources for effective secondary prevention through emergency response planning, heightened public awareness of cardiopulmonary resuscitation (CPR) and prompt deployment of AEDs.

Early recognition of SCA is the pivotal first step to an efficient emergency response. Delays may occur as SCA is often mistaken for epileptic seizures. Furthermore, agonal breathing during SCA may be interpreted as a normal breathing pattern, particularly following syncope in sport or apnoeic breathing at night [38].

After early recognition of SCA, the next step in the widely recognised 'chain of survival' is early CPR, which is improved through education and the development of policies and guidelines which aim to improve the survival of SCA by increasing the likelihood that victims receive effective bystander CPR and prompt defibrillation. Every educational and sports organisation is encouraged to have an emergency response plan for SCA, which is supported by written policies and procedures that promote a structured response to SCA [39, 40]. This is outlined in the ICC's minimum medical standard for major ICC events which requires the following:

1. An ambulance with an automated external defibrillator (AED) to be present, and stationed close to the playing area and dressing rooms, which is staffed by trained individuals capable of coping with SCA.
2. The host member to provide a protocol and chain of command in case of a medical emergency, including SCA.
3. An AED with manual override and monitor in the match day medical room.

The next step in the chain of survival is 'early defibrillation', which is the greatest factor affecting survival from SCA [41]. In a large study of exercise-related SCA, Drezner et al. reported 132 cases of young SCA, which occurred over a 2-year period. The majority (93%) of cases were witnessed with 83% surviving if a certified trainer was present at SCA, and 89% surviving if an AED was used [42]. These findings support the establishment of AED programmes and the potential for investment in improving facilities for effective CPR and early defibrillation.

Effective prevention measures require an understanding of the circumstances of young SCA. Data from Denmark, Australasia and the United Kingdom suggests that 40% to 70% of cases of young SCD occur at home [43–45]. Collectively, these studies suggest the majority of cases of young SCD are unlikely to be prevented by widespread AED programmes. For that reason, early identification of disease through primary preventative strategies (PPCS) appears to play an important role in reducing the overall burden of SCD in young individuals.

22.11 Future Considerations for PPCS

The great debate pertaining to what constitutes the most effective screening strategy is likely to continue when we consider no screening test is perfect, and a prospective controlled trial of adequate size and duration remains elusive. Efforts should therefore focus on maximising the efficiency of existing screening models.

The digital health revolution will play an important role in enhancing the effectiveness of future screening strategies, including the use of wireless telemonitoring technologies that have more recently enabled real-time ECG recording that can be viewed on tablets or smartphones [46]. Early data from studies using these novel ECG recording devices suggests they have the potential to identify cardiac conditions associated with SCD [47].

Using such telemonitoring technologies in athletes with established diseases reduces complications through enhanced, structured follow-up and also liberates them by reducing the frequency of travel, time off work and overall costs. The cost-effectiveness of screening models may also be enhanced by artificial intelligence, which is redefining ECG analysis through the application of machine learning and deep learning in ECG interpretation [48]. An on-site physician is often required to interpret findings from the HQ and ECG. The on-site physician is a costly, limited resource and compromises the cost-effectiveness of the screening protocol which in turn limits its application on a large-population scale. Advancements in Digital Health have enabled remote screening tools that can reduce assessment costs, making them especially valuable for sports organisations operating with limited financial resources.

References

1. Drezner JA, O'Connor FG, Harmon KG, et al. AMSSM position statement on cardiovascular preparticipation screening in athletes: current evidence, knowledge gaps, recommendations and future directions. Br J Sports Med. 2017;51(3):153–67.
2. Corrado D, Pelliccia A, Bjornstad HH, et al. Cardiovascular pre-participation screening of young competitive athletes for prevention of sudden death: proposal for a common European protocol. Consensus Statement of the Study Group of Sport Cardiology of the Working Group of Cardiac Rehabilitation and Exercise Physiology and the Working Group of Myocardial and Pericardial Diseases of the European Society of Cardiology. Eur Heart J. 2005;26(5):516–24.
3. Maron BJ, Levine BD, Washington RL, et al. Eligibility and disqualification recommendations for competitive athletes with cardiovascular abnormalities: task force 2: preparticipation screening for cardiovascular disease in competitive athletes: a scientific statement from the American Heart Association and American College of Cardiology. Circulation. 2015;132(22):e267–72.
4. Ljungqvist A, Jenoure P, Engebretsen L, et al. The International Olympic Committee (IOC) consensus statement on periodic health evaluation of elite athletes March 2009. Br J Sports Med. 2009;43(9):631–43.
5. International Cricket Council. Minimum Medical Standards for Major ICC Events. Available from: https://images.icc-cricket.com/image/upload/prd/h8forjrphtngdoktcmud.pdf. Accessed 6 Nov 2024.
6. Harmon KG, Asif IM, Maleszewski JJ, et al. Incidence, cause, and comparative frequency of sudden cardiac death in National Collegiate Athletic Association Athletes: a decade in review. Circulation. 2015;132(1):10–9.
7. Mohananey D, Masri A, Desai RM, et al. Global incidence of sports-related sudden cardiac death. J Am Coll Cardiol. 2017;69(21):2672–3.
8. Couper K, Putt O, Field R, et al. Incidence of sudden cardiac death in the young: a systematic review. BMJ Open. 2020;10(10):e040815.
9. Harmon KG, Asif IM, Klossner D, Drezner JA. Incidence of sudden cardiac death in National Collegiate Athletic Association athletes. Circulation. 2011;123(15):1594–600.
10. Maron BJ, Haas TS, Ahluwalia A, Murphy CJ, Garberich RF. Demographics and epidemiology of sudden deaths in young competitive athletes: from the United States National Registry. Am J Med. 2016;129(11):1170–7.
11. Malhotra A, Dhutia H, Finocchiaro G, et al. Outcomes of cardiac screening in adolescent soccer players. N Engl J Med. 2018;379(6):524–34.
12. Orchard JJ, Neubeck L, Orchard JW, et al. ECG-based cardiac screening programs: legal, ethi-

cal, and logistical considerations. Heart Rhythm. 2019;16(10):1584–91.
13. Orchard JJ, Orchard JW, Toresdahl B, et al. Cardiovascular screening of elite athletes by sporting organizations in Australia: a survey of chief medical officers. Clin J Sport Med. 2021;31(5):401–6.
14. Brukner P, Gara TJ, Fortington LV. Traumatic cricket-related fatalities in Australia: a historical review of media reports. Med J Aust. 2018;208(6):261–4.
15. James CA, Bhonsale A, Tichnell C, et al. Exercise increases age-related penetrance and arrhythmic risk in arrhythmogenic right ventricular dysplasia/cardiomyopathy-associated desmosomal mutation carriers. J Am Coll Cardiol. 2013;62(14):1290–7.
16. Saberniak J, Hasselberg NE, Borgquist R, et al. Vigorous physical activity impairs myocardial function in patients with arrhythmogenic right ventricular cardiomyopathy and in mutation positive family members. Eur J Heart Fail. 2014;16(12):1337–44.
17. Maron BJ, Zipes DP, Kovacs RJ. Eligibility and disqualification recommendations for competitive athletes with cardiovascular abnormalities: preamble, principles, and general considerations: a scientific statement from the American Heart Association and American College of Cardiology. J Am Coll Cardiol. 2015;66(21):2343–9.
18. Orchard JJ, Orchard JW, La Gerche A, Raju H, Semsarian C. Misclassification of cricket in the American College of Cardiology (ACC) Task Force classification of sports. Br J Sports Med. 2020;54(8):491–2.
19. Pelliccia A, Sharma S, Gati S, et al. 2020 ESC Guidelines on sports cardiology and exercise in patients with cardiovascular disease: the Task Force on sports cardiology and exercise in patients with cardiovascular disease of the European Society of Cardiology (ESC). Eur Heart J. 2021;42(1):17–96.
20. Lampert R, Olshansky B, Heidbuchel H, et al. Safety of sports for athletes with implantable cardioverter-defibrillators: results of a prospective, multinational registry. Circulation. 2013;127(20):2021–30.
21. Garraud T, Pomares G, Daley P, Menu P, Dauty M, Fouasson-Chailloux A. Thoracic outlet syndrome in sport: a systematic review. Front Physiol. 2022;13:838014.
22. Olshansky B, Atteya G, Cannom D, et al. Competitive athletes with implantable cardioverter-defibrillators-how to program? Data from the implantable cardioverter-defibrillator sports registry. Heart Rhythm. 2019;16(4):581–7.
23. Palacio LE, Link MS. Commotio cordis. Sports Health. 2009;1(2):174–9.
24. Brannan J. 20 year old Cricketer suffers Sudden Cardiac Arrest: https://www.defibshop.co.uk/blog/post/20-year-old-cricketer-suffers-sudden-cardiac-arrest. Accessed 27 June 2024.
25. 29 Year-Old Sunshine Coast Cricketer, Alecz Day, collapses with Sudden Cardiac Arrest at Training and is Saved By Team Mates2020:https://en.wikipedia.org/wiki/Wilf_Slack. Accessed 27 June 2024.
26. Spencer RJ, Sugumar H, Jones E, Farouque O. Commotio cordis: a case of ventricular fibrillation caused by a cricket ball strike to the chest. Lancet. 2014;383(9925):1358.
27. Dougles RJ. Sudden cardiac death following blunt chest trauma: commotio cordis. World J Emerg Med. 2011;2(3):234–6.
28. Orchard JJ, Orchard JW, La Gerche A, et al. Audit of a cardiac screening policy for elite Australian cricketers. J Sci Med Sport. 2020;23(6):541–7.
29. Drezner JA, Sharma S, Baggish A, et al. International criteria for electrocardiographic interpretation in athletes: consensus statement. Br J Sports Med. 2017;51(9):704–31.
30. Orchard J, Puranik R, Semsarian C, et al. Prevention of sudden cardiac death in cricketers. J Postgrad Med Educ Res. 2016;50(2):49–58.
31. Orchard JJ, Puranik R, Inge PJ, Golding L, Orchard JW. Cardiac screening and prevention of other cardiac emergencies in cricket. J Postgrad Med Educ Res. 2023;57(4):154–7.
32. MacLachlan H, Dhutia H, Bhatia R, et al. Results of a nationally implemented cardiac screening programme in elite cricket players in England and Wales. J Sci Med Sport. 2022;25(4):287–92.
33. Grazioli G, Merino B, Montserrat S, et al. Usefulness of echocardiography in preparticipation screening of competitive athletes. Revista Española de Cardiología (English Edition). 2014;67(09):701–5.
34. D'Ascenzi F, Anselmi F, Mondillo S, et al. The use of cardiac imaging in the evaluation of athletes in the clinical practice: a survey by the sports cardiology and exercise section of the European Association of Preventive Cardiology and University of Siena, in collaboration with the European Association of Cardiovascular Imaging, the European Heart Rhythm Association and the ESC Working Group on Myocardial and Pericardial Diseases. Eur J Prev Cardiol. 2021;28(10):1071–7.
35. Mitchell AR, Hurry R, Le Page P, MacLachlan H. Pre-participation cardiovascular screening: is community screening using hand-held cardiac ultrasound feasible? Echo Res Pract. 2015;2(2):49–55.
36. Wyman RA, Chiu RY, Rahko PS. The 5-minute screening echocardiogram for athletes. J Am Soc Echocardiogr. 2008;21(7):786–8.
37. De Silva YHS, De Silva OL, Thebuwanaarachchi ST, Gunawardane S, Mendis H. Medical problems detected during pre-participation physical evaluation of school athletes in the Galle District. J Postgrad Inst Med. 2017;4(1)
38. Ruppert M, Reith MW, Widmann JH, et al. Checking for breathing: evaluation of the diagnostic capability of emergency medical services personnel, physicians, medical students, and medical laypersons. Ann Emerg Med. 1999;34(6):720–9.
39. Drezner JA, Courson RW, Roberts WO, Mosesso VN, Link MS, Maron BJ. Inter-association Task Force recommendations on emergency preparedness and management of sudden cardiac arrest in high school

and college athletic programs: a consensus statement. J Athl Train. 2007;42(1):143–58.
40. Drezner JA, Heinz WM, Asif IM, et al. Cardiopulmonary considerations for high school student-athletes during the COVID-19 pandemic: update to the NFHS-AMSSM guidance statement. Sports Health. 2022;14(3):369–71.
41. Drezner JA, Rao AL, Heistand J, Bloomingdale MK, Harmon KG. Effectiveness of emergency response planning for sudden cardiac arrest in United States high schools with automated external defibrillators. Circulation. 2009;120(6):518–25.
42. Drezner JA, Peterson DF, Siebert DM, et al. Survival after exercise-related sudden cardiac arrest in young athletes: can we do better? Sports Health. 2019;11(1):91–8.
43. Bagnall RD, Weintraub RG, Ingles J, et al. A prospective study of sudden cardiac death among children and young adults. N Engl J Med. 2016;374(25):2441–52.
44. Finocchiaro G, Papadakis M, Robertus JL, et al. Etiology of sudden death in sports: insights from a United Kingdom Regional Registry. J Am Coll Cardiol. 2016;67(18):2108–15.
45. Winkel BG, Holst AG, Theilade J, et al. Nationwide study of sudden cardiac death in persons aged 1–35 years. Eur Heart J. 2011;32(8):983–90.
46. Chen W, Khurshid S, Singer DE, et al. Cost-effectiveness of screening for atrial fibrillation using wearable devices. JAMA Health Forum. 2022;3(8):e222419.
47. Nasarre M, Strik M, Daniel Ramirez F, et al. Using a smartwatch electrocardiogram to detect abnormalities associated with sudden cardiac arrest in young adults. Europace. 2022;24(3):406–12.
48. Smaranda AM, Dragoiu TS, Caramoci A, Afetelor AA, Ionescu AM, Badarau IA. Artificial intelligence in sports medicine: reshaping electrocardiogram analysis for athlete safety – a narrative review. Sports (Basel). 2024;12(6)
49. Davis AJ, Orchard JW, McGhie D, Broadbridge D, Raju H, La Gerche A, Puranik R, Gray B, De Jongh J, Driscoll T, Orchard JJ. Comparison of 6-lead smartphone ECG and 12-lead ECG in athletes and a genetic heart disease population. Expert Rev. Med. Devices. 2025;22(1):99–105. https://doi.org/10.1080/17434440.2024.2443113.
50. Orchard JJ, Orchard JW, Raju H, La Gerche A, Puranik R, Semsarian C. Comparison between a 6-lead smartphone ECG and 12-lead ECG in athletes. J. Electrocardiol. 2021;6695–97. https://doi.org/10.1016/j.jelectrocard.2021.03.008.

Environmental Safety Considerations in Cricket

23

John W. Orchard, Michelle Cort, and Ollie Jay

23.1 Is There a Risk of Death Due to Heat Stroke in Cricket?

Heat stroke in sport is a genuine risk that is dependent on environmental conditions (temperature, humidity, sun exposure, wind), the activity/sport being undertaken and any individual risk factors (permanent or situational). Having said that, heat stroke deaths are surprisingly rare, not only in cricket but also in the sister sports that are generally played in summer (baseball, tennis and golf). A Wikipedia list of prominent deaths on the field playing cricket only lists one case of heat stroke, ironically from cool-climate Surrey in 1881 [1]. A review of exertional heat stroke deaths in Australia over 20 years did not cite any deaths playing cricket [2]. There are rare isolated claims of heat stroke deaths in amateurs, for example, in a cricketer in Pakistan in 2022 [3], but these reports are relatively unusual given the number of matches played in hot conditions. Heat stroke deaths are particularly common in summer pre-season training in American football [4], and this probably relates to body shape (some American football players have a large muscular body mass index (BMI)), protective equipment, the presence of sickle cell trait in Black Americans, plus a combination of a modest heat acclimatisation status and high peak temperatures and humidity when training camps begin [5, 6]. By contrast, cricketers have lower metabolic heat production during match play and training, a leaner body type, and the fielders (with the greatest exposure) do not wear protective equipment. The wicketkeeper might be at the highest risk of the fielders due to protective equipment but does not run as much as the other players. Batters might also theoretically and in practice [7] be at risk due to the running and protective equipment requirements. There may be a self-limiting factor in that a batter might simply be quite likely to be dismissed if in the early stages of heat illness, as concentration and reaction time might deteriorate. The risk, hence, is certainly real but perhaps far lower than might be imagined in the first instance, given that there is not a single famous case from the history of the sport.

Hospitalisations from heat illness in cricket are far more recognised, and in Australia, were previously reported at a rate of 10.0 per 1,000,000 participants per year, making cricket the fourth

J. W. Orchard (✉)
School of Public Health, University of Sydney, Sydney, NSW, Australia
e-mail: john.orchard@sydney.edu.au

M. Cort
Cricket Australia, National Cricket Centre, Brisbane, QLD, Australia
e-mail: Michelle.cort@cricket.com.au

O. Jay
Heat and Health Research Centre, University of Sydney, Sydney, NSW, Australia
e-mail: ollie.jay@sydney.edu.au

B. Olivier, J. W. Orchard (eds.), *Cricket Sports Medicine*,
https://doi.org/10.1007/978-981-96-6321-7_23

highest risk sport in Australia [8]. The vast majority of players who are adversely affected by heat during play would not present to hospital, so the 'true' incidence of low-grade heat illness is unknown (but potentially very high).

It might be that heat stress is a relevant co-factor in deaths from other causes on the playing field, even though these are rare themselves. Raymond van Schoor, the Namibian captain, died from a vascular stroke sustained whilst playing in a game. Some media reports suggested that he reported a headache but continued to play, and it was assumed that perhaps the symptom was due to the day being hot [9]. His cause of death is certainly reported as 'stroke'. Perhaps the occasional cardiovascular death that occurs in cricket might be presumed to be more common on hot days, although the rarity of such events makes study difficult.

23.2 A Near-Miss Case?

Possibly the most famous case of heat illness in professional cricket was Dean Jones, who scored a double century for Australia in the Tied Test of 1986 at Chennai. India is notorious for having some of the hottest and most humid conditions in world cricket (Fig. 23.1). It was in an era when Australia travelled without a team doctor. It is hard to accurately ascertain how close he might have come to dying of heat stroke, but it is reported that he vomited multiple times, was dizzy and confused and had memory loss of the innings [10]. He was apparently taken to hospital after he was dismissed. The rarity of such an innings may relate to the unlikelihood of batting that long without getting dismissed with the symptoms described. Whilst it is now lauded as a legendary innings that personified bravery, it can be seen in hindsight as an 'exception that proves the rule'. Most of the time, batters suffering from excessive heat stress will be dismissed prior to any serious consequences. On the other side of the field, bowlers suffering from the ill effects of heat stress might be somewhat protected by being overlooked by the captain when their bowling capacity drops. Individual sports (such as trail walking and distance running events) where there is no ability to 'tag' with a teammate appear to have a higher risk of serious consequences related to the heat [2]. Cricket cannot be complacent just because of the rarity of severe heat stress cases in the past, as climate change is increasing the number of extreme heat days.

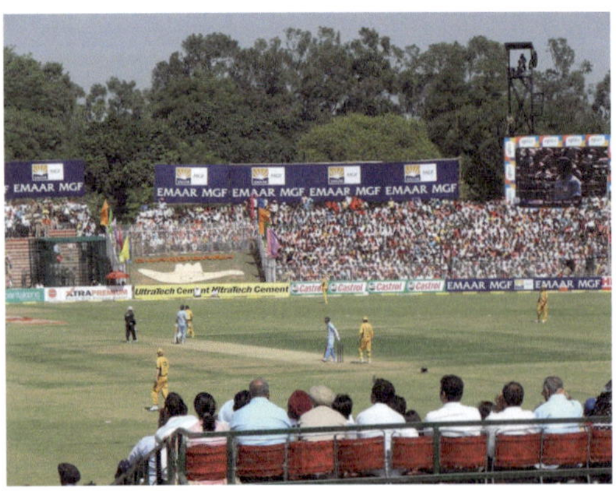

Fig. 23.1 Cricket in the Indian subcontinent is often played in extremely hot and humid conditions

23.3 The Interaction Between Infectious Illness and Heat Stroke

A less serious case from the modern era occurred to the England men's Test captain, Joe Root, in the Ashes Test in Sydney against Australia in January 2018 [11]. Conditions were extremely hot, with the temperature exceeding 40 °C during the match. However, Joe Root was the only player to suffer heat-related illness, and this was probably because he—like Dean Jones—was concurrently suffering from a viral gastrointestinal illness at the time. He is one of the very rare cases to have retired (ill) twice during the same innings. Both the Jones and Root histories emphasise that it might be the combination of very hot conditions and then individual additional factors, such as concurrent illness, which lead to the most severe heat-related illness cases in cricket. Therefore, in addition to the traditional measures used to prevent the negative impacts of heat stress (hydration, shading, ice packs), illness prevention is a further measure that can help (isolation of sick individuals, use of masks, vaccination).

23.4 The Historical Difference in Attitude Towards Heat Versus Rain and Poor Light

At the professional level, umpires and even both teams are loath to consider ever suspending a game because of heat. It is sometimes argued that it would be devastating for TV contracts and paying customers if a fixture was ever cancelled or suspended due to excessively hot conditions. By contrast, red ball cricket has a long tradition of suspending play when the most marginal of drizzle appears or the light drops below a dull level (even in stadiums where floodlights are available). This may be in part because objective readings of light have been available to umpires, whereas measurement of heat and humidity is more complicated (Fig. 23.2). Some of the reasoning behind this comparative decision-making is based on tradition: players come off in light rain and when light is borderline because they have always done so, and they don't come off in excessive heat because they have never done so. For red ball cricket, an eventual reset of the traditions is likely that it might occasionally be considered prudent to suspend play in extreme heat and, in the other direction, continue play in light drizzle or under floodlights for the sake of continuity of play.

The emergence of T20 cricket and the primacy of TV rights as the major revenue stream for the professional game have led to one fortunate change with respect to the risk of heat stress. The majority of T20 games are now played 'under lights' in the evening when more TV viewers are available to watch; this itself reduces the health risks due to heat stress to far lower levels. It is the day innings of 50-over matches and most multi-innings cricket (which is rarely played at night) where heat stress risks remain a consideration.

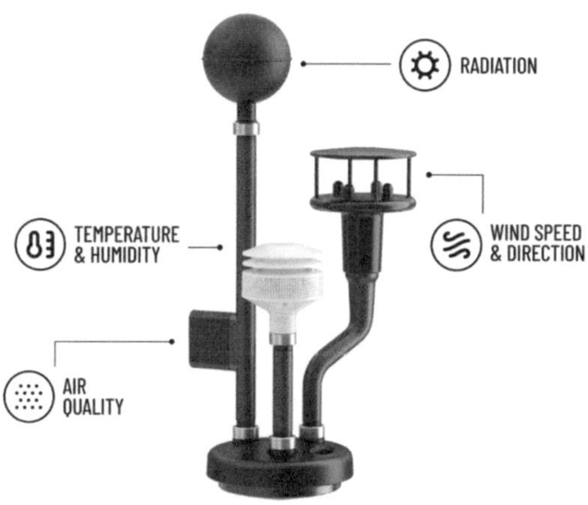

Fig. 23.2 A modern device used to measure heat stress index

23.5 Cancellation of Community Cricket

Common sense is more likely to prevail for community cricket and junior cricket, where there is no money on the line. However, the traditions of the game have a similar 'knock on' effect, where junior games which are cancelled due to rain do not raise any eyebrows at all, but it often becomes a matter of large controversy, even at the junior level, when play is suspended due to the heat. It should be remembered that for games where medical staff are not available and which are being played for enjoyment rather than for money, it would be sensible to err on the side of caution when considering the safety of junior and amateur cricket. It is also perhaps an easier but less painful decision to cancel in advance when weather conditions are forecast to be extremely oppressive. Once a match has commenced (and it is easier to start early in the morning when the heat will not be as bad), emotion comes into the decision as one team will be nominally leading by the time the day reaches its hottest point.

23.6 Is There a Risk of Death Due to Lightning Strike in Cricket?

Lightning is actually an environmental risk more likely to kill a cricketer, albeit still exceedingly low, with cricket historically being one of the most exposed sports to lightning [12]. Fortunately, the risk of lightning death has decreased substantially over the last century due to the increasing concentration of surrounding tall structures that attract lightning strikes [12], although some cricket

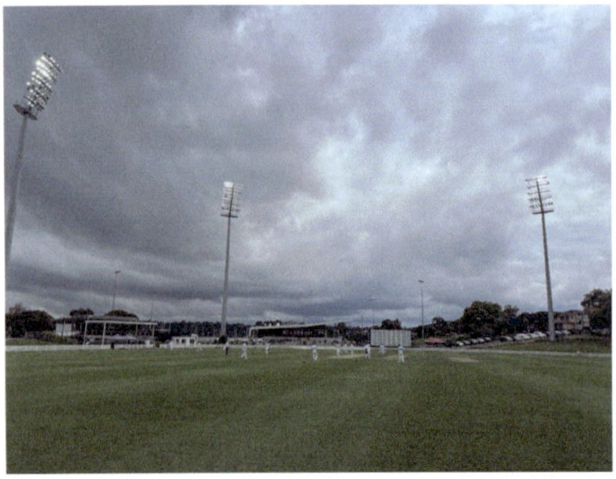

Fig. 23.3 Lightning is more of a risk at open grounds that have limited tree/grandstand fixtures (although the floodlights illustrated provide some protection)

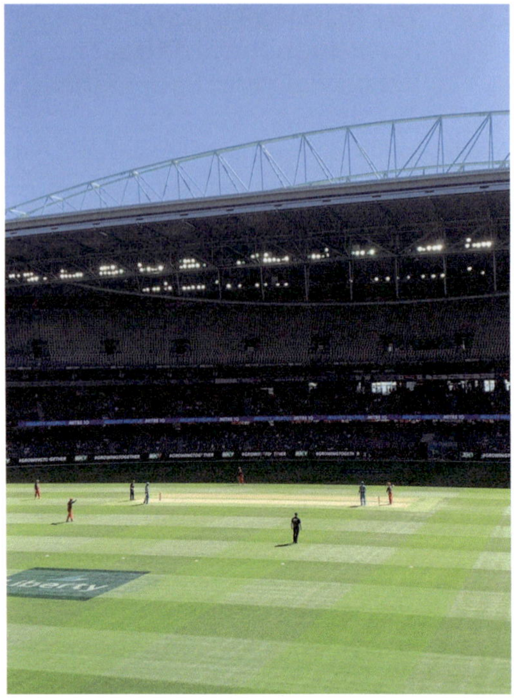

Fig. 23.4 Docklands (Marvel) Stadium in Melbourne has a retractable roof, making it very safe against lightning but perhaps still susceptible to conditions which might cause heat illness to occur

grounds retain an 'open' structure with some risk (Fig. 23.3). At the professional level, there is the best preparation against lightning strikes, but probably the least risk, as the presence of roofed grandstands (Fig. 23.4) almost certainly (but not absolutely) mitigates against much of the risk. Country/rural/provincial grounds would have higher risk than city and suburban grounds. A rare case of lightning strike at the elite level illustrates a historical disconnect between match suspension rules and actual safety considerations. In 2003, Mervyn Dillon and Fernix Thomas were both struck by lightning in a Red Stripe match in Jamaica [13]; despite this alarming incident, the match was not suspended, and Thomas returned to bowl two more overs after being struck. A belated decision was made to send the players to hospital for treatment after the match was suspended later on when the rain finally arrived. Lightning guidelines and surveillance would no doubt be more rigorous in contemporary times. The propensity for cricket play to be suspended even under mild drizzle means that the risk to players (slipping, for example) due to wet conditions is minimal. Perhaps the most realistic risk of playing on during light rain might be a pace bowler losing control of the ball during delivery and inadvertently bowling an above-the-waist full toss. The tradition of not playing on during rain is probably more grounded in competitive fairness, that the pitch and ground conditions would change too much from pre- and post-rain, rather than dire concerns about players' safety (albeit that the latter is a minor consideration). Occasional objections have been raised about the safety of batters and fielders being able to view the 'pink ball' in day-night Test cricket; very little research has been conducted on this to date, although there has not seemed to have been an obvious additional influx of injuries in batters in the limited number of 'pink ball' Tests played to date.

23.7 Guidelines for Cancellation and Extra Breaks in Elite Cricket

Considerations when deciding on whether conditions warrant additional drink break(s) or even suspension of play include the available weather data and the source of this data. To assess heat risk to players and officials with some accuracy, key parameters should include ambient air temperature in the shade, wind speed (in km/h), relative humidity (%) and black globe temperature

(Fig. 23.2). Using an official weather station or unofficial weather station (e.g. Weather Underground) will only provide some of this information. Another limiting factor to weather station data is that it is located a significant distance from the ground, and therefore, conditions will be different in both locations.

A tailor-made environmental measurement unit (EMU) [14] allows for measuring this data at the venue itself, which makes it highly reliable and useful when accurate data is required.

Cricket Australia currently uses a bespoke Heat Stress Risk Index (HSRI) [15] throughout its domestic cricket competitions to assess whether playing conditions should be changed. In addition to using the key weather parameters (mentioned above), the HSRI algorithm also incorporates data relating to player physiology and uniform. The HSRI is used in real time to provide information and recommendations to match officials as to whether extra drink breaks or a suspension of play is advisable.

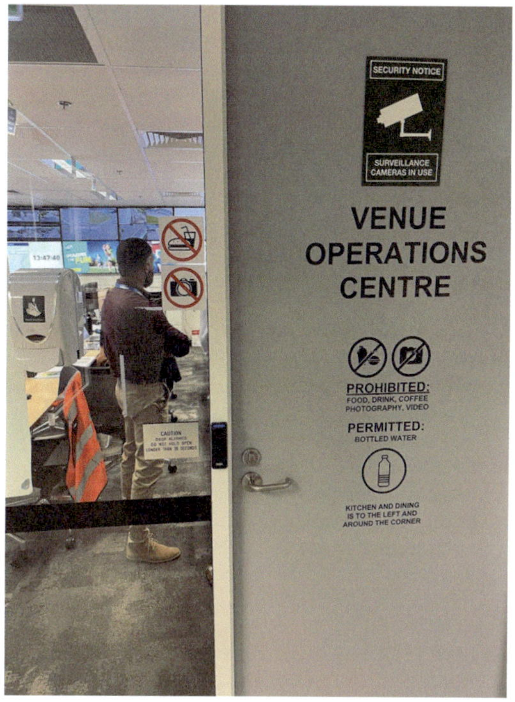
SECURITY NOTICE
SURVEILLANCE CAMERAS IN USE
VENUE OPERATIONS CENTRE
PROHIBITED:
FOOD, DRINK, COFFEE PHOTOGRAPHY, VIDEO
PERMITTED:
BOTTLED WATER
KITCHEN AND DINING IS TO THE LEFT AND AROUND THE CORNER

Fig. 23.5 At major professional stadiums, the Venue Operations Centre (VOC) is responsible for crowd safety and also monitoring weather conditions like approaching lightning

23.8 Crowd Considerations in the Heat in Professional Cricket

One reason for cancellation and rescheduling in extreme heat involves the crowd. A fortunate consequence of recent cricket revolving around TV schedules is that a much higher percentage of prime content has been shifted to evening fixtures (e.g. T20 cricket), where extreme heat is not a factor. However, Test cricket and ODIs for both sexes are played during the day.

A recent (non-cricket) tournament played in Australia (FIFW Women's World Cup 2023) had an approximate rate of stadium (crowd) ambulance transfers of 2–2.5/100,000 spectators per match. This rate was for a winter tournament where heat was not a factor and is very close to internationally published rates [16] and local ambulance service internal statistics. Feedback from local ambulance services is that this rate tends to increase two- to threefold on very hot days, supported by international data [16]. Although a concern, sporting events in the heat do not get anywhere near the ambulance transfer rates of music festivals, where the cultural propensity for the use of illicit drugs means that rates are often more than ten times higher than at sporting events. Similar to the players, there is very little published data (for example, crowd surveys) around the rate of 'mild' heat stress illness in crowd members [17], which would not prompt presentation to healthcare practitioners but might lead to customer dissatisfaction and avoidance of live cricket attendance in the future. The modern cricket stadium has sophisticated event planning (with a headquarters in the Venue Operations Centre (VOC)) that handles emergency response and issues within the crowd (Fig. 23.5).

References

1. List of Fatalities while playing cricket. https://en.wikipedia.org/wiki/List_of_fatalities_while_playing_cricket. Accessed 20/04/2024.

2. Fortington L, Gamage P, Cartwright A, Bugeja L. Exertional heat fatalities in Australian sport and recreation. J Sci Med Sport. 2021;24(8):787–92. https://doi.org/10.1016/j.jsams.2021.04.007.
3. Cricketer dies of heat stroke after back to back matches. The News International (Pakistan). https://www.thenews.com.pk/print/958112-cricketer-dies-of-heat-stroke-after-back-to-back-matches2022
4. Anderson SA, Eichner ER, Bennett S, Boden BP, Colgate B, Courson R, et al. Preventing exertional heat stroke in football: time for a paradigm shift. Sports Health. 2024;17:19417381241260045. https://doi.org/10.1177/19417381241260045.
5. Deren TM, Coris EE, Casa DJ, DeMartini JK, Bain AR, Walz SM, Jay O. Maximum heat loss potential is lower in football linemen during an NCAA summer training camp because of lower self-generated air flow. J Strength Cond Res. 2014;28(6):1656–63. https://doi.org/10.1519/jsc.0000000000000427.
6. Deren TM, Coris EE, Bain AR, Walz SM, Jay O. Sweating is greater in NCAA football linemen independently of heat production. Med Sci Sports Exerc. 2012;44(2):244–52. https://doi.org/10.1249/MSS.0b013e31822cb4e2.
7. Stay S, Cort M, Ward D, Kountouris A, Orchard J, Holland J, Saw A. Core temperature responses in elite cricket players during Australian summer conditions Sports (Basel, Switzerland). 2018;6(4). doi: https://doi.org/10.3390/sports6040164.
8. Driscoll TR, Cripps R, Brotherhood JR. Heat-related injuries resulting in hospitalisation in Australian sport. J Sci Med Sport. 2008;11(1):40–7. https://doi.org/10.1016/j.jsams.2007.04.003.
9. Namibian cricketer dies after stroke. https://www.cricket.com.au/news/3240773; 2015.
10. Parimal K. Dean Jones urinated, vomited, was dehydrated but he continued to battle on. https://www.cricketcountry.com/articles/india-vs-australia-1986-87-dean-jones-urinated-vomited-was-dehydrated--but-he-continued-to-battle-on-18060/; 2015.
11. Maasdorp J, Healy J. England captain Joe Root hospitalised with gastro. https://www.abc.net.au/news/2018-01-08/ashes-england-captain-joe-root-hospitalised-with-gastro/9310500; 2018.
12. Coates L, Blong R, Siciliano F. Lightning fatalities in Australia, 1824–1991. Nat Hazards. 1993;8(3):217–33. https://doi.org/10.1007/BF00690909.
13. Lightning strike fells Test star. https://www.espncricinfo.com/story/lightning-strike-fells-test-star-132767; 2005.
14. CSIRO: Environmental Measurement Units (EMU's). Accessed 2024.
15. Périard JD, DeGroot D, Jay O. Exertional heat stroke in sport and the military: epidemiology and mitigation. Exp Physiol. 2022;107(10):1111–21. https://doi.org/10.1113/ep090686.
16. Tajima T, Takazawa Y, Yamada M, Moriya T, Sato H, Higashihara J, et al. Spectator medicine at an international mega sports event: Rugby World Cup 2019 in Japan. Environ Health Prev Med. 2020;25(1):72. https://doi.org/10.1186/s12199-020-00914-0.
17. Khan Y, Leung GJ, Belanger P, Gournis E, Buckeridge DL, Liu L, et al. Comparing Twitter data to routine data sources in public health surveillance for the 2015 Pan/Parapan American Games: an ecological study. Can J Public Health. 2018;109(3):419–26. https://doi.org/10.17269/s41997-018-0059-0.

Visual Performance, Eye Diseases and Eye Protection in Cricket

24

Daya P. Sharma and Shanel Sharma

24.1 Visual Performance

Cricketing skills such as batting and catching are highly dependent on vision. To perform well, an early judgement about the speed & trajectory of the ball is required, combined with quick reactions with good timing [1]. This requires a reaction in less than 0.25 s, with excellent timing, especially for cross-batted shots, which require a more accurate judgement of the length of the ball [2].

Good batting and catching performance depend on a combination of visual factors, including static and dynamic visual acuity, saccades (fast and accurate eye movements) to the pitch of the ball, colour vision and contrast sensitivity. Static visual acuity refers to the standard high-contrast visual acuity tests with a stable target. Dynamic visual acuity is not a routine clinical test but measures the ability to resolve detail on a moving target. Colour vision deficiencies, especially red-green, can interfere with the ability to distinguish a red cricket ball against a green background and, therefore, can particularly affect fielding. Colour vision deficiencies are underrepresented in cricketers compared to the general population, but cricketers likely compensate for it. It is probably not necessary to screen for colour vision deficiency in selecting players [3]. Contrast sensitivity refers to the ability to distinguish details in dim conditions. This is especially relevant for day-night games and seeing the ball well in low-light conditions. The pink Test ball is harder to see than a red ball or a white ball, especially in dimmer conditions [4]. Some conditions, such as undercorrected myopia or astigmatism, will reduce contrast sensitivity.

Contrary to popular belief, batters do not 'keep their eye on the ball' at all times. The ball's motion is too fast to be able to follow it with 'smooth pursuit' eye movements. Batters judge the trajectory of the ball and then make a rapid movement (saccade) to where they judge that the ball is going to land. When a saccade occurs, vision is suppressed to avoid motion blur, so the saccade needs to be rapid and accurate. To make those accurate and early saccades to the predicted pitch of the ball, the player needs to swiftly judge the trajectory of the ball. After the ball bounces, the batter will track it off the pitch to make fine-tuning adjustments to their stroke. At the elite level, the batter often makes another saccade to where they predict the bat will hit the ball [5].

Some of the research on vision in cricket players can seem contradictory; explanations include the level of the cricketers studied and the testing conditions, such as thc use of a bowling machine and the speeds tested. For example, batting against a bowling machine at 120 km/h is far less

D. P. Sharma (✉) · S. Sharma
Eye & Laser Surgeons, Sydney, NSW, Australia
e-mail: daya@eyeandlaser.com.au; shanel@eyeandlaser.com.au

B. Olivier, J. W. Orchard (eds.), *Cricket Sports Medicine*,
https://doi.org/10.1007/978-981-96-6321-7_24

challenging than facing a fast bowler bowling at 140 km/h.

It is helpful to consider vision in baseball. The typical distance from the baseball pitcher's release point to a baseball batter (17.4 m) is similar to the typical distance from the bowler's release point to the batter (17.7 m). However, a baseball pitch is routinely significantly faster (average fastball speed 150 km/h; max 169 km/h) compared to a cricket delivery (a fast bowler bowls at >140 km/h; max 161 km/h). A slow pitch in baseball is around 105 km/h and a slow bowler in cricket bowls at 65-100 km/h. Although most deliveries hit the pitch and bounce in cricket, the batter has multiple options including playing a defensive shot, playing a straight-batted shot, or leaving a delivery wide of the stumps. In contrast, baseball swings require excellent timing, similar to a cross-batted shot in cricket. A fastball in baseball will reach the batter in 0.4 to 0.47 s, and the batter has about 0.125 s to decide whether or not to swing. For reference, a typical blink is between 0.1 and 0.4 s, in which vision is suppressed. A very fast delivery in cricket (161 km/h) will reach the batter in 0.4 s, with a fast delivery of 140 km/h reaching the batter in 0.46 s. A slow delivery in cricket will reach the batter in 0.65 to 1 s.

With the exception of baseball games with a designated hitter (DH), every player has to bat. Therefore, baseball players are likely self-selected to have 'supernormal' visual acuity. Professional hitters have better visual acuity and depth perception than professional pitchers [6]. Major League Baseball players typically have visual acuity better than 6/4 (normal is 6/6), and half the players of some teams have 6/3 visual acuity, which gives them a competitive advantage in batting performance [7].

Excellent dynamic visual acuity, a measure of how well the player can resolve the detail of a moving object, has been considered contributory to baseball batting success, helping a batter to 'read' a pitch. It is also likely relevant in cricket, as it is likely to relate to how quickly and well a batter can see the orientation and movement of the seam of the ball.

As a visual task, cricket batting has some distinct differences to baseball. Advance cues are available to the batter, including the type of bowler and the fielding positions (these are contextual advance cues). Contextual advance cues help the batter anticipate the delivery before there is any visual information about the delivery (kinematic cues such as wrist position and release point) [8]. It is likely that cricket batters need better visual acuity to play well against fast bowlers; however, a player has more defensive options and can avoid riskier and more difficult cross-batted shots.

One study found that batting performance was not significantly diminished by making batters myopic with contact lenses until they were −3.00D. This was done with a bowling machine at relatively slow speeds and with a consistent release point. It also eliminates kinematic information prior to the ball release [9]. Highly skilled players are better able to use kinematic cues (such as seam angle and spin) after the ball is released and prior to ball bounce in order to optimise ball contact. They are also better able to use visual information after the ball bounces to optimise contact.

Although specialist bowlers are often required to bat, they are not necessarily selected based on batting skills. Therefore, we should expect that cricket players would have more variability in their visual parameters than baseball players. Previous studies have a range of levels of cricket players, from grade to international, and are typically not stratified by performance.

Association studies can suggest various visual parameters are important for performance, but they don't inform us about performance in an individual. For example, an elite batter with mildly suboptimal visual acuity due to refractive error may be able to achieve improved performance with optimal refractive correction and improved visual acuity. When they were younger and coming up through the ranks, they may have had better vision and were able to develop the skills which allowed them to be selected. However, if vision deteriorates, their performance may deteriorate. This could occur without a reduction in vision being detected.

It is important to note that there are many conditions which can impact vision that develop through the teen years to young adulthood, which also highlights the benefit of screening professional players in order to maximise their vision to maximise their performance and prevent deterioration of vision.

24.2 Ocular Dominance and Hand Dominance

The dominant eye refers to the eye that is preferred for fixing on a target, and at a neurological level, it is the eye which has the most neural connections into the brain. The two eyes are not 'wired' equally. During childhood, the eyes compete with each other to form the most connections with the brain, and the eye which has the best vision wins. In some people, there is co-dominance.

In sports such as archery or shooting, adapting techniques according to ocular dominance and hand dominance is critical. In cricket, the role of ocular dominance is less clear [10, 11] and not routinely tested. If the dominant eye is facing forward, a batter may have an advantage in terms of the eye being forward, closer to the ball, and with less obstruction with head movement. However, the evidence is conflicting. It may be that if the dominant eye is behind, the batter can compensate for this by rotating the head and adopting a more front-on stance.

In cricket batting, a 'conventional stance' means having the dominant hand on the bottom of the bat, and a 'reversed stance' has the dominant hand on top. Some left-hand batters are naturally right-hand dominant, and vice versa. It is not clear why some players adopt a 'reversed stance'. A left-hand batting stance is over-represented in cricket teams compared to the general population (left handedness is around 11% of the population). In countries like Australia, a left-hand batting stance has an advantage against right-arm seam bowling because it reduces the chance of being dismissed LBW or bowled.

One potential explanation is that having a reverse stance may improve control when playing with a straight bat. One study found a strong association between reverse stance and professional batters (vs inexperienced batters) [11]. In our assessment of state-level professional cricketers, we found that the 'reversed stance' batting position was not found amongst any bowlers (0/17), but 6 of the 25 specialist batters had a reversed stance. Five of these six batted with their dominant eye facing forwards. Interestingly, Sachin Tendulkar bats, bowls and throws right-handed, but writes left-handed. He is left-eye dominant; therefore, he bats with his dominant eye forwards in the reversed stance. A right-handed batting stance confers an advantage against right-arm spin, which could be a factor. Natural left handers who bat right-handed are giving up an 'infrequency advantage' of bowlers being generally less used to bowling to left handers. Although batting stance is usually fixed early in the career, it is not clear how the decision is made regarding stance and whether or not ocular dominance may play a role in what stance a child takes up or if it is simply that they commence playing with their stronger arm that can lift the heavy bat determining how they hold their bat. This is an area of interest for further investigation.

24.3 Ocular Disease and Screening

Cricketers are selected and promoted based on sporting performance, which to some extent requires ongoing optimum vision. Therefore, it is surprising that many players have not had any eye examinations in the last 2–5 years, if at all [12]. This is a reflection of cricketing bodies not having uniform policies for ophthalmic assessment. Even if the player's vision is optimum when they commence as a junior cricketer, vision may be impacted later in their career. Myopia, keratoconus and pterygium are diseases that can develop and progress during teenage years and early adulthood and impact a player's vision. Players may compensate initially to some extent for blurred vision, especially if only one eye is affected. Players may be unaware of a gradual decline, but may have worse performance in dim conditions or under lights. They may not complain of reduced vision because they may perceive that it could affect their chance of selection.

Myopia (short-sightedness), for example, may not become visually significant until the late teenage years. If myopia progresses, it may lead to a reduction in their performance. In our screening of professional cricketers, many players had excellent unaided vision. Of those with refractive error, some played without correction, some wore soft contact lenses or glasses and one used orthokeratology (overnight hard lenses to reshape the eye). Players described playing with one contact lens having fallen out, difficulty seeing the ball in the evening as the effect of the orthokeratology had worn off, or difficulty seeing the ball on days 3–5 of a test match due to the contact lens becoming 'stuck' to the eye. Furthermore, a pterygium on the ocular surface makes contact lens wear more difficult.

A pterygium grows onto the cornea and develops secondary to chronic UV damage (Fig. 24.1). The prevalence of pterygium in Australia is 8.4%, and the risk increases with outdoor occupation and male sex [13]. A pterygium is associated with a 24% increased risk of skin melanoma [14]. Pterygia are often bilateral, making the eyes red and irritated and causing blurred vision by inducing astigmatism. The degree of blur can vary with the pupil size in different light levels. If large, pterygia can significantly impair vision by encroaching on the visual axis.

Keratoconus is a corneal disease that results in thinning and irregularity of the cornea. The cornea contributes 2/3 of the focusing power of the eye; hence, if it becomes irregular, the vision is blurred and typically worse at night. Keratoconus typically develops after puberty, and usually one eye is worse. It can be missed early, as vision is initially correctable with spectacles or soft contact lenses, but speciality hard contact lenses or surgery may be needed as the

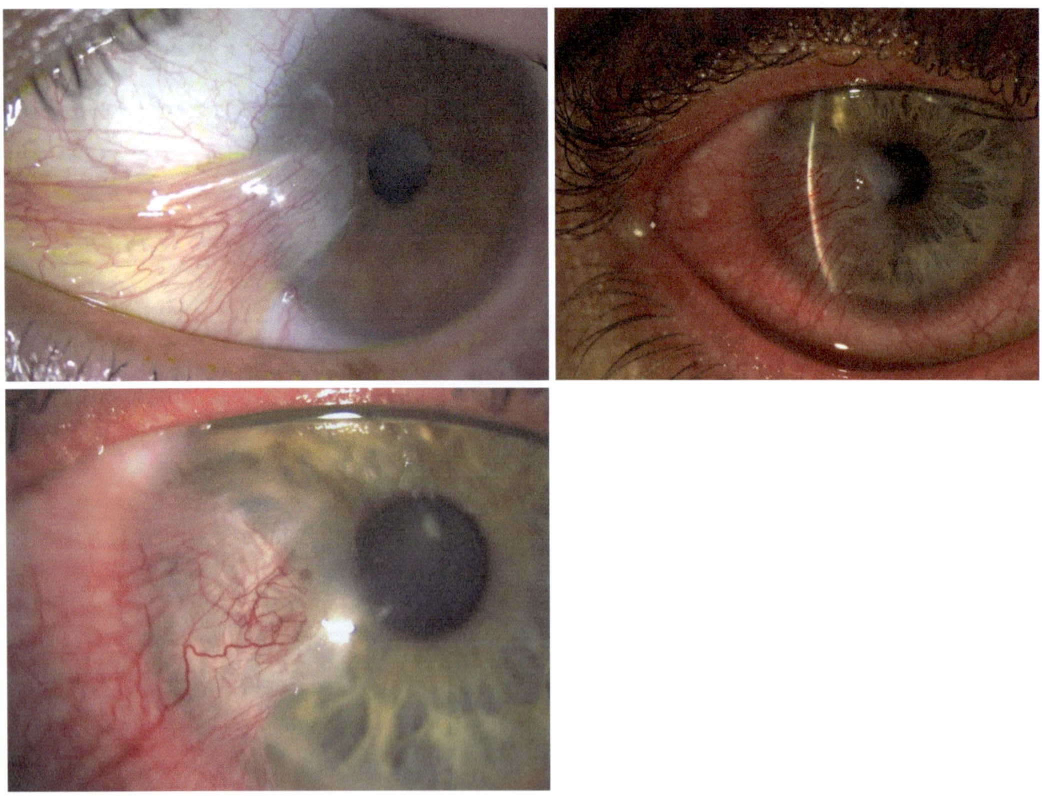

Fig. 24.1 Pterygium examples

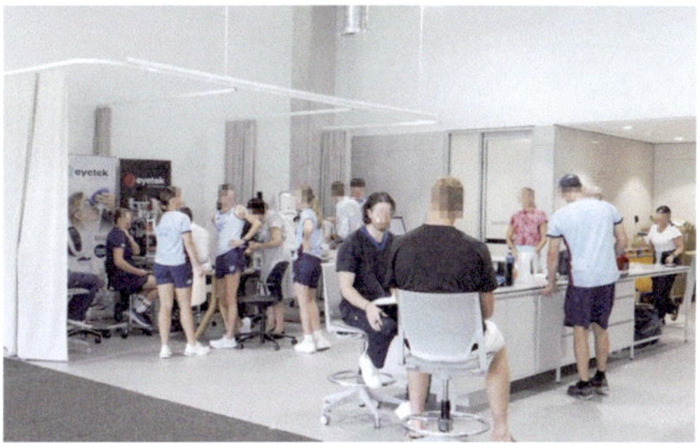

Fig. 24.2 Ophthalmic screening clinic at Cricket NSW

disease progresses. Early detection is important because early intervention can halt disease progression for many patients. A recent Australian study using corneal imaging for keratoconus screening found a prevalence of 1.2% in 20-year-olds, a much higher prevalence than anticipated [15].

Regular ophthalmic screening of cricketers would allow for early detection and timely treatment of ocular disease and prevent deterioration in performance caused by undetected reduced vision.

When we started an ophthalmology screening clinic (Fig. 24.2) for professional cricketers, we were all surprised that we detected significant ocular disease that could explain why some players hadn't progressed in their careers as had been expected. We also detected some conditions that could have an impact on future performance and on long-term eye health.

24.4 Ocular Injury and Protection

It is well recognised that the brain needs to be protected when playing cricket [16]. Similarly, the eyes & orbits are also vulnerable to injury. In a worst-case scenario, the potential for permanent loss of vision can't be discounted. Blunt trauma to the globe from a cricket ball can lead to retinal detachment, commotio retinae (bruising of the retina), hyphaema (bleeding in the anterior chamber of the eye which can rebleed and result in loss of vision), vitreous haemorrhage, lens subluxations, and corneal abrasions. In the longer term, the player would be at increased risk of developing glaucoma, cataract and retinal detachment [17]. Batters and wicketkeepers are the most likely to have a head or facial injury. Some players have been injured when a ball has passed between the peak and grille of a helmet, resulting in new ICC regulations for helmets [16]. It is important to note that some ocular injuries can be career-ending, hence the importance of wearing appropriate eye protection.

24.5 UV Protection

The dangers of ultraviolet radiation (UVR) are well understood. Sunscreen, arm sleeves and a hat are routinely utilised to protect the skin, and regular dermatology screening has been undertaken to understand the devastating impact UVR can have on the skin.

The damage of UVR on the eyes has not received the same profile as the skin. UV radiation-related eye diseases include pterygium, pinguecula, ocular surface tumours (Fig. 24.3) and cancers, cataracts, eyelid skin cancers (Fig. 24.4) and macular degeneration. Partly, this has been due to the effectiveness of ophthalmic surgeries that allow pterygia, cataracts, and ocular surface tumours to be surgically excised with good outcomes.

Skin cancers of the periorbital skin (skin around the eyes) account for 5–10% of all skin cancers and include basal cell carcinomas, squamous cell carcinomas and melanomas. Periorbital skin cancers occur in a region where wide excision is not readily practical due to the specialised nature of this skin. Reconstruction of an eyelid requires harvesting ear cartilage or hard palate and is frequently complicated by ongoing problems of trichiasis, ectropion, entropion and dry eye for the patient.

The periorbital skin is an area that is not able to be readily protected with sunscreen, as it gets into the tear film and causes stinging [18]. Furthermore, sunscreen manufacturers indicate that sunscreen should not be used around the eyes. The culture of UV-blocking wraparound sunglasses has not been routine for cricketers, umpires, spectators or junior players alike. Good

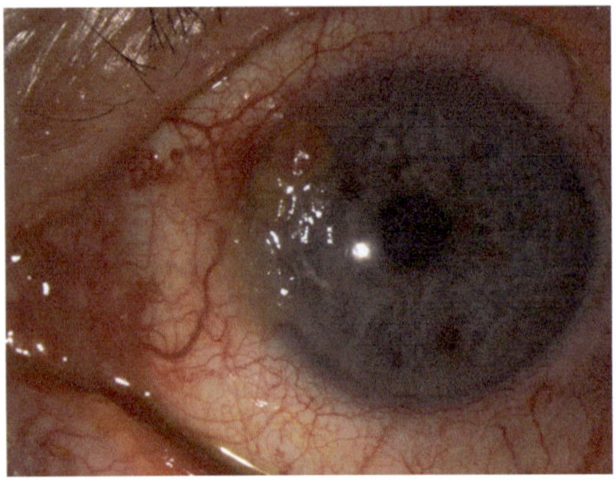

Fig. 24.3 Ocular surface precancerous lesion due to chronic UV exposure

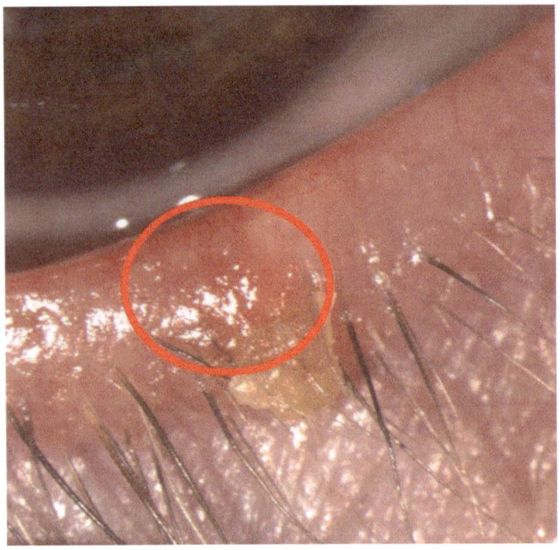

Fig. 24.4 BCC on the lower eyelid margin (it is an ulcerated eyelid lesion circled in red)

UV protection does not necessarily mean a dark tint; sunglasses can affect the vision if the tint is too dark for the conditions. A good pair of sunglasses will block UV light, especially from the sides. Many sunglasses do not provide adequate UV protection. Sunglasses without a wraparound design or wide sidearms allow light to hit the eyes from the sides, meaning there is damage from UV exposure but also glare as well (Fig. 24.5).

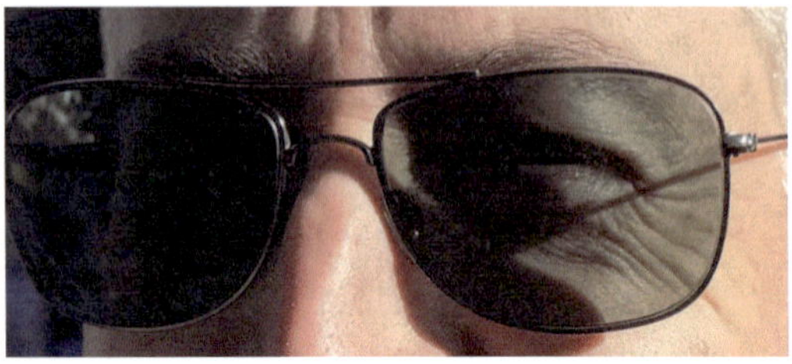

Fig. 24.5 Despite wearing UV-blocking, polarised sunglasses that meet all the standards for eye protection, the sun is visible, burning the periorbital skin and eyes of the wearer

References

1. Fogt JS, Fogt N. Studies of vision in cricket – a narrative review. Vision (Basel). 2023;7(3) https://doi.org/10.3390/vision7030057.
2. Regan D. Visual factors in hitting and catching. J Sports Sci. 1997;15(6):533–58.
3. Harris RW, Cole BL. Abnormal colour vision is a handicap to playing cricket but not an insurmountable one. Clin Exp Optom. 2007;90(6):451–6. https://doi.org/10.1111/j.1444-0938.2006.00180.x.
4. Maule JJ, Maguire R, Timmis MA, Runswick OR, Wilkins L, Mann DL, et al. Difficult at dusk? Illuminating the debate on cricket ball visibility. J Sci Med Sport. 2024;27(6):408–14. https://doi.org/10.1016/j.jsams.2024.02.004.
5. Vater C, Mann DL. Are predictive saccades linked to the processing of peripheral information? Psychol Res. 2023;87(5):1501–19. https://doi.org/10.1007/s00426-022-01743-2.
6. Klemish D, Ramger B, Vittetoe K, Reiter JP, Tokdar ST, Appelbaum LG. Visual abilities distinguish pitchers from hitters in professional baseball. J Sports Sci. 2018;36(2):171–9. https://doi.org/10.1080/02640414.2017.1288296.
7. Laby DM, Rosenbaum AL, Kirschen DG, Davidson JL, Rosenbaum LJ, Strasser C, et al. The visual function of professional baseball players. Am J Ophthalmol. 1996;122(4):476–85. https://doi.org/10.1016/s0002-9394(14)72106-3.
8. Muller S, Abernethy B. Batting with occluded vision: an in situ examination of the information pick-up and interceptive skills of high- and low-skilled cricket batsmen. J Sci Med Sport. 2006;9(6):446–58. https://doi.org/10.1016/j.jsams.2006.03.029.
9. Mann DL, Abernethy B, Farrow D. The resilience of natural interceptive actions to refractive blur. Hum Mov Sci. 2010;29(3):386–400. https://doi.org/10.1016/j.humov.2010.02.007.
10. Thomas NG, Harden LM, Rogers GG. Visual evoked potentials, reaction times and eye dominance in cricketers. J Sports Med Phys Fitness. 2005;45(3):428–33.

11. Mann DL, Runswick OR, Allen PM. Hand and eye dominance in sport: are cricket batters taught to bat back-to-front? Sports Med. 2016;46(9):1355–63. https://doi.org/10.1007/s40279-016-0516-y.
12. Barrett BT, Flavell JC, Bennett SJ, Cruickshank AG, Mankowska A, Harris JM, et al. Vision and visual history in elite/near-elite-level cricketers and Rugby-league players. Sports Med Open. 2017;3(1):39. https://doi.org/10.1186/s40798-017-0106-z.
13. Stevenson LJ, Mackey DA, Lingham G, Burton A, Brown H, Huynh E, et al. Has the sun protection campaign in Australia reduced the need for Pterygium surgery nationally? Ophthalmic Epidemiol. 2021;28(2):105–13. https://doi.org/10.1080/09286586.2020.1797120.
14. Crewe JM, Threlfall T, Clark A, Sanfilippo PG, Mackey DA. Pterygia are indicators of an increased risk of developing cutaneous melanomas. Br J Ophthalmol. 2018;102(4):496–501. https://doi.org/10.1136/bjophthalmol-2017-310686.
15. Chan E, Chong EW, Lingham G, Stevenson LJ, Sanfilippo PG, Hewitt AW, et al. Prevalence of keratoconus based on scheimpflug imaging: the Raine study. Ophthalmology. 2021;128(4):515–21. https://doi.org/10.1016/j.ophtha.2020.08.020.
16. Wilkins L, Mann D, Dain S, Hayward T, Allen P. Out with the old, in with the new: how changes in cricket helmet regulations affect the vision of batters. J Sports Sci. 2019;37(1):13–9. https://doi.org/10.1080/02640414.2018.1479944.
17. Mahapatra SK, Malhotra K, Mendke RG. A 3-year prospective study on ocular injuries with tennis or cricket ball while playing cricket: a case series. Indian J Ophthalmol. 2018;66(2):256–61. https://doi.org/10.4103/ijo.IJO_458_17.
18. Pratt H, Hassanin K, Troughton LD, Czanner G, Zheng Y, McCormick AG, et al. UV imaging reveals facial areas that are prone to skin cancer are disproportionately missed during sunscreen application. PLoS One. 2017;12(10):e0185297. https://doi.org/10.1371/journal.pone.0185297.

Management of Skin Conditions in Cricketers Including Screening for Skin Cancer

25

Alex Chamberlain, Lena Ly, Alicia O'Connor, David Orchard, and John W. Orchard

25.1 Disorders of the Skin and Nails on the Feet of Fast Bowlers

Cricketers, in particular fast bowlers, are at high risk for injuries to all components of the foot, not simply musculoskeletal. Traumatic skin and toenail injuries are not uncommon due to the repetitive nature of bowling. Batters and fielders required to sprint repetitively or who are struck on the foot by a ball are at risk, too, but less so.

A. Chamberlain (✉)
Victorian Melanoma Service, Paula Fox Melanoma and Cancer Centre, Alfred Health, Melbourne, VIC, Australia

School of Translational Medicine, Faculty of Medicine Nursing and Health Sciences, Monash University, Alfred Health, Melbourne, VIC, Australia
e-mail: alex.chamberlain@glenferriedermatology.com.au

L. Ly
Eastern Health Clinical School, Monash University, Melbourne, VIC, Australia

A. O'Connor
Eastern Suburbs Dermatology, Sydney, NSW, Australia

D. Orchard
Royal Children's Hospital, Melbourne, VIC, Australia
e-mail: David.Orchard@rch.org.au

J. W. Orchard
School of Public Health, University of Sydney, Sydney, NSW, Australia
e-mail: john.orchard@sydney.edu.au

The varying cutaneous injuries to plantar skin may be acute or chronic. Both friction blisters and subcorneal haemorrhage ('talon noir') are caused by extreme shearing forces on the skin resulting in diminished intercellular adhesion. Friction blisters may be exacerbated by hyperhidrosis especially affecting feet confined to damp shoes for long periods of exercise. Despite popular belief, blisters do not need active lancing unless tense and painful. "Talon noir" presents as a blackened macule or plaque on the sole, typically the heel and can occasionally be mistaken for melanoma but has distinct dermoscopic features (Fig. 25.1a, b) [1].

The colours of haemorrhage, ranging from red through purple and black, are usually seen with satellite or splatter globules at the margin. A capillary effect may also be observed at their periphery. These clear with superficial paring (Fig. 25.1c) using a 15 blade which is diagnostic. Calcaneal petechiae represent a variation of talon noir. These are multiple, small volumes and of sudden onset (Fig. 25.2a, b).

Typically, these haemorrhages cause minimal symptoms and do not require active management. Chronic pressure and friction may lead to callosities requiring active podiatric management. Callosities can be improved with paring or keratolytic creams (salicylic acid, 10–25% urea creams). These issues may still occur even where shoes are supportive and well-fitted. Callosities

B. Olivier, J. W. Orchard (eds.), *Cricket Sports Medicine*,
https://doi.org/10.1007/978-981-96-6321-7_25

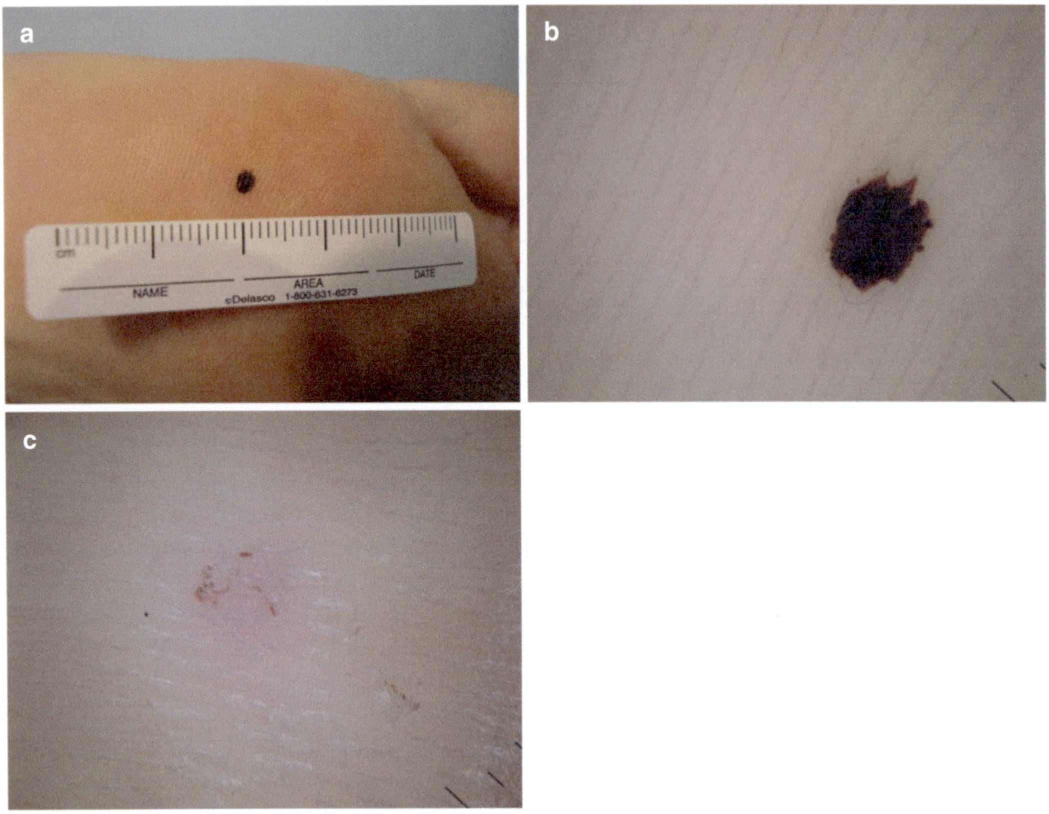

Fig. 25.1 (**a**) Talon noir on the weight bearing sole (**b**) Dermoscopy of talon noir showing red-black blotch with satellite/splatter globules (**c**) Dermoscopy post-paring of talon noir showing clearance

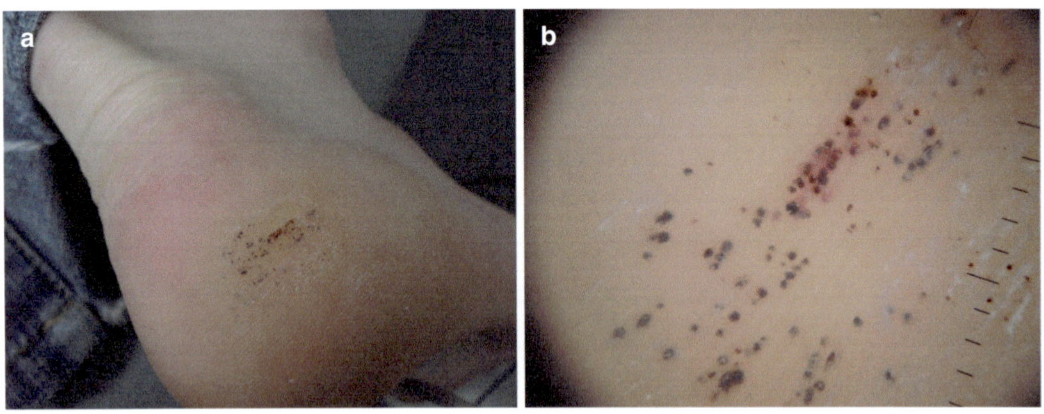

Fig. 25.2 (**a**) Calcaneal petechiae on the heel (**b**) Dermoscopy of calcaneal petechiae showing haemorrhagic "pebbles on the ridges"

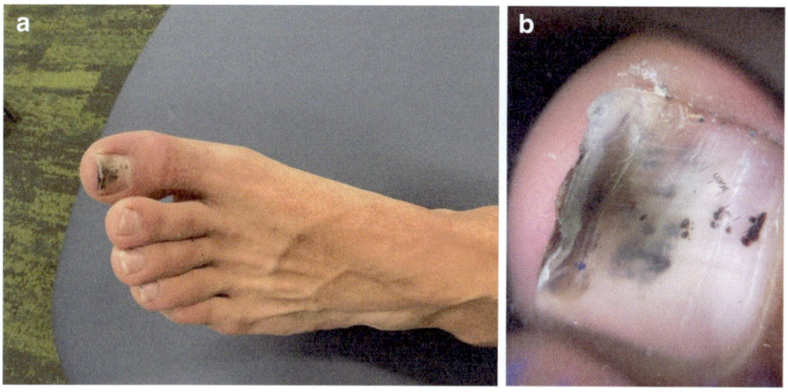

Fig. 25.3 (**a**) Subungual haemorrhage in a fast bowler; (**b**) Dermoscopy showing haemorrhagic purple globules and focal dystrophy/leukonychia. There is also some brown pigment, likely haemosiderin, especially involving the great toenail. This, too, may be mistaken for melanoma of the nail unit (Fig. 25.4)

don't have the thrombosed capillaries one sees in plantar warts [2].

Toenails are most at risk of traumatic pathology in cricketers. Pace bowlers in particular are prone to subungual haemorrhage (Fig. 25.3a, b).

As they are slow to clear and can appear very blackened, dermoscopy is key for diagnosis and distinguishing significant potential melanocytic pathology (Table 25.1) [3]. The dermoscopic hallmark of subungual or nail unit melanoma is varying bands of different colour, width, and spacing along with loss of parallelism (Fig. 25.4). The volume of benign haemorrhage does not need to be significant to appear dramatic. Slow colour change evolves over time from red purple through to black and then brown as the haemorrhage migrates out and resorbs. Sometimes micro-trauma will manifest as smaller "splinter haemorrhages" (Fig. 25.5a, b).

Subungual haemorrhage (Fig. 25.6) involving over 25% of the nail should prompt consideration of fracture of the distal phalanx (Fig. 25.7) where there is significant pain.

Fast bowlers may have nails avulse after the stress of prolonged bowling, so-called onychomadesis, when a deep split appears in the proximal nail plate prior to ultimately shedding. A partly detached nail is best kept in situ (even if requiring taping) rather than actively removed to minimise the discomfort of a raw nail bed. Short-lived inflammation or even bacterial infection within the nail folds may result from the trauma of bowling, otherwise known as acute paronychia. When purulent, anti-staphylococcal antibiotics are typically required.

Biomechanically, the great toenail or hallux and the second toenail are at highest risk as these bear the brunt of the repetitive pressure. This is especially so for the leading foot of a bowler. Chronic repetitive trauma may cause the nail to thicken, discolour, and develop a stepped surface (onychauxis) [2]. Stepped ridges may develop in affected toenails (Fig. 25.6), along with varying pigmentation and scarring (pterygium) [4]. Properly fitted shoes, an enlarged toe-box, and improved arch support may minimise the damaging impact [5].

Prolonged exposure to sweat may predispose to infections such as tinea and pitted keratolysis. Onycholytic or dystrophic toenails from repetitive trauma may be complicated by pseudomonal infection, which results in green colouration or chloronychia. More details on infections are covered elsewhere in this chapter.

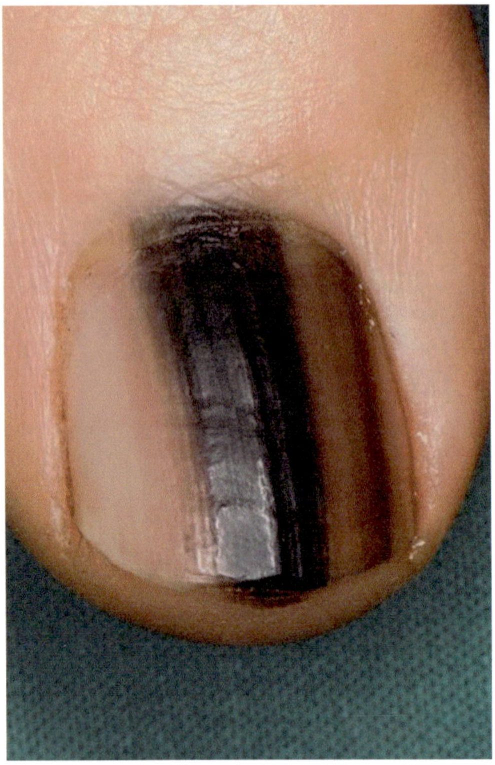

Fig. 25.4 Broad and blackened longitudinal melanonychia with Hutchinson's sign (periungual pigment involving the hyponychium) in keeping with nail unit melanoma (hallux)

Table 25.1 Contrasting dermoscopic features of subungual haemorrhage versus melanoma

Subungual haemorrhage	Subungual/nail unit melanoma
Irregularly shaped homogenous red and purple colour (brown later)	Banded brown to black pigmentation >3 mm
Distal spikes and globules	Varying colour, width, and spacing of parallel lines
Rounded proximal margin with clearance	Pigment spill onto nail fold (Hutchinsons's or micro-Hutchinson's sign)
Leukonychia	Band may be broader proximally (triangle sign)
	Nail dystrophy (advanced cases only)

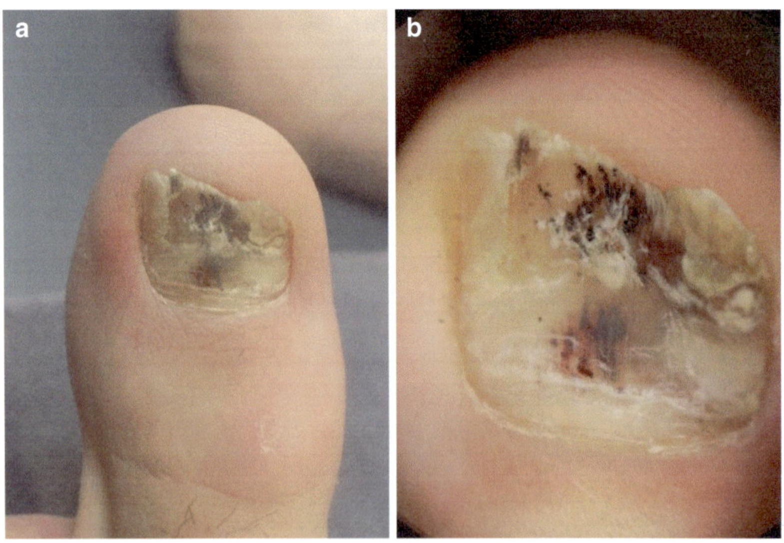

Fig. 25.5 (**a**) Partial regrowth of an avulsed and dystrophic toenail with haemorrhage. Mild callus can be seen over the R distal interphalangeal joint (**b**) Dermoscopy showing multiple blackened splinter haemorrhages (distally) and purplish linear haemorrhages proximally

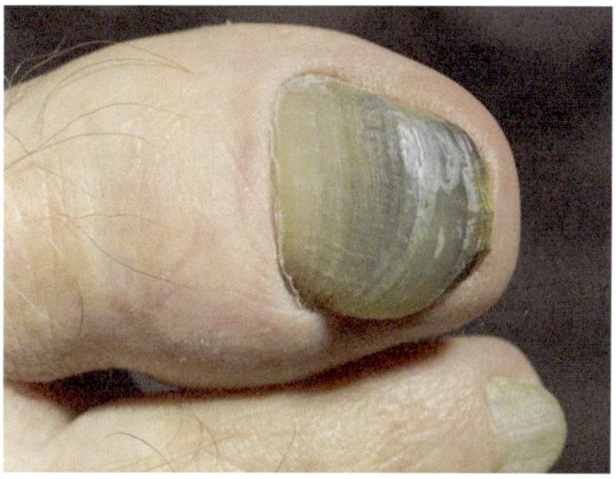

Fig. 25.6 Onychauxis related to chronic repetitive trauma to the great toe

25.2 General Inflammatory Dermatoses in Cricketers

The varying cutaneous pathologies seen in cricketers are primarily triggered by to UV irradiation, infection, sweat, trauma, and allergy.

Solar issues include sunburn (ranging from bright red erythema to blistering), chronic solar damage (actinic keratoses and photoaging), and skin cancers (mostly basal cell carcinoma, squamous cell carcinoma and melanoma). This higher occupational exposure to UV demands strict sun protection including a wide-brim hat of at least 10 cm, SPF50+ sunscreens (Fig. 25.8), long sleeve collared shirts and an annual skin check as the minimum requirement. Prolonged sun

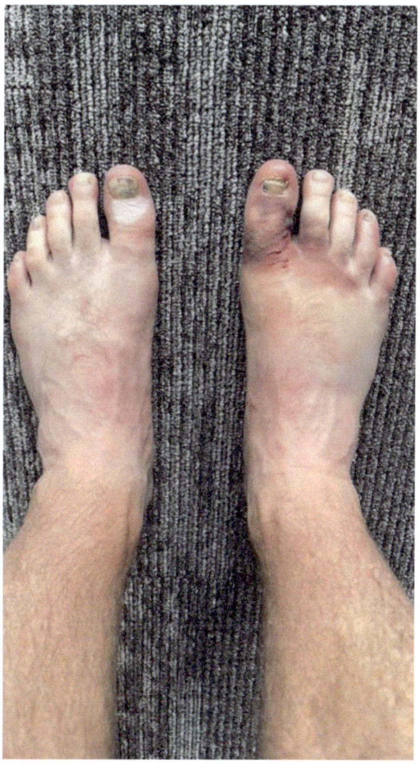

Fig. 25.7 Fracture of the distal phalanx of right big toe displaying swelling and ecchymosis

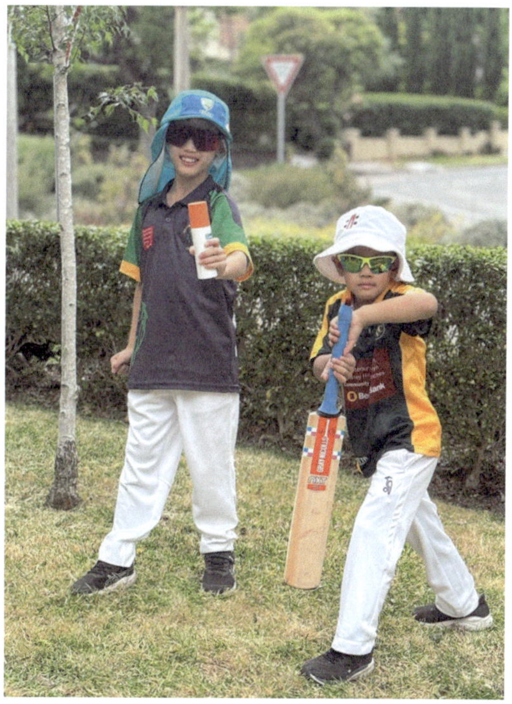

Fig. 25.8 Junior cricketers in Australia wearing broad brimmed hats, eye protection, sunscreen and a wide brim hat of at least 10 cm

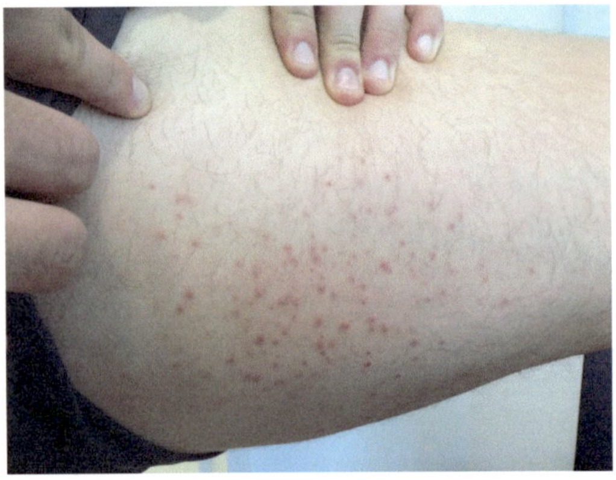

Fig. 25.9 Bacterial folliculitis affecting the medial thigh

exposure can also aggravate inflammatory skin conditions including rosacea (associated with flushing and fixed facial erythema) and dermatitis (associated with xerosis and pruritic plaques).

Cutaneous infections include impetigo (a bacterial infection commonly caused by Staphylococcal Aureus), thrush (a yeast infection from Candida species), tinea cruris or pedis (a fungal infection of the groin or feet), and shingles or localised HSV1 infection (viral infection caused by Varicella Zoster virus or Herpes Simplex virus respectively). Tight-fitting protective equipment and close contact in training sessions and change rooms can contribute to spread [6].

Increased and prolonged sweating can give rise to specific conditions in different regions of the body. Generalised conditions include folliculitis (Fig. 25.9), pityriasis versicolor, Grover's disease, and atopic dermatitis. There is a predilection for acne, seborrheic dermatitis, and rosacea on the head and neck. Pitted keratolysis can affect the soles of sweaty feet. Erythrasma (an axillary rash due to Corynebacterium), granular parakeratosis (scaly inflammatory dermatosis commonly from irritants including benzalkonium chloride exposure), and primary hyperhidrosis can also involve the flexures.

Traumatic and pressure injuries include general abrasions, minor cuts resulting in hypertrophic or keloidal scars, or post-inflammatory hyper- or hypopigmentation. Pressure urticaria (Fig. 25.10) or symptomatic dermographism can also occur. Psoriasis can involve scalp, hands, and feet and can arise in areas of trauma (so called Koebner phenomenon).

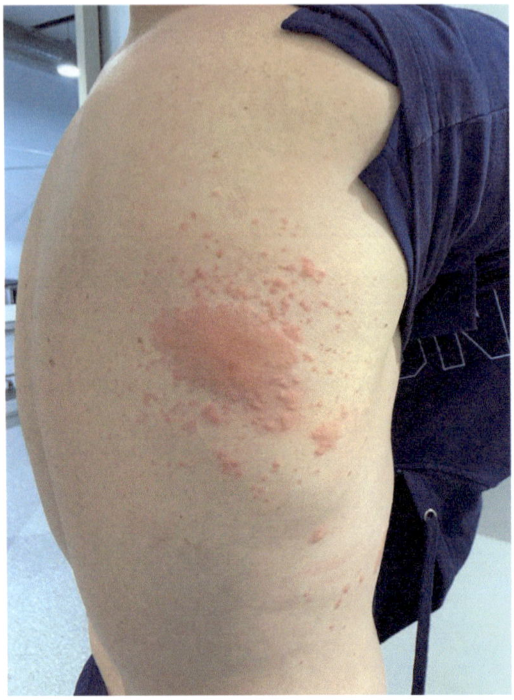

Fig. 25.10 Urticarial truncal rash with coalescing erythematous papules

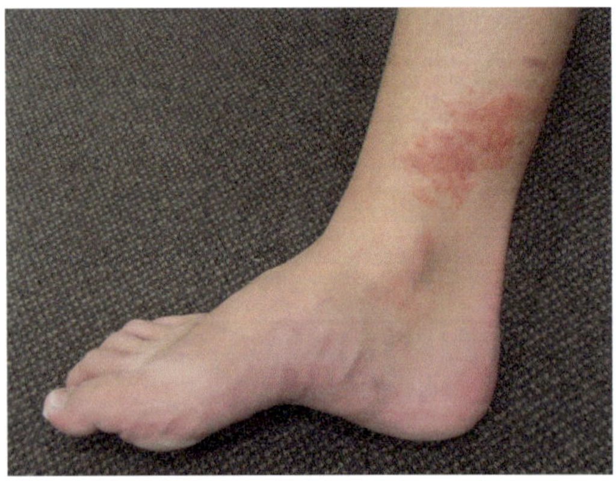

Fig. 25.11 Acute contact dermatitis from adhesive ankle strapping. This may be irritant or allergic in nature

Contact dermatitis (Fig. 25.11) is more commonly irritant (related to sweat, heat, and friction). Allergic contact dermatitis is less common but can develop due to components of the protective equipment and ball (rubber components comprise of 20% of contact allergy in student athletes). Other exposures specific to cricket players include cricket oil (linseed oil), glues (acrylates), and leather materials (chromates) [7]. Medicaments and cosmeceuticals used for massage can also contribute to contact allergy (benzocaine, topical non steroidals, and essential oils). Underlying atopy (the association of asthma, dermatitis, and allergic rhinitis) increases the risk of developing contact dermatitis. Hand dermatitis including dyshidrotic eczema can also develop in athletes. Airborne contact dermatitis is uncommon but allergic rhinitis to grasses can aggravate facial and eyelid dermatitis.

25.3 Management of Fungal Infections in Cricketers

25.3.1 Fungal Nail Infections (Onychomycosis)

Infection of toenails with dermatophyte, yeasts, and non-dermatophyte moulds is common amongst cricket players. Predisposing factors include heat, sweat, occlusive footwear, repetitive toe trauma, and shared change room facilities [8, 9]. Five clinical patterns of disease are recognised; these include distal lateral subungual onychomycosis, white superficial onychomycosis, proximal subungual onychomycosis, endonyx onychomycosis, and total dystrophic onychomycosis [10]. Dermoscopy may show the typical jagged edge with yellowish spikes or spears in early cases. Diagnosis should be confirmed by obtaining nail clippings or scrapings and sending these for fungal microscopy and culture. PCR is now available and highly sensitive for dermatophyte identification.

Prevention of onychomycosis is an important part of management. Cricket players should be educated on measures that reduce transmission. These include keeping nails short, wearing moisture-wicking socks, showering straight after competition or training, wearing flip flops in common wet areas, not sharing towels, socks, footwear, uniforms, hot washing socks at 60 °C daily, and using a separate towel to dry the feet [8].

Treatment selection should be based on the pathogenic organism, clinical pattern of disease, the number of nails affected, and patient comorbidities. Terbinafine, itraconazole, and fluconazole are commonly employed systemic antifungal medications. Laboratory monitoring of full blood count and liver function tests at baseline and part-way through treatment is prudent. Anti-fungal nail lacquers such ciclopirox and amorolfine are topical options. They are often desirable due to their limited adverse effects, lack of drug interactions, and avoidance of laboratory monitoring [10]. However, their efficacy is limited by their inability to penetrate the nail plate [10]. Moreover, in recent years, there has been increased reporting of both clinical and microbiological resistance to antifungal therapies [11].

25.3.2 Cutaneous Fungal Infections

Most cricket players, by virtue of their sport, have encountered either tinea pedis (foot), cruris (groin), or corporis (body). Cutaneous fungal infections are usually present as pruritic, erythematous plaques that exhibit central clearing, a raised border and a leading edge of scale [12]. When involving the feet, they can present as macerated, peeling, and sometimes malodorous skin between the toes or painful fissures (Fig. 25.12) (**a**, **b**) A skin scraping sent for fungal microscopy, culture and PCR confirms the diagnosis. Education and preventative measures are essential in preventing transmission to other body sites and teammates. Topical treatment is indicated for localised and recent-onset infections. These agents include terbinafine and imidazoles (ketoconazole, econazole, miconazole, clotrimazole, bifonazole). Systemic agents should be reserved for widespread, recalcitrant, and more severe presentations. Terbinafine, itraconazole, and fluconazole are the mainstays of such treatment. Griseofulvin is considered less effective. Elsewhere in the world, other topicals and oral therapies are available, such as ciclopirox and efinaconazole, along with voriconazole and posaconazole, respectively.

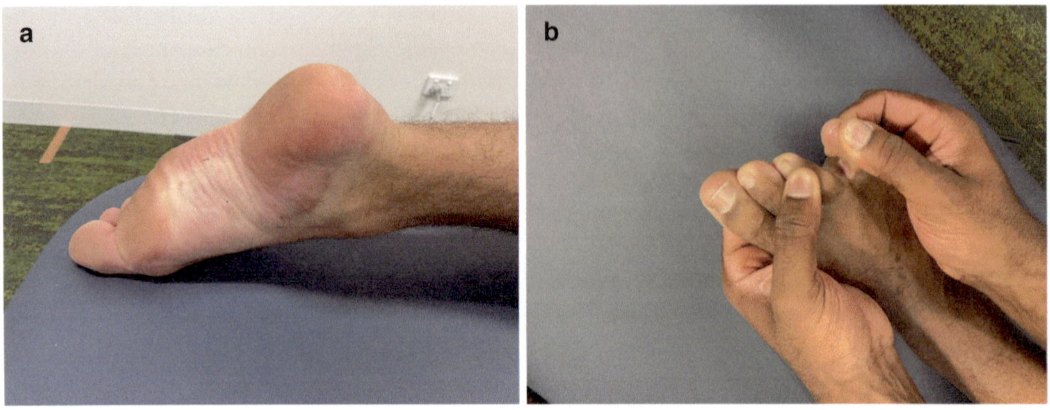

Fig. 25.12 (**a**, **b**) Examples of tinea pedis involving plantar surface and fissuring of the 3rd/4th web space

Fig. 25.13 (**a**, **b**) Initial presentation of melanoma in situ (Fig. 25.13a, b) on the medial leg of a female cricketer, which showed rapid growth before removal

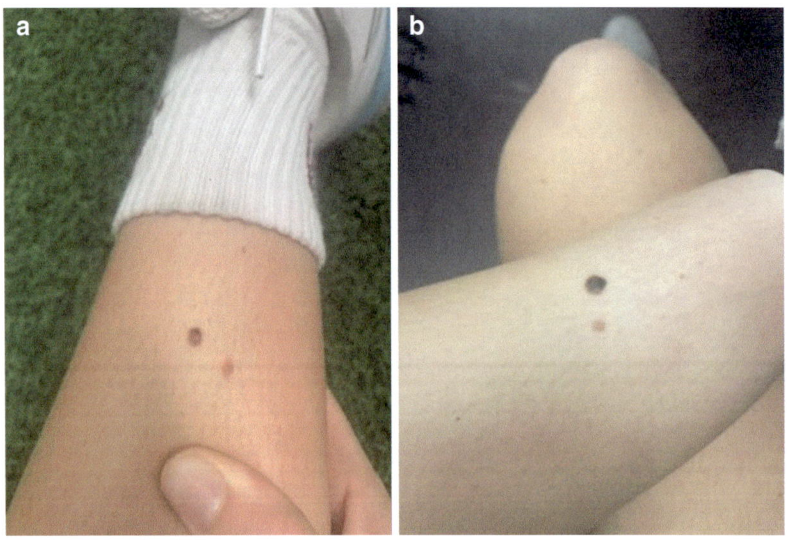

25.4 Skin Cancer in Cricketers

Compared to some other sports, cricket is considered a relatively safe pursuit, with the retired cricketer generally not fearing severe consequences resulting from their career [13]. Australian Sheffield Shield cricketers have recently been shown to live longer than the general Australian male population [14]. For cricketers with fair skin living in warm climates, it is perhaps the risk of developing skin cancer including melanoma that is one of their biggest concerns (Fig. 25.13). In Australia, most regular surveillance of elite players is directly organised by Cricket Australia, which occasionally reveals malignant lesions (Fig. 25.14a, b). However, historically the origin of targeted skin surveillance more than a decade ago was primarily a venture of the Australian Cricketers Association (ACA), the players association. This representative group had significant concerns and experience regarding the risks of skin cancer leading to organising and funding their own skin screening program. The Professional Cricketers Association (PCA) has had a similar program running in the UK.

For all the fears, there are not huge numbers of cricketers who have died of skin cancer, including melanoma. The tragic fate of Ken Wadsworth,

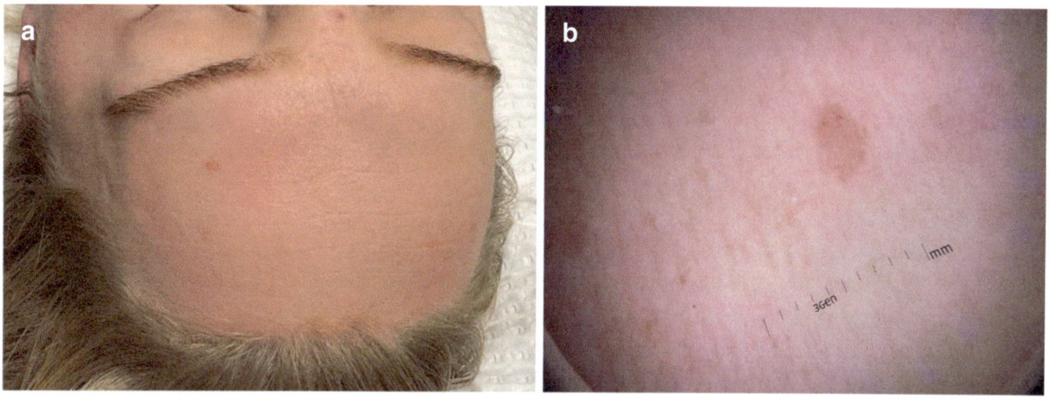

Fig. 25.14 (**a**, **b**) Macroscopic and dermoscopic appearance of a small superficial BCC on the forehead of a young female cricketer

former New Zealand men's Test wicketkeeper, is a somewhat sad story, dying of melanoma at the age of 29 in the late 1970s. Richie Benaud OBE, an ex-Australian Test captain and famous commentator, died of squamous cell carcinoma (keratinocyte cancer), but at the age of 84, slightly above the average life expectancy for an Australian male. Bruce Yardley is a former Australian cricketer who died of melanoma, at the age of 71. The list of cricketers who have publicly declared they have been treated for skin cancer, including melanoma, is much longer, with the implication being that most of them are being diagnosed at an early enough stage that treatment is usually successful. The number of active contracted players at Cricket Australia who have had a recent melanoma diagnosis is surprisingly high, numbering at least 5 (out of approximately 300 active players), although most of these diagnoses are melanoma-in-situ with an excellent prognosis.

Darker-skinned players have a much lower risk of skin cancer, although contrary to expectations, it is not zero. Although there is no famous cricketer from India, Sri Lanka, or the West Indies to have died of skin cancer, Bob Marley the Jamaican reggae singer died of acral melanoma at the age of 36.

Studies on the risk of cancer in physically active people show that exercise is strongly protective against the majority of cancer types [15]. Melanoma is an exception, with no protective association with exercise [16]. This may be a direct non-association [17], but is subject to the reverse confounder that physically active people are almost certainly more likely to have had high childhood exposure to the sun, a known strong risk factor for melanoma [18].

25.5 Is Annual Skin Cancer Screening Worthwhile?

Cancer screening is popular for many different types of cancer and is driven by at-risk populations and cancer frequency. The screening programs with most proven efficacy include smear tests for cervical cancer and faecal occult blood screening for colorectal cancer. Skin cancer screening is particularly popular, especially so given that it lacks proven evidence base for saving lives. Expert evidence-based advice supports regular self-examination and early presentation of changing skin lesions to doctors. However, it has not been established that adding a regular annual skin check to this advice actually leads to any survival advantage [19]. Perhaps further defining a population at higher risk may change this over time. Advocates of skin screening would argue that the risks and costs associated with excising a small skin lesion are preferable to investigating potential metastatic disease. All cancer screening programs would have significant numbers of false positives, but false positive skin lesions almost certainly wouldn't have negative implications on death rates [19]. This, unfortunately, cannot be said (that there are no substantial risks) about prostate or bowel cancer screening.

The unanswered question with our current state of knowledge is whether the rate of skin cancer in cricketers is high enough to warrant consideration of further studies of skin screening, including randomised trials with lengthy follow-ups. As a starting point, fair-skinned players who've experienced high recreational UV exposure, or anyone with a family history, would be a priority candidate for further study. Equally, players with large numbers of dysplastic/atypical naevi or with precancerous lesions, such as solar keratoses deserve attention. It can be assumed that there is unlikely to be any harm for these individuals to undertake regular skin screening by a medical practitioner, but the question of whether it is of major benefit or is cost-effective remains unanswered. A nuanced process of triage may be necessary to define those at truly highest risk.

References

1. Zalaudek I, Argenziano G, Soyer HP, Saurat JH, Braun RP. Dermoscopy of subcorneal hematoma. Dermatologic Surg. 2004;30(9):1229–32. https://doi.org/10.1111/j.1524-4725.2004.30381.x.
2. Farhadian JA, Tlougan BE, Adams BB, Leventhal JS, Sanchez MR. Skin conditions of baseball, cricket, and softball players. Sports Med. 2013;43(7):575–89. https://doi.org/10.1007/s40279-013-0022-4.
3. Bowling J, Paoli J, Chamberlain A. Chapter 7.3 Onychoscopy. In: Diagnostic dermoscopy. 2nd ed. Oxford: Wiley Blackwell; 2022. p. 183–98.
4. Mortimer PS, Dawber RP. Trauma to the nail unit including occupational sports injuries. Dermatol Clin. 1985;3(3):415–20.
5. Bolognia J, Schaeffer J, Cerroni L. Chapter 88: Environmental and sports-related skin diseases. In: Hannam S, Smith M, editors. Dermatology. 5th ed. Elsevier; 2024.
6. Pecci M, Comeau D, Chawla V. Skin conditions in the athlete. Am J Sports Med. 2009;37(2):406–18. https://doi.org/10.1177/0363546508325663.
7. Ventura MT, Dagnello M, Matino MG, Di Corato R, Giuliano G, Tursi A. Contact dermatitis in students practicing sports: incidence of rubber sensitisation. Br J Sports Med. 2001;35(2):100–2. https://doi.org/10.1136/bjsm.35.2.100.
8. Daggett C, Brodell RT, Daniel CR, Jackson J. Onychomycosis in athletes. Am J Clin Dermatol. 2019;20(5):691–8. https://doi.org/10.1007/s40257-019-00448-4.
9. Lipner SR, Scher RK. Onychomycosis: clinical overview and diagnosis. J Am Acad Dermatol. 2019;80(4):835–51. https://doi.org/10.1016/j.jaad.2018.03.062.
10. Lipner SR, Scher RK. Onychomycosis: treatment and prevention of recurrence. J Am Acad Dermatol. 2019;80(4):853–67. https://doi.org/10.1016/j.jaad.2018.05.1260.
11. Gupta AK, Venkataraman M, Renaud HJ, Summerbell R, Shear NH, Piguet V. A paradigm shift in the treatment and management of onychomycosis. Skin Appendage Disord. 2021;7(5):351–8. https://doi.org/10.1159/000516112.
12. Winokur RC, Dexter WW. Fungal infections and parasitic infestations in sports: expedient identification and treatment. Phys Sportsmed. 2004;32(10):23–33. https://doi.org/10.3810/psm.2004.10.601.
13. Jones ME, Davies MAM, Leyland KM, Delmestri A, Porter A, Ratcliffe J, et al. Osteoarthritis and other long-term health conditions in former elite cricketers. J Sci Med Sport. 2018;21(6):558–63. https://doi.org/10.1016/j.jsams.2017.10.013.
14. Luies N, Orchard JJ, Driscoll T, Sahdra SK, Cheng J, Davis A, et al. Sheffield shield cricketers live longer than the age-matched general Australian male population. Indian J Orthop. 2023;57:1613.
15. Rezende LFM, Sá TH, Markozannes G, Rey-López JP, Lee I-M, Tsilidis KK, et al. Physical activity and cancer: an umbrella review of the literature including 22 major anatomical sites and 770000 cancer cases. Br J Sports Med. 2018;52(13):826–33. https://doi.org/10.1136/bjsports-2017-098391.
16. Moore SC, Lee IM, Weiderpass E, Campbell PT, Sampson JN, Kitahara CM, et al. Association of leisure-time physical activity with risk of 26 types of cancer in 1.44 million adults. JAMA Intern Med. 2016;176(6):816–25. https://doi.org/10.1001/jamainternmed.2016.1548.
17. Perrier F, Ghiasvand R, Lergenmuller S, Robsahm TE, Green AC, Borch KB, et al. Physical activity and cutaneous melanoma risk: a Norwegian population-based cohort study. Prev Med. 2021;153:106556. https://doi.org/10.1016/j.ypmed.2021.106556.
18. Garbe C, Forsea AM, Amaral T, Arenberger P, Autier P, Berwick M, et al. Skin cancers are the most frequent cancers in fair-skinned populations, but we can prevent them. Eur J Cancer. 2024;204:114074. https://doi.org/10.1016/j.ejca.2024.114074.
19. Henrikson NB, Ivlev I, Blasi PR, Nguyen MB, Senger CA, Perdue LA, et al. U.S. Preventive Services Task Force evidence syntheses, formerly systematic evidence reviews. Screening for skin cancer: an evidence update for the US Preventive Services Task Force. Rockville: Agency for Healthcare Research and Quality (US); 2023.

Optimising Health and Performance During International Cricket Travel

26

Antonia Rossiter, Rónán Doherty,
Dina C. Janse van Rensburg (Christa),
Audrey Jansen van Rensburg,
and Brendan Connor

26.1 Introduction

Travel for training and competition is synonymous with elite sport. International cricket players spend much of their year travelling all over the globe to compete at various multi-format series and international World Cup events. International cricket is often played as tours, requiring intensive periods of travel and competition and extended periods away from home, which can last several weeks. Athletes and their support teams widely perceive international travel to cause substantial disturbance to physical and mental performance and increase the risk of illness and injury [1], which may result in under-recovery and reduced performance if left unchecked.

The travelling coaching and support staff are also susceptible to the detrimental effects of international travel. In modern-day elite sports, athletes generally receive some time to recover from the journey before they compete. However, the support staff must be ready to perform their role to the highest standards upon arrival. Thus, the challenges associated with international travel and the mitigating strategies are relevant to both the players and their travelling support staff.

Supplementary Information The online version contains supplementary material available at https://doi.org/10.1007/978-981-96-6321-7_26.

A. Rossiter (✉)
Sport Ireland Institute, National Sports Campus, Dublin, Ireland

Sport and Human Performance Research Centre Health Research Institute, University of Limerick, Limerick, Ireland
e-mail: arossiter@instituteofsport.ie

R. Doherty
Sport Ireland Institute, National Sports Campus, Dublin, Ireland

Atlantic Technological University, Donegal, Ireland
e-mail: ronan.doherty@atu.ie

D. C. Janse van Rensburg (Christa)
Section Sports Medicine, Faculty of Health Sciences, University of Pretoria, Pretoria, South Africa

Medical Advisory Panel, World Netball, Manchester, UK
e-mail: christa.jansevanrensburg@up.ac.za

A. J. van Rensburg
Section Sports Medicine, Faculty of Health Sciences, University of Pretoria, Pretoria, South Africa
e-mail: audrey.jansenvanrensburg@up.ac.za

B. Connor
Cricket Ireland, Cricket Ireland High Performance Training Centre, National Sports Campus, Dublin, Ireland
e-mail: Brendan.connor@cricketireland.ie

B. Olivier, J. W. Orchard (eds.), *Cricket Sports Medicine*,
https://doi.org/10.1007/978-981-96-6321-7_26

26.2 Challenges of International Travel

26.2.1 Travel Fatigue and Jet Lag

During any long journey, travel fatigue develops over time, irrespective of the mode or direction of travel [2]. It is experienced as general fatigue, weariness, and disorientation. Four areas should be considered when addressing travel fatigue: total distance travelled, time of travel, frequency of travel, and length of the season [3]. Travel fatigue is not only experienced after a single episode of travel but can also accumulate with multiple journeys due to congested competition schedules.

Disrupted sleep duration and quality are common due to travel schedules. On flights, factors such as dry, hypoxic cabin conditions; cramped seating; proximity to other passengers; noisy galleyways; aircraft vibrations; and lighting can severely affect comfort and passengers' ability to sleep. When sleep is reduced to <7 h, there is a detrimental impact on both cognitive and physical performance, while injury risk increases [4, 5]. Limited access to preferred food and fluid choices due to airline restrictions and added stressful situations like flight delays, missing baggage, and customs clearance further exacerbate weariness and fatigue. However, with careful planning and self-management, travel fatigue can be minimised. Recovery from travel fatigue usually occurs within a few days with adequate rest, sleep, and nutrition [2, 6].

Jet lag follows rapid travel across three or more time zones, resulting in the desynchronisation of the circadian system to the light/dark cycle of the destination. This can disrupt every system in the human body, including body temperature, hormonal release, and the sleep–wake cycle. The circadian system cannot immediately adjust to the new time zone, leading to the detrimental symptoms of jet lag. These symptoms include sleep disturbances, daytime sleepiness, difficulty sleeping at night, irritability, reduced motivation, gastrointestinal disruption and reduced cognitive and physical performance [2, 7]. The severity and duration of jet lag symptoms generally increase with the number of time zones crossed and tend to be more pronounced after eastward flights compared to westward flights. The circadian rhythm, also known as the human body clock, needs time to adjust gradually; consequently, the symptoms of jet lag will persist until the circadian rhythms shift to the new destination time. To resynchronise, the circadian system must be delayed when travelling West and advanced when travelling East. It is roughly estimated that resynchronising the body clock to the destination's time zone takes about 1 day per time zone crossed following travel East and half a day per time zone following travel West. It is important to note that there is a high degree of individual chronobiological variability in the severity and recovery of jet lag. Unless the negative effects of both travel fatigue and jet lag can be managed or minimised, athlete health, well-being, and performance are likely to suffer [8].

26.3 Travel and Nutrition

International travel poses significant challenges for cricket players in maintaining their regular diets, which are essential for achieving and sustaining peak physical health, performance, and overall well-being. When travelling internationally, players may encounter unfamiliar foods, differing food safety standards, and language barriers that may limit and disrupt their preferred nutritional plan. They may be unable to access familiar foods and supplements or those they rely on for performance. Travel fatigue and jet lag can disrupt normal meal schedules, metabolism, and digestion. Additionally, limited access to fluids while travelling, along with warmer environmental conditions and water safety concerns at their destination, can challenge proper hydration status.

26.4 Travel and Health

International travel can pose a risk to player health. Picking up an infectious illness while travelling can have severe consequences for a player, including failure to compete in total health. Being in crowded airports, planes, hotels, and competition venues increases the likelihood of exposure to various illnesses, including colds, flu, and other infections; however, communication and implementation of risk mitigation strategies have been shown to be a successful means of reducing infection [9]. Table 26.1 details some of the various methods of contracting illnesses during travel and the mitigation factors relevant to each form of spread. A two-to-threefold increase in the incidence of diseases, such as upper respiratory tract infection and gastrointestinal infection, has been reported in elite athletes who have travelled across >5 time zones [10].

During international travel, players may be exposed to unfamiliar foods, water sources, and lower standards of food safety and hygiene than they are accustomed to at home, leading to gastrointestinal issues if they are not adequately managed. Dehydration and restricted movement during long-haul air travel can lead to stiffness and soreness, potentially reducing the capacity and quality of training or competition performance. A more serious consequence of prolonged sitting and dehydration, particularly on flights of >8 h duration, is the increased risk of venous thromboembolism [11].

Table 26.1 Example of types of disease spread and specific mitigation factors (in addition to vaccination, which itself can reduce the risk of many diseases)

Type of spread	Example diseases	Mitigation strategies
Ingestion (food-borne)	Salmonella, Hepatitis A	Choice of quality food vendors/ restaurants; refrigeration, cooking at high temperatures
Fomites	Rotavirus, Norovirus	Handwashing
Body contact (e.g. sexual transmission)	Chlamydia, Gonorrhoea, HIV	Use condoms during sexual contact
Aerosol	COVID-19, Influenza, other respiratory viruses	N95 masking in crowded indoor situations
Vector (e.g. mosquito bite)	Malaria	Mosquito repellent, long-sleeved clothes

26.5 Strategies for International Travel

The symptoms of jet lag and travel fatigue are complex and often overlap, making them difficult to distinguish. Therefore, a multifaceted travel strategy that addresses both travel fatigue and jet lag is recommended. Travel strategies should consider various aspects, including the travel route and schedule, sleep hygiene, stress management, health protection, nutrition, hydration, and training for periods pre-, during, and post-travel [3, 12].

26.6 Resynchronising the Body Clock

In mammals, many cellular processes, physiological functions, and behaviours follow internally driven 24-h cyclic patterns called circadian rhythms, which synchronise through zeitgebers or time-givers. Zeitgebers are the cues (physiological, psychological, behavioural, pharmacological, and environmental) that entrain the phase of a biological rhythm [3]. The most important zeitgeber is natural sunlight, but lifestyle factors such as socialising, eating, and physical activity may also play a role [13], as well as some pharmacological treatments, such as exogenous melatonin [14].

Melatonin is a hormone released by the pineal gland during darkness. Exposure to bright light suppresses melatonin release (signalling the end of sleep and a rise in core body temperature), and darkness triggers melatonin release (inducing sleep and lowering core body temperature). Melatonin onset occurs approximately 2 h before habitual bedtime [15], and daily minimum core body temperature (CBTmin) occurs approximately 7 h later [16]. A person normally sleeping from 23:00 to 07:00 will have melatonin onset at approximately 21:00, CBTmin at 04:00, and maximum core body temperature at 16:00 [17].

The best way to alleviate jet lag is by resynchronising the body clock to the destination time as quickly as possible. Light exposure at appropriate times is the most powerful way of achieving this. However, other zeitgebers, such as social and physical activity and meals, deserve consideration, as combined strategies seem beneficial [17, 18].

Even with adherence to appropriate light exposure strategies on arrival, recovery from jet lag still takes a few days, particularly after travelling East. It is possible to partially pre-adjust the body clock 3–4 days before travel by gradually shifting sleep schedules and appropriately managing light exposure [18]. This can be particularly useful if your arrival date is close to the competition.

Notably, adjusting the body clock is often challenging for athletes due to training/competition commitments, social interference, and the risk of sleep disturbance. The following sections describe using light, physical training, and exogenous melatonin to promote an appropriate phase shift after travelling across time zones. However, it is advisable to seek assistance from a travel scientist to develop a strategy designed specifically for your journey.

Light exposure—Strategically managing light exposure can assist the body clock in adjusting to the new time zone and reduce the effects of jet lag. Light exposure after CBTmin shifts the circadian system forward (phase advance), and light exposure before CBTmin causes a shift back (phase delay). The largest shifts arise when light exposure occurs in the 0–3 h on either side of CBTmin [3]. Bright natural light (even on cloudy days) has the most significant impact on circadian rhythms. However, blue light [19] and even modest-intensity artificial light [20] can induce a shift in circadian rhythm.

Physical activity—If travelling across several time zones, the appropriate time to train after travel is the same as the recommended exposure to bright light. Coaches and athletes can use outdoor training sessions as a strategy to reduce the severity and duration of jet lag symptoms [3]. However, it is important to allow the body sufficient time to recover from the physical stress of travel, including any stiffness and soreness incurred on the journey. It is recommended to gradually increase the training load over the first few days after arrival, prioritising stretching and mobility during the first 24 h.

Melatonin supplementation—Exogenous melatonin is a drug with both hypnotic and chronobiotic effects. Thus, it helps alleviate the symptoms of jet lag [21, 22]. The regulation and availability of melatonin vary from country to country, and its effectiveness is highly dependent on the timing of administration. Therefore, players should exercise caution when using melatonin and clear its use with their team doctor. Melatonin taken in the afternoon and evening (before CBTmin) causes a phase advance, and taking it in the morning (after CBTmin) causes a phase delay [17, 22]. It has been recommended that doses of 2–3 mg of melatonin should be administered 4 h after CBTmin for westward travel and 11.5 h before CBTmin for eastward travel for up to 4 days after travel to alleviate the symptoms of jet lag [23].

Box 26.1 Example Strategies to Promote the Appropriate Shift in Body Clock Before and After Travel Across Three or More Time Zones

Example 1. Adjusting your body clock in advance of travel

(a) For 3–4 days before travelling east:

- Move your bedtime and wake-up time 30–60 min earlier each day.
- Expose yourself to bright natural light for 2–3 h after waking. Use a lightbox if natural bright light is unavailable.
- Supplement 3 mg of melatonin 7 h before desired bedtime.

(b) For 3–4 days before travelling west:

- Move your bedtime and wake-up time 30–60 min later each day.
- Expose yourself to bright natural light in the evening. Use a lightbox if natural light is unavailable.

(continued)

Box 26.1 (continued)

Example 2. Adjusting your body clock after travel

(a) For travelling east (across 6 time zones).

Time at which CBTmin occurs at destination: 10:00 (04:00 + 6 h)*

- Seek bright natural light and engage in physical training after 10:00.
- Avoid light and intense physical activity before 10:00.
- Supplement 3 mg of melatonin at 22:30.

(b) For westward travel (across 6 time zones).

Time at which CBTmin occurs at destination: 22:00 (04:00–6 h)*

- Seek bright natural light and engage in physical training before 22:00.
- Avoid light and intense physical activity after 22:00.

* assuming CBTmin normally occurs at 04:00

26.7 Practising Sleep Hygiene

Good sleep hygiene, i.e. habits that promote good sleep quality and daytime alertness, is vital to reducing the impact of travel fatigue and jet lag on athletes' sleep [24]. Common sleep hygiene strategies include strategic caffeine use (see Table 26.1), avoiding alcohol, not overeating close to bedtime (≥1 h), and a relaxing bedtime routine. The same sleep hygiene habits established and practised at home should be applied during international travel. Circadian disruption following East or West travel may cause sleep disruption. However, it is important to try to maintain your regular sleep schedule. Recent napping guidelines for athletes [25] recommend a 20-min nap before 16:00 to optimise recovery and performance. If significant sleep loss has been incurred, a 90-min nap can be taken. Players should allow a minimum of 30 min between waking and training or competition to reduce sleep inertia.

Box 26.2 Sleep Hygiene Tips for Travelling Players

Sleep hygiene items

- Sleep mask.
- Earplugs/earphones, depending on preference.
- Neck pillow/your own pillow for comfort.

Sleep hygiene practices

- Keep the bedroom cool and dark.
- Don't snooze your alarm.
- Seek sunlight in the morning*.
- Avoid electronic screen time 2 h before bed (if possible).
- Shower/bath 1–2 h before bed.
- Listen to music/podcasts/audiobooks/guided meditation.
- Appropriate nutrition practices (see Table 26.1).

*timing of light exposure may need to be adjusted following east or west travel

26.8 Minimising Stress

Increased stress levels in the days before international travel can contribute to the symptoms of travel fatigue. Planning and packing for the journey well in advance and researching the destination can help prevent last-minute panic, travel disruptions, and problems with accommodation and facilities on arrival.

- *Pack well in advance*—Compile a packing list, particularly for items you will need up to a few days before travel (*see downloadable Hand Luggage Packing List*).
- *Check important documentation*—In the weeks before travel, ensure that all important documentation required for your trip is up-to-

date and in order (e.g. passport, visa, travel insurance, therapeutic use exemptions).

- *Research the destination*—Do ample online research on the area, hotels, and food options at the destination. Check online reviews and speak to other athletes, coaches, or support staff who may have travelled there before. Familiarise yourself with the culture, language, and customs of the destination. Contact the competition organisers to determine the facilities available at the venue (i.e. safe drinking water and ice, fridge/freezer, etc.). You may consider bringing a cooler box and blender to help with food preparation. Research the destination's environment and consider acclimatising to a new time zone, warmer conditions, high altitude, etc., before leaving.
- *Research the journey*—Consider travel duration, travel direction, and number of time zones crossed to arrive at the destination. Choose a reputable airline, look for reviews and compare in-flight amenities. Opt for flights with minimal layovers and the shortest travel time, considering an arrival time that will maximise appropriate exposure to natural light on arrival.
- *Organise personal affairs*—Before an extended period away from home, getting affairs in order is crucial. Organise financial matters, such as paying upcoming bills and setting up automatic payments. Arrange for someone to care for your home, pets, and plants. Take time to visit family and close friends and consider that you may have media obligations on the days before travel. Finally, ensure all essential travel documents, medications, and emergency contacts are readily accessible.
- *Leave for the airport in plenty of time*—Allow more than enough time to arrive, check-in, and move through security.
- *Prepare for a relaxing flight*—Before you board your plane, move your flight essentials into a smaller bag to store at your feet and easily access during the flight. Before and during the flight, use meditation and relaxation apps to relax your body and mind.

26.9 Protecting Health

- *Contact your team doctor before travel*—It is advisable that medical and dental check-ups and vaccinations are up-to-date. Standard vaccinations, which are relevant for all countries and may require boosters, include Influenza, COVID-19, pertussis, tetanus, and Hepatitis B. Consider additional vaccinations that may be required for your destination, such as Hepatitis A and typhoid. A responsibility of the team doctor prior to travel is to assess the risks of the various diseases at the destination and prioritise prevention for those diseases if/when there are outbreaks known (e.g. malaria, Influenza, COVID-19, measles).
- *Protect immunity*—Take steps to protect the immune system in the weeks before international travel. Avoid sleep debt and stress, and practice good sleep hygiene in the weeks before travel. Maintain a balanced diet and ensure adequate hydration. If needed, consult a nutritionist or team doctor about supplements like vitamin D, zinc, or probiotics, which can support immune health, especially in cases of deficiencies.
- *Infection control*—Implementing some simple steps to prevent the spread of infection can help reduce the risk of illness. To reduce the risk of respiratory infection, wear an N95 face mask in crowded areas and on flights for as much time as possible. During travel, use disinfectant wipes to clean surfaces around your seat. Wash hands regularly with soap and water or hand sanitiser.
- *Regular movement and compression*—Reduce the risk of venous thromboembolism and mitigate reduced capacity and quality of training or competition performance after travelling by wearing compression garments (such as flight socks) for the flight duration [26]. Regular movement, such as walking up and down the cabin aisle and performing seated exercises, can be effective in a restricted space and help improve circulation. Wearing loose, comfortable clothing can help you move more easily and stay relaxed during the flight. If the budget allows, consider investing in business-

class seating for a more comfortable sleep environment and additional space to move around. In economy class, select seats in advance; for extra legroom, consider seats in the exit rows. Aisle seats provide easier access to move around, and window seats allow for easier sleeping and views.

- *Avoid gastrointestinal infection*—Some simple steps can reduce the risk of gastrointestinal complaints that often occur with international travel:
  - Educate athletes and support staff before travel.
  - Choose restaurants and food establishments with high food safety standards; avoid street food.
  - Avoid the local water supply in countries with a risk of illness.
  - Use bottled water to brush your teeth and make ice if necessary.
  - Beware of salads and peeled fruit washed in the local water supply.
  - Use high-quality probiotics and/or prebiotics before and during travel (bring a supply with you).
  - Eat food as soon as it is prepared.
  - Avoid raw/unpasteurised dairy products.

26.10 Following Nutrition Guidelines

An athlete's nutrition goals should be central to the travel strategy planning process. Maintaining a healthy diet that meets the players' performance needs while away from home can be challenging. A travel nutrition plan should consider the travel itinerary, training, and competition schedule. It should also consider meals, facilities (fridge, kettle, etc.), and food safety standards at the accommodation and competition venue.

Generally, there are limited meal options at airports and provided by airlines. Individuals often cannot get access to their preferred foods, and gut discomfort may arise during and after travel. Before you embark on your flight, choose a balanced meal rich in protein, healthy fats, and complex carbohydrates. Pack your own healthy snacks that are high in fibre for the flight (*see downloadable Hand Luggage Packing List*). Avoid excessively sugary and salty food options, as they can exacerbate bloating and gut discomfort. At the training/competition location, players may have to cook for themselves or eat in local buffets or restaurants. Box 26.3 outlines some simple tips for maintaining a healthy, balanced performance diet while away from home.

Nutrition strategies can also support sleep and recovery and help mitigate the effects of travel fatigue and jet lag. Table 26.2 summarises some practical recommendations based on the available evidence.

Table 26.2 Nutrition strategies to promote sleep and recovery

Nutrient/food	Strategy
Carbohydrate	A high glycaemic index carbohydrate (≥1 h before bed) can improve sleep latency, duration, and quality
Caffeine	Use caffeine to promote alertness, e.g. in the morning, before training, and before competition Avoid caffeine ≥6 h before bed when possible "Coffee nap" (150–200 mg caffeine pre-nap)
Creatine	Supplement with creatine to mitigate the cognitive symptoms associated with sleep loss
Kiwifruit	2 x kiwifruit (≥1 h before bed) may improve sleep duration and quality and reduce fatigue
Magnesium	Magnesium supplementation may improve sleep duration and quality, especially in those who are deficient
Meals	Combinations of carbohydrates and protein (≥1 h before bed) may improve sleep quality and duration
Nitrate (beetroot)	Nitrate supplementation may improve sleep quality
Protein	Tryptophan-rich protein can improve sleep quality Protein supplementation (whey or casein ≥1 h before bed) may improve sleep quality and duration
Tart cherry	Supplementation (30 ml morning and evening) may improve sleep quality, sleep duration, and/or recovery

(Adapted from: [27])

Box 26.3 Tips to Help Players Maintain a Healthy Diet While Away From Home

Self-catering (cooking)

- Research food availability before travel (local shops and opening times).
- Maintain your usual food hygiene standards.
- Stick to quick, familiar recipes (get advice from the team nutritionist).
- Batch cook where possible.

Eating out

- Check menus online before selecting a restaurant.
- Check online reviews (e.g. yelp, Google reviews, TripAdvisor).
- Contact the restaurants to discuss dietary requirements and pre-order if possible.

Buffet

- Check menus online before selecting a restaurant.
- Check online reviews (e.g. yelp, Google reviews, TripAdvisor).
- Contact the restaurants to discuss dietary requirements and pre-order if possible.
- Players should be familiar with their nutritional goals.
- Check what is available before deciding what to eat.
- Be selective rather than taking one of everything.
- Leave the dining hall/restaurant as soon as you finish your meal.

26.11 Hydration

- *Carry empty water bottles*—Bottled water can be expensive in some airports, and the water supply can be limited on flights. Refill bottles at water stations after passing through airport security to ensure you are prepared with plenty of water for the flight.
- *Rehydrate on the flight*—Recent guidelines recommend that athletes aim to consume 100–300 ml of fluids per hour during a long-haul flight [28].
- *Avoid beverages with diuretic effects*—Avoid alcohol and excessive caffeine, which can cause you to pass urine more frequently, increasing the risk of dehydration and sleep disruption.
- *Supplement electrolytes*—Supplementation with electrolytes can be a simple and effective means of rehydrating while travelling.

References

1. Rossiter A, Comyns TM, Sherwin I, Nevill AM, Warrington GD. Elite athletes' and support staffs' experiences and perceptions of long-haul travel, and the self-management strategies they use. Int J Sports Sci Coach. 2024;19:698–709.
2. Samuels CH. Jet lag and travel fatigue: a comprehensive management plan for sport medicine physicians and high-performance support teams. Clin J Sport Med. 2012;3:268–73.
3. Janse van Rensburg DC (Christa), Jansen van Rensburg A, Fowler PM, et al. Managing travel fatigue and jet lag in athletes: a review and consensus statement. Sports Med. 2021;51:2029–50.
4. Laux P, Krumm B, Diers M, Flor H. Recovery–stress balance and injury risk in professional football players: a prospective study. J Sports Sci. 2015;33:2140–8.
5. Charest J, Grandner MA. Sleep and athletic performance. Sleep Med Clin. 2020;15:41–57.
6. Sack RL. The pathophysiology of jet lag. Travel Med Infect Dis. 2009;7:102–10.

7. Waterhouse J, Reilly T, Edwards B. The stress of travel. J Sports Sci. 2004;22:946–66.
8. Fowler P, Knez W, Thornton HR, Sargent C, Mendham AE, Crowcroft S, Miller J, Halson S, Duffield R. Sleep hygiene and light exposure can improve performance following long-haul air travel. Int J Sports Physiol Perform. 2021;16:517–26.
9. Jooste M, Schwellnus M. Countermeasures to reduce the risk of infections at the 2024 Olympic and Paralympic games—a balancing act. J Sport Health Sci. 2024;13:722–5.
10. Schwellnus MP, Derman WE, Jordaan E, et al. Elite athletes travelling to international destinations >5 time zone differences from their home country have a 2-3-fold increased risk of illness. Br J Sports Med. 2012;46:816–21.
11. Silverman D, Gendreau M. Medical issues associated with commercial flights. Lancet. 2009;373:2067–77.
12. Janse van Rensburg DC (Christa), Jansen Van Rensburg A, Fowler P, et al. How to manage travel fatigue and jet lag in athletes? A systematic review of interventions. Br J Sports Med. 2020;54:960–8.
13. Mistlberger RE, Skene DJ. Nonphotic entrainment in humans? J Biol Rhythm. 2005;20:339–52.
14. Arendt J. Melatonin: characteristics, concerns, and prospects. J Biol Rhythm. 2005;20:291–303.
15. Burgess HJ, Savic N, Sletten T, Roach G, Gilbert SS, Dawson D. The relationship between the dim light melatonin onset and sleep on a regular schedule in young healthy adults. Behav Sleep Med. 2003;1:102–14.
16. Eastman CI, Gazda CJ, Burgess HJ, Crowley SJ, Fogg LF. Advancing circadian rhythms before eastward flight: a strategy to prevent or reduce jet lag. Sleep. 2005;28(1):33–44.
17. Roach GD, Sargent C. Interventions to minimize jet lag after westward and eastward flight. Front Physiol. 2019;10:1–11.
18. Revell VL, Eastman CI. Jet lag and its prevention. In: Blumer J, Lockley SW, Schenck CH, editors. Therapy in sleep medicine. Philadelphia: Elsevier Saunders; 2012. p. 390–401.
19. Geerdink M, Walbeek TJ, Beersma DGM, Hommes V, Gordijn MCM. Short blue light pulses (30 min) in the morning support a sleep-advancing protocol in a home setting. J Biol Rhythm. 2016;31:483–97.
20. Sack RL, Auckley D, Auger RR, Carskadon MA, Wright KPJ, Vitiello MV, Zhdanova IV. Circadian rhythm sleep disorders: part I, basic principles, shift work and jet lag: an American Academy of sleep medicine review. Sleep. 2007;30:1460–83.
21. Herxheimer A, Waterhouse J. The prevention and treatment of jet lag. Br Med J. 2003;326:296–7.
22. Arendt J. Approaches to the pharmacological management of jet lag. Drugs. 2018;78:1419–31.
23. Herxheimer A, Petrie KJ. Melatonin for the prevention and treatment of jet lag. Cochrane Database Syst Rev. 2002:1–18.
24. Walsh NP, Halson SL, Sargent C, et al. Sleep and the athlete: narrative review and 2021 expert consensus recommendations. Br J Sports Med. 2021;55:356–68.
25. Lastella M, Halson SL, Vitale JA, Memon AR, Vincent GE. To nap or not to nap? A systematic review evaluating napping behavior in athletes and the impact on various measures of athletic performance. Nat Sci Sleep. 2021;13:841–62.
26. Broatch JR, Bishop DJ, Zadow EK, Halson S. Effects of sports compression socks on performance, physiological, and hematological alterations after long-haul air travel in elite female volleyballers. J Strength Cond Res. 2008;24:91–101.
27. Doherty R, Madigan S, Warrington G, Ellis JG. Sleep and nutrition in athletes. Current Sleep Medicine Reports. 2023;9(1):82–89.
28. Zubac D, Buoite Stella A, Morrison SA. Up in the air: evidence of dehydration risk and long-haul flight on athletic performance. Nutrients. 2020;12:1–15.

Part III

Lumbar Stress Fractures – The Signature Injury of Bowlers in Cricket

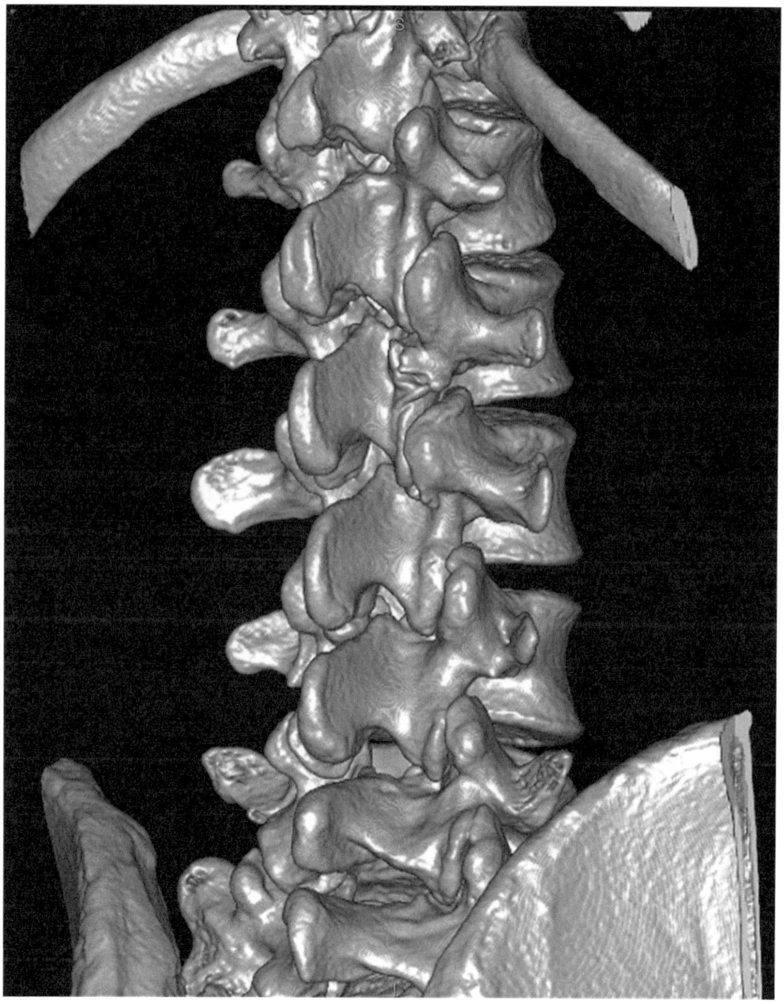

A 3-D CT reconstruction showing a pars defect at L2 level

27 Lumbar Stress Fractures Prevention

Angela Jackson

27.1 Prevention of Lumbar Bone Stress Injuries

There are multiple physical and mental health benefits to participating in sports, especially during adolescence. However, there is also a negative aspect associated with a risk of injury. Injuries such as lumbar bone stress injuries (LBSI) require prolonged time off from the game, resulting in a high financial burden to the athlete and their club, high dropout rates from the sport, a greater risk of future injury, and a negative impact on the athlete's mental health [1].

As such, many sporting organisations have allocated considerable resources to injury prevention strategies to reduce the risk of injuries. Injury prediction is not an exact science, and multiple injury prevention models have failed in their ability to predict injury. What is clear is that prior to implementing an injury prevention programme (IPP), the following factors need to be considered based on The Translating Research into Injury Prevention Practice (TRIPP) framework [2]:

1. Injury surveillance to identify injury prevalence, incidence and population groups most at risk adopting robust methodology
2. Injury mechanism
3. Risk factors associated with injury
4. Development of an effective programme
5. An implementation strategy to ensure the programme is adopted

27.2 Which Injuries Have the Highest Incidence and Burden?

Injury prevalence within cricket is high but varies between adult and junior settings, formats of the game, playing standard, player position and between genders, so it is important when planning injury prevention strategies that research performed in one population is not extrapolated to another [3]. In addition, particularly when considering LBSI, differences in anatomy, intensity, skill level and volume may not be comparable, and therefore, tissue adaptations may not have developed in the same way that offer protective qualities against injury [4].

Fast bowlers are more susceptible to injury than other player positions due to the highly dynamic, multi-planar motion involved in the bowling action. The injury that creates the highest time loss injury in fast bowlers is a lumbar bone stress injury (LBSI), particularly in adolescents and 18–23-year-olds [5], although these are also observed in spin bowlers and in adolescent multisport athletes. The expected rehabilitation

A. Jackson (✉)
Kids Back 2 Sport Limited, Manchester, UK
e-mail: info@kidsback2sport.com

B. Olivier, J. W. Orchard (eds.), *Cricket Sports Medicine*,
https://doi.org/10.1007/978-981-96-6321-7_27

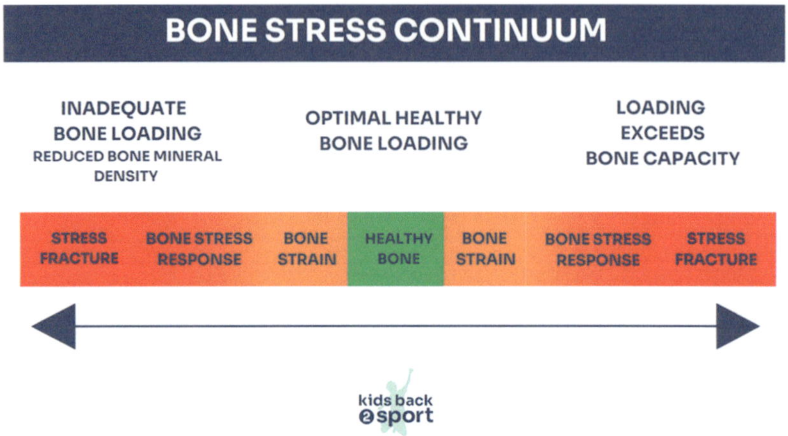

Fig. 27.1 Bone stress injury continuum

periods of these injuries often exceed 6–9 months depending on the severity of the injury, meaning this injury can cause the loss of a full season depending on the timing of the injury and the potential for the player to drop out of the game.

LBSI occur along a spectrum, ranging from an asymptomatic bone stress response to a complete stress fracture, which may become chronic with minimal potential for healing (Fig. 27.1).

Repetitive mechanical loading produced during the bowling action stresses the posterior area of the posterior neural arch region of the vertebrae, most commonly at L4 and L5 [6]. This region of the bone does not achieve peak bone mineral density (BMD) or skeletal ossification until the ages of 23.6 years in males and 20.1 years in females [7], potentially making it more susceptible to injury.

In junior athletes with just a 2-week history of low back pain during sporting activity, at least 40% had already developed an LBSI on imaging [8], highlighting the need for early recognition at the very first signs of low back pain. A delay in diagnosis can reduce the potential for healing, and whilst 98% of players will return to play at pre-participation levels after an LBSI, the long-term impact of playing with a non-united fracture is not known. What has been observed is that, anecdotally, at the professional level, players whose LBSI healed and those who avoided sustaining the injury early in their careers appear to have longer test careers than those who did not [9]. Priority is therefore firmly around preventing these injuries progressing from an acute to chronic injury through early identification and appropriate management to ensure bony union where possible. An urgent campaign is needed within all levels of cricket worldwide to raise awareness of the risks associated with players under the age of 23 participating with the presence of low back pain (LBP) and to emphasise the importance of early removal from play and appropriate rehabilitation to allow the bone to adapt and get strong enough to tolerate higher loads.

> **Key Message**
>
> To empower parents and players to report all low back pain immediately and start an immediate period of rest for a minimum of 2 weeks followed by a graduated return to play to allow for bone adaptation to occur.

27.3 What Are the Risk Factors for Injuries in Cricket?

Over the past two decades, despite improvements in technology to better evaluate the multiaxial motion of the bowling action, much remains unknown. However, if technical dysfunctions were solely to blame for injury, why would every player with a mixed action or excessive degree of lateral flexion not be injured?

27.3.1 There Is No One-Size-Fits-All Approach to Injury Prediction or Prevention

A recent systematic review [10] highlighted the large discrepancies that exist in the cricket-related literature regarding the risk factors associated with LBSI in pace bowlers. Individuals differ anatomically, and their capacity to tolerate the demands of fast bowling fluctuates, making injury prediction and injury prevention a challenge. At any given time, an athlete may display certain risk factors for a specific injury, but the human body and the interactions between multiple systems are complex and dynamic and interact in an unpredictable manner [11]. Having a high-risk profile is not a predictor of injury; an inciting event must occur before, on any given day, an athlete may sustain a non-contact injury [12] (Fig. 27.2).

The more common risk factors for bone stress injuries reported in the literature are outlined in Table 27.1. Some of these factors may be modifiable, such as sleep quantity or nutritional intake, whilst others, such as sex, growth and genetics, are non-modifiable. When considering injury reduction from a biopsychosocial perspective, identifying modifiable risk factors may be helpful to address the athlete as a whole, not just the injury itself, and can be integrated into player education injury prevention programmes (IPPs). Using a pre-participation questionnaire can be a highly effective tool to develop a cumulative risk profile of each player [13] and may identify those players who might need more specific individual interventions and rehabilitation programmes.

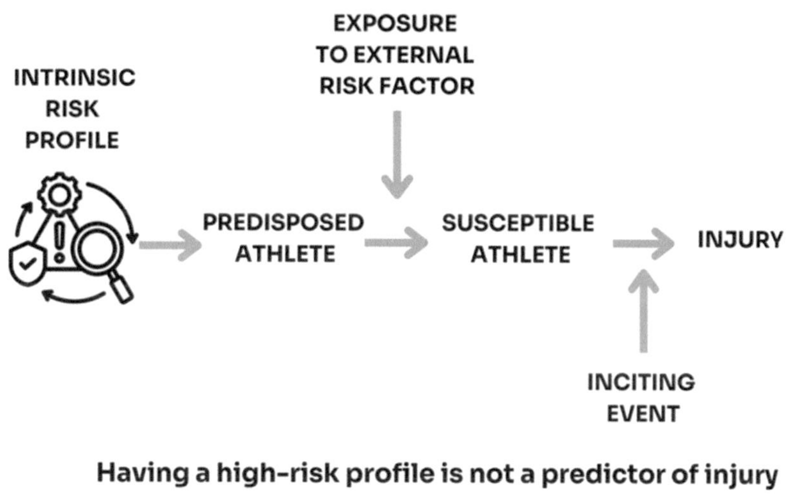

Fig. 27.2 A schematic diagram illustrating the complex relationship between the presence of intrinsic and extrinsic risk factors and the need for an inciting event to induce injury

Table 27.1 Potential risk factors associated with bone stress injuries

Intrinsic modifiable	Intrinsic non-modifiable	Extrinsic modifiable
Low energy availability	Gut health	Bowling workloads
Poor sleep quality	Food allergies or intolerances	Indoor nets
Low vitamin D or iron levels	Hypermobility	Duration of bowling history
Nutrition	Growth rate	Match formats
Fatigue	Maturation	Footwear
Psychologically perceived stress	Height	Surface
Muscle strength and endurance	Genetics	Bowling technique
Poor neuromuscular control	Medications	Training monotony
Nicotine	Low bone mineral density	
	Hormonal imbalances	
	Metabolic disorders	

27.4 Development of an Effective Injury Prevention Programme

There have been different approaches adopted when designing programmes to mitigate injury risk. Amongst the most popular approaches have been:

1. Musculoskeletal screening
2. Imaging to increase early identification of bone stress
3. Neuromuscular training injury prevention programmes (IPPs)
4. Fast bowling guidelines
5. Education of players and stakeholders

27.5 Can We Screen Players to Identify Those Most at Risk of Injury?

Many cricketers now turn to social media to seek techniques to increase their performance. Trends such as bracing the front leg or creating a pre-turn may work for some players, but not all players have the physical attributes to absorb the forces generated by the fast-bowling action, and excessive strain may be placed on the immature vertebral arch causing injury. In addition, there are anatomical differences between individuals and within individuals. Some players may have congenital or acquired asymmetries in hip or shoulder rotation, which render them unable to achieve the "desired" bowling action, and coaches need to be aware of these factors.

Musculoskeletal screening may not be able to accurately predict injury, but it can help to highlight some of these individual variants and highlight any strength deficits to ensure any technical changes are within the capabilities of the player. Many of the objective screening tests previously used have poor sensitivity, and determining a reliable threshold for each test and population group is difficult.

Musculoskeletal screening is not without limitations. It is both time-consuming and requires specialist knowledge, which excludes its suitability within community settings. It does enable the collection of baseline data over time that might inform and build knowledge around injury risk reduction for future generations. In the community setting, coaches should be aware that in players who seem to struggle to adopt coaching cues, a physical rather than technical restriction may be present, and if pain is present, the player should be advised to consult a health professional.

27.6 Should All Bowlers Have a Pre-Season MRI Scan?

The gold standard for identifying early-stage LBSI is a magnetic resonance imaging (MRI) scan. If cost were not a barrier to regular MRI scanning of both fast and spin bowlers, imaging may support early diagnosis of an LBSI and limit the progression of injuries to a grade that may not heal. To date, there have only been small studies published where pre-season and within-season MRI scans were performed across a group of players. The results in 65 adolescent fast bowlers highlighted bone marrow oedema (BMO) in asymptomatic players ahead of them developing symptoms [14]. In contrast, the imaging results in 22 adult male professional fast bowlers reported BMO in pre-season, and yet only one player developed a stress reaction [15]. The difference may be related to BMD being greater in older players who may have developed greater resilience to bowling and highlights the need for more research.

27.7 Is Bowling Too Much the Problem?

When managing training load, it is important to remember that it is a combination of both the sport-related and non-sport-related loads that contributes to maintaining a player's physical and mental wellness. Historically, non-contact injuries in youth athletes were just thought to be due to doing too much. This led to the creation of fast bowling guidelines for junior cricketers by many National Governing Bodies (NGBs) with subtle regional variations. They promote maximum "safe" bowling levels for each junior age group but fail to account for low bowling volumes that pose an injury risk too.

Bone can adapt to increased stresses placed upon it by laying down new bone to reinforce the area under the greatest stress, but this immature bone takes time to become strong enough to withstand high loads. Lumbar bone stress injuries (LBSI) occur when the capacity of the bone is exceeded either through a change in load or a drop in the capacity of the individual to tolerate that load. Regular loading is required to maintain bone density (BMD); so where there is inadequate loading, such as during the off-season or following LBSI, the bone can "decondition" within as little as 8 weeks [16], and become more vulnerable to injury. It may, therefore, be sensible to advocate for a maintenance level of bowling at lower intensities throughout the year rather than giving amateur players a complete shutdown over the winter.

The excitement of the new season and a lack of awareness about the risks can cause some players to exceed their capacity by bowling high volumes at high intensities in week one of the season. These sudden "spikes" in workload at a level not trained for are amongst the most cited risk factors for LBSI [5]. Some of the more common causes of spikes in load are described in Table 27.2. It is essential to identify times in the year when spikes in load might be anticipated so that players can prepare through a graduated build-up in tolerance.

In the Australian, English and New Zealand fast-bowling guidelines, a period of progressive loading is advised pre-season. An education campaign is needed to make sure that parents, coaches and players are aware that where there has been inadequate preparation from insufficient bowling pre-season, a reduced volume and intensity of bowling in the early weeks of the season is recommended with adequate recovery between sessions to allow for musculoskeletal adaptations.

Table 27.2 External risk factors associated with changes in load that have the potential to increase injury potential

Factors associated with low chronic load	Factors associated with spikes in activity
Post-long holidays	Holiday camps
Post-injury or illness	Start of a new season
Off-season	Overlapping seasons
New to sport	Calendar congestion
	Playing for multiple teams
	Sports tours & festivals
	Changes to technique

Key Messages
After a period of rest and at the start of the season, adopt a graduated, progressive buildup in bowling volume and intensity. Identify potential spikes in activity across the year and plan to build up resilience.

27.8 Athlete Development Is Not Athlete Restriction

We do not want to demonise high bowling volumes as there are significant protective benefits to appropriate loading of the skeleton, especially during adolescence. That is, providing it is coupled with a progressive build-up in volume and intensity, adequate sleep, recovery and a positive energy balance. If players are adequately prepared and coping well with their current training load, have a longer training history in the game, are not in their adolescent growth spurt and are more skeletally mature [17], there is no physiological reason to limit them. Indeed, exposing them to higher loads during adolescence may generate significant osteogenic potential that cannot be achieved outside this hormonal window, better preparing them for the transition to adult cricket and reducing the incidence of LBSI in 18–23-year-olds.

Adolescents who grow faster and by more than 7–8 cm per annum are at greater risk of injury [18]. In response to these findings, the England and Wales Cricket Board (ECB) has produced a supplementary document, the ECB Recreational Fast Bowling Guidance, to support the ECB Bowling Directives, suggesting that players who are growing at greater than 7 cm a year could adopt the guidelines from the age group below.

> **Key Message**
> Track growth in adolescents and report to coaches' periods of accelerated growth.

This is a positive step forward but does not make provision for the children with delayed maturation, who may be up to 3 years behind (late developers) their peers of the same age [19].

For example, in an under-13 age group, some children will have the skeletal age of a 10-year-old, whilst others may be up to 3 years ahead of their peers and already have the body of a 16-year-old. Men against boys!

Most fast-bowling directives and guidelines are based on grouping players according to chronological age (a player's date of birth), not skeletal maturation (skeletal age). In other sports, bio-banding is used to group children based on their skeletal age rather than their chronological age, using calculations such as the Khamis–Roche method to ensure that they are not being exposed to inappropriate loads for their maturation status. This approach may hold the key to protecting late developers from injury by ensuring that late developers or smaller players are not working at excessively high intensities in a bid to keep up with more mature peers. To date, bio-banding has only been reported in the literature in one study of 57 boys attending a 3-day regional under-14 boys' cricket development camp in New Zealand. The player's maturity status was assessed, and a series of cricket and strength-related tests were performed, and whilst this is a step forward to creating more individualised approaches to training, more work is needed to assess if this approach could reduce injury rates [20]. Coach education is needed to ensure that coaches are aware of the differences in maturation between individuals and the need to modify the training load for late-maturing players and for players who develop a temporary loss in coordination and capacity around the time of the peak adolescent growth spurt.

LBSI are not limited to fast bowlers, with spin bowlers also sustaining these injuries too. Anecdotally, all players exposed to spikes in workload not trained are at risk of an LBSI, and more work is needed to establish if spin bowlers would also benefit from specific bowling guidelines before and around puberty.

27.9 Not All Sessions Are Equal

Just like sprinting is more demanding than jogging, bowling at maximal intensity has a greater metabolic and physical impact on the body, requiring greater recovery and energy intake when compared to a mixture of high- and low-intensity efforts. Increases in bowling workload and intensity were associated with increased rates of LBSI in 40 male 14–18-year-old fast bowlers as they progressed towards senior and elite cricket [21]. Younger bowlers are eager to improve and impress selectors, and their peers are often unaware of the cost of bowling at 100% effort at all opportunities, frequently exceeding their current capacity by regularly training at or near their limits.

New Zealand Cricket (NZC) [22] advocates a F.I.R.S.T approach in their Youth Pace Bowling Guidelines to account for not just the volume but also the intensity of each bowling session. See Table 27.3.

They describe an "Intensity Guide" with scores from 0 to 3 encouraging players to vary the intensity by adjusting the length of the run-up depending on the setting. Care should be taken; however, reducing the length of the run-up may not prevent a less experienced bowler from still trying to bowl at maximal effort, and without the benefit of momentum from a longer, quicker run-up, this may inadvertently increase the load through the spine. Elite, experienced fast bowlers have been shown to be able to adjust their bowling intensity accurately and still achieve near-maximal ball release speeds (BRS) at sub-maximal intensities [23]; however, younger

Table 27.3 A F.I.R.S.T approach implemented by New Zealand Cricket [22] to account for not just the volume but also the intensity of each bowling session

F	Frequency—sessions per week
I	Intensity—effort level
R	Rest and recovery required
S	Surface—indoor vs outdoor vs artificial wickets
T	Type of training—technical, tactical, training and competition

and less experienced bowlers may struggle to identify how a 50 or 60% effort should feel.

Key Message

Teach players the benefits of performance of varying intensity of bowling across the week and increase both recovery and energy intake following higher intensity periods.

27.10 How Well Is the Player Coping?

Whilst there is little doubt that participating in a load not trained for is likely to result in a load that exceeds the current capacity of the tissues, it fails to explain why in a squad of players who, for example, all attend a cricket festival and who are all exposed to similar training loads, do not all get injured at the same time. Each player has their individual capacity, which fluctuates from day to day due to illness, a lack of sleep, nutrition, or perhaps a spike in stress levels or a growth spurt. The cumulative effect of these different stressors can reduce an individual's tolerance to load [24], blunt the benefits of exercise and leave them at greater risk of injury.

Measuring the response of the body to training (internal load) is reported to give a more accurate assessment of the individual's response to training stress [25], and yet, the majority of bowling guidelines only consider bowling volume (external load), without taking into account individual differences in run-up distance, intensity, speed, maturation, height and mass that will ultimately influence fatigue and readiness to bowl.

Failure to factor in sufficient recovery time can lead to the development of fatigue, injury and illness [26]. The England and Wales Cricket Board (ECB) [27] have encouraged junior bowlers to observe no greater than 2 consecutive days of fast bowling and no greater than four sessions of bowling in every 7-day rolling period, whilst Cricket Australia (CA) [28] and New Zealand Cricket (NZC) [22] advocate a day off between each bowling session for specific age groups. They ECB also encourage fast bowlers to plan a light (50% volume) bowling week every 4–5 weeks and a full week off without bowling every 10–12 weeks to facilitate bony adaptation.

Cricket is a time-consuming game that can leave players time-poor. Junior and youth players are often juggling the demands of academia and sporting commitments with schedules that can impact sleep quality. Training late at night, sharing rooms when travelling to away games, and jetlag when travelling abroad on tour can leave players fatigued [29]. A reduction in sleep volume coupled with a sudden increase in training volume and intensity was associated with a 2.3-fold higher injury risk [30]. Players need to be educated about the benefits of sleep and, when needed, prescribed greater recovery time.

27.11 Do They Eat Enough for What They Do?

Maintaining a positive energy balance between energy intake versus energy expenditure is crucial for injury prevention, wellness and optimal performance. Low energy availability (LEA) can trigger a downregulation of non-essential hormonal processes [31], which can impact multiple bodily systems and cause Relative Energy Deficiency in Sports (REDs) [32]. This cascade of hormonal reactions can affect bone synthesis, making the player more susceptible to bone stress injuries. In certain individuals, low levels of iron and vitamin D can also increase the risk of LBSI. Coaches, parents and health professionals should be alert to athletes who may develop LEA through skipping

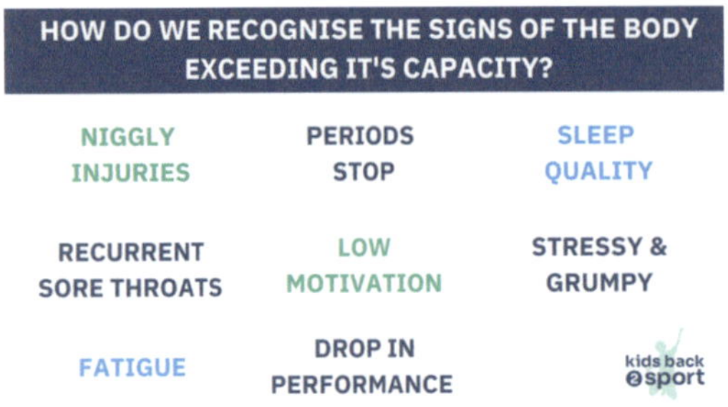

Fig. 27.3 The early signs of a player who may be at risk of developing Relative Energy Deficiency in Sports

breakfast, having specific dietary needs, having an apparent poor relationship with food, or appearing to be overly concerned with body image. Education is needed around the importance of fuelling for wellness and performance and awareness of the early symptoms of REDs. These are summarised in Fig. 27.3.

27.12 Stress, Perfectionism and Injury

There is no current evidence citing stress or anxiety as a direct risk factor for LBSI; however, stress can trigger a very similar cascade of hormonal changes to LEA, and bone health may be adversely affected. Those players who display maladaptive perfectionist responses to failure with high levels of anxiety and low levels of self-esteem may be at greater risk [33]. In pursuit of "flawless" performances, players may push themselves harder and risk overtraining, illness and injury [33]. Coaches need to be trained to recognise these traits and adapt training loads during times of higher perceived stress. Parents and coaches need to understand the heightened risk of injury associated with placing excessively high expectations on children, especially during the peak adolescent growth spurt when self-esteem often drops and performances may falter. Creating positive learning environments with less pressure on results and embracing mistakes as development opportunities can address many of the performance anxieties exhibited in many players and may ultimately protect them from injury.

27.13 Successful Load Management

Monitoring load can give an understanding of current performance and wellness levels and identify if training load adjustments are required. At the elite level, the use of GPS and accelerometry microtechnology units helps provide more accurate feedback on bowling volume and intensity. In academy settings, bowling diaries can be monitored and current week bowling volumes and intensities prescribed. However, in community settings, monitoring load in those who play more than one sport or play for multiple teams may be more challenging. Ultimately, responsibility will lie with the player to self-report and for parents to be empowered to introduce greater recovery when they sense a drop in capacity. Younger players may underreport their bowling volume, failing to record "fun" net sessions or hiding their volume for fear of being not allowed to bowl again that week.

Monitoring player wellness is an essential part of load management. Understanding how well the player is coping can identify when the capacity to tolerate load may be compromised. Prior to training, parents and athletes can be taught to use athlete self-report measures (ASRM) to assess response to training and current levels of fatigue. These are often complex questionnaires but can be simplified to assess factors such as daily soreness, fatigue, sleep quality and stress levels (Table 27.4).

If a player reports high levels of soreness, tiredness or stress, it may be better for them to miss a training session and focus on recovery, rather than risk an injury that could result in the loss of an entire season. Moderate scores might indicate that the training focus should be on more tactical and technical bowling skills at lower intensities, and on days when their "battery" is full, they can go hard and maximise training gains (see Fig. 27.4). This enables a dialogue between the player–coach and parent to ensure the player does not get overtrained or injured and promotes how to listen to their body and train appropriately.

Table 27.4 Example of a simplified wellness score questionnaire using a 1–5 scale where 5 indicates readiness to train and 1 indicates a need for greater recovery

	1	2	3	4	5
SORENESS					
FATIGUE					
STRESS					

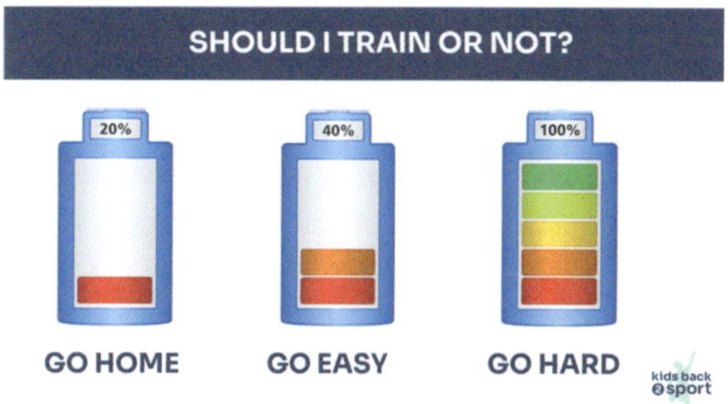

Fig. 27.4 Parents and players need to learn to assess readiness to train to reduce the risk of injury and illness

> **Key Message**
>
> To understand the importance of tracking both internal and external load and how to recognise the early signs of a drop in capacity and adjust training load accordingly. Players can boost their capacity to tolerate greater loads through a well-balanced diet, vitamin D supplementation, good quality sleep, and taking time out for recovery and relaxation.

27.14 Injury Prevention Programme (IPP)

To tolerate the demands of the fast-bowling action, adequate neuromuscular control and strength are required. There is evidence to support that the inclusion of targeted resistance training programmes in youth athletes may reduce injury rates by as much as 50% [34]. Whilst there is little research to support specific exercise interventions within cricket, lower levels of single-leg strength and trunk control may be associated with a greater risk of developing an LBSI [35]. In 39 elite fast bowlers, aged 16–22, moderate correlations were found between rear hip flexion angle at BFC with the side plank endurance test and the lumbopelvic stability test [36], supporting exercise intervention in theory.

The back extensor muscles maintain a more vertical trunk alignment during the ground contact phases of the bowling action [37]. Greater fatigue and a drop-off in endurance capacity in young adults with low back pain have been reported [38], suggesting exercise interventions that increase endurance capacity of the back and hip extensor muscles might mitigate LBSI risk in some players.

Exercise-based IPPs are an inexpensive means of implementing "neuromuscular training" to increase resilience to injury and improve balance, agility and strength. Specifically, chosen exercises can be integrated into a warm-up or cool-down to address known injury risk factors within a population group and prepare the athlete for play. The FIFA (Fédération Internationale de Football Association) 11+ programme has been shown to reduce the risk of injury by 35% [39] when performed 2–3 times per week; however, there have been challenges around uptake and adherence.

Successful programmes to be effective are said to be the ones that athletes do [40], emphasising the need to implement a top-down approach from NGBs to fund coach and player education to ensure the programme becomes an integral part of all training settings, not just those under coach supervision. All too often, junior players faced with barriers such as time constraints, lack of knowledge and peer pressure neglect this essential part of injury prevention and preparation. Explaining why the programme is important, along with its benefits for performance and enhanced player availability, can increase adoption. Programmes should be simple, fun, relevant

Table 27.5 Details of existing cricket-specific injury prevention programmes

Cricket Injury Prevention Programme: CIPP 14 drills—beginner & advanced [43]	Multilevel IPP community level, pace bowlers aged 14–17 [44]
Dynamic stretch and running	A dynamic warm-up
Strength and agility	Strength-based exercises
Balance and core strength	Dynamic neuromuscular control
Game-based exercises	Muscular endurance exercises

and time efficient, requiring no specialist equipment. They should be introduced at a grassroots level to develop physical literacy in the key cricket movement patterns and establish good habits at an early age. Critically, they need to support coaches to develop the confidence to teach correct exercise execution, ensure all drills are performed pain-free, and be able to modify exercises to meet individual needs.

Despite the high prevalence and recurrence rates of lumbar bone stress injuries in fast bowlers and the injury burden these injuries create in time lost from the sport, there is no internationally adopted community-based IPP in cricket. Within the literature, there have only been two protocols described designed to be integrated within training sessions twice a week taking around 15 minutes to complete. These are outlined in Table 27.5. Small cohort studies have been performed using these programmes, reporting fewer injuries and increases in strength and endurance [41, 42]; however, to date, there has not been a large-scale, high-level quality review of the efficacy of either programme in a community-based setting.

Key Message
To implement a consistent strength-based warm-up into every cricket setting and provide high quality educational resources about injury prevention to all levels.

History supports, however, that simply making athletes stronger with better biomechanics is not predictive of who will and won't get injured. When planning and implementing an IPP, one of the key components is player education [45], which needs to be made available to community-based players at an early age; do not wait until players achieve representative levels before introducing it. The sparsity of accessible community-based education and exercise-based programmes for club cricket coaches led the author to create a programme called Ready 4 Cricket [46] for use within a junior club and county cricket setting. It includes both an exercise-based programme and an online education module for parents, players and coaches. If players understand why the programme is important and what benefit there might be to the player in enhancing performance and reducing injury risk, compliance rates increase. To date, this programme has not been externally validated but provides a framework for future development.

27.15 Future Considerations and Recommendations

It is not known how many players are lost to the game through LBSI, but the cost and time commitment of rehabilitation, along with the relatively high rates of recurrence, present significant barriers to a return to play. Much investment is needed to find more effective injury prevention approaches to reduce the incidence of injury and also limit progression to a more impactful injury, but these will take time to implement. Early diagnosis of LBSI is key to better outcomes, and this can only be achieved through awareness amongst the whole cricket community. A quick and effective solution is to provide high-quality online educational platforms with easy access for players of all ages and abilities to deliver key messages around how to mitigate injury risk and be proactive in managing workload and boosting their capacity to tolerate more.

References

1. Williams A, Peirce N, McKay C, Stokes K, Williams S. The financial cost of injuries in elite cricket in England and Wales: a retrospective study of seven years of insurance claims. Br J Sports Med. 2024;58:A52.1.
2. Finch CF. A new framework for research leading to sports injury prevention. J Sci Med Sport. 2006;9(1–2):3–9.
3. Gamage PJ, Fortington LV, Kountouris A, Finch CF. Match injuries in Sri Lankan junior cricket: a prospective, longitudinal study. JSAMS. 2019;22(6):647–52.
4. McLeod G, O'Connor S, Morgan D, Kountouris A, Finch CF, Fortington LV. Prospective reporting of injury in community-lev cricket: a systematic review to identify research priorities. J Sci Med Sport. 2020;23(11):1028–43.
5. Alway P, Brooke-Wavell K, Langley B, King M, Peirce N. Incidence and prevalence of lumbar stress fracture in English county cricket fast bowlers, association with bowling workload and seasonal variation. BMJ Open Sport Exerc Med. 2019;5(1):e000529.
6. Alway P, Felton P, Brooke-Wavell K, Peirce N, King M. Cricket fast bowling technique and lumbar bone stress injury. Med Sci Sports Exerc. 2021;53(3):581–9.
7. Xue S, Kemal O, Lu M, Lix LM, Leslie WD, Yang S. Age at attainment of peak bone mineral density and its associated factors: the National Health and Nutrition Examination Survey 2005–2014. Bone. 2020;131:115163.
8. Nitta A, Sakai T, Goda Y, et al. Prevalence of symptomatic lumbar spondylolysis in pediatric patients. Orthopedics. 2016;39(3):e434–7.
9. Orchard JW, Saw R, Kountouris A, Redrup D, Farhart P, Sims K. Management of lumbar bone stress injury in cricket fast bowlers and other athletes. South Afr J Sports Med. 2023;35(1):v35i1a15172.
10. Farhart P, Beakley D, Diwan A, Duffield R, Rodriguez EP, Chamoli U, Watsford M. Intrinsic variables associated with low back pain and lumbar spine injury in fast bowlers in cricket: a systematic review. BMC Sports Sci Med Rehabil. 2023;15:202.
11. Bittencourt NF, Meeuwisse WH, Mendonça LD, et al. Complex systems approach for sports injuries: moving from risk factor identification to injury pattern recognition-narrative review and new concept. Br J Sports Med. 2016;50:1309–14.
12. Ruddy JD, Cormack SJ, Whiteley R, Williams MD, Timmins RG, Opar DA. Modeling the risk of team sport injuries: a narrative review of different statistical approaches. Front Physiol. 2019;10:829.
13. Hamstra-Wright KL, HuxelBliven KC, Napier C. Training load capacity, cumulative risk, and bone stress injuries: a narrative review of a holistic approach. Front Sport Act Liv. 2021;3:665683.
14. Kountouris A, Sims K, Beakley D, Saw AE, Orchard J, Rotstein A, Cook JL. MRI bone marrow oedema precedes lumbar bone stress injury diagnosis in junior elite cricket fast bowlers. Br J Sports Med. 2019;53(19):1236–9.
15. Bell AJ, Nunnerley JL, Shackel DF, Coates MH, Campbell RG, Frampton CM, Schouten R. Is MRI screening for bone marrow oedema useful in predicting lumbar bone stress injuries in adult male professional cricketers? A New Zealand pilot study. J Sci Med Sport. 2023;26(8):410–4.
16. Alway P, Peirce N, Johnson W, King M, Kerslake R, Brooke-Wavell K. Activity specific areal bone mineral density is reduced in athletes with stress fracture and requires profound recovery time: a study of lumbar stress fracture in elite cricket fast bowlers. J Sci Med Sport. 2022;25(10):828–33.
17. Jayanthi N, Schley S, Cumming SP, Myer GD, Saffel H, Hartwig T, Gabbett TJ. Developmental training model for the sport specialized youth athlete: a dynamic strategy for individualizing load-response during maturation. Sports Health. 2022;14(1):142–53.
18. Monasterio X, Cumming S, Larruskain J, Johnson DM, Gil SM, Bidaurrazaga-Letona I, Lekue JA, Diaz-Beitia G, Santisteban JM, Williams S. The combined effects of growth and maturity status on injury risk in an elite football academy. Biol Sport. 2024;41(1):235–44.
19. Johnson A, Doherty PJ, Freemont A. Investigation of growth, development, and factors associated with injury in elite schoolboy footballers: prospective study. BMJ. 2009;27:338.
20. Walters SR, Renshaw IA, Whatman C, Zoellner A, Harrison C, Millar S, Pithey R. Maturity status, relative age and bio-banding in youth cricket. New Z Cric Rep. 2021;48:66–75.
21. Keylock L, Alway P, Felton P, McCaig S, Brooke-Wavell K, King M, et al. Lumbar bone stress injuries and risk factors in adolescent cricket fast bowlers. J Sports Sci. 2022;40(12):1336–42.
22. Cricket, New Zealand. Youth Pace Bowling Recommendations. New Zealand Cricket. [Online], 2021. https://www.nzc.nz/media/18857/youth-pace-bowling-recommendations.pdf.
23. Feros SA, Bednarski DA, Kremer PJ. The relationship between prescribed, perceived, and actual delivery intensity in cricket pace bowling. Int J Sports Physiol Perform. 2021;16(5):731–4.
24. Puga TB, Mazumder RM, Ruan T, Scigliano N, Thiel GE, Treffer K. Sleep, nutrition, hydration and rest: the equal importance of external factors outside of training and practice for sports injury prevention. Sci J Sport Perform. 2023;2(4):428–38.
25. Impellizzeri FM, Marcora SM, Coutts AJ. Internal and external training load: 15 years on. Int J Sports Physiol Perform. 2019;14(2):270–3.
26. Schwellnus M, Soligard T, Alonso JM, Bahr R, Clarsen B, Dijkstra HP, Gabbett TJ, Gleeson M, Hägglund M, Hutchinson MR, Van Rensburg CJ. How much is too much?(part 2) International Olympic Committee consensus statement on load in sport and risk of illness. Br J Sports Med. 2016;50(17):1043–52.
27. Cricket, England. Recreational fast bowling guidance. England and Wales Cricket Board.

[Online], 2024. https://resources.ecb.co.uk/ecb/document/2024/06/14/292038a2-ac47-4655-bdf7-454c79d285eb/Recreational-Fast-Bowling-Guidance-2024.pdf.
28. Cricket, Australia. Youth pace bowling guidelines. Cricket Australia. [Online] 2017. http://community.cricket.com.au/clubs/youth-pace-bowling-guidelines.
29. Peacock C, Mena M, Sanders G, Silver T, Kalman D, Antonio J. Sleep data, physical performance, and injuries in preparation for professional mixed martial arts. Sports. 2018;7(1):1.
30. Von Rosen P, Frohm A, Kottorp A, Fridén C, Heijne A. Multiple factors explain injury risk in adolescent elite athletes: applying a biopsychosocial perspective. Scand J Med Sci Sports. 2017;27:2059–69.
31. Shirley MK, Longman DP, Elliott-Sale KJ, Hackney AC, Sale C, Dolan E. A life history perspective on athletes with low energy availability. Sports Med. 2022;52(6):1223–34.
32. Mountjoy M, Ackerman KE, Bailey DM, Burke LM, Constantini N, Hackney AC, Heikura IA, Melin A, Pensgaard AM, Stellingwerff T, Sundgot-Borgen JK. International Olympic Committee's (IOC) consensus statement on relative energy deficiency in sport (REDs). Br J Sports Med. 2023;57(17):1073–97.
33. Madigan DJ, Stoeber J, Forsdyke D, et al. Perfectionism predicts injury in junior athletes: preliminary evidence from a prospective study. J Sports Sci. 2018;36:545–50.
34. Lloyd RS, Cronin JB, Faigenbaum AD, et al. National Strength and Conditioning Association position statement on long-term athletic development. J Strength Cond Res. 2016;30:1491–509.
35. Bayne H, Elliott B, Campbell A, Alderson J. Lumbar load in adolescent fast bowlers: a prospective injury study. J Sci Med Sport. 2016;19(2):117–22.
36. Worsdale S, King M, Brooke-Wavell K, Ahmun R, Griffin S, Etherington C, Alway P. Physical characteristics associated with lumbar bone stress injury related technique in male fast bowlers. ISBS Proc Arch. 2024;42(1):1030.
37. Johnstone JA, Mitchell AC, Hughes G, Watson T, Ford PA, Garrett AT. The athletic profile of fast bowling in cricket: a review. J Strength Cond Res. 2014;28(5):1465–73.
38. Shaw J, Jacobs JV, Van Dillen LR, Beneck GJ, Smith JA. Understanding the Biering-Sørensen test: contributors to extensor endurance in young adults with and without a history of low back pain. J Electromyogr Kinesiol. 2024;74:1028.
39. Al Attar WSA, Soomro N, Pappas E, et al. How effective are F-MARC injury prevention programs for soccer players? A systematic review and meta-analysis. Sports Med. 2016;46:205–17.
40. Finch CF. No longer lost in translation: the art and science of sports injury prevention implementation research. Br J Sports Med. 2011;45(16):1253–7.
41. Afzal MF, Imran A, Arif A, Memon AG, Sarfraz K, Javaid HM. Comparison of injury prevention program on physical fitness among cricketers in warm-up and cool-down phases. Rehabil J. 2021;5(02):239–4.
42. Forrest MR, Hebert JJ, Scott BR, Dempsey AR. Exercise-based injury prevention for community-level adolescent cricket pace bowlers: a cluster-randomised controlled trial. J Sci Med Sport. 2020;23(5):475–80.
43. Soomro N, Chua N, Freeston J, Ferdinands RE, Sanders R. Cluster randomised control trial for cricket injury prevention programme (CIPP): a protocol paper. Inj Prev. 2019;25(3):166–74.
44. Forrest MR, Scott BR, Hebert JJ, Dempsey AR. Injury prevention strategies for adolescent cricket pace bowlers. Sports Med. 2018;48(11):2449–61.
45. Mendonça LM, Schuermans J, Denolf S, Napier C, Bittencourt NFN, Romanuk A, Tak I, Thorborg K, Bizzini M, Ramponi C, Paterson C, Hägglund M, Malisoux L, Al Attar WSA, Samukawa M, Esteve E, Bakare U, Constantinou M, Schneiders A, Cavallieri Gomes A, Florent. Sports injury prevention programmes from the sports physical therapist's perspective: an international expert Delphi approach. Phys Ther Sport. 2022;55:146–54.
46. Jackson A. Ready 4 Cricket. [Online] Kids Back 2. Sport Limited; 2022. https://angelajacksonphysio.thinkific.com/courses/ready-4-cricket.

Lumbar Stress Fractures Imaging

28

Mitchell Yam, Eugene Ng, Ashton Reeve, and James M. Linklater

28.1 Introduction

Imaging is indispensable in the diagnosis of lumbar pars bone stress injury due to the limited sensitivity of clinical history and physical examination. Its use has evolved over the decades from plain radiography and bone scintigraphy to a combination of computed tomography and SPECT and/or MRI, but increasingly MRI alone. MRI, which avoids ionising radiation, a crucial factor to consider when imaging the young athlete, is now the modality of choice (if appropriate sequences are utilised). It has a validated multifunctional role in assessing for clinically relevant bone stress, identifying incomplete and complete fractures, distinguishing between active and chronic lesions, and in the assessment of bone healing. Early identification of lumbar bone stress injury, with appropriate modification of training, can positively influence the trajectory of the condition and assist in hastening return to play and minimising long-term impairment. Late diagnosis increases the risk of pars fracture non-union, need for surgical intervention and prolonged rehabilitation. Here, we review the literature and present our approach to the imaging of lumbar bone stress injury.

M. Yam · E. Ng · A. Reeve · J. M. Linklater (✉)
Castlereagh Imaging, Westmead, Sydney, NSW, Australia
e-mail: MitchellYam@casimaging.com; EugeneNg2@casimaging.com; AshtonReeve@casimaging.com; JamesLinklater@casimaging.com

28.2 Stage and Pattern of Pars Bone Stress Injury

Pars bone stress injury on imaging is purported to progress, if left untreated, along a continuum beginning with early evidence of bone stress in the absence of a fracture line, then active bone stress with a complicating incomplete or complete fracture line, and culmination in either fracture healing or chronic non-union.

Typical fractures originate at the inferomedial or inferior cortex and propagate posterosuperiorly or superiorly [1]. Pars bone stress fractures with bone defects that differ in shape and course are considered atypical, one type of which is where there is a vertical line at the inferolateral part of the pars and a horizontal line at the superomedial part through the lamina [2]. Complete unilateral fractures of the pars interarticularis alter loadbearing through the spine and predispose to fractures of the contralateral side. This may eventually result in spondylolisthesis, defined as the anterior shift of the affected vertebra relative to the vertebra immediately inferior to it [3, 4].

Posterior element vertebral bone stress injury does not occur exclusively at the pars interarticu-

B. Olivier, J. W. Orchard (eds.), *Cricket Sports Medicine*,
https://doi.org/10.1007/978-981-96-6321-7_28

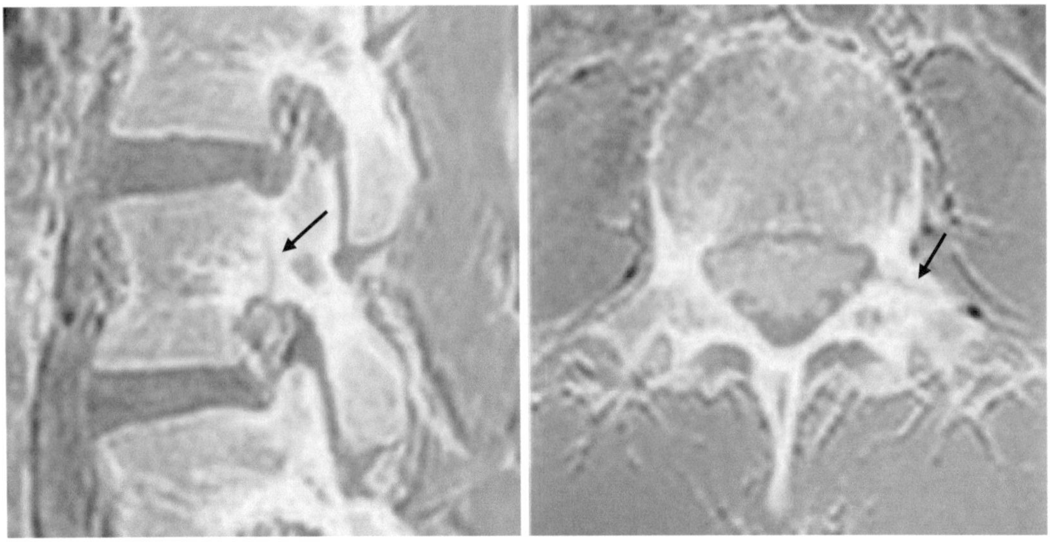

Fig. 28.1 Sagittal oblique and axial oblique reconstructed MRI fat-suppressed, balanced volumetric T1 gradient echo sequence (inverted grayscale) demonstrating an incomplete left pedicle stress fracture (black arrows)

laris. Other sites of potential bone stress injury include the pedicle (retrosomatic; Fig. 28.1) and lamina (retroisthmic; Fig. 28.8) locations but are less common than at the pars interarticularis. Pedicle lesions are more common in the presence of a non-union or fibrous union of the contralateral pars. A study of elite Australian cricket players demonstrated a frequency of pedicular bone stress injury of 38%, either in isolation or in conjunction with involvement of other portions of the posterior vertebra, amongst players with posterior element vertebral bone stress injury. Involvement of the lamina, transverse process or articular process demonstrated a frequency of 9% [5].

28.3 Imaging Modalities

The various imaging modalities have differing abilities to detect the morphological and physiological changes of bone stress injury at its various stages.

28.4 Historical

28.4.1 Radiography

Radiographs are often used in the initial assessment of low back pain. Routine views of the spine can readily identify spondylolisthesis, but pars fracture alone can be difficult to identify (Fig. 28.2). Additional views, including 45° lateral oblique, which theoretically best profiles the typical pars fracture line, 40° lateral oblique with 30° cranial angulation and anteroposterior with 30° cranial angulation projections, can potentially increase the sensitivity of pars fracture identification to approximately 32% [6], though additional projections increase the radiation dose per study and overall sensitivity remains low. Non-structural changes, such as bone marrow oedema and osteoblastic activity, cannot be assessed on radiographs, and therefore these cannot identify early-stage pars bone stress injury nor distinguish active stress response around a fracture line from chronic quiescent non-union [7].

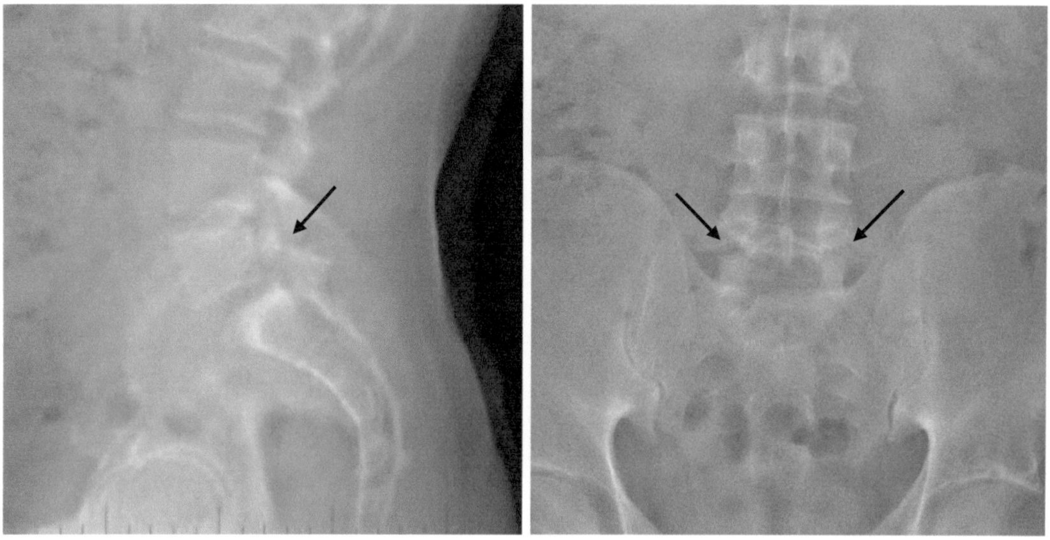

Fig. 28.2 Anteroposterior and lateral x-ray views of the lumbar spine demonstrating bilateral complete L5 pars defects with grade 1 anterolisthesis

28.4.2 Bone Scan/SPECT

Historically, nuclear scintigraphy (bone scan) has been used to supplement some of the shortcomings of radiography. Radiopharmaceuticals targeting sites of osteoblastic activity within bone, and the resultant planar images they produce, can be used to infer the presence of bone stress and thereby identify potential early bone stress injury when there is no perceptible fracture on radiographs or CT, or distinguish active disease from chronic quiescent non-union when a fracture line is present. The introduction of single-photon emission tomography (SPECT) produced 3-dimensional data, improving sensitivity and localisation. The metabolic abnormality identified by bone scan and SPECT, however, is a nonspecific feature and can occur with other disease processes. These imaging methods alone also cannot be used to characterise the morphology of a fracture if present and are limited in the assessment for chronic lesions and alternative causes of low back pain. Supplementing SPECT with concurrent CT imaging enables greater accuracy for disease localisation and allows characterisation and a degree of injury prognostication. A positive SPECT study without a fracture on CT can be interpreted as an early stress reaction and has a favourable prognosis, while a negative SPECT study with a pars fracture line on CT can be interpreted as chronic fracture non-union with limited propensity to heal. The exposure to ionising radiation renders nuclear imaging undesirable in the evaluation of young athletes.

When comparing SPECT to MRI, it has been demonstrated that in 8–10% of cases where SPECT is positive, MRI can be negative, which has led some authors to suggest that SPECT may have higher sensitivity than MRI. However, this should be interpreted with caution as positive SPECT imaging has been documented in asymptomatic athletes and may be attributable to physiologic stress reaction that would not naturally progress to symptomatic bone stress [8]. Bone scan and SPECT have essentially been superseded by MRI, except for cases where MRI is contraindicated or nondiagnostic, or not readily available.

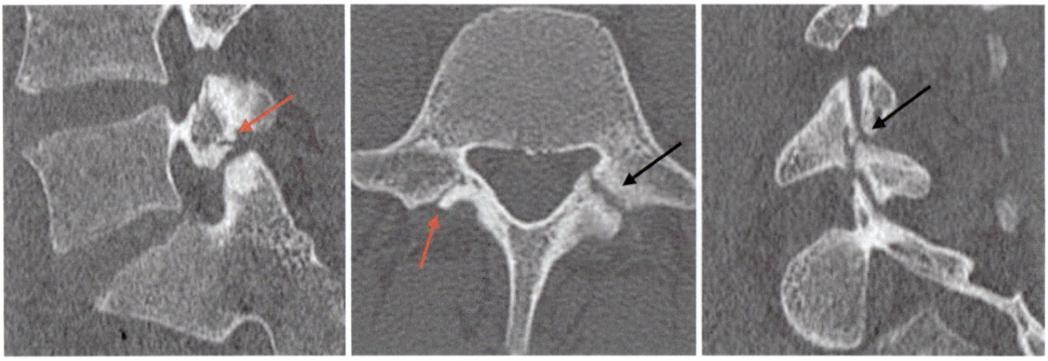

Fig. 28.3 Sagittal oblique and axial oblique reconstructed CT images of a subacute complete L5 pars fracture on the left (black arrows). Note the nutrient foramen at the pars interarticularis region on the right (red arrow), which can mimic the appearance of an incomplete pars fracture

28.4.3 Computed Tomography

Computed tomography (CT) provides high-resolution imaging that can be reconstructed in multiple planes and is often considered the gold standard for the assessment of traumatic bone injuries, allowing the identification and characterisation of subtle fractures and the assessment of new bone bridging and callus formation during healing. For the detection of early-stage pars defects on CT, oblique sagittal reconstructions are optimal due to improved visualisation of defects isolated to the anterior-inferior aspect of the pars.

Although CT is unable to distinguish pars fractures with underlying active bone stress from chronic non-union, it can still provide valuable information for prognostic purposes: a narrow pars defect with non-corticated margins suggests an acute-subacute fracture with favourable healing potential when managed appropriately (Fig. 28.3); while a fracture with measurable gapping between sclerotic margins suggests progression towards chronic non-union and a lower propensity to heal with conservative treatment.

With its strengths lying in structural assessment, CT has limited utility in the identification of early bone stress injury without fracture and, therefore, in early diagnosis. In addition to this, a principal disadvantage is radiation exposure, especially when imaging may be needed on multiple occasions for initial investigation and follow-up. Lifetime cancer and mortality risks attributable to the stochastic effects of radiation from serial paediatric CT examinations are estimated to be much higher than for adults, given the additional years of life these patients live subsequent to their imaging studies, which is particularly relevant in the context of bone stress injuries given their commonly young age at presentation [9, 10].

28.5 Magnetic Resonance Imaging

Traditional lumbar spine MRI protocols producing 4-mm thick slice images with T1 and T2 weighting in the sagittal and axial plane are commonly used in the assessment of low back pain and are insensitive for diagnosing pars bone stress injury, though they are effective in identifying other potential causes of pain such as from intervertebral disc and facet joint pathology. The addition of fluid-sensitive, fat-suppressed sequences facilitates improved detection of bone marrow oedema, such as in the setting of pars bone stress injury, and presents a viable alternative to bone scintigraphy/SPECT. The lower spatial resolution of conventional 2D MRI sequencing relative to CT, however, meant that CT historically remained more accurate in identifying and characterising pars fractures and often resulted in the use of a combination of MRI and CT imaging. In more recent years, as well as becoming more readily available, MRI assessment has further evolved with the development of isotropic volumetric acquisition fat-suppressed, balanced T1 gradient echo sequences to assess for pars bone stress fractures, with comparable sensitivity and specificity to CT [11]. 3T MRI, with its greater magnetic field strength and often equipped with other more advanced technologies, compared to 1.5T MRI generates higher quality images with increased spatial and contrast resolution [12]. Its superior features can be harnessed in a manner, which shortens examination time and, amongst other benefits, can lead to less motion artefact. Given its lack of ionising radiation, MRI is now considered the imaging modality of choice in the evaluation of pars bone stress injury, with an all-encompassing ability to assess for clinically relevant bone stress, identify incomplete and complete fractures, distinguish between active and chronic injuries, and assess for bone healing [7].

28.5.1 Fat Suppression Techniques

To readily detect bone marrow oedema, fat suppression techniques must be included in MRI imaging protocols. The most common techniques for fat suppression in 3T musculoskeletal MRI imaging include chemical shift selective fat suppression (CHESS), inversion recovery pulse sequences (STIR) and DIXON techniques. A description of the differences in these techniques is detailed in the sections below.

MRI signal is generated through the manipulation of hydrogen nuclei based on its spin properties. In the human body, it is the hydrogen nuclei within water and fat that contribute most to the signal. Fat suppression techniques aim to minimise the MR signal contribution of fat whilst not substantially affecting the contribution of water. This can be achieved by exploiting the two main differences in MR properties of fat and water, namely precession frequency and T1 relaxation time.

28.5.2 Chemical Shift Selective Fat Suppression

The precession frequency of hydrogen nuclei differs depending on the chemical nature of the molecule in which the hydrogen nuclei reside. These differences are referred to as chemical shifts. In frequency selective fat suppression, the signal contribution of fat is nulled through a series of steps that begins with an excitation pulse with a narrow bandwidth centred on the resonance frequency of fat [13].

Some key considerations which can affect the effectiveness of chemical shift selective fat suppression imaging are outlined in Table 28.1 [13].

Table 28.1 Impact of technical/clinical factors on the chemical shift selective fat suppression technique

Factor	Impact
Magnetic field strength	The difference in resonance frequency peaks of fat and water increases with greater magnetic field strength. As such, more selective fat suppression can be achieved with 3T MRI. At lower magnetic field strengths, where the resonance frequency peaks tend to converge, fat suppression may be inhomogeneous
B0 homogeneity	B0 heterogeneity can alter the water and fat resonance frequency peaks so that the fat-saturation excitation radiofrequency pulse lies outside of the fat frequency range, resulting in failed fat suppression. The off-centre position of the lumbar spine, where there is higher B0 heterogeneity, can contribute to this, as can using a large field of view
Susceptibility artefact	Chemical shift selective fat suppression leads to increased susceptibility artefact and therefore is suboptimal for patients with metallic implants

28.5.3 Short Tau Inversion Recovery (STIR)

Inversion recovery techniques utilise the difference in the T1 relaxation time of the tissues being imaged. Following a 180-degree inversion radiofrequency pulse, the longitudinal magnetisation of fat is allowed to recover to the zero line (i.e. no net magnetisation) for a period of time (inversion time), before a 90° acquisition pulse is then applied to produce a fat-free signal [13].

Whilst imaging time may be longer, the STIR technique can achieve more uniform fat suppression compared to the CHESS technique as outlined in Table 28.2 [13].

The utility of STIR imaging, however, is limited by its low signal-to-noise ratio and high specific absorption rate. In addition, STIR is not a fat-specific suppression technique because other tissues with a short T1 relaxation time such as methaemoglobin, mucoid tissue, proteinaceous material, and melanin, will be affected in a similar manner to fat. For the same reason, the STIR technique is not suitable for contrast-enhanced imaging, as contrast shortens the T1 relaxation time of enhanced tissue.

28.5.4 Dixon Method

Due to the differing precession frequencies of water and fat, their magnetisation vectors rotate relative to each other such that they will, at various stages, be 'in-phase' (i.e. vectors pointing in the same direction) and 'out-of-phase' (i.e. vectors pointing in opposite directions). Images are acquired at these 'in-phase' and 'out-of-phase' stages, which are then used to generate pure water images with fat suppression and pure fat images with water suppression.

B0 heterogeneity, which can result in unwanted components being suppressed (known as fat-water swapping), is a problem affecting the Dixon method. To mitigate against its effects, various methods, such as unwrapping reconstruction algorithms, have needed to be developed and applied (Table 28.3) [13].

The technique can be used with MRI sequences, including T1 and T2 weighted fast spin echo, and gradient echo.

Table 28.2 Impact of technical/clinical factors on the short tau inversion recovery technique

Factor	Impact
Magnetic field strength	With increasing magnetic field strength, T1 relaxation time increases, and therefore inversion time and imaging time also increase
B0 homogeneity	Due to insensitivity to B0 inhomogeneity, STIR imaging can achieve better fat suppression in off-centre and large field-of-view imaging
Susceptibility artefact	There is minimal impact of metallic implants on the homogeneity of fat suppression with STIR imaging

Table 28.3 Impact of technical/clinical factors on the Dixon method technique

Factor	Impact
Magnetic field strength	More selective fat suppression can be achieved at greater magnetic field strengths. Increasing magnetic field strength, however, also increases B0 inhomogeneity [14]
B0 homogeneity	B0 heterogeneity can alter the fat and water precession frequency peaks resulting in fat-water swapping. Methods, such as unwrapping reconstruction algorithms, however, can counteract this. As such, Dixon imaging is relatively insensitive to B0 inhomogeneity
Susceptibility artefact	There is minimal impact of metallic implants on the homogeneity of fat suppression with Dixon imaging

28.5.5 Summary

The main clinically relevant features of the fat suppression techniques described are summarised in Table 28.4.

28.5.6 MRI Detection and Quantification of Bone Marrow Oedema in Pars Bone Stress

The detection of bone marrow oedema using MRI is analogous to the detection of increased osteoblastic activity on bone scan, and in the setting of a stress injury with no detectable fracture on CT, allows the diagnosis of early pars bone stress injury. Bone marrow oedema in the pars interarticularis is an early imaging indicator of bone stress and is also a positive predictor of healing in those injuries with a fracture (Fig. 28.4). In athletes who perform movements resulting in high repetitive loading of the spine, it is, however, important to note that bone marrow oedema does not necessarily equate to symptomatic pars bone stress injury, as has been demonstrated in a study of 65 junior cricket players where 58% had MRI detected bone marrow oedema [15]. In this study, 39% of those with bone marrow oedema developed a clinical bone stress injury during the season, 37% had persistent bone marrow oedema without symptoms at the end of the season and 24% had resolution during the season. This study highlighted the continuum of increased physiologic bone turnover and pathologic bone stress, and the need to incorporate clinical judgement when interpreting radiological findings.

A systematic review comparing 1T and 1.5T MRI against SPECT-CT as a reference standard in the detection of pars bone stress demonstrated MRI sensitivity and specificity of 80% and 100% in one study [16] and MRI sensitivity 88% and specificity of 97% in another [8] and concluded

Table 28.4 Summary of the main clinically relevant features of commonly used fat suppression techniques

Technique	Imaging time	Signal-to-noise ratio	Specific absorption rate	Effect of metal	B0 sensitivity	Preferred field strength
Chemical shift selective fat suppression	Short	High	Medium	Sensitive	Sensitive	High
STIR	Long	Low	High	Minimal	Insensitive	Indifferent
Dixon	Long	High	Low	Minimal	Insensitive	Medium

Adapted from [13]

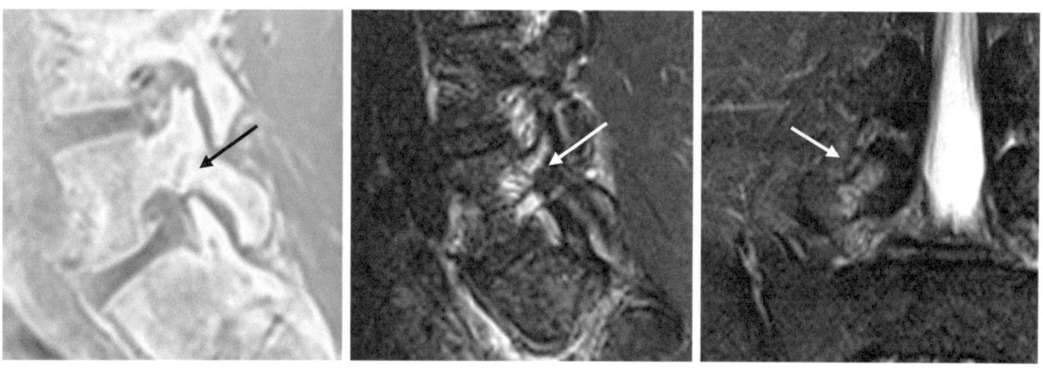

Fig. 28.4 Sagittal oblique reconstructed MRI fat-suppressed, balanced volumetric T1 gradient echo sequence with inverted grayscale demonstrating an incomplete right L5 pars fracture (black arrow). Sagittal and coronal MRI STIR sequence demonstrating associated bone marrow oedema (white arrows)

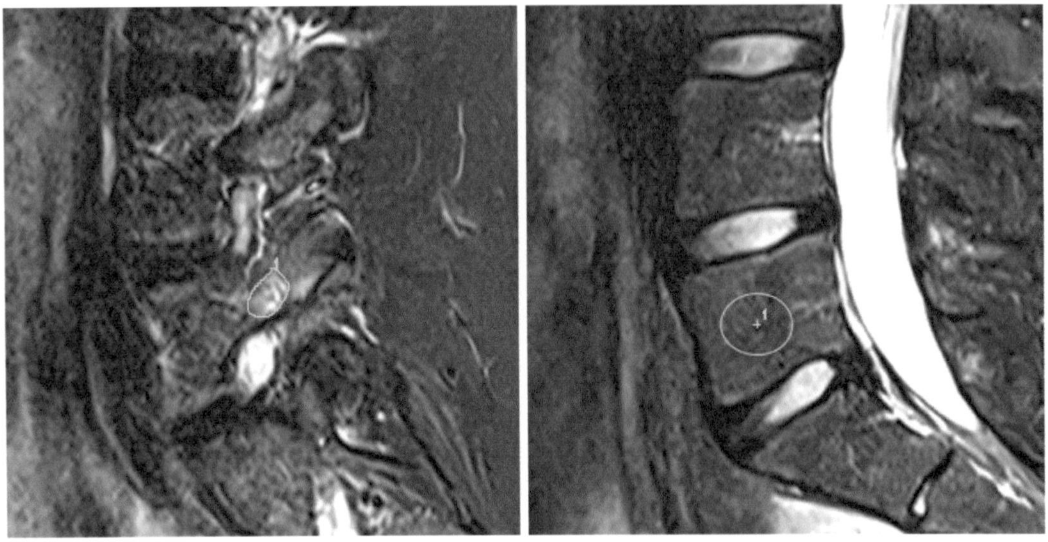

Fig. 28.5 Sagittal MRI STIR sequence demonstrating the measurement of STIR signal intensity at the right L5 pars and L5 vertebral body using 'region of interest' tool for calculating the STIR signal intensity ratio

MRI was consistent with SPECT-CT for diagnosing posterior element bone stress injury, but the clinical value of cases where MRI had false negatives remained uncertain due to possible oversensitivity by SPECT-CT [10].

Although the intensity of bone marrow oedema on MRI cannot be directly quantified in a reproducible way between scans, it can be indirectly quantified and compared by creating a ratio of STIR signal intensity at the area of pars bone stress relative to normal bone marrow within the corresponding vertebral body utilising the methodology outlined below (Fig. 28.5):

- STIR signal intensity is measured at the site of maximal signal at the area of bone stress by using a 'region of interest' tool, with the area measured approximating 0.4 cm^2
- STIR signal intensity is then measured within the central vertebral body at the same vertebral level with the 'region of interest' tool, incorporating a larger area approximating 2.5 cm^2 on the closest sagittal image to the midline where measurement is not hampered by the basi-vertebral artery [17, 18]
- The ratio of the first to the second measurements is calculated

It is worth noting that due to closer proximity to the receiver coil of the pars interarticularis when compared to the vertebral body, the baseline STIR signal intensity ratio will be greater than 1.0. It has been suggested that an STIR signal intensity ratio must be at least greater than 2 to be of clinical relevance. At less than a ratio of 3, patients will frequently be asymptomatic [19]. A ratio greater than 3 will usually be associated with symptoms, albeit with some exceptions.

Less frequently in literature, the degree of bone marrow oedema has also been quantified by expressing the measured T2-fat-suppressed signal intensity as a ratio of T2-fat-suppressed signal intensity at the T12 level spinal cord and adjacent normal pedicle [20].

The extent of bone marrow oedema in the posterior vertebral arch should be described. In literature, the extent of involvement has been quantified by dividing the posterior vertebral arch into seven anatomical zones and totalling the number of involved zones [21], though this can often prove impractical in daily practice and a brief anatomical description may suffice.

28.5.7 MRI Detection of Pars Stress Fractures

Volumetric fat-suppressed balanced T1 gradient echo sequences have the advantage of improving spatial resolution compared to traditional lumbar MRI sequences and can be used to generate thin slice, high-resolution multiplanar images analogous to CT [10]. Contrast resolution relies on the high intrinsic tissue contrast between cortical bone and fatty marrow, and between cortical bone and mineralising callus/fibrous tissue. This results in high overall sensitivity and specificity for fracture detection. On volumetric fat-suppressed balanced T1 gradient echo sequences, a fracture line will appear as linear high signal intensity breaching the cortical bone, with or without involving cancellous bone. MR image greyscale can be inverted so that it resembles the attenuation pattern of CT, which can increase the conspicuity of pars fracture lines (Figs. 28.6 and 28.7).

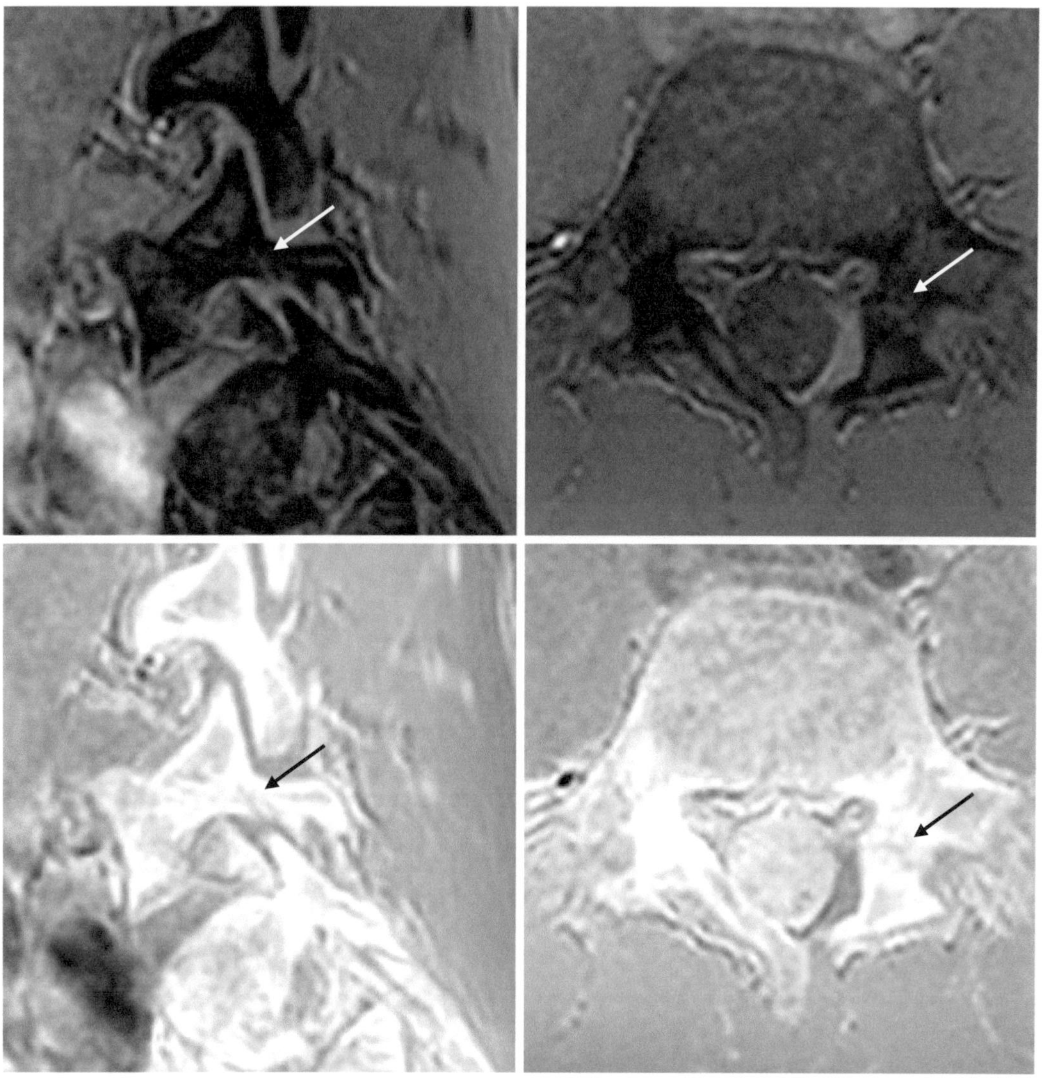

Fig. 28.6 Sagittal oblique and axial oblique reconstructed MRI fat-suppressed, balanced volumetric T1 gradient echo sequence demonstrating incomplete left L5 pars stress fracture, without (white arrows) and with inverted grayscale (black arrows)

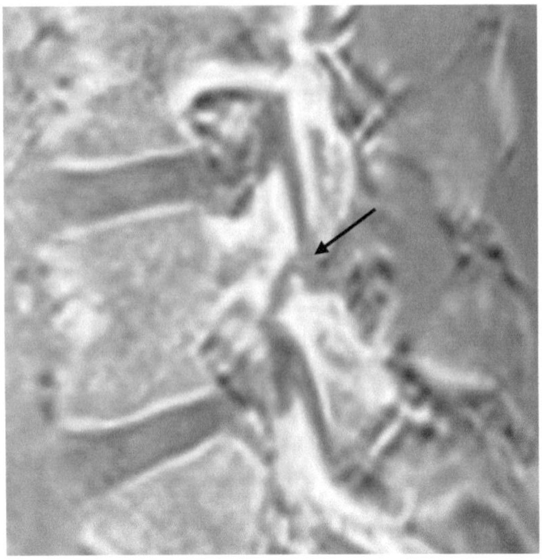

Fig. 28.7 Sagittal oblique reconstructed MRI fat-suppressed, balanced volumetric T1 gradient echo sequence with inverted grayscale demonstrating complete right L5 pars stress fracture (black arrow) with sclerotic margins of established non-union

The fat-suppressed, balanced volumetric T1 gradient echo sequence is known by different vendor-specific monikers: VIBE (Siemens), LAVA (GE), THRIVE (Philips), 3D Quick (Toshiba) and TIGRE (Hitachi). A typical sequence is acquired in the sagittal plane, with slice thickness of 0.8 mm, matrix 320 x 320, TR 6.1 ms and TE 2.4 ms, flip angle of 12°, with a small field of view of 23 cm. Acquisition of this sequence in the coronal plane decreases the utility of the sequence in demonstrating and characterising incomplete pars stress fractures because of the limited number of images acquired through the typically coronally oriented fracture line, when compared to a sagittal acquisition, particularly if the sequence is non-isotropic.

3T MRI with fat-suppressed, balanced volumetric T1 gradient echo sequencing can reach sensitivity, specificity and accuracy of 97.7%, 92.3% and 95.7%, respectively, in detecting pars fractures, and 100% accuracy for complete pars fractures [11], and can obviate the need for supplementary CT imaging, particularly in a young cohort. Measurements of the dimensions of the fracture line are best performed on oblique axial and oblique sagittal images reconstructed to be perpendicular to the fracture line.

28.5.8 A Suggested MRI Lumbar Spine Pars Bone Stress Injury Protocol

SIEMENS MAGNETOM 3.0T

Coronal STIR: slice thickness 3.0 mm, FOV 300 mm, TE 49 ms, TR 3000 ms

Sagittal STIR: slice thickness 3.0 mm, FOV 300 mm, TE 77 ms, TR 3200 ms

Sagittal T2: slice thickness 3.0 mm, FOV 280 mm, TE 101 ms, TR 3030 ms

Sagittal T1 VIBE fat suppressed: slice thickness 0.8 mm, FOV 260 mm, TE, 2.46 ms, TR 7 ms, flip angle

12 degrees, SPAIR for fat-water contrast

Axial T2: slice thickness 4.0 mm, FOV 200 mm, TE 100 ms, TR 5240 ms

Axial T2 fat suppressed: slice thickness 4.0 mm, FOV 200 mm, TE 100 ms, TR 5500 ms

28.5.9 MRI Stage of Pars Bone Stress Injury

Pars interarticularis stress injuries typically progress through early to late stages as follows:

1. Isolated stress reaction: Cortical and/or cancellous bone marrow oedema on sagittal STIR sequence, with no fracture line on sagittal fat-suppressed, balanced volumetric T1 gradient echo sequence
2. Active bone stress with a complicating fracture: Bone marrow oedema on sagittal STIR images, and a fracture line (incomplete or complete) on sagittal fat-suppressed, balanced volumetric T1 gradient echo sequence images, demonstrating indistinct non-corticated margins
3. Chronic fracture without stress reaction: Fracture line on sagittal fat-suppressed, balanced volumetric T1 gradient echo sequence images, demonstrating sclerotic margins without underlying bone marrow oedema on sagittal STIR sequence [17]
4. Progression to bilaterality if rotational loading continues on the background of a unilateral fibrous union
5. Spondylolisthesis if rotational loading continues with bilateral complete fracture

28.5.10 MRI Pitfalls in Assessment of Bone Stress Injuries

Bone marrow oedema can be mimicked by nutrient vessels passing through the region of interest, inherent signal heterogeneity in haematopoietic marrow and intraosseous hemangiomas.

Fracture lines can be mimicked by developmental clefts in the medial margin of the cortex, nutrient vessels (Fig. 28.2) and marginal osteophytes from adjacent superior articular facets. Multiplanar reconstructions of the volumetric 3D sequencing can be helpful in distinguishing these [22].

28.5.11 Progress MRI for Bone Stress Injury

Symptom-based assessment in deciding return to play remains inexact. Millson et al. (2004) postulate that pain is felt during the earlier stages of pars bone stress injury, but that pain may resolve when the injury progresses to a complete fracture incorporating both cortical fracture start and cortical fracture endpoints [23]. Additionally, imaging evidence of a healed pars bone stress injury may not necessarily correspond with symptom resolution [24].

Progress can be classified, like diagnosis, based on bone marrow oedema assessed on sagittal STIR and fracture extent assessed on sagittal fat-suppressed, balanced volumetric T1 gradient echo sequence images (Table 28.5) [17].

Fracture healing occurs in the reverse direction to fracture propagation [1], and complete bone healing can take 6–7 months (Fig. 28.8) [25]. It is however important to note that the resolution of bone marrow oedema and fracture healing can be disparate (Figs. 28.8 and 28.9). With deloading, in the early phase of healing, bone marrow oedema may decrease or resolve, but the fracture line may paradoxically increase in extent due to relative delay in resolution of the bony resorption when compared to the resolution of bone marrow oedema [26].

Incomplete stress fractures have greater potential for healing when compared to complete fractures [24, 27]. Within the subset of complete fracture, there is a greater potential for healing if there is surrounding bone marrow oedema (Fig. 28.10), relatively narrow fracture width, and no spondylolisthesis [26–28].

Fracture morphology also affects the potential for healing with Watura et al. (2024) demonstrating better fracture healing outcomes with fractures that were oriented more vertically than horizontally, postulated to be due to the horizontal vector of biomechanical stress leading to greater multidirectional instability with horizontally oriented fractures [17, 25].

Table 28.5 Classification of progress of bone stress injury on MRI

Progress	Bone marrow oedema on STIR sequence	Fracture extent on fat-suppressed balanced volumetric T1 gradient echo sequence
Worsened	Increased bone marrow oedema signal	Increased extent of the fracture line
Stable	No change in bone marrow oedema signal	No change in fracture morphology
Improved	Reduced bone marrow oedema signal	Increased ground glass bridging at fracture line, consolidation of margins and/or reduction in dimensions of fracture line
Healed (Fig. 28.8)	Resolution of bone marrow oedema signal	Fracture line is no longer visible
Chronic non-union (Fig. 28.6)	Resolution of bone marrow oedema signal	Corticated fracture margins No progressive bony bridging

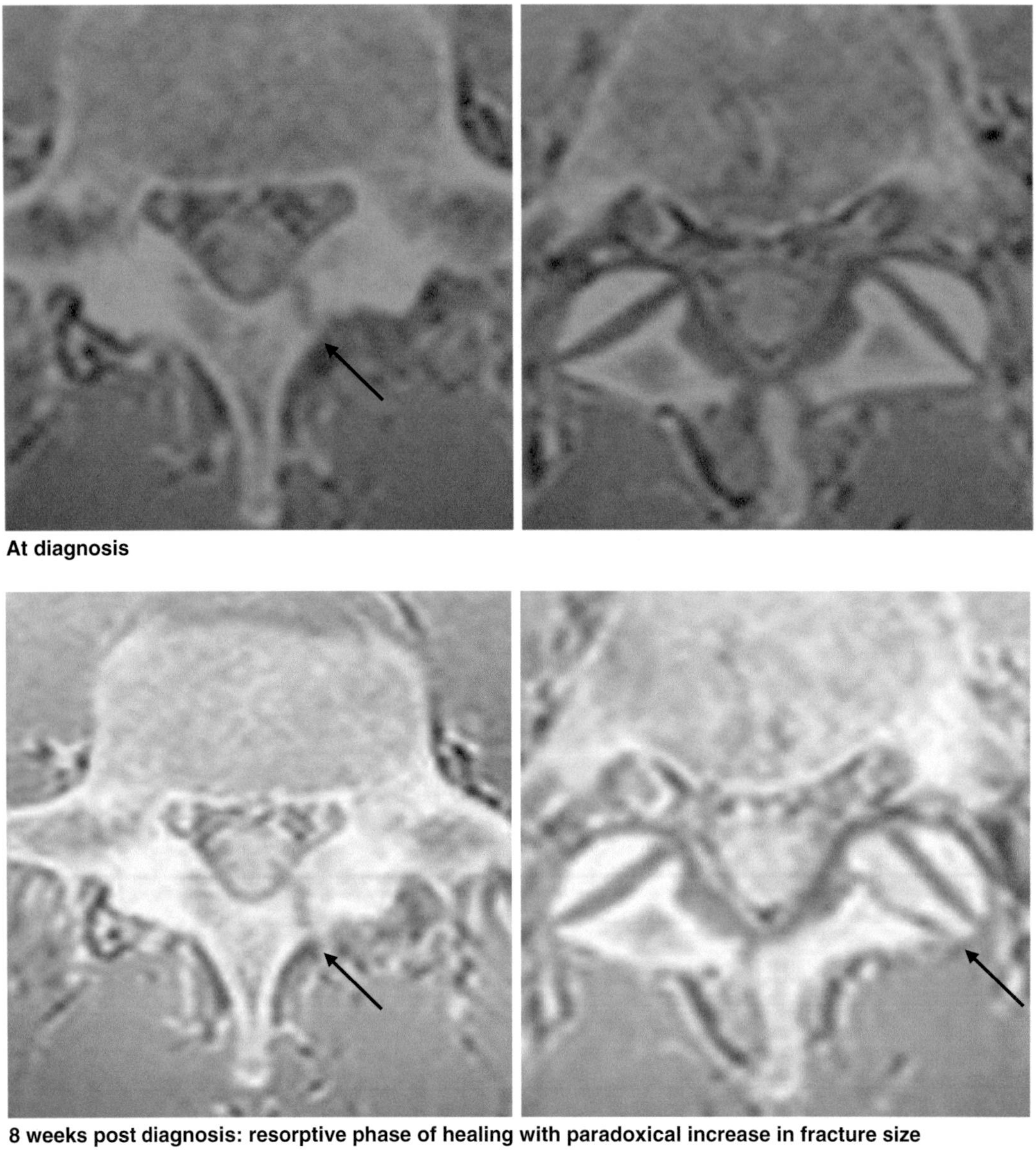

Fig. 28.8 Sequential axial MRI fat-suppressed, balanced volumetric T1 gradient echo sequence (inverted grayscale) demonstrating the progress of a complete left L5 lamina fracture to mature union (black arrows) over 6 months

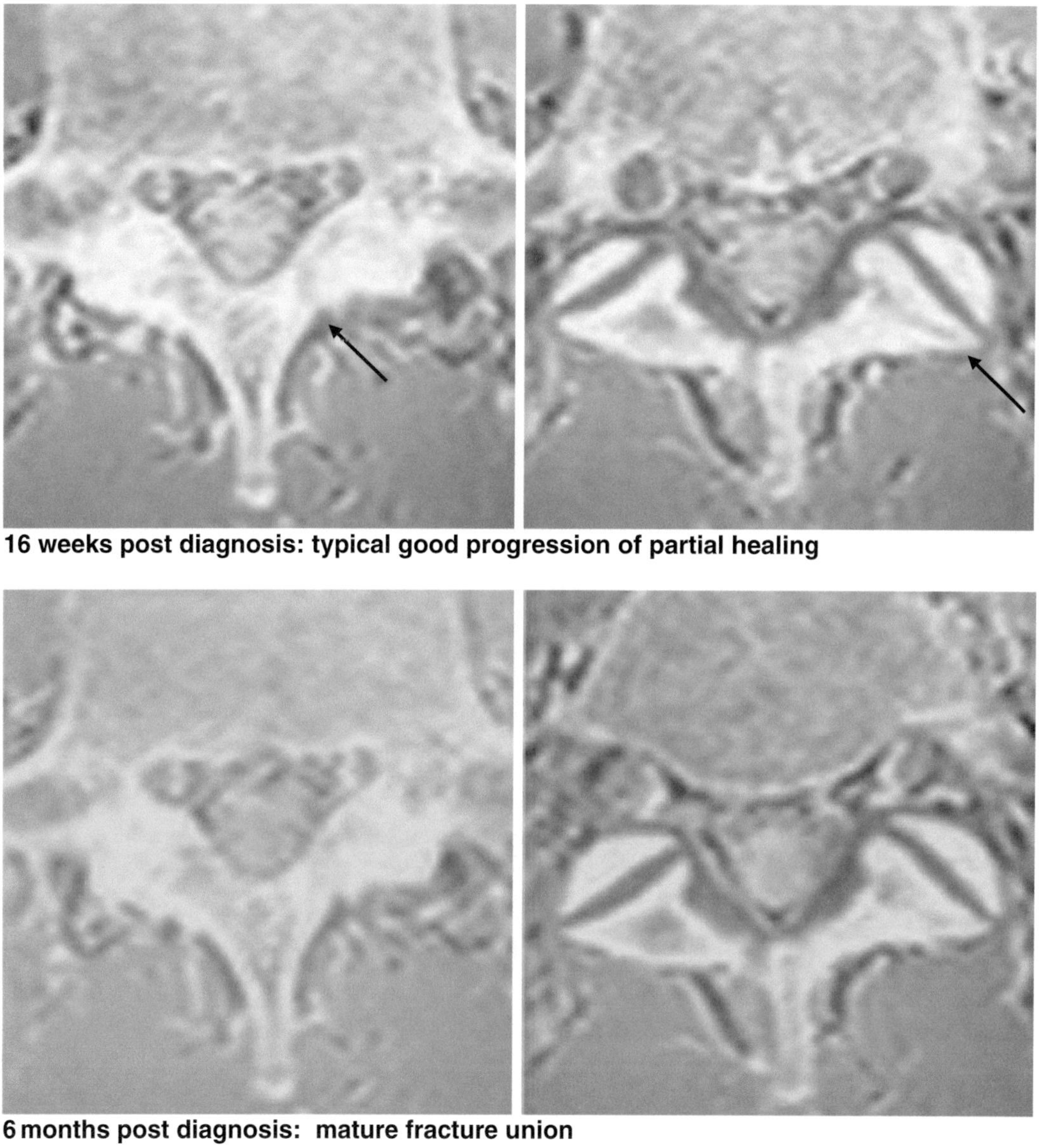

Fig. 28.8 (continued)

28.5.12 MRI Follow-up of Fracture Healing

Table 28.6 provides an example of management of lumbar pars bone stress injury in elite fast bowlers which for the timing of imaging can be summarised into MRI progress scans at 8 weeks (early reloading phase) and 16 weeks (return to skills training phase). However, variations in individual cases may warrant variations in the timing of the follow-up MRI scans.

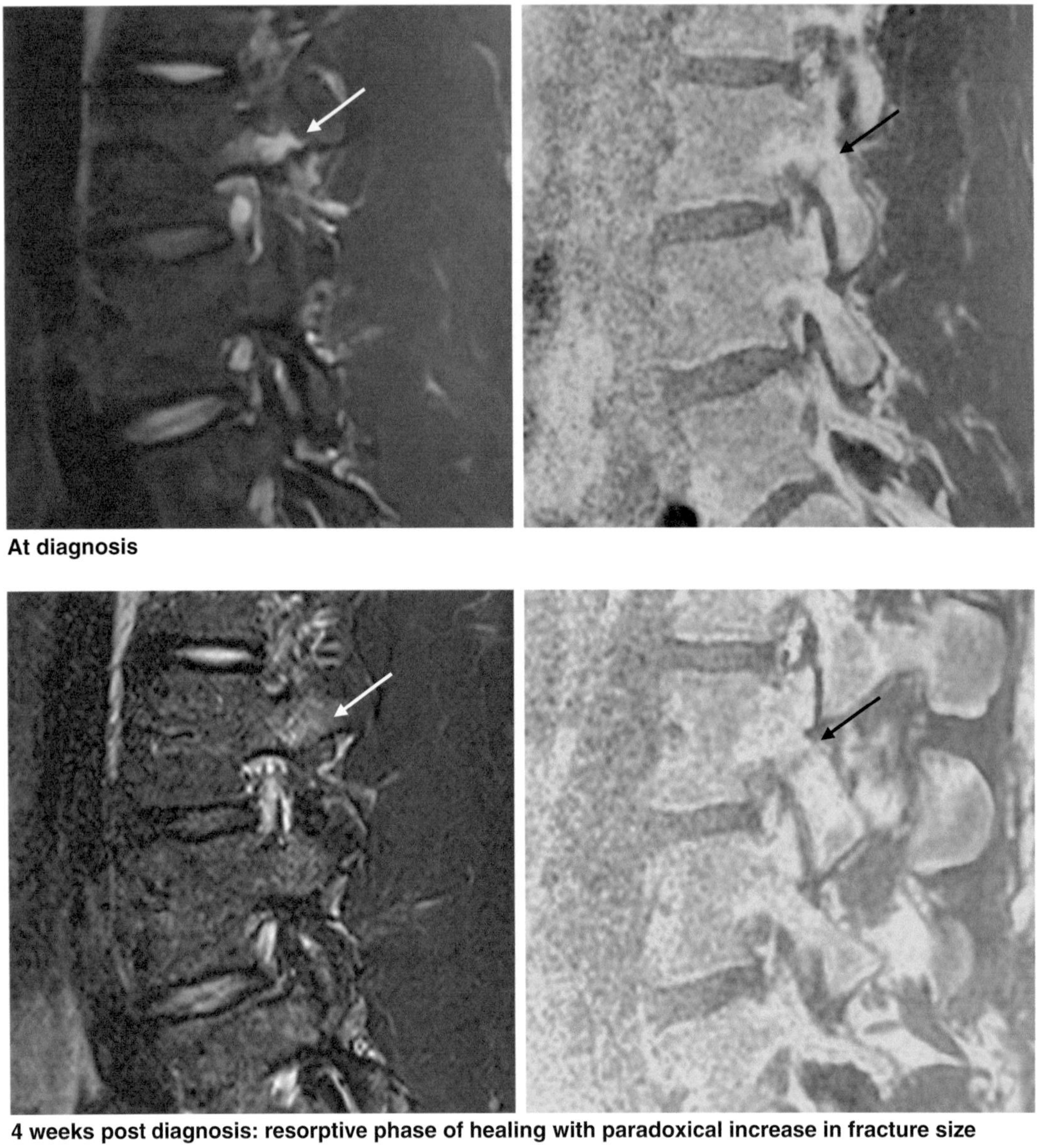

Fig. 28.9 Sequential sagittal MRI STIR sequence and sagittal oblique reconstructed MRI fat-suppressed, balanced volumetric T1 gradient echo sequence (inverted grayscale) demonstrating the progress of an incomplete right L3 pars fracture to mature union (black arrows), with gradual reduction in associated bone marrow oedema (white arrows)

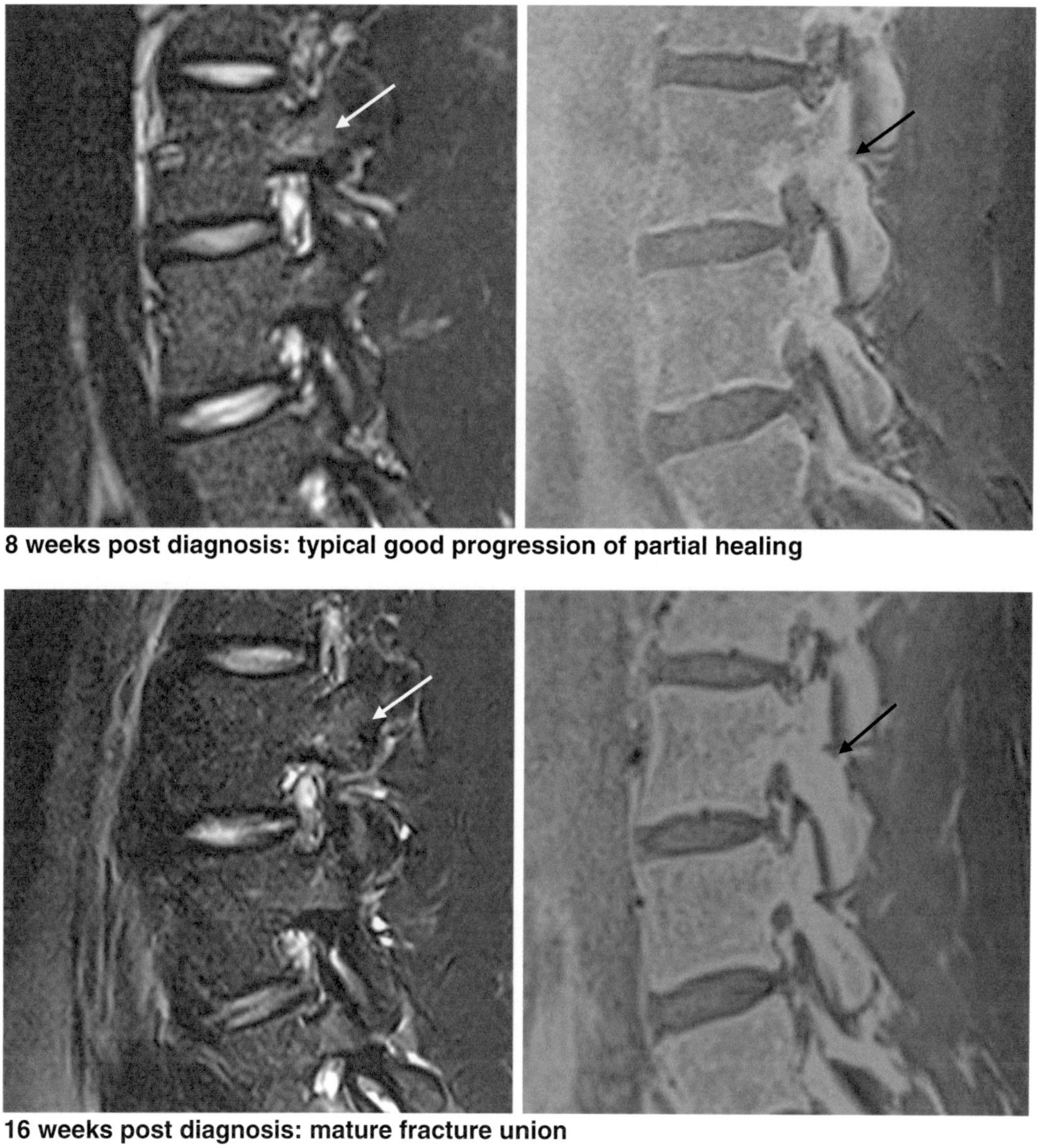

Fig. 28.9 (continued)

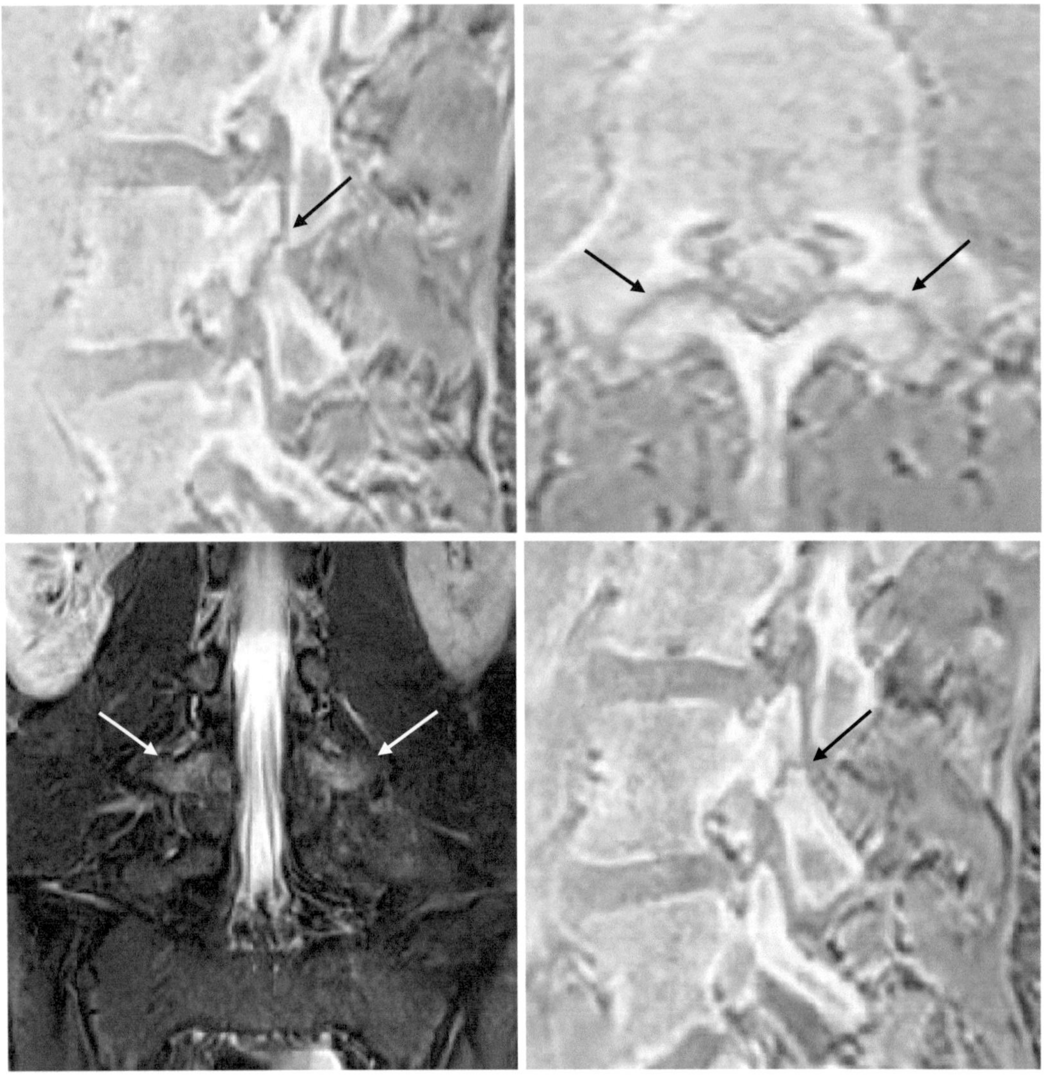

Fig. 28.10 Sagittal oblique and axial reconstructed MRI fat-suppressed, balanced volumetric T1 gradient echo sequence with inverted grayscale demonstrating subacute complete bilateral L4 pars fractures (black arrows). Coronal MRI STIR sequence demonstrating associated bilateral bone marrow oedema (white arrows)

28.5.13 Pre-season Screening MRI for Pars Bone Stress Injury

Preliminary imaging studies have found that up to 67% of bowlers with pre-season asymptomatic bone marrow oedema on MRI subsequently sustained a lumbar bone stress injury during the playing season, equating to a 4.8× increased risk versus those without pre-season bone marrow oedema on MRI [29]. Close clinical monitoring and regulation of training volumes of those with asymptomatic bone marrow oedema on pre-season screening MRI come at the expense of those players with asymptomatic bone marrow oedema who do not progress to symptomatic pars bone stress injury. The threshold STIR signal intensity ratio for significant bone marrow oedema in this clinical setting has not yet been well defined or validated.

Association of asymmetry in lumbar paraspinal musculature, including the quadratus lumborum, with predisposition to pars bone stress

Table 28.6 Clinical guidelines for the management of lumbar pars bone stress injury in elite fast bowlers

Phase 1 (week 1–4): Protect	First 2 weeks (focus on unload) Avoid hyperextension, twisting, axial/impact forces Consider brace if patient adopts these positions/movements in ADL Week 3–4 Resume walking alternate days (pain free) Low-level trunk muscle activation Mobility—hips, low back
Phase 2 (week 5–8): Increase Activity	Avoid hyperextension/rotation/impact/axial load Add bodyweight resisted exercise with the limitations above Progress walking (faster 5–6 km/h) Progress mobility (Tx extension & rotation supervised) *MRI at 8 weeks*
Phase 3 (week 9–12): Add load	MONITOR: less concern about extension & rotation if MRI good ADD: add loads to BW exercise drills (use DBs and avoid axial load from bar) PROGRESS: progress trunk muscle activation START: start running twice per week—shorter distances on repeat initially
Phase 4 (week 13–16): Prepare to Return to Skills Training	ADD: add axial loading to gym (carefully) RUNNING: progress running START: start medball bowling-specific drills START: start shadow bowling and technical drills *ASSESS: assess MRI at week 16 to determine readiness to resume normal training*

injury in adolescents is contentious [30], and whilst muscular asymmetry may be noted, the clinical utility and application of this knowledge are limited.

28.6 Conclusion

Magnetic resonance imaging performed at 3T incorporating STIR and fat-suppressed, balanced volumetric T1 gradient echo sequences is a radiation-free and accurate technique to diagnose and monitor pars bone stress injuries and healing in both adult and adolescent athletes and represents the current gold standard in imaging.

References

1. Murthy NS. Imaging of stress fractures of the spine. Radiol Clin North Am. 2012;50(4):799–821. https://doi.org/10.1016/j.rcl.2012.04.009.
2. Nakayama T, Ehara S. Spondylolytic spondylolisthesis: various imaging features and natural courses. Jpn J Radiol. 2015;33(1):3–12. https://doi.org/10.1007/s11604-014-0371-4.
3. Chosa E, Totoribe K, Tajima N. A biomechanical study of lumbar spondylolysis based on a three-dimensional finite element method. J Orthop Res. 2004;22(1):158–63. https://doi.org/10.1016/S0736-0266(03)00160-8.
4. Dietrich M, Kurowski P. The importance of mechanical factors in the etiology of spondylolysis. A model analysis of loads and stresses in human lumbar spine. Spine (Phila Pa 1976). 1985;10(6):532–42. https://doi.org/10.1097/00007632-198507000-00007.
5. Saw A, Eales B, Jones N, Obst A, Smith M, Kountouris A, et al. Lumbar bone stress injuries and nonunited defects in elite Australian Cricket players. Clin J Sport Med. 2024;34(1):44–51. https://doi.org/10.1097/JSM.0000000000001132.
6. Saifuddin A, White J, Tucker S, Taylor BA. Orientation of lumbar pars defects: implications for radiological detection and surgical management. J Bone Joint Surg Br. 1998;80(2):208–11. https://doi.org/10.1302/0301-620x.80b2.8219.
7. Mushtaq R, Porrino J, Guzman Perez-Carrillo GJ. Imaging of spondylolysis: the evolving role of magnetic resonance imaging. PM R. 2018;10(6):675–80. https://doi.org/10.1016/j.pmrj.2018.02.001.
8. Campbell RS, Grainger AJ, Hide IG, Papastefanou S, Greenough CG. Juvenile spondylolysis: a comparative analysis of CT. SPECT MRI Skelet Radiol. 2005;34(2):63–73. https://doi.org/10.1007/s00256-004-0878-3.
9. Chodick G, Kim KP, Shwarz M, Horev G, Shalev V, Ron E. Radiation risks from pediatric computed tomography scanning. Pediatr Endocrinol Rev. 2009;7(2):29–36.
10. Esh R, Grodahl LHJ, Kerslake R, Strachan K, Spencer S, Fawcett L, et al. Diagnostic accuracy of MRI for identifying posterior element bone stress injury in athletes with low back pain: a systematic review and narrative synthesis. BMJ Open Sport Exerc

Med. 2020;6(1):e000764. https://doi.org/10.1136/bmjsem-2020-000764.
11. Ang EC, Robertson AF, Malara FA, O'Shea T, Roebert JK, Schneider ME, et al. Diagnostic accuracy of 3-T magnetic resonance imaging with 3D T1 VIBE versus computer tomography in pars stress fracture of the lumbar spine. Skeletal Radiol. 2016;45(11):1533–40. https://doi.org/10.1007/s00256-016-2475-7.
12. Khodarahmi I, Fritz J. The value of 3 Tesla field strength for musculoskeletal magnetic resonance imaging. Investig Radiol. 2021;56(11):749–63. https://doi.org/10.1097/RLI.0000000000000801.
13. Del Grande F, Santini F, Herzka DA, Aro MR, Dean CW, Gold GE, et al. Fat-suppression techniques for 3-T MR imaging of the musculoskeletal system. Radiographics. 2014;34(1):217–33. https://doi.org/10.1148/rg.341135130.
14. Farrelly C, Shah S, Davarpanah A, Keeling AN, Carr JC. ECG-gated multiecho Dixon fat-water separation in cardiac MRI: advantages over conventional fat-saturated imaging. AJR Am J Roentgenol. 2012;199(1):W74–83. https://doi.org/10.2214/AJR.11.7759.
15. Kountouris A, Sims K, Beakley D, Saw AE, Orchard J, Rotstein A, et al. MRI bone marrow oedema precedes lumbar bone stress injury diagnosis in junior elite cricket fast bowlers. Br J Sports Med. 2019;53(19):1236–9. https://doi.org/10.1136/bjsports-2017-097930.
16. Masci L, Pike J, Malara F, Phillips B, Bennell K, Brukner P. Use of the one-legged hyperextension test and magnetic resonance imaging in the diagnosis of active spondylolysis. Br J Sports Med. 2006;40(11):940–6; discussion 6. https://doi.org/10.1136/bjsm.2006.030023.
17. Watura C, Mitchell AWM, Fahy D, Houghton J, Kang S, Lee JC. T1-VIBE and STIR MRI of lumbar pars interarticularis injuries in elite athletes: fracture characterisation and potential prognostic indicators. Skeletal Radiol. 2024;53(3):489–97. https://doi.org/10.1007/s00256-023-04437-x.
18. Bell AJ, Nunnerley JL, Shackel DF, Coates MH, Campbell RG, Frampton CM, et al. Is MRI screening for bone marrow oedema useful in predicting lumbar bone stress injuries in adult male professional cricketers? A New Zealand pilot study. J Sci Med Sport. 2023;26(8):410–4. https://doi.org/10.1016/j.jsams.2023.06.013.
19. Sims K, Kountouris A, Stegeman JR, Rotstein AH, Beakley D, Saw AE, et al. MRI bone marrow Edema signal intensity: a reliable and valid measure of lumbar bone stress injury in elite junior fast bowlers. Spine (Phila Pa 1976). 2020;45(18):E1166–E71. https://doi.org/10.1097/BRS.0000000000003277.
20. Nakamae T, Kamei N, Tamura T, Kanda T, Nakanishi K, Adachi N. Quantitative assessment of bone marrow Edema in adolescent athletes with lumbar spondylolysis using contrast ratio on magnetic resonance imaging. Asian Spine J. 2021;15(5):682–7. https://doi.org/10.31616/asj.2020.0173.
21. Borg B, Modic MT, Obuchowski N, Cheah G. Pedicle marrow signal hyperintensity on short tau inversion recovery- and t2-weighted images: prevalence and relationship to clinical symptoms. AJNR Am J Neuroradiol. 2011;32(9):1624–31. https://doi.org/10.3174/ajnr.A2588.
22. Smith E, Nischal N, Murphy J, Azzopardi C, Iyengar KP, Haleem S, et al. Does chemical shift magnetic resonance imaging improve visualization of pars interarticularis defect? Indian J Radiol Imaging. 2023;33(3):327–31. https://doi.org/10.1055/s-0043-1764490.
23. Millson HB, Gray J, Stretch RA, Lambert MI. Dissociation between back pain and bone stress reaction as measured by CT scan in young cricket fast bowlers. Br J Sports Med. 2004;38(5):586–91. https://doi.org/10.1136/bjsm.2003.006585.
24. Sundell CGJH, Adin L, Larsen K. Stress fractures of pars interarticularis in adolescent athletes: a classification system with MRI and CT enabling evaluation of the healing process. J Exer Sports Orthop. 2018;5(1):1–6. https://doi.org/10.15226/2374-6904/5/1/00169.
25. Singh SP, Rotstein AH, Saw AE, Saw R, Kountouris A, James T. Radiological healing of lumbar spine stress fractures in elite cricket fast bowlers. J Sci Med Sport. 2021;24(2):112–5. https://doi.org/10.1016/j.jsams.2020.06.018.
26. Sairyo K, Sakai T, Yasui N. Conservative treatment of lumbar spondylolysis in childhood and adolescence: the radiological signs which predict healing. J Bone Joint Surg Br. 2009;91(2):206–9. https://doi.org/10.1302/0301-620X.91B2.21256.
27. Fujii K, Katoh S, Sairyo K, Ikata T, Yasui N. Union of defects in the pars interarticularis of the lumbar spine in children and adolescents. The radiological outcome after conservative treatment. J Bone Joint Surg Br. 2004;86(2):225–31. https://doi.org/10.1302/0301-620x.86b2.14339.
28. Cheung KK, Dhawan RT, Wilson LF, Peirce NS, Rajeswaran G. Pars interarticularis injury in elite athletes - the role of imaging in diagnosis and management. Eur J Radiol. 2018;108:28–42. https://doi.org/10.1016/j.ejrad.2018.08.029.
29. Kountouris A, Portus M, Cook J. Cricket fast bowlers without low back pain have larger quadratus lumborum asymmetry than injured bowlers. Clin J Sport Med. 2013;23(4):300–4. https://doi.org/10.1097/JSM.0b013e318280ac88.
30. Kountouris A, Portus M, Cook J. Quadratus lumborum asymmetry and lumbar spine injury in cricket fast bowlers. J Sci Med Sport. 2012;15(5):393–7. https://doi.org/10.1016/j.jsams.2012.03.012.

Lumbar Stress Fractures Clinical Management

29

Patrick Farhart, Peter Alway, and Dayle Shackel

29.1 Introduction

Non-surgical treatment is the foundation of clinical management of bowlers with lumbar bone stress injuries (LBSI). Management strategies are influenced by player age, injury history, bowling speed, skill level, injury characteristics, and access to radiological imaging. There is a fundamental distinction between treating LBSI functionally (allowing return to activities as soon as pain allows) and structurally (aiming to achieve resolution of bony abnormalities, including fracture union, before recommencing bowling) [1]. Functional approaches may be suitable for lower demand bowlers, those in the latter stages of playing careers, or bowlers with chronic defects [2], where bone healing may not be deemed realistic or necessary. The main advantage of a functional approach is a faster return to play, although this is usually a trade-off against higher rates of recurrence in both the short and long term.

Functional approaches may not be suitable for high-level young fast bowlers, as acute LBSI in bowlers can achieve bone healing [3], which is associated with superior long-term fast bowling performance and career trajectories [2]. Injuries that do not achieve bone healing may recur and cause ongoing pain and contralateral LBSI [4], potentially reducing opportunities for skill development and acquiring resilience to the stresses of fast bowling. The availability of MRI utilising VIBE sequences for accurate cortical and trabecular bone assessment allows a structural approach with bone healing as a critical outcome to be the current gold standard [5] in managing LBSI in bowlers. Clinical management described hereafter will primarily detail a structural management approach to the spectrum of acute symptomatic LBSI, spanning stress reactions, incomplete unilateral stress fractures, complete unilateral stress fractures, and bilateral injuries.

29.2 Physical Assessment

A high index of suspicion for LBSI is advised in bowlers who experience bowling-related lumbopelvic stiffness or pain, particularly if symptoms are contralateral to the bowling arm [2]. Single-leg lumbar hyperextension, lumbar quadrant, and

P. Farhart (✉)
School of Sport, Exercise and Rehabilitation, Faculty of Health, Human Performance Research Centre, University of Technology Sydney, Ultimo, NSW, Australia
e-mail: patrick.j.farhart@student.uts.edu.au

P. Alway
England and Wales Cricket Board, London, UK
e-mail: Peter.Alway@ecb.co.uk

D. Shackel
New Zealand Cricket, High Performance Centre, Burt Sutcliffe Pavilion, Lincoln, New Zealand
e-mail: dayle.shackel@nzc.nz

B. Olivier, J. W. Orchard (eds.), *Cricket Sports Medicine*,
https://doi.org/10.1007/978-981-96-6321-7_29

lumbar lateral flexion tests are neither sensitive nor specific for detecting LBSI [6–8], and symptomatic bowlers should undergo MRI scanning if a clinician wishes to confidently determine LBSI presence or absence [9]. The key goals of imaging are to determine the presence of a clinically relevant LBSI, to understand whether a cortical breach is present, to distinguish between active bone stress and chronic injuries, and to assess bone healing during rehabilitation [10].

Along with radiological findings, detailed assessment incorporating the following is essential in planning the clinical management of bowlers with LBSI:

(a) Evaluation of bowling speed; recent and career training and match bowling loads; injury history; bowling technique; and metrics related to running, strength and conditioning loads, and other sports.
(b) Motor control as this may be integral in LBSI development [11]:
    - Lumbar lordosis; thoracic kyphosis; trunk anterior, posterior and frontal plane displacement relative to the pelvis; hip and knee alignment; anterior, posterior and lateral pelvic tilt. These variables should be assessed in standing, single-leg stance, bilateral and single leg squat, open and closed-chain hip flexion, lunging, running, and back foot contact (BFC) and front foot contact (FFC) bowling positions if practical.
    - Alignment during lumbopelvic stability testing [12] that may relate to insufficient stabiliser recruitment/strength or excessive co-contraction.
    - Lumbopelvic, thoracic, and hip and knee displacement during bilateral and single-leg landings to examine segmental stiffness.
    - Lower limb propulsive force/impulse, reactive strength index, landing force/impulse, and asymmetries related to these metrics derived from force plate technologies.
(c) Ranges of motion:
    - Bowling shoulder external rotation (ER) and total arc of rotation [13].
    - Lumbar spine: Restriction and symptoms associated with lumbar extension, flexion, rotation, and lateral flexion.
    - Thoracic spine: Rib cage motion and thoracic lateral flexion, rotation, flexion, and extension.
    - Hip and thigh: Hip flexion/extension, hip rotation at 0°/90° of hip flexion, hip flexor length, quadriceps length, hamstring length at 90°/maximal hip flexion.
    - Ankle: Plantarflexion and open/closed-chain dorsiflexion as this may impact the ability of calf musculature to mitigate ground reaction forces (GRF).
(d) Sacroiliac joint (SIJ) function: Unidirectional pelvic shear and torsional forces associated with high impact and repetitive front foot landings during bowling may increase the potential for SIJ dysfunction [14].
(e) Muscle strength and endurance: Hip extensor, hip abductor, hamstring, calf, quadricep and abdominal/trunk strength, lumbar extensor endurance if deemed suitable to assess [15].

29.3 Rehabilitation Considerations

Rehabilitation should address findings identified during examination, and a comprehensive physical therapy and exercise programme is fundamental to this [16]. Progressions based on achieving specific criteria as opposed to time-based protocols are recommended [1], as bowlers are high risk athletes for LBSI complications and recurrence [2]. Bone healing and restoration of bone strength are important criteria to consider alongside clinical, functional, workload, and technical variables [17].

Male fast bowlers below 22 years of age possess the highest risk of sustaining LBSI [18], and this is associated with lower skeletal robustness [19]. In a large general population study, the age of attainment of peak lumbar bone mineral density (BMD) was described as 20.1 years in females and 23.6 years in males [20], and this was reported as 24 years in a cohort of 91 male fast bowlers [19]. Risk of LBSI for bowlers is probably at its greatest when they start competing at senior levels [19], as this often coincides with increased bowling loads, participation in multiple teams, and increases in strength, mass, and height which likely increase forces transmitted to the lumbar spine. This combination of relative lumbar skeletal weakness, increasing workload, and increases in force must be considered during rehabilitation and return to play.

LBSI occurrence in spin bowlers is not rare, and in elite Australian bowlers monitored over 13 seasons, 8% of all recorded LBSI occurred in spin bowlers [4]. For spin bowlers in this cohort, return to bowling occurred at a mean of 81 days compared to 154 days for fast bowlers, accompanied by an absence of bone healing in 13% of spin bowlers and 7% of fast bowlers [4]. This may be due to bone healing not being deemed a priority for spin bowlers, and whilst we do not advocate this approach, there may exist a subset of spin bowlers who are able to return to play successfully with less emphasis placed upon this milestone.

Manual therapy aimed at improving thoracic spine and rib cage mobility is beneficial, as increases in thoracic flexibility may reduce lumbar loading and prevent stress-related disorders of the lumbar spine [21]. Further to this, increases in thoracic rotation range between BFC and FFC are associated with reduced lumbar pain in young fast bowlers [22].

The optimisation of SIJ function should be considered, as reduced SIJ form/force closure can increase moments at the L4 and L5 vertebrae [23]. Reduced hip internal rotation (IR) range is associated with non-dominant side LBSI in rotation-related sports [24], and improving this may reduce lumbar loads in bowlers as the trunk rotates over a fixed front hip during FFC of bowling [25]. Manual therapy of the lumbar spine can commence once bone healing has been established, and thrust manipulative techniques are not recommended in bowlers recovering from LBSI [1].

Whilst non-steroidal anti-inflammatory drugs (NSAIDS) have been recommended in the management of young athletes with acute LBSI [15], we do not endorse this approach, as NSAIDS are linked to inhibitions in adaptive bone formation that may reduce bone healing capacity [26]. Low-intensity pulsed ultrasound may be safely utilised to enhance bone healing and has been demonstrated to significantly reduce pain and functional disability in early-stage LBSI [27]. No high-quality evidence exists to support parathyroid hormone use in bowlers with LBSI; however, its administration is occasionally considered in professional cricket environments, even as clinicians await results of trials examining its efficacy.

Female bowlers with menstrual irregularity may possess increased risk of LBSI, and if present, then BMD testing and an endocrine workup should be considered [28]. Bowlers with multiple LBSI should undergo testing for vitamin D and calcium levels, and if levels are deficient, then supplementation is recommended [29]. Relative energy deficiency in sport (RED-S) can be associated with LBSI incidence in male and female bowlers, and if established, a multidisciplinary approach utilising endocrinology, nutrition, and occasionally psychiatry is required [1].

LBSI are typically viewed through a biomedical lens, but a range of psychosocial factors are important for clinicians to consider and address throughout rehabilitation [1]. Injured bowlers are often unable to participate in cricket for months, and transparent communication, setting of expectations and psychological support can improve rehabilitation compliance and return to play outcomes.

Consideration of injury characteristics is necessary, as previous research demonstrated that bowlers with stress reactions returned to competition 150 days post-injury, whereas those with incomplete cortical breaches in the presence of bone healing (229 days) and partial/no healing (217 days) returned later [4]. Bone healing occurred in all stress reactions, in 82% of incomplete stress fractures and in 53% of complete stress fractures [4]. In Australian bowlers, fractures occurring at the same site as a previously united fracture took a median of 276 days to achieve bone healing in comparison with 114 days for index fractures [3], and recurrent injuries took longer than index injuries to return to bowling (165 vs 130 days) and competition (217 vs 171 days). Elsewhere it has been reported that more vertically orientated cortical breaches situated above a longer superior articular facet are more likely to heal than horizontally projecting fractures [5].

In symptomatic fast bowlers with a chronic unilateral defect, MRI to establish either an acute contralateral pars interarticularis/pedicle injury, or ongoing symptoms at the site of the defect [4] is recommended. Clinical management in the absence of an acute contralateral injury or in the case of a chronic bilateral injury is essentially symptom-based, as there is little prospect for bone healing of a chronic defect with conservative management [10]. These cases often require a short period of unloading from bowling, with NSAIDS and/or guided corticosteroid infiltration providing symptom resolution and functional restoration [30]. The presence of an acute contralateral injury requires a structural management approach.

29.4 Clinical Management

Clinical management described hereafter will focus on a structural approach divided into four phases: unloading and protection, integrated reloading, return to high-intensity bowling, and return to competition, and these are summarised in Table 29.1.

Table 29.1 Summary of structural rehabilitation programme post-LBSI

Phase	1. Unloading and protection	2. Integrated reloading	3. Return to high-intensity bowling	4. Return to competition
Length	6 weeks or more dependent upon injury characteristics	6 weeks +	Up to 12 weeks or more	Ongoing
Objectives	Early bone healing, prevent LBSI progression. Training of lumbo-pelvic stabilisers	Integrate progressed lumbo-pelvic stabilisation into unsupported resistance training	Multiplanar strengthening within a high-performance framework. Return to high-intensity bowling	Maintain fast bowling technique, speed and skill. Prevention of recurrence of LBSI
Avoid	Swimming, running, jumping, resistance training, cricket, painful lumbar movement or therapeutic exercise	Excessive axial lumbar loading and trunk rigidity, painful lumbar extension, rotation, or lateral flexion	Lumbar symptoms during, after and the day following loading, rapid increases in bowling volume and intensity	Physical impairments and functional/skill limitations that may develop following return to match play
Interventions	Education re-injury and aggravating factors, optimise movement to unload vertebral arch, lumbo-pelvic stabilisation, stretching, possible use of bracing	Progress lumbo-pelvic stabilisation, upper body strengthening, lower body resistance training, multiplanar gluteal strengthening, return to running	Rotational power training, high-speed running, plyometrics, bowling prehab, technical bowling focus, progressive increments of bowling volume and intensity	Continue strength and conditioning, monitor bowling technique, coach and player education, management of bowling loads
Criteria to progress to next stage	Pain-free lumbar range and activities of daily living, neutral spine during exercises. MRI: reduced BMO intensity and distribution, progress towards cortical breach healing	Pain-free lumbar movement, tolerance of strength program, optimal movement patterns in resistance training. MRI: complete BMO resolution and advanced cortical breach healing	No lumbar symptoms, maintenance of optimal bowling technique under fatigue, attainment of high volume and intensity bowling loads over extended period	Ongoing multidisciplinary support, consideration of career workloads to prevent recurrent injury

29.4.1 Phase 1: Unloading and Protection

This typically involves a minimum of six weeks duration and is often extended with cortical breach LBSI. The goals of management during this phase are to prevent LBSI progression and maximise early bone healing. Whilst absence from cricket and potentially aggravating loading is imperative, full participation in pain-free activities of daily living is beneficial to recovery. The injured bowler should be educated about specific movements and activities that may aggravate symptoms and the implications of injury non-healing or progression. The avoidance of provocative lumbar extension, flexion, rotation, and lateral flexion is paramount, as are combinations of these movements. Therapeutic exercise causing pain, swimming, running, jumping, and resistance training should be avoided.

The value of thoracolumbar spine bracing in bowlers with LBSI is debatable, and whilst bracing to limit lumbar extension and rotation theoretically should promote bone healing, no evidence supports this [2]. Bowlers who may benefit from bracing include those with complete acute cortical disruptions, clinical factors that may delay or prevent bone union, an exaggerated lumbar lordosis, or those who require enforced unloading from activity and/or experience persistent symptoms at rest [2]. Bracing may also be of value in the management of children of school age to prevent them from participating in other sports, including casual activities during breaks.

Bowlers who experience lumbar symptoms at rest and during activities of daily living should be provided with strategies to optimise postural and movement patterns to unload the lumbar vertebral arch [31]. This may involve cues and education to relax abdominal musculature and train active posterior tilt of the pelvis to reduce lordotic tendencies of the lumbar spine [31].

Lumbopelvic stabilisation training with transversus abdominis and multifidus contraction emphasising neutral lumbo-pelvic position and retraining of lumbopelvic dissociation [32] is a major focus, and spinal control and stability requirements must be balanced with minimising excessive compression forces [33]. Training can commence in supine and be incorporated into exercises including leg slides, basic single arm and leg dead bug progressions, hundreds, and quadruped hip extension and abduction exercises. Practitioners should be cautious about including bridging (particularly single leg), as this may aggravate symptoms in this phase.

Bowlers with stress reactions and minor cortical disruptions can integrate lumbopelvic stabilisation training into standing exercises and stationary cycling at low to moderate intensities if these activities are pain-free. Unloaded squat, step-up, and forward lunging are suitable if lumbar lordosis can be controlled through posterior pelvic tilt and recruitment of hip abductors and extensors [31]. We do not advocate upper body resistance training during this phase due to axial loading and spinal compression concerns, even in neutral lumbar spine.

Stretching and mobility exercises can be commenced providing the bowler is able to maintain a neutral spine position. Whilst there is a tendency for practitioners to recommend hip flexor stretching in the management of LBSI, this intervention must be based on the results of physical assessment. Young bowlers presenting with a "sway back" posture will often display lengthened hip flexors accompanied by a lordosis that extends into the mid-thoracic spine, and hip flexor stretching for these bowlers may increase loading of the lumbar spine [34].

Criteria to progress to Phase 2 include pain-free and full lumbar range of motion, minimal pain on provocative testing, pain-free activities of daily living, and maintenance of a neutral lumbo-pelvic position during exercises. Reduced intensity and distribution of bone marrow oedema (BMO), and progress towards cortical breach healing on MRI are necessary if using a structural approach to dictate progression. Six weeks is proposed between initial and subsequent MRI scans for stress reactions, eight to ten weeks for incomplete unilateral stress fractures, and ten to twelve weeks for unilateral complete stress fractures and acute bilateral LBSI.

29.4.2 Phase 2: Integrated Reloading

This can range from six weeks upwards and integrates progressed lumbopelvic stabilisation training into standing and resistance training. Pain-free, low-velocity, single-plane activities such as squatting, step-up, forward/lateral lunging, and Romanian deadlift can commence. Single-leg closed chain front leg hip flexion and single-leg back leg squat training in bowling-specific positions can be progressed with resistance bands and weights. The control of lumbopelvic extension, anterior pelvic tilt, ipsilateral pelvic drop, and frontal plane movement of the lumbar spine in single-leg stance should be highlighted as these have been linked to LBSI development [11].

Whilst resistance training provides a mechanical loading stimulus that may improve bone formation and fracture healing [35], it is important to avoid excessive axial lumbar loading and trunk rigidity, as well as symptomatic lumbar flexion, extension, rotation, or lateral flexion. Lumbar extensor endurance training can begin, and symptom response and degree of extension during this exercise should be closely monitored.

Posterior oblique, anterior oblique, and posterior longitudinal sling strengthening is recommended, as activation of these systems may optimise SIJ force closure [36]. Endurance training of lumbopelvic stabilisers can be accompanied by internal oblique, external oblique, and rectus abdominis strengthening, as these muscles are integral to axial torque resistance and generation [37]. This could involve advanced dead bug exercises utilising ipsilateral, contralateral, single, and double arm/leg variations with and without band resistance; front and side planks with and without arm and hip movements; and straight/oblique abdominal curls with bent and straight knees.

Multiplanar strength and endurance training targeting deep hip ER, gluteus medius, and gluteus maximus musculature can improve insufficient pelvifemoral control which is associated with excessive hip flexion at BFC [11]. This could include clamshell progressions, pelvic drops, sidelying hip abduction, double and single-leg bridging, lateral step-ups, and skater squats [38]. Bowling-specific pull through strengthening in single-leg stance will target posterior oblique sling fascial connections between latissimus dorsi and the contralateral gluteus maximus [36].

Upper body and overhead loading can commence, provided the lumbar spine is in neutral and symptom free. Based on assessment, interventions to maximise shoulder ER and total rotation arc range may be valuable as shoulder range limitations are reported to be associated with bowlers adopting potentially injurious movement strategies in the bowling action [13].

Swimming should be introduced cautiously, as it may aggravate symptoms due to repetitive lumbar extension and rotation, particularly in non-competent swimmers. The introduction of low to moderate intensity running may provide an osteogenic stimulus [17], but widely cited guidelines for increasing running distance and intensity [39] may not be suitable for all bowlers. More conservative progressions may be required in bowlers with lordotic postures during running, and those who possess poor lower limb strength, non-optimal kinetic chain function, and reduced capacity for impact absorption.

Criteria to progress to Phase 3 include pain-free lumbar movements and provocative testing, tolerance of consistent strength programming, and maintenance of optimal movement patterns during resistance training [17]. MRI should ideally demonstrate complete BMO resolution and advanced or complete cortical breach healing; however, attainment of healing may be prolonged in bowlers with substantial cortical breaches.

29.4.3 Phase 3: Return to High-Intensity Bowling

This may last twelve weeks or more and is aimed at achieving a safe return to high-intensity fast bowling through a multidisciplinary approach. Continued development of multiplanar lumbar spine, pelvic, and hip control is integrated within a high-performance training framework that includes rotational power training, high-speed running, lower limb plyometrics, bowling prehab activities, and a return to bowling programme.

Development of lumbar spine resilience is required, and exposure to lumbar flexion, extension, rotation and lateral flexion movements and loads is essential, as these are inevitable during fast bowling. A variety of diagonal, rotational slam, and trunk flexion exercises using medicine balls, cables, bands, and weight plates can be performed in standing, lunging, and kneeling positions to develop dynamic trunk stability and power. Increasing complexity, speed, and resistance of these exercises can occur as capacity and competency allow.

Whilst early-stage running may have an endurance focus, transitions to high-intensity running are central to performance recovery. Fast bowling techniques linked to increased ball release speed involve efficient transfer of linear momentum of the centre of mass generated during the run-up to angular momentum of distal body segments [40]. Running programmes should consider repeated sprint performance, acceleration/deceleration abilities, and demands that a fast bowler is likely to experience when returning to competition. Returning to basic fielding (in the absence of diving) and defensive batting drills are appropriate at this stage. These normally can be progressed quickly into full fielding and batting activities, and this would coincide with match play without bowling.

Plyometric training is proposed to contribute to reduced LBSI risk through improved capacity to dissipate GRF on FFC [41]. Low-intensity and high-volume programming is suitable and can comprise vertical hops and jumps, squat jumps, bounding, and counter movement hurdle jumps and hops [41]. Plyometrics can facilitate more knee extended positions during FFC, and this may enhance transfers of whole-body linear momentum into angular momentum [42]. Increasing back foot ankle stiffness and reactive strength may control prolonged and excessive ankle dorsiflexion and subsequent increased rear hip and knee flexion during BFC.

Fast bowling prehabilitation (Prehab) challenges components and patterning of the bowling action related to lumbar loading, technical development, power, strength, and dissipation of GRF [43]. Key priorities can relate to increasing ankle stiffness at BFC, rapid shifts of momentum in transitions from BFC to FFC, and the control of excessive frontal plane lumbar motion in single-leg stance. Medicine ball slams with and without trunk rotation in kneeling, standing, and from BFC to FFC to follow-through can be progressed with run ups, resistance bands, hopping, and landing from heights. Furthermore, a mini trampoline can assist development of BFC and FFC shock attenuation, proprioception, and control.

Stationary bowling alignment drills are an ideal starting point for technical coaching, and these can be progressed to bowling walkthroughs, bowling on shortened pitch lengths and low/moderate intensity bowling over a full-length pitch. Initial technical interventions to optimise rear hip flexion at BFC, lumbopelvic extension at FFC and lumbopelvic lateral flexion away from the bowling arm at BR are valuable as these variables are associated with LBSI in fast bowlers [11]. Coaching should facilitate development of a bowler's momentum in the direction of a batter, emphasise hip and shoulder alignment that promotes technical efficiency, improve stability during BFC and FFC, train effective use of the non-dominant arm, and encourage completion of the bowling action with an effective follow-through. Multidisciplinary input is required throughout this process, as a bowler's ranges of motion, motor control, and strength are important considerations in understanding whether that bowler can safely attain positions and alignments recommended during coaching.

A return to high-intensity bowling is best achieved in a structured yet agile programme that features gradual increases in bowling volume and intensity, as a prolonged break from bowling has negative effects on BMD and bone strength of the lumbar spine [44]. Furthermore, changes in bowling mechanics are accompanied by altered lumbar loading patterns that may require extended periods to adapt to, and lumbar loading from all bowling related activities, even those as simple as bowling walkthroughs, should be considered. The presence of recovery days between bowling sessions is important to allow bone adaptation and minimise risk of excessive bone stress, particularly following high volume or high-intensity bowling days [10], and the use of lower load weeks at 4-to-5-week intervals during return to bowl programmes is advised.

The monitoring of running and strength training loads is also necessary as these may contribute to total lumbar load and affect tolerance of the lumbar spine to fast bowling. The adage of optimal loading during BSI rehabilitation being symptom-driven [45] should be adhered to, and the only acceptable lumbar pain level when managing LBSI is 0/10 during, after, and the day following loading. Shortened run-ups whilst bowling with maximal effort can be used to manipulate lumbar loads, as this causes small reductions in ball speed (3.5%) but disproportionately large reductions (44%) in lumbar loading [46]. This presents an alternative to reducing the number of deliveries bowled, as optimal strategies for load management must balance the need to maintain levels of performance during return to play programmes [46].

No consensus exists on optimal timelines to facilitate a successful return to high-intensity bowling or whether increases in bowling volumes should precede increases in bowling intensities or vice-versa. Returning to bowling at 16 weeks post-LBSI is associated with increased recurrence in comparison with bowlers returning at 21 weeks [4], and this may be due to truncated rehabilitation, inadequate bone healing, or decreases in BMD that can take up to 52 weeks to return to baseline [44]. Whilst attaining bone healing is central to structural LBSI rehabilitation objectives, it is not a statistically significant factor with respect to return to bowling times or injury recurrence [47].

Even in the presence of radiological resolution, progressive increments of bowling volume and intensity over a prolonged period are required to facilitate adequate lumbar spine BMD recovery and adaptation contralateral to the bowling arm to accomplish resilience to resist recurrent LBSI [44]. The prolonged nature of rehabilitation in comparison with other LBSI incident sports is partly due to the need to rebuild this adaptation. Current return to play programmes may not reflect this, and we have provided an example of a successful return to bowling programme for a fast bowler aged 18 years who commenced bowling at 24 weeks post-cortical breach LBSI and returned to competition at 45 weeks post-injury (Table 29.2).

Criteria to progress to Phase 4 include no lumbar symptoms, maintenance of optimal bowling technique under fatigue, and attainment of high volume and high-intensity bowling loads over an extended period that adequately prepare a fast bowler to cope with the repetitive high force demands of fast bowling in competition environments.

29.4.4 Phase 4: Return to Competition

The objectives of this phase are to maintain high-performance technical, speed, and skill outcomes related to fast bowling following return to competition whilst preventing injury recurrences. LBSI recurrence rates in bowlers are reported as 22% in females and as high as 53% in males, and median time for recurrences is 313 days post-injury and 171 days post-return to match availability [4]. Even in the presence of bone healing, clinicians, coaches, and bowlers should be aware that recurrence risk is high, and that careful and well-planned management following return to competition is required to help prevent recurrences.

In addition to factors associated with BMD, high recurrence rates may be associated with physical impairments and functional/skill limitations that predated or developed following return to match play. Index and recurrent LBSI in bowlers are associated with multiple intrinsic and extrinsic risk factors [48], and previously described rehabilitation strategies highlight the widespread nature of interventions required to facilitate full recovery. Following return to competition, bowlers may receive limited clinical

Table 29.2 Return to bowling programme for a fast bowler aged 18 post-cortical breach LBSI

Week 24 post-injury	Session 1	Session 2	Session 3	Total deliveries	Week 35 post-injury	Session 1	Session 2	Session 3	Total deliveries
Volume	12	0	12	24	Volume	30	24	30	84
Intensity	25%		25%		Intensity	70%	80%	80%	
Week 25 post-injury	Session 1	Session 2	Session 3	Total deliveries	Week 36 post-injury	Session 1	Session 2	Session 3	Total deliveries
Volume	12	0	16	28	Volume	30	30	36	96
Intensity	35%		35%		Intensity	80%	80%	80%	
Week 26 post-injury	Session 1	Session 2	Session 3	Total deliveries	Week 37 post-injury	Session 1	Session 2	Session 3	Total deliveries
Volume	12	18	12	42	Volume	0	0	36	36
Intensity	35%	35%	50%		Intensity			80%	
Week 27 post-injury	Session 1	Session 2	Session 3	Total deliveries	Week 38 post-injury	Session 1	Session 2	Session 3	Total deliveries
Volume	0	0	18	18	Volume	36	36	36	108
Intensity			50%		Intensity	85%	85%	90%	
Week 28 post-injury	Session 1	Session 2	Session 3	Total deliveries	Week 39 post-injury	Session 1	Session 2	Session 3	Total deliveries
Volume	18	18	18	54	Volume	36	36	36	108
Intensity	50%	50%	50%		Intensity	90%	90%	90%	
Week 29 post-injury	Session 1	Session 2	Session 3	Total deliveries	Week 40 post-injury	Session 1	Session 2	Session 3	Total deliveries
Volume	18	24	18	60	Volume	42	36	42	120
Intensity	50%	50%	60%		Intensity	90%	90%	90%	
Week 30 post-injury	Session 1	Session 2	Session 3	Total deliveries	Week 41 post-injury	Session 1	Session 2	Session 3	Total deliveries
Volume	24	18	24	66	Volume	0	0	42	42
Intensity	60%	60%	60%		Intensity			90%	
Week 31 post-injury	Session 1	Session 2	Session 3	Total deliveries	Week 42 post-injury	Session 1	Session 2	Session 3	Total deliveries
Volume	24	24	24	72	Volume	42	36	42	120
Intensity	60%	60%	70%		Intensity	90%	100%	100%	
Week 32 post-injury	Session 1	Session 2	Session 3	Total deliveries	Week 40 post-injury	Session 1	Session 2	Session 3	Total deliveries
Volume	0	0	24	24	Volume	42	42	42	126
Intensity			70%		Intensity	100%	90%	100%	
Week 33 post-injury	Session 1	Session 2	Session 3	Total deliveries	Week 43 post-injury	Session 1	Session 2	Session 3	Total deliveries
Volume	24	30	24	78	Volume	48	42	48	138
Intensity	70%	60%	70%		Intensity	100%	100%	100%	
Week 34 post-injury	Session 1	Session 2	Session 3	Total deliveries	Week 44 post-injury	Session 1	Session 2	Session 3	Total deliveries
Volume	24	30	24	78	Volume	48	48	48	144
Intensity	70%	70%	70%		Intensity	100%	100%	100%	

management and performance support in comparison with what they experienced during rehabilitation, and it is vital that direction regarding strength and conditioning, bowling technique, and management of bowling workloads continues at this time.

Well-planned bowling workloads that consider bowling intensity, volume, and adequate recovery are the simplest and possibly most important step that bowlers can take to reduce risk of recurrence post-return to competition, and players and coaches require ongoing education regarding the potential benefits of this initiative. This applies to all fast bowlers returning from LBSI, regardless of their access to high-quality physical therapy, strength and conditioning, sports science, and technical coaching support.

Cricket Australia and the England and Wales Cricket Board (ECB) have been at the forefront of developing fast bowling guidelines for young players that aim to develop protective bone strength and reduce the risk of index and recurrent LBSI. Whilst some differences exist between the guidelines provided by these organisations, both have proposed carefully managed workloads specific to different age groups [49, 50].

Some features of Cricket Australia's guidelines include a 10-week pre-season gradual build up in bowling, with a bowler attaining expected match intensities and weekly volumes in the month preceding a season [49]. During a season, under-17 bowlers should aim to bowl 100 to 120 deliveries per week, have at least 1 day off between bowling days, and bowl a maximum of 3 days per week and a maximum of 30 deliveries in each bowling spell [49]. Under-19 bowlers should aim to bowl 120 to 140 deliveries per week, not bowl more than 2 days in a row, and bowl a maximum of 4 days per week and a maximum of 36 deliveries in each bowling spell [49].

Furthermore, the ECB recommends that young fast bowlers undergo a 7- to 10-day bowling break during the middle of the season, a low bowling volume week every 4 to 5 weeks, a post-season 4-week bowling break, and the avoidance of long periods of not bowling to maintain BMD [50]. In addition to the planning of bowling workloads on a daily, weekly, and monthly basis, consideration of career workloads is required to prevent recurrent injury. High career workloads appear to be protective against LBSI [51], as older fast bowlers are likely to have developed tolerance to the stresses of fast bowling in addition to the substantial skeletal adaptations that allow them to be significantly more robust than their younger counterparts [19].

29.5 Conclusion

High incidences of index and recurrent LBSI continue to challenge clinicians, coaches, and bowlers. Accurate diagnosis of these injuries is integral to informed decision-making, and clinical management is influenced by player age, injury history, bowling speed, player skill level, injury characteristics, and access to radiological imaging. Whilst bone healing is not associated with time to return to bowling and recurrence in fast bowlers with LBSI, it, along with recovery of BMD, is a critical factor in a structural approach to managing bowlers with LBSI.

Optimising movement, control, and loading patterns that aim to reduce risk of LBSI progression and enhance bone healing are a priority during early stages of rehabilitation. Subsequent strength, power, and plyometric training within a high-performance framework, as well as attention to technical aspects of bowling, and incremental progressions in bowling volume and intensity are required to improve resilience to fast bowling stresses and reduce risk of recurrence. Rehabilitation recommendations in this chapter are based on expert opinion and research conducted in fast bowling cohorts, and we believe that they will be of assistance in establishing effective approaches for the clinical management of bowlers with LBSI.

References

1. Selhorst M, Allen M, McHugh R, MacDonald J. Rehabilitation considerations for spondylolysis in the youth athlete. Int J Sports Phys Ther. 2020;15(2):287.
2. Orchard JW, Saw R, Kountouris A, Redrup D, Farhart P, Sims K. Management of lumbar bone stress injury in cricket fast bowlers and other athletes. South African. J Sports Med. 2023;35(1):v35i1a15172.
3. Singh SP, Rotstein AH, Saw AE, Saw R, Kountouris A, James T. Radiological healing of lumbar spine stress fractures in elite cricket fast bowlers. J Sci Med Sport. 2021;24(2):112–5.
4. Saw A, Eales B, Jones N, Obst A, Smith M, Kountouris A, Saw R. Lumbar bone stress injuries and nonunited defects in Elite Australian cricket players. Clin J Sport Med. 2024;34(1):44–51.

5. Watura C, Mitchell AW, Fahy D, Houghton J, Kang S, Lee JC. T1-VIBE and STIR MRI of lumbar pars interarticularis injuries in elite athletes: fracture characterisation and potential prognostic indicators. Skeletal Radiol. 2024;53(3):489–97.
6. Masci L, Pike J, Malara F, Phillips B, Bennell K, Brukner P. Use of the one-legged hyperextension test and magnetic resonance imaging in the diagnosis of active spondylolysis. Br J Sports Med. 2006;40(11):940–6.
7. Grødahl LH, Fawcett L, Nazareth M, Smith R, Spencer S, Heneghan N, Rushton A. Diagnostic utility of patient history and physical examination data to detect spondylolysis and spondylolisthesis in athletes with low back pain: a systematic review. Man Ther. 2016;24:7–17.
8. Sugiura S, Aoki Y, Toyooka T, Shiga T, Takato O, Ishizaki T, Omori Y, Takata A, Kiguchi Y, Tsukioka A, Okamoto Y. Lateral bending differentiates early-stage spondylolysis from nonspecific low back pain in adolescents. Musculoskelet Sci Pract. 2022;58:102526.
9. Alqarni AM, Schneiders AG, Cook CE, Hendrick PA. Clinical tests to diagnose lumbar spondylolysis and spondylolisthesis: a systematic review. Phys Ther Sport. 2015;16(3):268–75.
10. Kountouris A, Saw R, Saw A. Management of lumbar spondylolysis in athletes: role of imaging. Curr Radiol Rep. 2018;6:1–2.
11. Alway P, Felton P, Brooke-Wavell K, Peirce N, King M. Cricket fast bowling technique and lumbar bone stress injury. Med Sci Sports Exerc. 2021;53(3):581–9.
12. Sahrmann S. Diagnosis and treatment of movement impairment syndromes-e-book. Elsevier Health Sciences; 2001.
13. Felton PJ, McCaig S, King MA. Cricket fast bowling: the relationship between range of motion and key performance and injury technique characteristics. J Sports Sci. 2023;41(2):112–20.
14. Fortin JD. Enigmatic causes of spine pain in athletes. In: Watkins RG, editor. The spine in sports. Chicago: Mosby Year-Book; 1994.
15. Goetzinger S, Courtney S, Yee K, Welz M, Kalani M, Neal M. Spondylolysis in young athletes: an overview emphasizing nonoperative management. J Sports Med. 2020;2020(1):9235958.
16. Grazina R, Andrade R, Santos FL, Marinhas J, Pereira R, Bastos R, Espregueira-Mendes J. Return to play after conservative and surgical treatment in athletes with spondylolysis: a systematic review. Phys Ther Sport. 2019;37:34–43.
17. Sims K. Rehabilitation of lumbar bone stress injuries in Tennis players. Aspetar Sports Med J. 2024;Targeted Topic - Sports Medicine in Tennis 13:316–22.
18. Alway P, Brooke-Wavell K, Langley B, King M, Peirce N. Incidence and prevalence of lumbar stress fracture in English County Cricket fast bowlers, association with bowling workload and seasonal variation. BMJ Open Sport Exerc Med. 2019;5(1):e000529.
19. Keylock L, Alway P, Johnson W, Crabtree N, King M, Peirce N, Brooke-Wavell K. Lumbar spine bone mineral adaptation: cricket fast bowlers versus controls. BMJ Open Sport Exerc Med. 2023;9(2):e001481.
20. Xue S, Kemal O, Lu M, Lix LM, Leslie WD, Yang S. Age at attainment of peak bone mineral density and its associated factors: the National Health and Nutrition Examination Survey 2005–2014. Bone. 2020;131:115163.
21. Morimoto M, Tripathi S, Kodigudla M, Motohashi E, Fujitani J, Goel VK, Sairyo K. Biomechanical effects of thoracic flexibility and stiffness on lumbar spine loading: a finite element analysis study. World Neurosurg. 2024;184:e282–90.
22. Senington B, Lee RY, Williams JM. Biomechanical risk factors of lower back pain in cricket fast bowlers using inertial measurement units: a prospective and retrospective investigation. BMJ Open Sport Exerc Med. 2020;6(1):e000818.
23. Aihara T, Takahashi K, Yamagata M, Moriya H, Tamaki T. Biomechanical functions of the iliolumbar ligament in L5 spondylolysis. J Orthop Sci. 2000;5(3):238–42.
24. Nagamoto H, Abe M, Konashi Y, Kimura R, Takahashi M, Oizumi A. Rotation-related sports players demonstrate rotation-type lumbar spondylolysis fracture angle and decreased hip internal rotation range of motion. J Orthop. 2021;28:101–6.
25. Keylock L, Alway P, Felton P, McCaig S, Brooke-Wavell K, King M, Peirce N. Lumbar bone stress injuries and risk factors in adolescent cricket fast bowlers. J Sports Sci. 2022;40(12):1336–42.
26. Staab JS, Kolb AL, Tomlinson RE, Pajevic PD, Matheny RW Jr, Hughes JM. Emerging evidence that adaptive bone formation inhibition by non-steroidal anti-inflammatory drugs increases stress fracture risk. Exp Biol Med. 2021;246(9):1104–11.
27. Tanveer F, Arslan SA, Darain H, Ahmad A, Gilani SA, Hanif A. Effects of low-intensity pulsed ultrasound on pain and functional disability in patients with early-stage lumbar spondylolysis: a randomized controlled trial. J Bodyw Mov Ther. 2022;30:125–31.
28. Kiel J, Kaiser K. Stress reaction and fractures. In: StatPearls [Internet]. Treasure Island: StatPearls Publishing; 2023.
29. Knechtle B, Jastrzębski Z, Hill L, Nikolaidis PT. Vitamin D and stress fractures in sport: preventive and therapeutic measures—a narrative review. Medicina. 2021;57(3):223.
30. Sairyo K, Sakai T, Mase Y, Kon T, Shibuya I, Kanamori Y, Kosugi T, Dezawa A. Painful lumbar spondylolysis among pediatric sports players: a pilot MRI study. Arch Orthop Trauma Surg. 2011;131:1485–9.
31. Mitchell T, O'Sullivan P, Burnett A. Motor control retraining in athletes with low back pain. Aspetar Sports Med J. 2015;1:144–51.
32. Hides J, Stanton W, McMahon S, Sims K, Richardson C. Effect of stabilization training on multifidus muscle cross-sectional area among young elite cricketers with low back pain. J Orthop Sports Phys Ther. 2008;38(3):101–8.

33. Parkinson RJ, Callaghan JP. The role of dynamic flexion in spine injury is altered by increasing dynamic load magnitude. Clin Biomech. 2009;24(2):148–54.
34. Norris CM. Chapter 13 - the lumbar spine. In: Norris CM, editor. Managing sports injuries. 4th ed. Churchill Livingstone; 2011. p. 257–91. ISBN 9780702034732.
35. Ma Q, Miri Z, Haugen HJ, Moghanian A, Loca D. Significance of mechanical loading in bone fracture healing, bone regeneration, and vascularization. J Tissue Eng. 2023;14:20417314231172573.
36. Pool-Goudzwaard AL, Vleeming A, Stoeckart R, Snijders CJ, Mens JM. Insufficient lumbopelvic stability: a clinical, anatomical and biomechanical approach to 'a-specific' low back pain. Man Ther. 1998;3(1):12–20.
37. Ng JK, Parnianpour M, Richardson CA, Kippers V. Functional roles of abdominal and back muscles during isometric axial rotation of the trunk. J Orthop Res. 2001;19(3):463–71.
38. Boren K, Conrey C, Le Coguic J, Paprocki L, Voight M, Robinson TK. Electromyographic analysis of gluteus medius and gluteus maximus during rehabilitation exercises. Int J Sports Phys Ther. 2011;6(3):206.
39. George ER, Sheerin KR, Reid D. Criteria and guidelines for returning to running following a tibial bone stress injury: a scoping review. Sports Med. 2024;54(9):2247–65.
40. Bhandurge S, Alway P, Allen S, Blenkinsop G, King M. Technique variables associated with fast bowling performance: a systematic-narrative review. Appl Sci. 2024;14(15):6752.
41. Krishna SA, Alwar TK, Sibeko S, Ranjit S, Sivaraman A. Plyometric-based training for isokinetic knee strength and jump performance in cricket fast bowlers. Int J Sports Med. 2019;40(11):704–10.
42. Felton PJ, Shine KJ, Yeadon MR, King MA. Optimal initial position and technique for the front foot contact phase of cricket fast bowling: commonalities between individual-specific simulations of elite bowlers. J Biomech. 2023;158:111765.
43. Hartwich K. 'Bowling Prehab': an innovative approach to injury prevention and rehabilitation for fast bowlers. Sport Health. 2009;27(4):23–7.
44. Alway P, Peirce N, Johnson W, King M, Kerslake R, Brooke-Wavell K. Activity specific areal bone mineral density is reduced in athletes with stress fracture and requires profound recovery time: a study of lumbar stress fracture in elite cricket fast bowlers. J Sci Med Sport. 2022;25(10):828–33.
45. Warden SJ, Edwards WB, Willy RW. Optimal load for managing low-risk tibial and metatarsal bone stress injuries in runners: the science behind the clinical reasoning. J Orthop Sports Phys Ther. 2021;51(7):322–30.
46. Greig M, Child B. Submaximal cricket fast bowling offers a disproportionate reduction in loading versus performance: an alternative workload intervention. J Sport Rehabil. 2019;29(4):483–7.
47. Eales B, Jones N, Saw A, Obst A, Smith M, Kountouris A, Saw R. Lumbar bone stress injuries in elite Australian cricket players: a comprehensive case series. J Sci Med Sport. 2022;25:S79.
48. Olivier B, Taljaard T, Burger E, Brukner P, Orchard J, Gray J, Botha N, Stewart A, Mckinon W. Which extrinsic and intrinsic factors are associated with non-contact injuries in adult cricket fast bowlers? Sports Med. 2016;46:79–101.
49. Cricket Australia. Cricket Australia junior bowling guidelines [Internet]. Melbourne (Australia): [updated July 2023; cited 2024 Nov 23]. Available from: https://play.cricket.com.au/community/clubs/managing-your-club/youth-pace-bowling-guidelines.
50. England and Wales Cricket Board. Recreational junior fast bowling guidance 2024 [Internet]. Loughborough (United Kingdom): [updated 2024; cited 2024 Nov 23]. Available from: https://resources.ecb.co.uk/ecb/document/2024/06/14/292038a2-ac47-4655-bdf7-454c79d285eb/Recreational-Fast-Bowling-Guidance-2024.pdf.
51. Orchard JW, Blanch P, Paoloni J, Kountouris A, Sims K, Orchard JJ, Brukner P. Cricket fast bowling workload patterns as risk factors for tendon, muscle, bone and joint injuries. Br J Sports Med. 2015;49(16):1064–8.

Lumbar Stress Fractures Surgery

30

Rowan Schouten and Dayle Shackel

30.1 Introduction

Lumbar stress injuries (LSI) are a significant concern for cricketers, often impacting their performance and career longevity. For the vast majority of acute lumbar stress injuries in cricketers, non-operative treatment is favoured. This chapter explores the indications for surgery, various surgical techniques, and the outcomes and rehabilitation protocols associated with lumbar stress fracture injuries in cricketers. Understanding these can help healthcare professionals support athletes in returning to their pre-injury performance levels.

30.2 What Are the Goals of Treatment of Lumbar Stress Injuries in Cricketers?

It makes sense to start by defining 'success' in regard to the treatment of LSI. The goal is to ensure cricketers can promptly return to play at their pre-injury athletic performance level without discomfort and further interruption from recurrences.

If a lumbar stress injury is chronic or longstanding, then bony healing is considered unattainable and treatment is focused on symptom resolution and an early graduated return to play. However, for acute fractures, the prevailing opinion amongst healthcare professionals managing cricketers is that a successful outcome is more likely if complete bony healing is achieved, particularly for fast bowlers wanting to play red ball cricket.

A further objective of treatment is to avoid potential later sequelae of these injuries, the most significant of which is the development of spondylolisthesis. Spondylolisthesis refers to the forward slip of one vertebra relative to the vertebra below. Studies have documented that 43–74% of those with bilateral chronic (un-united) pars defects will progress to develop a subsequent spondylolisthesis, whereas those with unilateral defects have a significantly lower risk [1]. The consequences of spondylolisthesis vary; many remain clinically silent; however, a significant proportion develop lumbar pain and neurological symptoms later in life (typically between 40 and 60 years of age), which may require a surgical solution.

R. Schouten (✉)
Forte Orthopaedics, Christchurch, New Zealand

D. Shackel
New Zealand Cricket, High Performance Centre, Burt Sutcliffe Pavilion, Lincoln, New Zealand
e-mail: dayle.shackel@nzc.nz

B. Olivier, J. W. Orchard (eds.), *Cricket Sports Medicine*,
https://doi.org/10.1007/978-981-96-6321-7_30

30.3 When Should Surgery Be Considered for Lumbar Stress Fractures?

With the goals of treatment defined for acute fractures, when is surgery considered the best option to achieve these goals? As is the case across all sporting cohorts, it's universally recommended that almost all first-time lumbar stress injuries in cricketers should initially be treated non-surgically. As highlighted elsewhere in this book, this involves a range of interventions, including rest and targeted rehabilitation, as well as a review and optimisation of aspects such as bowling biomechanics, bowling workloads and bone health.

In reality, surgery is rarely needed and is typically only considered when initial non-surgical care has failed to achieve these goals of care, albeit with some exceptions. In this setting, 'failure' can take one of many forms. It may involve a symptomatic non-union, either from long-standing established pars defects or an acute stress fracture or fractures that fail to unite. More commonly, 'failure' of non-surgical care relates to a fracture that initially unites but then reoccurs at the same level and location when a cricketer returns to play, i.e. a 'recurrence'.

30.3.1 Recurrent Lumbar Stress Injuries

So, what are the rates and risk factors associated with a recurrence of LSI following non-surgical care in cricketers? While most experts believe the fast-bowling group is at particular risk, currently the best-published data providing insights into this essential question involves a case study involving all adult Australian professional cricketers over a 13-year period (2009–2022) [2]. Within this cohort of elite cricketers, 101 individuals developed a lumbar stress injury and were managed non-surgically. Following a return to match availability, 22% (4 of 18) of females and 52% (43 of 83) of males developed a recurrence. Of the injury characteristics studied, none significantly differed between those with recurrent and non-recurrent LSI.

Following a 'failure' of initial non-surgical care, the choice then centres around the potential of surgical intervention versus the option of repeating a further period of non-surgical care. If initial non-surgical care has been unsuccessful, then subsequent non-surgical care should, in principle, involve additional measures if a more successful outcome is to be expected. This often entails a longer spell of rest and rehabilitation, often extending to periods of 9–12 months.

Some unfortunate cricketers can experience one or multiple serial recurrences that can significantly interrupt their playing careers. These are the cohorts most suited to surgical consideration.

There are some exceptions to the philosophy of initial non-surgical care. In rare circumstances, surgical care can also be considered pre-emptively for injuries with a high chance of failure from non-surgical care. In this scenario, two specific injury patterns deserve a mention. Firstly, lumbar stress fractures can occasionally involve the pedicle. Pedicle stress injuries typically develop on the contralateral side in individuals with a pre-existing chronic unilateral spondylolysis of the pars or lamina. The low incidence of this injury combination makes it difficult to develop treatment guidelines, but published case reports and anecdotal experience suggest that they represent a particularly high-risk injury combination prone to recurrence and persistent symptoms following non-operative care (Fig. 30.1). Secondly, neurological symptoms may develop due to impingement of the adjacent nerve root by a 'hook-like' osteophyte from an established spondylolysis (Fig. 30.2). In both these scenarios, early surgical consultation is advised.

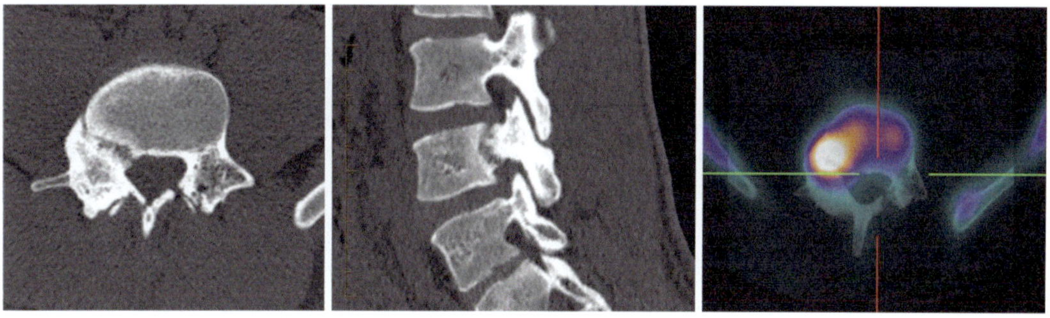

Fig. 30.1 An international right-arm fast bowler with a recurrent fracture through a hypertrophied right pedicle, with corresponding increased uptake noted on CT SPECT scanning, combined with a contralateral long-standing non-united left lamina fracture

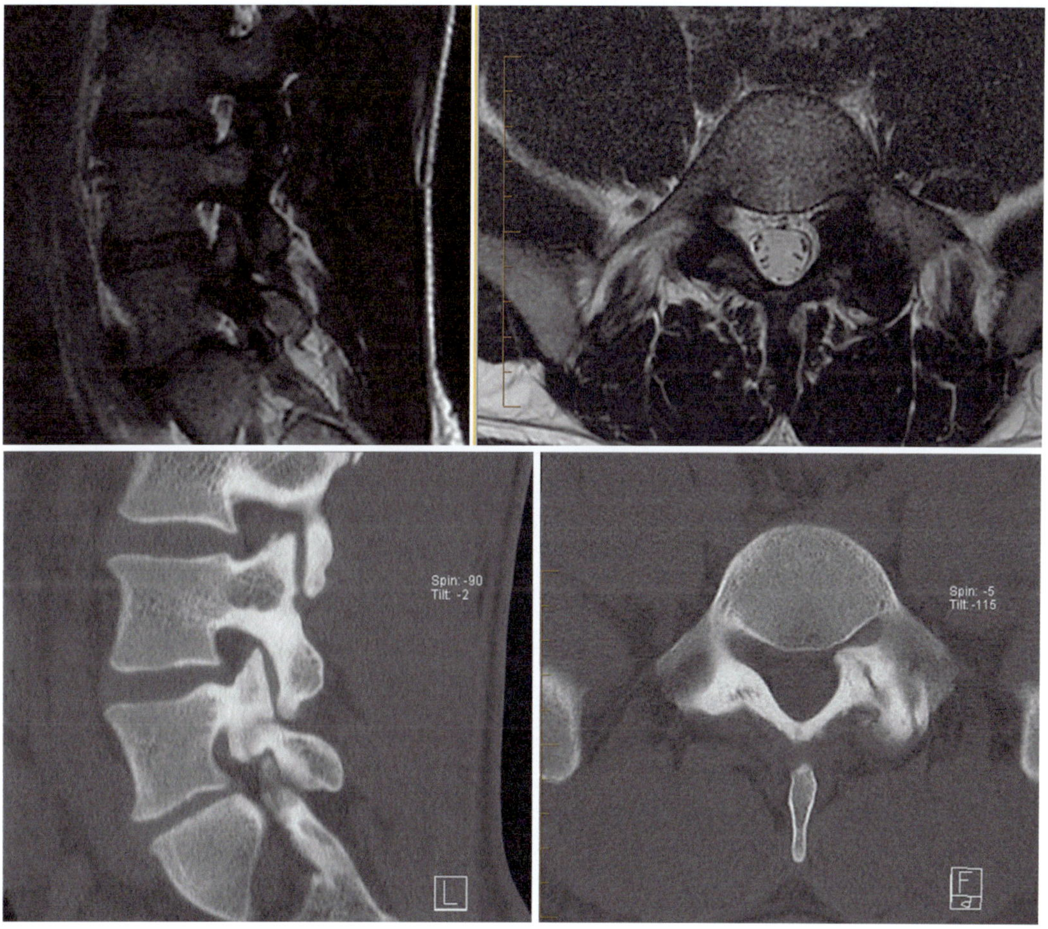

Fig. 30.2 An international right-arm fast bowler with a left L5 chronic hypertrophic non-united pars fracture involving a 'hook-like' osteophyte causing compression of the left L5 nerve root

30.4 Surgical Intervention: How, When and What Are the Outcomes?

How effective is the surgical alternative in achieving the goals of bony healing, timely return to play and avoiding any later consequences? The remainder of this chapter will review the current surgical techniques, the expected outcomes and the potential complications to further analyse the option of surgical repair of lumbar stress injuries in cricketers.

30.4.1 What Surgical Techniques Are Currently in Use?

When surgery is preferred, one of the many available techniques to repair lumbar stress injuries needs to be selected. While they vary in their structure and composition, all the options in current use share the same primary anatomical goal of adding stability and applying compression across the fracture to promote robust and resilient bony healing and, in the process, restore integrity to the posterior vertebral bony arch.

Importantly, all of these techniques do not involve a 'spinal fusion'. That is, they do not fixate one vertebral level to another, allowing normal motion and avoidance of any disruption to the normal spinal biomechanics so essential to cricketers, particularly fast bowlers.

Popular surgical techniques in widespread use include the single lag-screw fixation ('Buck's repair' [3]) and varying pedicle screw-based implant combinations (Fig. 30.3.) [4]. The implants employed are commonly made of titanium due to less post-operative imaging distortion compared with stainless-steel implants.

Buck's repair is still the most popular procedure used worldwide across a range of sporting cohorts [5]. This involves stabilisation and direct compression of the fracture by a single screw placed across (and ideally perpendicular) to the fracture. Typically, in this technique, a guide wire is first inserted under image guidance. Once the guide wire is ideally positioned, a cannulated screw is advanced over it. Tightening of the screw 'squeezes' (or 'lags') the fracture. Thereafter the guide wire is removed. Given the fracture morphology in cricketers can vary, challenges with this technique include accurate placement of the screw, particularly across a small fracture surface area that is often surrounded by hard cortical bone.

The other prevalent surgical techniques use a common anchor point—one or two pedicle screws [4]. These screws do not typically cross the pars fracture but instead pass lateral to them. The lumbar stress fractures can then be indirectly compressed and stabilised using various constructs anchored to this base, including titanium cables passed around the posterior vertebra arch in varying configurations (screw-cable fixation (Fig. 30.3b) [6]); implants that hook under the lamina (screw-lamina fixation (Fig. 30.3c)); or U-shaped rods placed under the spinous process (screw-rod fixation (Fig. 30.3d)).

Occasionally, when a lumbar stress injury involves a pedicle fracture and a contralateral pars/lamina fracture, a hybrid version of these various techniques can be used (Fig. 30.4.). In one option, two pedicle screws are used, with one directed across the pedicle fracture to directly compress it, while the other forms the second part of the base for a screw-cable construct that indirectly compresses the contralateral pars/lamina fracture.

With all techniques, debridement of fibrous tissue within the fracture site, freshening and decorticating of the fracture ends, and packing of the defect with bone graft are also commonly performed when the fracture site is accessible. To expose the fracture, an osteotomy of the tip of the inferior facet of the vertebra above may be a necessary step. Cancellous bone, with its superior osteogenic potential, can be locally harvested from the patient's posterior iliac crest. Alternatively, to minimise additional donor site morbidity, cadaveric allograft or synthetic bone graft substitutes and growth factors (e.g. bone morphogenic proteins) can be employed.

The potential benefits of spinal navigation systems and minimally invasive techniques are

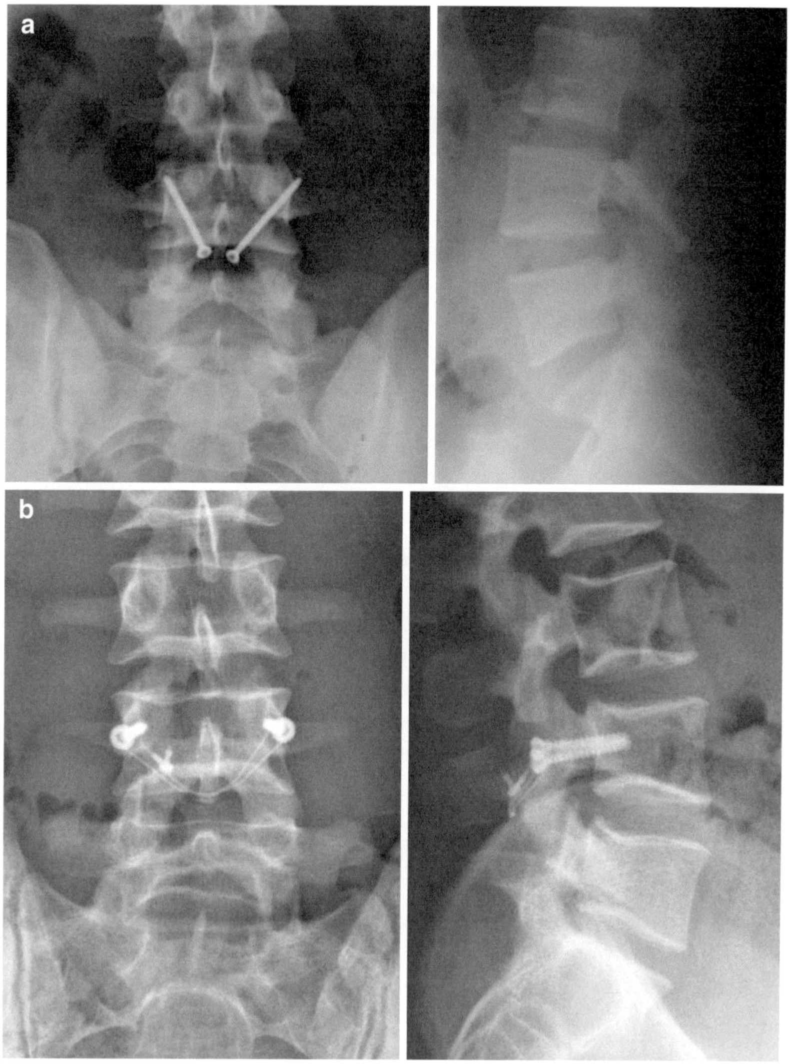

Fig. 30.3 Examples of common surgical techniques used to repair lumbar stress fractures. (**a**) Buck's repair (courtesy of Peter Robertson). (**b**) Pedicle screw and cable. (**c**) Pedicle screw and laminar hook (courtesy of Antony Field). (**d**) Pedicle screw and U shaped rod (courtesy of Kristian Dalzell).

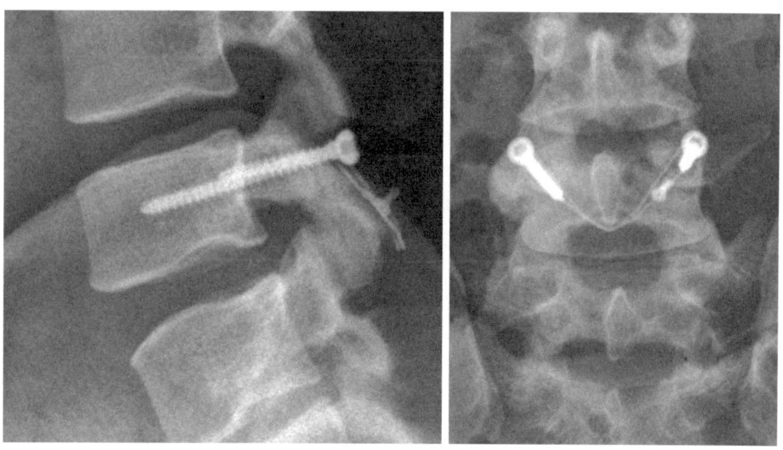

Fig. 30.4 Plain radiographs to demonstrate the hybrid surgical technique used to repair the case illustrated in Fig. 30.1. The right pedicle fracture is directly lagged by a longer pedicle screw. This then forms one anchor point for a cable-screw construct that indirectly compresses the non-united left-sided pars/lamina fracture

being explored by modifying these established surgical techniques. Intra-operative scanning of patients coupled with 3D stereotactic navigation systems can assist in achieving accurate screw placement, which is particularly critical for the success of the single lag-screw (Buck's repair) technique. Performing the surgery through small incisions or 'percutaneously' are hallmarks of 'minimally invasive techniques' which aim to limit the disruption to the surrounding paraspinal muscles [7]. These muscle-sparing principles have been associated with decreased levels of post-operative pain and a potentially faster functional recovery.

30.5 Who Are the Best Surgical Candidates?

The ideal surgical candidate is typically of younger age, has an acute re-fracture rather than a chronic established pars defect and has no significant herniation or degeneration in the adjacent disc.

Currently, there is no published literature on the results of surgical intervention of lumbar stress injuries in female cricketers. However, based on anecdotal evidence, the factors influencing the decision to operate on female and male cricketers are currently equivalent.

30.6 Are There Any Contraindications to Pars Repair Surgery?

The most important contraindication to attempting pars repair surgery is the presence of spondylolisthesis. Once spondylolisthesis exists, it's difficult to promote bony bridging across a large fracture gap using motion-sparing techniques. In these scenarios, surgical interventions involving fusion are the only option. The ability of a cricketer to return to their previous performance level following a fusion is considered more uncertain.

30.7 What Are the Expected Outcomes of Surgical Intervention?

Published studies of athletes involved in a variety of sports have shown the operative interventions in current practice are similarly effective in getting >90% of athletes back to play at their previous performance at intervals of 5–12 months post-surgery [4]. One meta-analysis comparison of techniques concluded that the pedicle-screw-based procedures achieved the most favourable fusion and lowest complication rates [8]. Given largely comparable outcomes, the selected technique is based more on the surgeon's familiarity with each surgical option coupled with an appreciation of the anatomical variations present.

The literature reporting on the results of surgical pars repair performed specifically in cricketers is currently sparse, but the technique has shown to be a reliable option. The merged results from four published studies involving a combined cohort of 36 elite male cricketers reported 35 returned to play competitive cricket [6, 9–11]. While 3 of these studies (a total of 23 players) involved Buck's technique, the largest and latest case series show equivalent results when a pedicle screw/titanium cable construct (Inglis technique) was used in a multinational cohort of 13 professional cricketers.

30.8 What Are the Potential Complications of Surgery?

While modern techniques that avoid fusions are considered low-risk surgical options, a variety of potential complications can occur. Superficial infections are typically managed successfully by simple wound care, antibiotics and a delay in rehabilitation. Hardware failure with pedicle-screw-based procedures, including pedicle screw or cable breakage or screw pull-out, is uncommon; however, drill, guide wire or screw breakage and suboptimal screw position are recognised challenges associated with the Buck's repair technique.

While failure of the lumbar stress fractures to heal after surgery can be evident on post-operative imaging, the clinical consequences of these bony non-unions can be variable. While some studies suggest non-fusion patients after pars repair have inferior clinical results, other studies have detailed players being able to return to play despite a lack of radiological bony healing.

Despite initial fracture healing after surgical stabilisation, a recurrence of a lumbar stress fracture is still possible in cricketers following a return to play (~10% personal experience rate). This is a clear reminder that surgical intervention cannot claim to be universally successful in creating resilient and durable healing in these highly stressed anatomical environments.

30.9 What Are the Unique Considerations for Post-surgical Rehabilitation?

Post-surgical rehabilitation has similarities to standard non-surgical protocols, albeit with some notable differences.

The rehabilitation protocol can be broken down into several distinct phases with clear objectives defined for each phase which will prepare the athlete for transition to the next one (Table 30.1.)

One of the primary differences between surgical and non-surgical management is the first 2–4 weeks post-surgery versus those of non-surgical management. In a non-surgical setting, the initial symptoms of the acute injury are often minimal after the first 48–72 h, and the athlete can resume most activities without symptoms apart from bowling. In the surgical setting, Phase 1 is centred around wound care and pain management, both of which are sometimes underestimated prior to surgery. The presence of an infection or elevated pain levels will need specific management and delay the transition to the more active phases until they are under control.

Once the wound has healed satisfactorily and the pain has stabilised, the active Phases 2 to 6 can begin. These are based around progressions of load, which are thought to be safe based on accepted healing times for the muscle and bone affected during the surgical process. These active phases are the same as for the non-surgical man-

Table 30.1 Typical phases of a post-surgical rehabilitation protocol [6]

Phase (weeks)	Objective	Activities	Avoid/precautions
Phase 1 (Weeks 0–2)	Wound care/pain management	Regain functional ROM ADL	Wound infection Over exertion (range of movement, ADL, i.e. lifting)
Phase 2 (Weeks 2–6)	Muscle and bone healing	Lower abdominal activation Mobility patterns (neutral spine) Non-axial leg strength Fitness (non-weight bearing)	End range extension Increased ground reaction forces, i.e. running
Phase 3 (Weeks 6–10)	Trunk and leg strength	Lower limb strengthening Multi-joint strength Anti-rotation strength Off-feet conditioning (Alter-G, X-trainer)	End range extension Lumbar spine rotation Increased ground reaction forces, i.e. running
Phase 4 (Weeks 10–16)	Running	Trunk rotation strength Plyometrics Interval running (progression of intensity is the focus)	Combined rotation and ground reaction forces, i.e. bowling
Phase 5 (Weeks 16+)	Bowling	Gradual progression of bowling load, frequency, and intensity	Accelerated loading programme
Phase 6 (TBC)	Playing	Progression of playing intensities back to the original level of competition	Accelerated playing programme, i.e. multi-day games as first game time

agement process. The balance required is to prevent deconditioning by increasing load as quickly as possible without jeopardising the healing/integrity of the surgical site, thus returning the athlete to bowling as quickly and as safely as possible.

Post-surgical radiological imaging of the surgical site is restricted to plain radiographs and Computed Tomography (CT) scans, as the implants used generate metal artefacts that degrade the imaging detail obtainable from subsequent MRI scans. As these imaging techniques expose the individual to ionising radiation, their use is restricted. A plain radiograph is typically used to provide an overall assessment of the position of the surgical construct post-surgery. A CT scan is commonly employed 3–6 months post-surgery to confirm progression towards union.

The timing of a return to unrestricted playing following surgical stabilisation varies depending on multiple factors, including radiological progress, post-operative complications, avoidance of other non-spine-related injuries and any important scheduling priorities for that player. A typical rehabilitation protocol targets a return to full-intensity playing 6–8 months post-op; however, bespoke accelerated rehabilitation programmes have been successful in allowing an earlier return to play (i.e. within 4–5 months) if key games, selection deadlines or, for the professionals, key international series or World Cups are critical to the player's career.

As with players whose injuries have been managed non-surgically, bowling action analysis and bowling load management are also key considerations.

30.10 Illustrative Case Study

A 26-year-old professional international left-arm bowling all-rounder presented with a recurrent right L3 complete pars lumbar stress fracture with corresponding high bone marrow oedema noted on MRI (Fig. 30.5a-c). He had normal disc morphology but did have established long-standing bilateral L5 pars defects with no associated spondylolisthesis or bone marrow oedema. In the preceding 3 years, he had undergone two full non-surgical rehabilitation programmes for recurrent injuries in the same (right L3) location. He elected to proceed with surgical repair in an attempt to achieve a more robust and resilient healing response instead of a further (third) cycle of non-surgical care.

Surgical intervention involved a bilateral L3 pedicle screw-cable construct with curettage of the fracture site and bone grafting harvested from the posterior iliac crest (Fig. 30.5d-e). Post-operatively he developed a superficial wound infection that resolved with oral antibiotics and dressings. His rehabilitation protocol was deferred until the infection had resolved.

Thereafter he progressed through the phases of his post-surgical rehabilitation protocol. Bony union was confirmed on imaging taken 5 months post-surgery (Fig. 30.5f). He returned to play state-level cricket 6 months after surgery, made his return to international cricket 14 months post-operatively and continues to play international white ball cricket 7 years on from his procedure. He has had no further interruption to his playing career due to the same or other lumbar spinal issues.

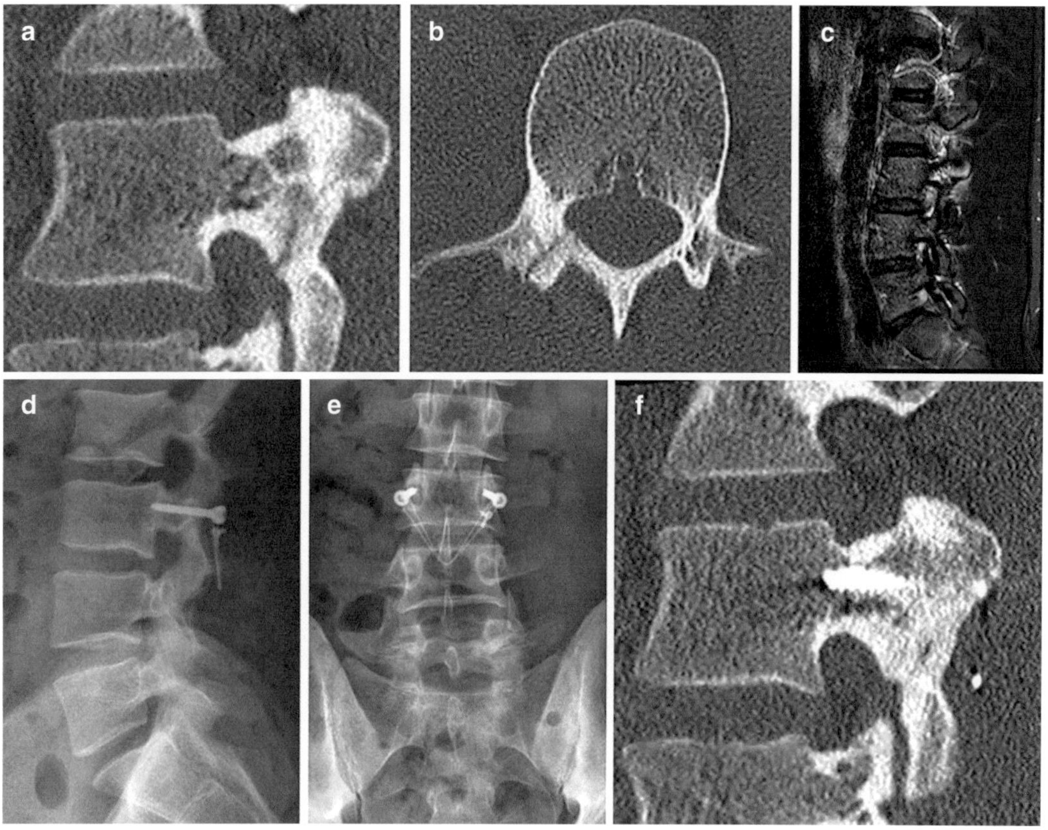

Fig. 30.5 Case study of an international left arm all-rounder with a recurrent right L3 lumbar stress injury, with associated bone marrow oedema (**a**-**c**), treated with an L3 cable-screw construct (**d**, **e**), with post-operative union, confirmed on CT taken 5 months post-surgery (**f**) and successful return to play

30.11 Conclusion

While rarely required, for cricketers with lumbar stress fractures that have failed non-surgical treatment, modern direct surgical repair techniques have been shown to be highly effective. Factors that influence the decision to operate are evolving. A better understanding of those injuries at high risk of recurrence may allow earlier surgical consideration.

References

1. Crawford CH, Ledonio CGT, Bess RS, Buchowski JM, Burton DC, Hu SS, et al. Current evidence regarding the etiology, prevalence, natural history, and prognosis of pediatric lumbar spondylolysis: a report from the Scoliosis Research Society evidence-based medicine committee. Spine Deform. 2015;3(1):12–29.
2. Saw A, Eales B, Jones N, Obst A, Smith M, Kountouris A, et al. Lumbar bone stress injuries and nonunited defects in elite Australian cricket players. Clin J Sport Med. 2024;34(1):44–51.
3. Buck JE. Direct repair of the defect in spondylolisthesis. Preliminary report. J Bone Joint Surg. 1970;52-B:432–7.
4. Drazin D, Shirzadi A, Jeswani S, Ching H, Rosner J, Rasouli A, et al. Direct surgical repair of spondylolysis in athletes: indications, techniques, and outcomes. Neurosurg Focus. 2011;31(5):E9.
5. Panteliadis P, Nagra NS, Edwards KL, Behrbalk E, Boszczyk B. Athletic population with spondylolysis: review of outcomes following surgical repair or conservative management. vol. 6, Global Spine Journal. Thieme Medical Publishers, Inc.; 2016. p. 615–25.
6. Schouten R, Shackel D, Inglis G. Surgical repair of lumbar stress fractures in professional cricketers. J Spine Surg. 2021;7(3):385–93.

7. Wilson L, Altaf F, Tyler P. Percutaneous pars interarticularis screw fixation: a technical note. Eur Spine J. 2016;25(6):1651–4.
8. Mohammed N, Patra DP, Narayan V, Savardekar AR, Dossani RH, Bollam P, et al. A comparison of the techniques of direct pars interarticularis repairs for spondylolysis and low-grade spondylolisthesis: a meta-analysis. Neurosurg Focus. 2018;44(1):E10.
9. Hardcastle PH. The journal of bone and joint surgery repair of spondylolysis in young fast bowlers.
10. Debnath UK, Freeman BJC, Gregory P, de la Harpe D, Kerslake RW, Webb JK. Clinical outcome and return to sport after the surgical treatment of spondylolysis in young athletes. J Bone Joint Surg B. 2003;85(2):244–9.
11. Ranawat VS, Dowell JK, Heywood-Waddington MB. Stress fractures of the lumbar pars interarticularis in athletes: a review based on long-term results of 18 professional cricketers. Injury. 2003;34(12):915–9.

31 Personal Reflections on the Emergence of Cricket Sports Medicine and Lumbar Stress Fracture Management in Australia

John W. Orchard

31.1 Introduction

The history of cricket in Australia goes back to at least the mid-nineteenth century [1]. The history of cricket in England possibly starts 200 years before this, but the history of fast bowling with an overarm action starts in the 1860s, close to the time when England started to tour Australia and play matches against the colonies such as Victoria and New South Wales. One of the most influential books of Australian sporting history, perhaps Australian history in general, is 'Tom Wills: the first hard man of Australian sport' by Sydney psychiatrist and historian Greg de Moore [1], who has written the foreword for this textbook. The true and complete history of Australia is that Indigenous Australians lived for many thousands of years prior to white European appearance (which is legitimately both considered settlement from one perspective and invasion from the equally valid alternate perspective). Modern Australian history is that we (along with perhaps the USA) are both one of the world's greatest immigrant nations and one of the world's greatest sporting nations. Our national semi-Indigenous sport is Australian (Rules) Football, but perhaps our true national sport is cricket, in that it is at least the second most popular sport in every state and territory in Australia. The history of the development of Australian Football and cricket in Australia intersect remarkably, with Tom Wills being the centre point of that intersection, detailed in Greg de Moore's wonderful book [1].

The so-called 'Big 3' countries in cricket are England, Australia and India. England and Australia share the longest history with India usurping both as the modern superpower of the game. India is the world home of spin (slow) bowling, which is most suited to the dry pitches prepared in the subcontinent. England is the home of swing and seam bowling, with the combination of the Dukes ball, moist rye-grass pitches and prevailing overcast humid weather meaning that pace bowlers can weave magic with the ball. Australia is the spiritual home of pure fast bowling, with hard and true pitches that suit batting and generally make life tough for all but the quickest bowlers. Without the same movement in the air and off the seam as occurs in England, the prime way that the fast bowler can beat the batters in Australia is with true air speed. But because fast bowlers must bowl so many deliveries at pace (particularly in the traditional red ball format of cricket), overuse injury is common and nowhere more so than the lumbar spine.

Our modern understanding is that lumbar stress fractures in cricket would have been occurring in the nineteenth century, as whenever bowlers deliver at pace using an overarm action, there will be the tendency to overload the spine.

J. W. Orchard (✉)
School of Public Health, University of Sydney, Sydney, NSW, Australia
e-mail: john.orchard@sydney.edu.au

B. Olivier, J. W. Orchard (eds.), *Cricket Sports Medicine*,
https://doi.org/10.1007/978-981-96-6321-7_31

31.2 The Early West Australian Influence

Spondylolisthesis (and spondylolysis) have been known medical diagnoses shortly after the development of X-ray in the early twentieth century, although initially, the lesions were thought to occur primarily in childhood [2]. Lumbar stress fractures were perhaps first 'discovered' as a diagnosis in fast bowlers in Australia in the early 1970s, when young Australian fast bowler, Dennis Lillee, was diagnosed with one by his medical and fitness team in Perth, Western Australia. This hub quickly became the Australian and perhaps the world centre of excellence in the management of lumbar stress fractures for a 25-year period from the mid-1970s, with the first Australia proliferation of scientific publications [3–10].

As per Dennis Lillee's documented history [11], his team in Perth gave him an extended period of time away from bowling in the winter of 1973 during which he wore a plaster cast for 6 weeks. This is likely the first documented case of lengthy non-surgical rehab for an elite fast bowler in Australia. Apparently in John Snow's biography, he made the comment that he thought that Dennis Lillee had been overbowled by Western Australia and Australia between 1971 and 1973 and it reduced Lillee's effectiveness [11]. As will be a recurring theme in this chapter, this is the glass half empty view (that he may have maintained express pace for longer if he had bowled fewer overs earlier). The glass half full view is that Dennis Lillee had taken the second highest number of wickets in Tests by an Australian fast bowler (at 355) up until 2024, when he was finally overtaken by Mitchell Starc. Only Glenn McGrath currently stands above these two in terms of all-time Test wickets from an Australian pace bowler. It should be very hard, in hindsight, to criticise the overall management of Dennis Lillee, one of the all-time greats of fast bowling. The counterargument, therefore, is that the repetition of skill development was critical in Lillee attaining his prowess and that stress fractures were an almost necessary side effect.

The other major development out of Western Australia which emerged in the 1980s was the view that lumbar stress fractures could be prevented by amending the bowling action. The culprit bowling technique was the 'mixed' action, halfway between the classic side-on bowling action (for which Lillee was the prototype, Fig. 31.1) and the front-on bowling action (typified in the 1980s by Bob Willis of England and then later Glenn McGrath himself). The West Australian view prevailed as, allegedly, the primary way to prevent stress fractures was to modify one's action to either be side-on or front-on, but not in between, and this was meant to be a way to avoid stress fractures.

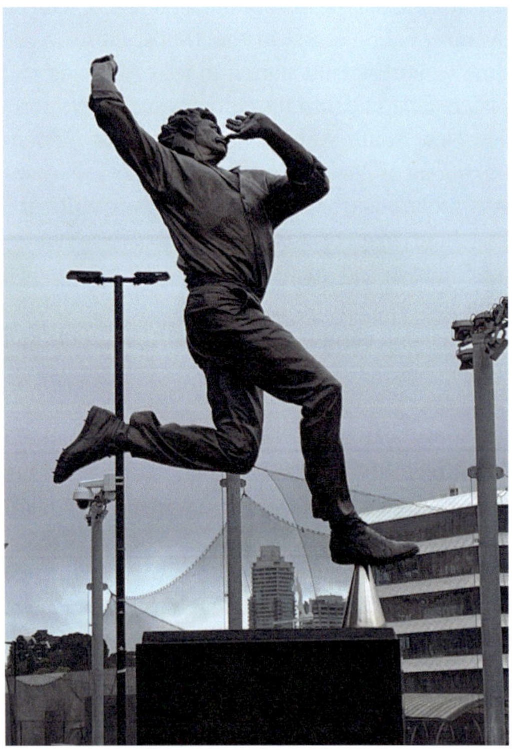

Fig. 31.1 The statue of Dennis Lillee outside the MCG members, showing his famous side-on action

31.3 Melbourne in the Early 1980s

In Melbourne in the early to mid-1980s, a young doctor named Greg Hoy, who would go on to become one of the city's top upper limb and shoulder surgeons, gathered together data he'd been working on as the Victorian Sheffield Shield cricket team doctor and as part of a Fellowship in Surgery he was doing at Monash University over the previous few years.

We are blessed 40 years later to have this data available as a time capsule. It may or may not surprise you to read that the vast majority of pace bowlers had both chronic back pain and X-ray evidence of unhealed (spondylolisthesis or pars defect) stress fractures of the lumbar spine (Table 31.1 and Fig. 31.2). Stress fractures not only did not stop you from making it as a fast bowler in the Victorian Shield team; it almost seemed as if they were essential! That is, until you realise that correlation is not causation. The repetition of bowling thousands of deliveries was the essential part, and the stress fractures were the seemingly inevitable side effect of the former. The Greg Hoy data would precede but be very similar to the Western Australia data published a few years later [3, 6, 7].

Greg Hoy would not go on to specialise in the lumbar spine (he had perhaps seen enough to learn that this would not be a wise choice), but he did decide to become a surgeon. A colleague and friend of his in Melbourne, Trefor James, would choose a career step far more radical at the time in choosing to specialise in sports medicine (an almost yet-to-be-created speciality). Trefor would go on to be the most influential sports physician in cricket in Australia in the 1990s and 2000s, being appointed as the official doctor for the Victorian Cricket Association (VCA) in 1990.

Meanwhile, I was a 15-year-old studying Year 11 at school in 1982. On December 30, I took the train down to the MCG to watch Allan Border and Jeff Thomson try to win an Ashes Test by breaking the all-time tenth wicket partnership. They failed by three runs, but seeing the excitement live may have turned me into a cricket fan

Table 31.1 Victorian Sheffield Shield squad pace bowlers of the early 1980s

Case number	Position type	History and symptoms	Finding on X-ray
1	Fast bowler	Lumbar pain 80–81	No stress fractures seen
2	Fast bowler	Chronic back pain	Spondylolisthesis x 2 on X-ray, multiple stress fractures, scoliosis
3	Fast bowler	Lumbar pain 82–83	Spondylolisthesis on X-ray
4	Fast bowler	No back pain	No indication of an X-ray
5	Pace all-rounder	Chronic lumbar pain	? Discogenic (? No X-ray)
6	Fast bowler	Chronic lumbar pain	Spondylolisthesis on X-ray
7	Fast bowler	Lumbar pain 1982	Spondylolysis on X-ray
8	Fast bowler, retired 1982	Chronic lumbar pain	Spondylolysis on X-ray
9	Fast bowler	Back pain	Spondylolisthesis L4/5 on X-ray
10	Fast bowler	Back pain	No X-ray
11	Fast bowler	Back pain	Spondylolysis on X-ray 79–80
12	Ex-pace all-rounder now batsman	Retired from pace bowling due to injuries	Spondylolysis on X-ray 1981
13	Pace all-rounder	Back pain	Spondylolisthesis L5/S1 on X-ray
14	Pace all-rounder	Chronic lumbar pain	No X-ray
15	Ex-junior pace bowler now batsman	Chronic lumbar pain	Spondylolisthesis on X-ray
16	Pace all-rounder	Back pain 2 years	No X-ray

Data courtesy of Greg Hoy

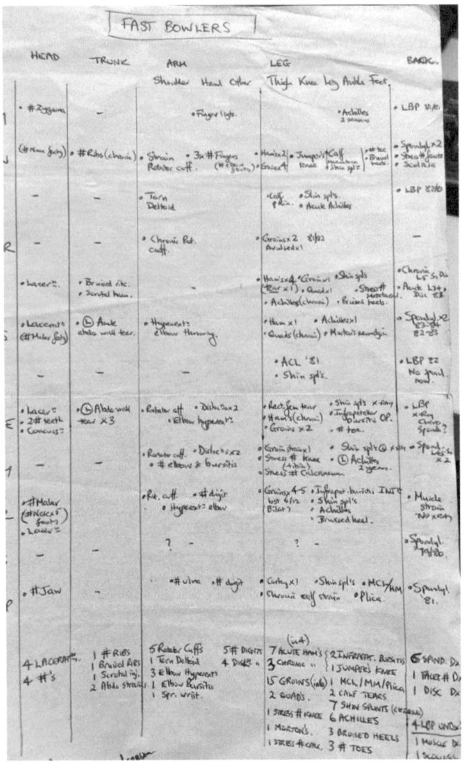

Fig. 31.2 Some of Greg Hoy's handwritten notes from the mid-1980s

for life. After the match, I managed to get my autograph book signed by Geoff Lawson, who would go on to be the best fast bowler in the country during the 1980s. His crowning glory was to lead the bowling attack on the successful 1989 Ashes tour, which regained the trophy in England, setting Australia up for 15 years of dominance of this famous series. He later revealed that he battled stress fractures in the back for most of his career, taking the viewpoint that they were inevitable and you needed to keep bowling and be tough enough to play through them [12]. From the data of the era from both Victoria and WA, he was in good company.

31.4 Increasing Professionalism in the Late 1990s

In the 1990s, most of the domestic teams started to appoint physiotherapists who were close to full-time during the summer months. Pat Farhart was one of these working with the NSWCA (New South Wales Cricket Association). The Australian Test team already had a full-time physiotherapist in Errol Alcott. Pat helped a young fast bowler—Brett Lee—take a substantial amount of time off to recover from lumbar stress fractures a la Dennis Lillee, and as it turned out, he didn't seem to have lost any pace on his eventual return. I first met Pat in 1996, when I was working as the doctor for the Sydney Swans (having moved to Sydney to take up this job offer in late 1994), who were co-tenants of NSW Cricket at the Sydney Cricket Ground.

On December 2, 1996, Australia played the West Indies in a Test match at the SCG. The Australian opener, Matthew Elliott, seriously injured a knee colliding mid-pitch with his batting partner Mark Waugh. Errol Alcott, the physio, was looking for a doctor, but the only doctor at the ground was an honorary (unpaid) appointment of the NSWCA, who had been watching the game from the top tier and enjoying the excellent-quality French red available in the board room. At the time, I was working at a sports medicine clinic in Anzac Parade, only 3 km away, and Errol called me and asked if I could come up to the SCG dressing room to assist with the player, which I did.

By mid-1997, the Australian Cricket Board (ACB) had decided this amateur medical set-up needed to be upgraded, and they invited the impressive VCA doctor, Trefor James, to become the official ACB doctor as well, which he accepted. One of his early and most important achievements was that there should be paid medical staff at the grounds for all First Class matches, with the expectation that, whilst being paid, the doctors should be attentive and ready to react to injuries and illnesses at all times, as they would be for professional football matches. Another of his decisions was that the ACB should institute an injury surveillance programme, and he/they invited me to run it, as I had been doing similar work for the Australian Football League (AFL) at the time [13]. It wasn't too long before our first major publication [14]. Fast bowlers slowly started presenting with back pain to team physiotherapists and had access to team doctors, usually sports physicians or GPs with a sports interest, and they were getting their backs scanned and often being advised to rest to allow the pain from stress fractures to reduce [15].

31.5 Workload Studies in the 2000s

A research team of Pat Farhart's (along with PhD student Rebecca Dennis, working under Caroline Finch) led the first few studies on workload and its relationship to injury in fast bowlers in the early 2000s [16–18]. These studies led to Cricket Australia first publishing workload guidelines for junior fast bowlers in the mid-2000s. Pat also assisted a medical student, Richard Saw, who later would become the men's Test team doctor, to do a study of throwing workload and shoulder pain [19]. This set of research kicked off a flurry of workload studies over the next decade [20–26]. Trying to change fast bowlers away from having mixed actions didn't seem to be solving the stress fracture issue, and we thought perhaps workload studies might eventually have more success.

In addition to continuing my role as injury surveillance co-ordinator with Cricket Australia (CA), I did a tour to India with the national team in 2007 (the first time in over 20 years that they had taken a doctor on tour, where I worked with the new men's team physiotherapist, Alex Kountouris) [27] and I took on the role of the State Medical Officer for CNSW in 2008.

31.6 A Home Ashes Loss and a Domestic T20 Match Which Changed Everything

Cricket Australia's men's Test team reached a nadir point in the home summer of 2010–11, in which the visiting England team thrashed the Australians 3-1. We had been out-batted, out-bowled and out-fielded, with England shining briefly as the best team in the world. There were massive recriminations, and an 'Argus report' was commissioned to find out what had gone wrong. It took a few years for Australia to rise again, but the green shoots were visible soon after that Ashes loss. In what was apparently a meaningless domestic T20 match on January 19, 2011, at Stadium Australia between Tasmania and NSW, a young player named Pat Cummins made his professional debut. I remember getting a text, as I watched from the bench, from Alex Kountouris asking 'who is this young kid? He is bowling absolute rockets!' My reply was prescient: 'I think you'll know him very well soon. They are already talking about picking him in the Test team, so you'll probably be looking after his stress fractures before too long'. None of this was exaggeration. Within 2 months, Pat Cummins had his first lumbar stress fracture (after bowling 65 overs in the Shield final in March), and within 10 months, he made his Test debut on a tour of South Africa. The most important outcome, by far, was that the selectors for the mediocre Australian squad decided that they had to invest in youth, and within 12 months Pat Cummins had an official Cricket Australia contract, alongside two of the other promising young fast bowlers from the same state, Josh Hazlewood and Mitchell Starc. The implication of this decision was—in hindsight—earth-shattering. The central contracts meant that Cricket Australia was the primary contracting body for these three fast bowlers, not Cricket NSW. So when all three of these fast bowlers soon developed lumbar stress fractures (and it would be on multiple occasions for Cummins and Hazlewood), CA led the management, not CNSW. Alex Kountouris—backed by his new bosses Pat Howard and Peter Blanch—insisted that whenever these young fast bowlers were diagnosed with a stress fracture, they wouldn't bowl until the fractures had completely healed on scans [28]. This didn't always suit the NSW coaching staff, who were deprived of their best young bowlers much of the time in the early 2010s and had lived through the prevailing culture that it was OK to keep bowling with stress fractures if the pain wasn't bad enough. Cricket Australia just backed the advice of their lead physio that it was in the long-term interests of CA to preserve the lumbar anatomy of their most promising fast bowlers. I was part of the team at the coalface in Sydney, along with physios Murray Ryan and Danny Redrup, instructed to hold the line on keeping the bowlers in the rehab room until their stress fractures had healed. We managed to, despite occasional attacks in the media questioning the strategy [29], perhaps to be expected when you are trying to achieve a paradigm shift.

Alex Kountouris went even further with a study showing how common it was for junior fast bowlers to have asymptomatic bone stress which often led to later stress fractures [30]. Andrew Rotstein in Melbourne led a group of radiologists around Australia developing a technique of imaging stress fractures using MRI, which did not involve radiation [28]. This led to a strategy of end-of-season asymptomatic screening of junior fast bowlers. This process, eventually, reduced playing time missed through back injuries [31], but also now proof that the average lumbar stress fracture in an Australian elite fast bowler heals (>80% of the time in the 2010s, compared to almost never back in the 1980s) [32]. The ultimate vindication is that the modern Australian men's Test bowling attack (Cummins, Starc, Hazlewood and Lyon) is the most successful and resilient of all time (the only quartet of bowlers to have played together, all having taken 250 Test wickets, and having taken the most wickets in Tests of all-time playing as a foursome).

31.7 From 'Can You Be an International Fast Bowler Without Stress Fractures?' to 'Can You Be One with Unhealed Stress Fractures'?

The only disserve done by the Cummins, Hazlewood and Starc cartel is any suggestion that we've finally 'beaten' stress fractures. It was a rare alignment of the planets that allowed these three modern greats the luxury of time to get their bodies right before the pressure was truly on to win Test matches for Australia. Many aspiring fast bowlers aren't good enough early enough to have that luxury of time. A comparison of two of the great understudies to the 'Big 3' shows the trade-off that still exists for all young fast bowlers. These two other excellent bowlers of the same generation who would have played more Tests, were it not for the 'Big 3', are James Pattinson and Michael Neser. James Pattinson's career preparation was out of the old-school textbook. He suffered stress fractures when very young and sometimes played through them. Born in the same year as Mitchell Starc, Pattinson had played the majority of his 21 Tests before Pat Cummins had even played his second Test for Australia. Injury (most often recurrent back injuries) [33] and the eventual emergence of the Big 3 cost him greater representation, but he should look back proudly on his career as being an awesome one. Another terrific fast bowler born in the same year as Pattinson and Starc (1990) is Michael Neser. Neser took the more modern approach to lumbar bone stress in his teenage years, although not initially because of insistence of his state cricket programme. Neser's father Chris is actually a spinal orthopaedic surgeon, and he strongly urged his son to temporarily avoid pace bowling after his first stress fracture at age 15 and concentrate on batting and off-spin until his lumbar bones had strengthened [34]. Michael Neser's career has already lasted longer than James Pattinson's, primarily due to having fewer injuries, but being stuck behind the Big 3 it is unlikely that Neser will go close to matching even Pattinson's number of Test caps. So, of the two approaches: Neser vs Pattinson, who has ended up with the more successful career? The answer must be that they've both had outstanding careers, they are both capped Test cricketers and should be very proud of their achievements and not regret a single thing.

The trade-off of optimum long-term management of lumbar stress fractures versus not jeopardising what might be a narrow window to achieve a professional cricket career is a real one. On the day of the WBBL03 (Women's Big Bash League) final in Perth in 2018, a Sydney Sixer international academy player, Irishwoman Kim Garth, revealed to the team physio that mild back pain she had been reporting might be worse than first thought, and she'd like to get a scan the day after the match. It turned out she had played the whole tournament—successfully—with a lumbar stress fracture [35]. In this instance, the opportunity to go from essentially being an amateur player in Ireland to having a fully professional career playing cricket in Australia was too good to pass up for Kim. The window to impress teams in Australia was so narrow that if she had missed the WBBL03 tournament with lumbar stress fractures, she may never have fulfilled her dream of being paid a living wage to play full-time professional cricket. The 'old-school' approach was certainly the right one for her, at the right time, showing that even in the modern era the management of these injuries must be situational.

It is worth briefly noting that in female fast bowlers (and female players in general), there are more lower limb stress fractures than lumbar spine stress fractures [31]. The primary cause of the latter is high workloads of pace bowling, with the rotational element being the key mechanism. Female fast bowlers bowl fewer overs than males (because they don't play nearly as much red ball cricket), but they are now running as much in training for general fitness, leading to relatively more lower limb stress fractures.

Much as some people would hate the analogy, I liken Australia's COVID strategy to our lumbar bone stress strategy. When fast bowlers are young, it is generally preferable to maintain a 'zero tolerance' strategy to lumbar bone stress, if possible, just as we tried to maintain a zero COVID strategy in Australia (as did New Zealand) prior to vaccination becoming available. When a fast bowler hits the age of perhaps 23 or 24 (when bone density finally peaks), that is the age analogous to COVID vaccination when you can shift attitude from 'zero tolerance' of lumbar bone stress to a far less cautious and interventional attitude. There is some evidence that lumbar bone stress is more benign (less likely to lead to complete stress fracture) in adult fast bowlers [36] than juniors [30].

It is also worth noting that the research centre of the cricket world may have recently shifted somewhat from Melbourne, Sydney and Brisbane [37] to Loughborough in the UK. The ECB has already heavily invested in PhD students to learn more about lumbar spine injuries and continue to tackle the biggest problem in cricket [38–43].

In conclusion, we haven't solved the problem of lumbar stress fracture in fast bowlers in cricket, as the majority of elite junior pace bowlers will eventually develop bone stress. What we have done in the modern era is give junior fast bowlers an option: the old-school management or modern management (which is usually, but not always, a better option for aspiring elite bowlers). It is possible to reach adult mid-20s with a completely intact lumbar spine and be an elite fast bowler, and it is desirable; this strategy however will often lead to regular downtime in the junior years, which represents a challenging trade-off. It has been a privilege to be part of a medical and physiotherapy team in Australia which has navigated this paradigm shift over the past 40 years.

31.8 Postscript

Shortly after finalising this chapter, like many others, I was fascinated by the case of the gruesome murder of United Healthcare's CEO Brian Thompson in New York. The alleged assassin, Luigi Mangione, has already had plentiful details of his life published in the mainstream media as commentators search for motives for the killing. The first eye-catching detail was that he had apparently suffered from chronic back pain for many years due to sports-related spondylolisthesis. This is a reminder of the potential severe effect on mental health of the combination of pain from a chronic back injury and also the inability to keep playing sports/exercising, which for many young people is one of the most important factors protecting mental health. The second detail is that from social media postings, it appeared as if Luigi Mangione held a grudge against the US healthcare system, particularly its propensity to deny funding for healthcare treatments. This extra point was a reminder to me that I needed to 'record our privilege' about everything detailed in the chapter above. At the elite level in sport in Australia, we are very well funded and can afford and order as many lumbar MRI scans as we need to best manage our players. At the community level, even in Australia, and certainly in many of the other cricket-mad countries, it may not be financially realistic to order preventive scans, follow-up scans, and have dozens of physiotherapy appointments during rehabilitation. Management of lumbar bone stress in athletes is extremely challenging *before* you take into account financial considerations, which themselves only add to the challenge. Maintaining good mental health during lengthy rehabilitation and making choices which appropriately weigh up short-term and long-term concerns are dilemmas in both well-funded elite programmes and in community-level sports.

References

1. de Moore G. Tom Wills: first wild man of Australian sport. Sydney: Allen & Unwin; 2008.
2. Lu Y, Le VH, Lebwohl NH. Spondylolisthesis: a historical perspective on etiology, diagnosis, and treatment. In: Wollowick AL, Sarwahi V, editors. Spondylolisthesis: diagnosis, non-surgical management, and surgical techniques. Cham: Springer International Publishing; 2023. p. 3–17.
3. Annear PT, Chakera TM, Foster DH, Hardcastle PH. Pars interarticularis stress and disc degeneration in cricket's potent strike force: the fast bowler. Aust N Z J Surg. 1992;62(10):768–73.
4. Elliott B, Foster D, Blanksby B. Send the stumps flying: the science of fast bowling. Perth: University of Western Australia; 1989.
5. Elliott BC. Back injuries and the fast bowler in cricket. J Sports Sci. 2000;18(12):983–91. https://doi.org/10.1080/026404100446784.
6. Elliott BC, Davis JW, Khangure MS, Hardcastle P, Foster D. Disc degeneration and the young fast bowler in cricket. Clin Biomech. 1993;8:227–34.
7. Elliott BC, Hardcastle PH, Burnett AE, Foster DH. The influence of fast bowling and physical factors on radiologic features in high performance young fast bowlers. Sports Med Train Rehabil. 1992;3(2):113–30.
8. Hardcastle P. Lumbar pain in fast bowlers. Aust Fam Physician. 1991;20(7):943, 6–51.
9. Hardcastle P, Annear P, Foster DH, Chakera TM, McCormick C, Khangure M, et al. Spinal abnormalities in young fast bowlers. J Bone Joint Surg Br. 1992;74(3):421–5.
10. Hardcastle PH. Repair of spondylolysis in young fast bowlers. J Bone Joint Surg Br. 1993;75(3):398–402.
11. Dennis Lillee. Accessed https://en.wikipedia.org/wiki/Dennis_Lillee
12. Lane D. Feeling the stress: why young bowlers face fractures caused by perils of pace. Sydney Morning Herald. 2012. https://www.smh.com.au/sport/cricket/feeling-the-stress-why-young-bowlers-face-fractures-caused-by-perils-of-pace-20121117-29ixc.html
13. Orchard J, Seward H, Brukner P. Comparison of injury profiles in the professional football codes played in Australia. Med Sci Sports Exerc. 1993;25(5 SUPPL).:S50–S. https://doi.org/10.1249/00005768-199305001-00276.
14. Orchard J, James T, Alcott E, Carter S, Farhart P. Injuries in Australian cricket at first class level 1995/96 to 2000/2001. Br J Sports Med. 2002;36:270–5.
15. Orchard J, Saw R, Kountouris A, Redrup D, Farhart P, Sims K. Management of lumbar bone stress injury in cricket fast bowlers and other athletes. S Afr J Sports Med. 2023;35(1). https://doi.org/10.17159/2078-516X/2023/v35i1a15172.
16. Dennis R. Australian cricket board national fast bowling workload and injury study 2000–2002. In: Noakes T, Stretch RA, Vaughan CL (Eds.). Second world congress of science and medicine in cricket. Cape Town. 2003;81–2. ComPress, South Africa
17. Dennis R, Farhart P, Goumas C, Orchard J. Bowling workload and the risk of injury in elite cricket fast bowlers. J Sci Med Sport. 2003;6(3):359–67.
18. Dennis R, Finch C, Farhart P. Is bowling workload a risk factor for injury to Australian junior cricket fast bowlers? Br J Sports Med. 2005;39:843–6.
19. Saw R, Dennis R, Bentley D, Farhart P. Throwing workload and injury risk in elite cricketers. Br J Sports Med. 2011;45(10):805–8.
20. Blanch P, Gabbett TJ. Has the athlete trained enough to return to play safely? The acute: chronic workload ratio permits clinicians to quantify a player's risk of subsequent injury. Br J Sports Med. 2016;50(8):471–5. https://doi.org/10.1136/bjsports-2015-095445.
21. Blanch P, Orchard J, Kountouris A, Sims K, Beakley D. Different tissue type categories of overuse injuries to cricket fast bowlers have different severity and incidence which varies with age. S Afr J Sports Med. 2015;27(4):108–13.
22. Hulin B, Gabbett T, Blanch P, Chapman P, Bailey D, Orchard J. Spikes in acute workload are associated with increased injury risk in elite cricket fast bowlers. Br J Sports Med. 2014;48:708–12.
23. Hulin B, Gabbett T, Lawson D, Caputi P, Sampson J. The acute:chronic workload ratio predicts injury: high chronic workload may decrease injury risk in elite rugby league players. Br J Sports Med. 2016;50(4):231–6.
24. Orchard J, Blanch P, Paoloni J, Kountouris A, Sims K, Orchard J, et al. Cricket fast bowling workload patterns as risk factors for tendon, muscle, bone and joint injuries. Br J Sports Med. 2015;49(16):1064–8.
25. Orchard J, Blanch P, Paoloni J, Kountouris A, Sims K, Orchard J, et al. Fast bowling match workloads over 5–26 days and risk of injury in the following month. J Sci Med Sport. 2015;18:26–30.
26. Orchard J, James T, Portus M, Kountouris A, Dennis R. Fast bowlers in cricket demonstrate up to 3- to

4-week delay between high workloads and increased risk of injury. Am J Sports Med. 2009;37:1186–92.
27. Orchard J. Aspects of medical care for Australian athletes competing in the Indian subcontinent. Sports Health. 2008;26(3):34–7.
28. Singh SP, Rotstein AH, Saw AE, Saw R, Kountouris A, James T. Radiological healing of lumbar spine stress fractures in elite cricket fast bowlers. J Sci Med Sport. 2021;24(2):112–5. https://doi.org/10.1016/j.jsams.2020.06.018.
29. Haigh G. How cricket's 'workload management' is poisoning the game and its players. The Australian. 2018.
30. Kountouris A, Sims K, Beakley D, Saw AE, Orchard J, Rotstein A, et al. MRI bone marrow oedema precedes lumbar bone stress injury diagnosis in junior elite cricket fast bowlers. Br J Sports Med. 2019;53(19):1236–9. https://doi.org/10.1136/bjsports-2017-097930.
31. Orchard JW, Inge P, Sims K, Kountouris A, Saw AE, Saw R, et al. Comparison of injury profiles between elite Australian male and female cricket players. J Sci Med Sport. 2023;26(1):19–24. https://doi.org/10.1016/j.jsams.2022.12.002.
32. Saw A, Eales B, Jones N, Obst A, Smith M, Kountouris A, et al. Lumbar bone stress injuries and nonunited defects in elite Australian cricket players. Clin J Sport Med. 2023. https://doi.org/10.1097/jsm.0000000000001132.
33. AAP. James Pattinson's shocking injury history. 2017. Accessed https://www.sbs.com.au/news/article/james-pattinsons-shocking-injury-history/zy7nfxy42
34. Harper T. Quit fast bowling in year 9, and suffered IPL debut disaster: Michael Neser's journey to the baggy green. 2021. Accessed https://www.theroar.com.au/2021/12/16/michael-nesers-long-road-to-the-baggy-green/
35. ICC. Kim Garth: 'we can take confidence from our preparation'. 2018. Accessed https://www.icc-cricket.com/news/kim-garth-we-can-take-confidence-from-our-preparation
36. Bell AJ, Nunnerley JL, Shackel DF, Coates MH, Campbell RG, Frampton CM, et al. Is MRI screening for bone marrow oedema useful in predicting lumbar bone stress injuries in adult male professional cricketers? A New Zealand pilot study. J Sci Med Sport. 2023;26(8):410–4. https://doi.org/10.1016/j.jsams.2023.06.013.
37. Dhillon MS, Patel S, Sharma S. Beyond the boundary: a bibliometric analysis of the published research on injuries in cricket. Indian J Orthop. 2023. https://doi.org/10.1007/s43465-023-00973-9.
38. Alway P, Felton P, Brooke-Wavell K, Peirce N, King M. Cricket fast bowling technique and lumbar bone stress injury. Med Sci Sports Exerc. 2021;53(3):581–9. https://doi.org/10.1249/mss.0000000000002512.
39. Alway P, Peirce N, Johnson W, King M, Kerslake R, Brooke-Wavell K. Activity specific areal bone mineral density is reduced in athletes with stress fracture and requires profound recovery time: a study of lumbar stress fracture in elite cricket fast bowlers. J Sci Med Sport. 2022;25(10):828–33. https://doi.org/10.1016/j.jsams.2022.08.006.
40. Alway P, Wedatilake T, Peirce N, Warren A, King M, Brooke-Wavell K. Bone health and asymmetry in elite female cricketers. Eur J Sport Sci. 2023;23(5):667–75. https://doi.org/10.1080/17461391.2022.2065929.
41. Keylock L, Alway P, Felton P, McCaig S, Brooke-Wavell K, King M, et al. Lumbar bone stress injuries and risk factors in adolescent cricket fast bowlers. J Sports Sci. 2022;40(12):1336–42. https://doi.org/10.1080/02640414.2022.2080161.
42. Keylock L, Alway P, Johnson W, Crabtree N, King M, Peirce N, et al. Lumbar spine bone mineral adaptation: cricket fast bowlers versus controls. BMJ Open Sport Exerc Med. 2023;9(2):e001481. https://doi.org/10.1136/bmjsem-2022-001481.
43. Keylock L, Felton P, Alway P, Brooke-Wavell K, Peirce N, King M. Lumbar bone mineral adaptation: the effect of fast bowling technique in adolescent cricketers. Med Sci Sports Exerc. 2022;54(3):438–46. https://doi.org/10.1249/mss.0000000000002820.

Part IV

Management of Common Cricket Injuries

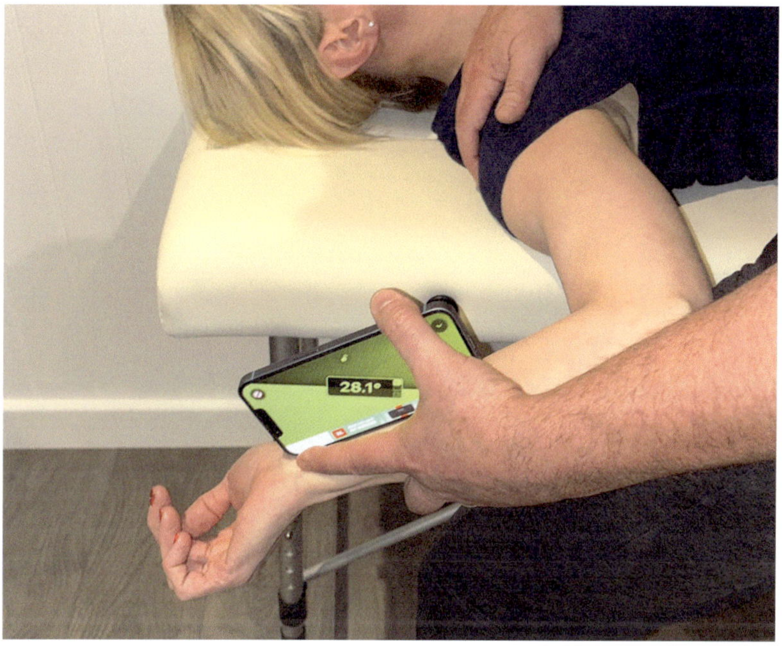

Measuring external range of motion of the shoulder in supine

Concussion in Cricket: Risk, Mechanism, Identification and Return to Play

32

Leigh Golding, John W. Orchard, and Martin Swan

32.1 Importance of Identifying Concussion

Historically, concussion was a rarely diagnosed injury in the context of competitive cricket. Thankfully, in recent years, this has changed and now concussions are assessed for and identified more readily. This is likely due to:

- New research highlighting a potential association between concussion history in sports and long-term neurocognitive problems
- Concussion identification procedures changing in other major sports
- Increased media attention for concussion cases
- The introduction of a concussion substitute in cricket by the international cricket council (ICC)

It is imperative that concussion cases are assessed for and diagnosed in a timely fashion for the following reasons:

L. Golding (✉)
Cricket Australia, Melbourne, Australia
e-mail: Leigh.golding@cricket.com.au

J. W. Orchard
School of Public Health, University of Sydney, Sydney, NSW, Australia
e-mail: John.orchard@sydney.edu.au

M. Swan
New Zealand Cricket, Auckland, New Zealand
e-mail: Martin.swan@nzc.nz

32.1.1 Missed Concussion Cases Increase the Risk of More Severe Symptoms and Prolonged Recovery

If a concussion is not diagnosed in the immediate period after the head impact, there is a significant risk that a player will provoke symptoms by continuing to undertake high-intensity exercise, leading to a recovery that is more difficult and protracted than it otherwise might have been. If the player sustains another head impact during this period, they are also more likely to have more severe symptoms and a more prolonged recovery [1].

32.1.2 Missed Concussion Cases may Increase the Risk of Poor Cricket Performance and Injury

Given that concussion is a mild traumatic brain injury (mTBI) that results in a degree of neurological impairment that may include disturbances to reaction time, balance, visual disturbance and cognitive function, it should not be surprising that cricket performance may be compromised if a concussion is not diagnosed and a player continues to play. There may also be an increased risk of the player sustaining an injury to another body part in these circumstances. Research conducted in England demonstrated a potential link between head impacts that were not diagnosed as concussion and reduced performance outcomes in cricket [2].

B. Olivier, J. W. Orchard (eds.), *Cricket Sports Medicine*,
https://doi.org/10.1007/978-981-96-6321-7_32

32.1.3 Cumulative Concussion Cases may Increase the Risk of Premature Long-Term Neurocognitive Decline

In players who sustain a concussion but are not diagnosed, there is a risk that a second impact may occur prior to recovery from the index injury. It is thought that these circumstances may increase the risk of developing long-term neurodegenerative outcomes such as memory impairment, mood disorders and personality change [3]. This link is theoretically applicable to cricket, although in practice with players averaging approximately one head impact per season or less [4], the risk is far lower than in collision or combat sports. Ongoing high-quality prospective research is required in this area; however, given the potential links, it is prudent for all healthcare practitioners to err on the side of caution when assessing for the presence of a potential concussion case.

32.1.4 The Gold Standard for Identification of Concussion in Other Professional Sports is Changing Rapidly

Other professional sports such as Rugby Union, Rugby League, Australian football, netball, American football, football (soccer), ice hockey and others have introduced more robust systems in recent years to ensure head impacts with the potential to result in a concussion are identified so that concussion can be assessed for in the most timely possible fashion. This may include measures such as dedicated 'concussion spotters' at the stadium, a mandate for independent match day medical staff to conduct all concussion assessments and match day return-to-play decisions or full head injury video surveillance systems that are either pitch side or remote in a television studio. Rugby union has successfully trialled instrumented mouthguards measuring collision impact forces. The collision sports have both far greater incidence of head trauma and a greater likelihood of missed incidents (as 'off the ball' collisions can be missed). Medical staff working in professional cricket should be aware of these gold-standard innovations when planning for and then attempting to identify concussion cases in cricket. This is challenging as the number of head impacts with high likelihood of concussion (in terms of signs on video replay) is relatively small in cricket, and to date this has not justified the introduction of dedicated video spotters.

32.1.5 There are Medicolegal Risks in Certain Countries if Concussion is not Adequately Identified

At the time of writing, there are currently active or presumptive class action concussion-related lawsuits in sports such as Rugby Union, Rugby League, Australian Rules football and football (soccer), as well as other sports, particularly in the United Kingdom, United States and Australia. Some of the allegations are that sporting bodies, or the practitioners involved in providing care, failed to adequately assess for and identify concussions in an appropriate manner and that the athletes may have suffered harm as a consequence. It is imperative that all medical staff working in cricket take as much care as possible to ensure that cases of concussion are not missed.

32.2 Concussion Incidence and Mechanism in Cricket

Approximately 0.5 concussions occur on average for every 1000 player-match hours played for females and 0.4 concussions per 1000 player-match hours played for males in Australian elite cricket [4]. Although there are fewer head impacts per hour of match exposure for female cricket players, for each head impact that occurs, there is a greater chance of a concussion being sustained in female cricket players compared to their male counterparts [4]. The reasons for this are not well understood; however, the data is similar in this regard across many sports.

T20 and 50-over cricket have higher rates of concussion per hour played compared to red ball cricket, possibly because there is less of an option to evade (as opposed to attack) in white ball cricket. The majority of concussions sustained during a match are a result of batters being struck by a pace delivery. Occasionally but less commonly, batters can sustain a concussion after being struck directly by a spin delivery. Deflection off the bat during an attempted shot is likely to increase the ball speed and, hence, increase the risk of sustaining a concussion. Batters can also be struck by the ball after throws from attempted run outs and can collide with other players while running.

The typical mechanism for fielders sustaining a concussion during a match is head contact with the ground while attempting a catch. There is commonly a 'whiplash' injury associated with this mechanism. Fielders can also sustain a head impact after being struck by the ball while attempting a catch. This is a high-risk mechanism for concussion and other associated head/neck injuries, as is any head impact where the player is not wearing a helmet. Finally, although rare, severe head injuries and concussions can occur if fielders collide with each other running in from opposite directions.

32.3 Identification of Concussion: Video Signs

After sustaining a head impact, there are a number of immediate signs that persons can display that are either immediately diagnostic of concussion or suggest that there is a significant likelihood that a concussion may have occurred. These are referred to as observed or video signs. There is a gold-standard consensus amongst sports and practitioners with regard to these signs and the appropriate action concerning diagnosing or assessing for a concussion [5]. Video replay, when available, should be viewed from as many angles as possible following a head impact to assess for the presence of these video signs that may not have been apparent when watching the incident live initially.

Category 1 video or observed signs (sometimes referred to as criteria 1 signs) are immediately diagnostic of concussion as follows:

- Loss of consciousness (confirmed or suspected)
- Tonic posturing
- Seizure/convulsion
- Clear confusion / clear behavioural change
- Motor incoordination

Category 2 video or observed signs (sometimes referred to as criteria 2 signs) suggest that there is a significant likelihood that a concussion may have occurred. The player should be *immediately removed* from play for an off-field concussion assessment. Category 2 signs are as follows:

- Possible loss of consciousness
- Possible tonic posturing
- Possible seizure / convulsion
- Possible confusion / behavioural change
- Possible motor incoordination
- Any other response or behaviour that raises the suspicion of a concussion

Although the rate of concussion is probably lower in community cricket (compared to professional cricket), concussion is still possible, and video replay and medical staff assessment are unlikely to be available. Education to teach players, umpires and team managers about the signs of potential concussion is important even at community level to ensure that removal from play is the standard response even when video replay and medical staff are not available.

32.4 Identification of Concussion: On-field Assessment

If a head impact with a significant enough force to cause a concussion has occurred and no Category 1 or 2 video or observed signs were present, then an on-field assessment should be conducted.

Concussion in cricket commonly occurs in the absence of video or observed signs compared to other sports, where concussion is more often diagnosed in the presence of these signs.

Mechanisms that are significant enough to cause a concussion include a direct impact from a pace delivery, a shot that is deflected off the bat or any player sustaining a ball impact to an unprotected head or a head impact with the ground (commonly when attempting a catch).

At elite level, the on-field assessment is likely best made by the team doctor if one is present as they are able to quickly respond to an evolving emergency and are well suited to assess for subtle cognitive impairment. Signs and symptoms that should alert a clinician to an evolving emergency include impairment of consciousness, agitation, severe or increasing headache, vomiting or focal neurological deficit. A physiotherapist with sufficient experience in assessing for concussion on-field may be a suitable alternative, particularly if they know the player well.

If it is clear that there is no immediate emergency, the player's cognitive state should be assessed by asking modified Maddocks questions for cricket:

- What venue are we at today?
- Which session of the game are we in?
- Who is bowling/batting at the moment in this game?
- What team did you play last week/game?
- What was the approximate score/your score in the last game?

The objective of asking the Maddocks questions is primarily to assess if the player is oriented to time, person and place and if they are as logical and coherent as you would expect them to be. In order to further assess, players can be asked to provide a description of the head impact event, and this can be compared to what was witnessed by the assessing practitioner. The player should be screened for any symptoms and specifically should be asked for the presence of the common symptoms of concussion which include headache, dizziness, difficulty concentrating or focusing, feeling nauseous or generally not themselves.

If the practitioner suspects that any aspect of the above assessment is unsatisfactory, then the player should be removed for an official off-field assessment. It may be clear from the on-field assessment that a concussion can immediately be diagnosed, e.g. if they are not able to correctly identify the venue or if they have reported new symptoms since the head impact that were not present prior.

32.5 Identification of Concussion: Off-field Assessment (Initial)

The off-field assessment should be a thorough and comprehensive evaluation to assess for the presence of concussion. This should be completed immediately if there is a category 2 video or observed sign or if the on-field assessment is unsatisfactory. It may also be completed at the discretion of the treating clinician in the absence of these scenarios if the impact was substantial enough for the clinician to want to undertake further assessment.

The gold-standard tool for assessing for concussion is the SCAT6 [6]. This tool should not be relied upon in isolation, and clinicians are empowered to make a diagnosis of concussion if they suspect it in the absence of an abnormal SCAT6 test.

The test should take around 15 minutes and should be conducted in a quiet area, where there is a low risk of interruptions or distractions. Ideally, all athletes should have a baseline SCAT6 test that can be used for comparison, but if this is not available then their performance should be assessed against how the clinician might expect the athlete to have performed. A clinician who is experienced in conducting the SCAT6 test is well placed to make these judgements. Some normative data on SCAT baselines have been published for various populations [7], but no baseline normative SCAT data have been published for cricket-only populations at the time of writing. A baseline SCAT6 can also identify athletes that are at increased risk of sustaining a concussion or at risk of a protracted recovery.

Specific attention should be paid to the reporting of symptoms during the SCAT6 test, as concussions are frequently associated with the reporting of symptoms. If symptoms are identified, attention should be paid to whether the athletes have significant cervicogenic (neck related), vestibular ocular motor (VOM) or cognitive symptoms. Identifying if athletes have a predominant symptom burden in these categories allows for targeted interventions during the rehabilitation process.

In addition to baseline SCAT6 tests, it can also be beneficial to have a computerised neurocognitive test for athletes. This is useful as it is able to assess different neurocognitive domains from the SCAT6 (such as reaction time). It can provide additional reassurance that an athlete has sufficiently recovered from their concussion before being considered fit to return to play.

32.6 Identification of Concussion: Off-field Assessment (Subsequent)

It is not uncommon in cricket for concussions to be diagnosed after satisfactory initial on-field and off-field assessments. Sometimes athletes will present well on the day of injury but will develop symptoms over the subsequent 72 h or so. It is, therefore, imperative to undertake a subsequent off-field assessment if the first off-field assessment was satisfactory. This should be completed either a few hours prior to the next planned match or training involvement or 2 days following the head impact (i.e. after the athlete has had two nights of sleep post injury), whichever comes sooner.

32.7 Return-to-Play Protocols and How They Might Be Tailored to Cricket

Once a concussion has been diagnosed, the athlete should not return to playing or training until they have successfully completed the required stages of a graduated return-to-play protocol [8] (see Table 32.1). Athletes can start step 1 (symptom-limited activity such as walking) as early as the day following the head impact, even if some symptoms are still present. They are able

Table 32.1 Return-to-sport (RTS) strategy

Step	Exercise strategy	Activity at each step	Cricket specific	Goal
1	Symptom-limited activity	Daily activities that do not exacerbate symptoms (e.g. walking)	N/A	Gradual reintroduction of work/school
2	Aerobic exercise **2A—light** (up to approximately 55% max HR) **then 2B—moderate** (up to approximately 70% max HR)	Stationary cycling or walking at slow to medium pace. May start light resistance training	An exercise tolerance test can be performed at this stage to establish an exercise tolerance threshold	Increase heart rate
3	Individual sport-specific exercise. Note: If sport-specific training involves any risk of inadvertent head impact, medical clearance should occur prior to step 3	Sport-specific training away from the team environment (e.g. running, change of direction and/or individual training drills). No activities at risk of head impact	Activities with no risk of head impact, e.g. ground fielding/throwing drills	Add movement, change of direction
	Steps 4–6 should begin after the resolution of any symptoms, abnormalities in cognitive function and any other clinical findings related to the current concussion, including with and after physical exertion.			
4	Non-contact training drills	Exercise to high intensity including more challenging training drills	Activities with low risk of head impact, e.g. boundary catches/batting to low-risk throwdowns and spin	Resume usual intensity of exercise, coordination and increased thinking
5	Full contact practice	Participate in normal training activities	Facing full pace sidearm and bowled deliveries	Restore confidence and assess functional skills by coaching staff
6	Return to sport	Normal game play		

Note: A minimum of 24 hours should elapse between each step

to progress to the subsequent two steps (2 and 3) even if exercise exacerbates their symptoms. They should only be permitted to progress if the exacerbation of symptoms is mild (up to two points worse than baseline on a ten-point scale) and brief (the exacerbation lasts no longer than 1 h). If the exacerbation is more than mild or brief then the athlete should stop exercise and attempt the step again the following day. Progression to stages 4 to 6 should occur only after full symptom resolution has occurred. A formal medical review by a doctor should occur following step 5 in order to provide clearance to return to full practice (i.e. batters facing pace balls). Full clearance to return to sport should only be provided once the athlete has participated in at least one full session of normal training activities without a recurrence of any symptoms.

32.8 Difficult Cases Requiring Specific Rehabilitation

In cases where athletes have any symptoms at 72 h post-head impact a SCOAT6 [9] can be conducted. This is a tool that is better suited to evaluating specific areas for potential targeted intervention as well as monitoring the recovery of athletes in the subacute phase of their concussion. Athletes with prominent vestibulocochlear deficits should receive specific rehabilitative input to address these deficits. This is best provided by a practitioner with suitable experience or expertise in this area. Similarly, athletes with prominent neck pain or other common post-concussive symptoms should be directed to a practitioner who can provide suitable targeted interventions to address these during this rehabilitative phase. Athletes with symptoms that have not resolved within 14–21 days should be referred to a medical practitioner with experience in managing complex concussion cases. This is often a neurologist or specialist Sports and Exercise Medicine physician.

32.9 The Athlete with Repeated or Complicated Concussions

A medical practitioner with experience in managing complex concussion cases should also be involved in providing care where any of the following are present:

- More than four career concussions
- A previous concussion that was complicated by psychological issues
- A previous concussion where recovery was prolonged (e.g. >21 days)
- Concussions that appear to be occurring with reduced impact thresholds

The above can be difficult to manage, and return-to-play decisions are often best made by convening a panel of medical practitioners with suitable experience to provide consensus on these cases. Very occasionally (in cricket), a difficult decision is required to decide between continued participation in cricket (with awareness of the risks associated) and retirement from the game in order to eliminate exposure from further head trauma. As per many of the other notes in this chapter, this type of dilemma is far more common in the collision sports, but it should not be assumed that cricket is immune from ever needing to consider such cases.

References

1. McCrea M, Guskiewicz KM, Marshall SW, Barr W, Randolph C, Cantu RC, et al. Acute effects and recovery time following concussion in collegiate football players: the NCAA concussion study. JAMA. 2003;290(19):2556–63. https://doi.org/10.1001/jama.290.19.2556.
2. O'Halloran P, Goggins L, Peirce N. Observable player behaviours and playing performance following helmet strikes in elite cricket. BMJ Open Sport Exerc Med. 2021;7(4):e001128. https://doi.org/10.1136/bmjsem-2021-001128.
3. Iverson GL, Castellani RJ, Cassidy JD, Schneider GM, Schneider KJ, Echemendia RJ, et al. Examining later-in-life health risks associated with sport-related concussion and repetitive head impacts: a systematic review of case-control and cohort studies. Br J Sports

Med. 2023;57(12):810–21. https://doi.org/10.1136/bjsports-2023-106890.
4. Hill T, Orchard J, Kountouris A. Incidence of concussion and head impacts in Australian elite-level male and female cricketers after head impact protocol modifications. Sports Health. 2019;11(2):180–5. https://doi.org/10.1177/1941738118811315.
5. Davis GA, Makdissi M, Bloomfield P, Clifton P, Echemendia RJ, Falvey ÉC, et al. International consensus definitions of video signs of concussion in professional sports. Br J Sports Med. 2019;53(20):1264–7. https://doi.org/10.1136/bjsports-2019-100628.
6. Echemendia RJ, Brett BL, Broglio S, Davis GA, Giza CC, Guskiewicz KM, et al. Sport concussion assessment tool™ – 6 (SCAT6). Br J Sports Med. 2023;57(11):622–31. https://doi.org/10.1136/bjsports-2023-107036.
7. Fuller GW, Govind O, Tucker R, Raftery M. Sport concussion assessment tool-third edition normative reference values for professional Rugby union players. J Sci Med Sport. 2018;21(4):347–51. https://doi.org/10.1016/j.jsams.2017.07.025.
8. Patricios JS, Schneider KJ, Dvorak J, Ahmed OH, Blauwet C, Cantu RC, et al. Consensus statement on concussion in sport: the 6th international conference on concussion in sport-Amsterdam, October 2022. Br J Sports Med. 2023;57(11):695–711. https://doi.org/10.1136/bjsports-2023-106898.
9. Echemendia RJ, Brett BL, Broglio S, Davis GA, Giza CC, Guskiewicz KM, et al. Introducing the sport concussion assessment tool 6 (SCAT6). Br J Sports Med. 2023;57(11):619–21. https://doi.org/10.1136/bjsports-2023-106849.

33 Shoulder Injuries in Cricket

Kevin Sims, Sibi Walter,
and Kushalappa Subbiah

33.1 Introduction

Injuries to the 'shoulder complex' are suitably, inherently complex. The shoulder complex contributes to all cricketing activities and, depending on the bowling style, fielding position and game format, is subjected to varying loading intensities and volume.

Although there is a relatively high prevalence of shoulder pain among elite and amateur cricketers, the incidence rates vary because most shoulder pain-related conditions do not lead to time loss. In comparison with batting or bowling activities, shoulder pain is commonly reported following fielding-throwing. Therefore, a player's primary skill (batting or bowling) may be unaffected even if their ability to throw is compromised. To offset this, a player with shoulder pain may be positioned within the inner circle where the throwing intensity is less due to the distance. This leads to a mismatch in the reported time-loss and non-time-loss shoulder pain incidence in cricket, with shoulder pain symptoms less likely to be reported and recorded in both amateur and elite cricket. In many instances, only when the shoulder pain symptoms are severe enough to affect training or match performance, do players report and seek medical advice. This may make it harder to establish the primary injury cause as many associated musculoskeletal adaptations occur within the time. This chapter will review what is known about the incidence of shoulder pain in cricketers, common pathologies, injury mechanisms and management approaches.

33.2 Epidemiology

Cricket injury surveillance studies from the last 10 years have reported varying levels of shoulder injury rates. Of the three key cricket skills, shoulder injury impacts fielding more than batting and bowling [1, 2]. In elite Australian cricketers, the incidence of match time-loss shoulder injury per 100 players per season is 3.8 and 2.8 in males and females, respectively [3]. However, if the definition of injury is expanded to include non-time-loss injury then the incidence increases to 25.3 in male and 36.9 in females [3]. Similarly, the majority (69%) of elite male English cricketers with shoulder injury did not miss any match time, but 63% reported a negative impact on fielding

K. Sims (✉)
Tennis Australia, University of Queensland, Queensland Sports Medicine Centre, Brisbane, QLD, Australia
e-mail: k.sims@qsmc.net.au

S. Walter
Faculty of Health, University of Canterbury, Christchurch, New Zealand
e-mail: sibiboycott.noelwalter@canterbury.ac.nz

K. Subbiah
Consultant Shoulder, Elbow & Sports Surgeon, Narayana Health City, Bangalore, India

B. Olivier, J. W. Orchard (eds.), *Cricket Sports Medicine*,
https://doi.org/10.1007/978-981-96-6321-7_33

performance [1], while only 32% of elite male South African players with shoulder injury experienced match or training time loss [4]. In a single season among elite fast bowlers in New Zealand, the shoulder was the fourth most injury-prone area (13%), but the time loss due to it was the lowest (0.2%) [5].

More recently, the advent of T20 cricket has elevated the injury profile of the shoulder with greater match injury incidence in both male [6] and female [7] players. This is likely the result of higher intensity of fielding (more injuries happen during fielding than bowling in T20 cricket [6]) requiring harder throws and a greater emphasis on diving to save runs.

Shoulder injury rates are also high below the elite level. In a 12-year period among community-level cricketers in New Zealand, the shoulder was the fourth most injury-prone body area with 7.0 shoulder injuries being reported for every 1000 participants [8]. In South African subelite female cricketers, the shoulder was also the fourth most injury-prone body area, with 9.9 injuries reported for every 1000 player match days in a single season [9].

33.3 Pathology

The act of throwing and bowling exposes the shoulder joint structures to high forces. Explosive throwing and bowling actions involve rapid glenohumeral movements elicited by the strong deltoid and pectoral muscles, which must be counterbalanced by the rotator cuff muscles, glenohumeral ligaments and capsule to maintain joint stability [10].

For example, just after ball release, there is a shoulder distraction force greater than 1 x the body weight [11, 12] which must be resisted by the rotator cuff. Additionally, large shoulder distraction forces are also associated with fast bowling [13]. Additionally, significant forces act on the front (during arm cocking) and back of the shoulder (after ball release) during the throwing motion [11] which again load the active muscular restraints. It is, therefore, not surprising that commonly diagnosed pathologies in cricketers include rotator cuff tendinopathy and strain [4], and in baseball pitchers, there is a demonstrable link between rotator cuff tears and pitching volumes [14].

High rotational workload of the glenohumeral joint during the throwing action leads to repetitive strain on the glenohumeral stabilising structures and may cause weakness and fatigue of the external rotators and scapular stabilisers [15]. This may lead to pathologies such as subacromial impingement, secondary to anterior-superior translation of the humeral head (thought to be a result of rotator cuff injury or fatigue) or a loss of scapula upward rotation [16]. This may lead to an irritation of structures in the subacromial space [17], but it is less likely that rotator cuff tears in throwing athletes occur by this mechanism as tears are typically on the articular side (undersurface) of the rotator cuff. An internal impingement, where the undersurface of the rotator cuff is compressed between the greater tuberosity and the posterior-superior aspect of the glenoid (and labrum) in a shoulder abduction and external rotation position [18] (the cocking position of a throw), is more likely to be associated with rotator cuff tears occurring by an impingement mechanism.

Repetitive throwing may lead to increased motion of the glenohumeral joint [19] which may lead to excessive translation of the humeral head. Both excessive anterior [20] and posterior [21] translation may occur. In the throwing athlete, the translation may be subtle and termed microinstability [22]. This may contribute to other pathologies such as impingement, superior labrum anterior to posterior (SLAP) tears or rotator cuff overload [23]. At the other end of the spectrum, a diving-related injury mechanism can cause gross instability leading to subluxations or dislocations of the glenohumeral joint.

33.4 Injury Management

Throwing subjects the shoulder to extreme ranges of motion and high forces and is a very common injury mechanism in cricket [4, 24]. There is evidence supporting reduced injury incidence in players with interventions addressing shoulder mobility (specifically internal rotation), shoulder strength (specifically external rotation) and lower extremity mobility (specifically hip range of motion [ROM]) [25].

33.5 Shoulder Strength

It makes intuitive sense that the rotator cuff strength is necessary to counter the very high shoulder distraction (up to 1.5 times body weight) and shear forces with throwing. There is also some evidence to suggest that throwers with reduced shoulder external rotation strength are less load-tolerant [26] and those with better strength less likely to be injured [25]. A study of cricketers found weakness of both the shoulder internal and external rotation groups compared to athletes in other overhead-throwing sports [27]. Overhead-throwing athletes exhibit stronger internal rotators in comparison with external rotators, and it has been recommended to incorporate only external rotator eccentric strengthening exercises to maintain the muscle strength ratio between the internal and external rotators and minimise impingement symptoms [28–30].

It is our experience that cricketers often default to higher reps and lower load 'activation' focus on shoulder exercise that may not stimulate sufficient strength and endurance capacity to control the high throwing forces. Shoulder strength training should therefore include a consistent rotator cuff resistance component (lower reps and higher loads) due to the high shoulder distraction forces at ball release. Rotator cuff endurance is also important as fatigue may lead to alterations in the ability to control shoulder motion when throwing [31], and fatigue is linked to shoulder injury in adolescent baseball pitchers [32]. While doing rotator cuff exercises, it is recommended that the load is progressively increased and controlled eccentric rotational movements are performed [33]. Exercises incorporating multiplanar movements using clubbells have been shown to improve the rotator cuff strength of pace bowlers within 6 weeks [34].

Table 33.1 lists some practical strength targets. Within a cricket population, the shoulder ER isometric strength is commonly within 90–100% of shoulder IR (Cricket Australia internal data) and ratios of 1:1 have been advocated in female cricketers [24].

Table 33.1 Practical shoulder strength targets

ER:IR ratio (using a handheld dynamometer)	ER within 75–100% of IR [35]
Shoulder endurance test (ER in abd/ER) [36]	No published cricket normative values
Isometric strength relative to body weight	>25% body weight (Cricket Australia internal data)

33.6 Shoulder Range of Motion

A common finding in the shoulder of a throwing athlete is an increase in external rotation and a reduction in internal rotation due to soft tissue [20] and bony adaptation [37] (humeral retroversion). However, the external rotation gain has not been identified in cricketers, potentially due to a lack of consistent throwing through the adolescent years when bony adaptation takes place [27]. The loss of internal rotation is based on observations of thickening of the posterior capsule, which is considered a key feature in the development of shoulder pathology in throwing athletes [38]. Posterior rotator cuff overload may also restrict motion, evidenced by transient loss of internal rotation associated with high throwing loads [39]. However, it has been observed that at the early stages of shoulder pain symptoms, pace bowlers do not exhibit a range of motion deficit [30].

If the loss of internal rotation range of motion is >20 degrees compared to the other arm and there is a total loss of rotation range of motion >10 degrees [35], then manual therapy [40] and/or a stretching programme may be warranted to improve shoulder internal rotation. However, the basis and effectiveness of stretching this region have been questioned more recently [41]. In many cases, the loss of motion may be due to posterior muscle overload (where strengthening of the posterior rotator cuff may reduce the loss of range of motion over time), and in some cases, there may be an underlying posterior instability [21], which may not respond well to strong posterior capsule stretching.

33.7 Screening

Musculoskeletal screening to predict injury is a vexed issue as it has been argued that the multifactorial nature of injury in an individual cannot be captured by a single physical measurement at a moment in time often far removed from the injury occurrence [42]. However, although prediction of injury is inaccurate, physical screening remains beneficial in terms of comparing results to normative values and setting up strength and mobility programmes, which may lead to improved performance and a role in injury prevention [43]. Weakness of the shoulder external rotators has been linked to shoulder overuse injury [44], but as has been previously described, this measure is prone to variation depending on physical use prior to testing [39]. Therefore, monitoring of relevant individual strength measurements over multiple time points may play a role in injury prevention [45] and potentially improved performance.

Range of motion measurements that may be appropriate to include in a screening battery would include shoulder external rotation, as there is evidence to suggest that a reduced range is associated with injury in throwing athletes [46]. The evidence supporting the measurement of shoulder internal rotation is not as clear [47], but there is face validity to monitoring this measure. Finally, the use of patient-reported outcome measures such as the Kerlan-Jobe Orthopaedic Clinic (KJOC) score has shown promise as measure of shoulder function [48–50] with a score of less than 90 suggestive of abnormal function.

33.8 Workload

As in any repetitive activity, there is likely to be a throwing volume beyond which the risk of shoulder injury increases. Risk factors for shoulder injury in cricket players have included throwing on average greater than 75 throws per week, more than 40 throws per day and higher volume and frequency in the week before injury [51]. Handballers who had a 60% spike in weekly volume relative to the previous months' volume had higher shoulder injury rates [26]. In baseball, more than 75 pitches in a match and pitching while fatigued were risk factors for shoulder pain [52]. In reality, specific throwing volume tolerance will vary from individual to individual and depend on factors such as recovery, fatigue, throwing efficiency, consistent throwing volumes, shoulder strength and range of motion.

A simple way to capture the individual response to throwing load is to ask them to rate the session on a scale of 1–10 in terms of difficulty [53]. This may be particularly relevant as a subjective rating of shoulder health has also been related to throwing-related injury [54]. Other monitoring options are described in Table 33.2. In an ideal world recording volume, intensity and type (e.g. off-balance throw) of throw would be optimal [55].

Table 33.2 Monitoring throwing workload in cricket

Peak Motus Sleeve [56]	Count and intensity of throws
Calculate throws per minute in often used fielding drills (video or manual count of one session)	When drill used subsequently can estimate throwing volumes for the group
Individual rating of session intensity [53]	Individual response to throwing

There is likely to be a U-shaped relationship between injury and load [57] whereby too little and too much throwing are both risk factors. Training should ensure the number of throws per week and the number of throws per month (based on a rolling 4-week average of throwing count) remain in a consistent window.

33.9 Planning Sessions

In practical terms, training should avoid sudden increases in throwing volume and intensity. This requires an understanding from coaching and Sports Science and Sports Medicine (SSSM) staff on throwing volumes and response over the past 2–3 months using some of the options outlined in the previous section.

A common scenario in cricket leading to shoulder injury is a training camp where players have not been throwing regularly beforehand and

Table 33.3 Planning of fielding training

Fielding drills	Throwing focus
Short catching	Nil
Boundary catching	Variable intensity—Can underarm if shoulder is fatigued
Mid-range (catching and ground fielding)	Variable intensity—Can focus on technique and footwork to get in good positions
Team drills	Higher intensity throwing at stump or to keeper

are then required to throw high volumes and intensity over 2–3 consecutive days. Therefore, it is recommended that cricketers keep a consistent throwing volume through the season or undertake a 3–4 week gradual progression prior to an out of season camp before trying to throw at full intensity. A useful maxim is that 'you need to earn the right to throw hard'.

When devising fielding training, it is also useful to have multiple stations (e.g. 5 min per station) with different throwing requirements (see Table 33.3).

The aim is for throwing to be spread over 30 min so there is recovery time between throwing bouts and for not every throw to be at full intensity. Anecdotal evidence suggests that baseballers perform fewer high intensity throws than cricketers during training sessions and are more particular about emphasising footwork to be in a good position to throw accurately.

33.10 Throwing Technique

Throwing involves the entire kinetic chain, and over 50% of the energy imparted to the hand is from the legs and trunk [58]. If the chain is not working efficiently, then more pressure may be placed on the shoulder to generate the forces required [59]. Therefore, it is important to practise good footwork and efficient throwing mechanics whenever possible. While off-balance throws are part of the game, it is suggested that they be used and practised sparingly to reduce shoulder overload. In many cases, taking an extra step to be able to use the kinetic chain more effectively may result in a stronger more accurate throw.

Table 33.4 Throwing technique considerations

Technical advice	Rationale
Use legs and trunk to develop power	Poor leg and trunk contribution may overload shoulder [59]
Alignment of front leg towards target at ball release	Aiming towards target stops opening up trunk too early and reduces load on shoulder [60]
Get over front leg during follow through	Dissipation of loads through posterior shoulder musculature over a larger range of motion

In addition, an adequate follow through over the front leg helps to dissipate the deceleration of the throwing arm over a larger range of motion taking some of the load off the posterior shoulder muscles. A summary of some throwing technical advice is in Table 33.4.

33.11 Diving

Diving in the field is an increasingly common injury mechanism [2] causing approximately 20% of shoulder injuries (CA injury data—unpublished) and significant damage to the capsular/ligamentous support structures of the shoulder leading to frank subluxation or dislocation. The injuries appear to be most significant when the player lands on a flexed elbow creating a superiorly directed force coupled with either an anterior or posterior bias depending on the alignment of the glenohumeral joint at elbow impact.

The risks can potentially be reduced with education and training on diving technique. Wicketkeepers learn this skill from a young age, and ideally, this early training should involve all players. Being able to dive laterally (with either a forward or a backward bias), incorporating a roll or diving forward incorporating a slide on outstretched arms should be key fielding skills that are practised regularly.

In addition, there is a risk of injury any time a player leaves their feet in the field, so fielding training should also emphasise good footwork to potentially reduce the need to dive. This can be augmented with consistent physical training incorporating flexibility and strength, particularly of the lower limb and the ability to function well in squat positions.

33.12 Surgical Consideration

Shoulder instability occurring in cricket is essentially because of a fall on an outstretched arm which is seen while diving in the field. Cricket being a non-contact sport with relatively controlled risk factors allows for a certain degree of flexibility when it comes to decision-making for definitive care.

33.13 Soft Tissue Procedure

In an essential Bankart lesion (Fig. 33.1a-c), there is disruption of the anterior inferior capsulolabral complex which leads to a loss of static restraint to the anterior dislocation of the humeral head. This most notably occurs in an abduction external rotation position (ABER)/cocking phase for throwing.

The risk of recurrent shoulder instability is dependent on the role of the player. As highlighted earlier, this arises mainly with throwing and not necessarily while batting or bowling. During bowling, the arm travels through a circumduction movement which is generally well tolerated. The exception for this might arise

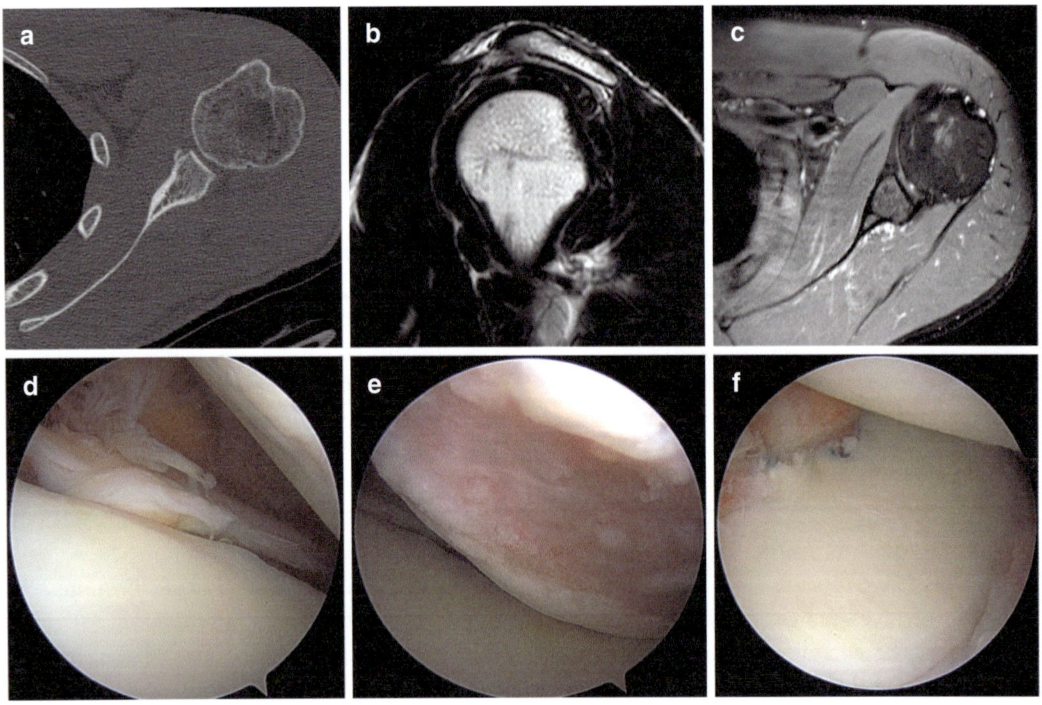

Fig. 33.1 (**a**) Axial section of a CT image showing an anterior glenoid bone fragment (Bony Bankart). (**b**): Sagittal section of T1-weighted MRI image showing posterior flattening of the humeral head (Hill-Sachs). (**c**): Axial section of T2-weighted MRI image showing blunting of anterior glenoid rim (Bankart lesion). (**d**): Intra-op image viewing from posterior portal showing disruption of labral tissue from anterior glenoid rim. (**e**): Intra-op image viewing from posterior portal showing Hill-Sachs defect in the posterior humeral head. (**f**): Intra-op image viewing from anterior-superior showing repair of Bankart lesion onto the anterior glenoid rim with centred humeral head

while dealing with a bowler who has more of a side sling style of ball delivery. When considering the batter, most, if not all, cricketing shots have the arms below shoulder height, which is a relatively safe position.

Arthroscopic Bankart repair (Fig. 33.1d-f) has become the gold standard of care for anterior shoulder instability in the non-contact athlete. It is a minimally invasive procedure where the anatomic disruption secondary to a dislocation event is repaired with the help of suture anchors onto the rim of the glenoid. Comparative studies in non-contact athletes have shown a low recurrence rate, better return to sport (RTS) and better range of motion (ROM) in throwing position compared to bony reconstruction [51]. Added remplissage procedure can be undertaken in situations of bipolar bone loss with an engaging lesion. Remplissage fills in the humeral head defect and provides a capsulotenodesis effect which utilises the posterior-superior capsule and infraspinatus [52]. Outcome studies have shown a 95.5% return to sport (RTS) with 65.5% of throwing athletes complaining of reduced ROM. Objective assessment showed an average loss of 5.3 degrees of external rotation [53].

33.14 Bony Procedure

Latarjet has shown success as a primary management option for recurrent instability and as a revision option in cases of failed soft tissue surgical management. When considering the cohort of contact sport athletes, there is a viable argument to consider this as a first line of care. Latarjet is considered a non-anatomic procedure where the coracoid along with its strap muscle attachment and coracoacromial ligament is osteotomised and fixed on the anterior aspect of the glenoid. This is achieved with screws/buttons, which can be done as an open/arthroscopic procedure. The access to the anterior glenoid is done through a split in the subscapularis muscle.

Biomechanically, the muscular sling formed by the lower portion of the subscapularis helps dynamically restrain the shoulder from anterior dislocation when in the ABER position. In cases with significant glenoid bone loss, Latarjet procedure has been shown to have a lower recurrence rate when compared to soft tissue procedures [54]. Being a bony procedure, the union rate is more predictable and easily assessed prior to a return to sport. Additionally, an open Latarjet procedure (Fig. 33.2) is more cost-effective; the fixation is achieved with two stainless steel screws which are in common use within the orthopaedic practice. This, when compared to an arthroscopic Latarjet/Bankart repair, which requires arthroscopic infrastructure along with suture anchors, might need to be considered in regions with limited resources.

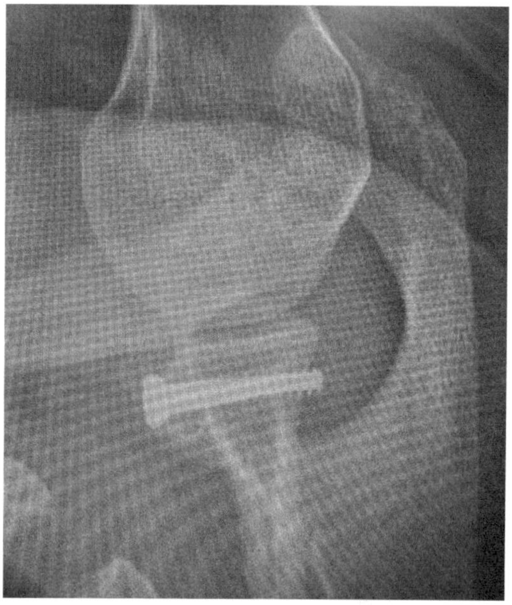

Fig. 33.2 Post-operative radiograph (Bernageau view) showing a healed coracoid to the anterior glenoid rim with stainless steel screw parallel to the joint surface

A systematic review of return to sport data shows the highest rates of return to sport amongst arthroscopic Bankart repair with shortest return to sport amongst Latarjet cohort. Return to pre-injury level was highest in the Bankart group with lowest in arthroscopic Latarjet group [55].

33.15 Atypical Instability

Considering the biomechanics of injury to the shoulder occurring while diving to the side, there is forceful adduction to an abducted and externally rotated shoulder which can result in a glenoid labrum articular disruption (GLAD lesion) [56]. These lesions result in instability and an articular defect at the edge of the capsulolabral disruption [57]. Management is aimed at addressing the instability and the articular defect—with a soft tissue procedure, the defect can be made well contained and secondary cartilage procedures performed (microfracture).

Posterior instability in isolation is a rare occurrence in the non-contact throwing athlete and when diagnosed is generally managed conservatively with surgical repair indicated only after failure of rehabilitation [58]. This may be provoked in flexion, adduction and internal rotation.

Microinstability is a condition associated with a subluxation of the humeral head, and unlike traumatic dislocations, it can be seen across all the roles in cricket. It is mostly a result of muscular fatigue from overuse, leading to loss of dynamic restraint. This typically is managed conservatively without needing surgical intervention.

33.16 Minimising Shoulder Injury Risk

Due to the lack of high-quality evidence in minimising shoulder injury risk in cricket, recommendations are made through expert consensus [55]. Table 33.5 provides a summary of some suggested recommendations. Coaches must encourage cricketers to report any symptom of shoulder pain regardless of severity so that training can be modified and early intervention implemented; throwing with pain should be avoided. Once pain has settled, throwing should be reintroduced by progressively increasing the throwing volume and intensity.

Table 33.5 Shoulder health recommendations

The Cricket First XI for shoulder health	
Throw regularly	3–4 sessions per week
Earn the right to throw hard	3–4 weeks of preparation
Not every throw needs to be high intensity	Fluctuate within a session
Use lower body to generate force	Tap into the kinetic chain
Regular shoulder strength and endurance exercise	Two strength sessions with external rotation focus per week
Practise diving but stay on feet if possible	Regular practice to reinforce safe diving
When diving do not land on elbow	Creates high load on the shoulder
Monitor throwing loads	Allows planning and modification of training
Consider throwing loads in the design of fielding sessions	Allows recovery within a fielding session
Monitor shoulder strength	Regular strength measures over the season
Monitor shoulder health	Use KJOC <90; do not throw with shoulder pain

References

1. Ranson C, Gregory P. Shoulder injury in professional cricketers. Phys Ther Sport. 2008;9(1):34–9.
2. Goggins L, Williams S, Griffin S, Langley B, Newman D, Peirce N. English and welsh men's domestic cricket injury risk by activity and cricket type: a retrospective cohort study from 2010 to 2019. J Sci Med Sport. 2024;27(1):25–9. https://doi.org/10.1016/j.jsams.2023.07.013.
3. Orchard JW, Inge P, Sims K, Kountouris A, Saw AE, Saw R, et al. Comparison of injury profiles between elite Australian male and female cricket players. J Sci Med Sport. 2023;26(1):19–24. https://doi.org/10.1016/j.jsams.2022.12.002.
4. Dutton M, Tam N, Gray J. Incidence and impact of time loss and non-time-loss shoulder injury in elite south African cricketers: a one-season, prospective cohort study. J Sci Med Sport. 2019;22(11):1200–5. https://doi.org/10.1016/j.jsams.2019.05.006.
5. Walter S, Peterson C, Basu A. Quantifying injuries among New Zealand cricket fast bowlers: a 12-month retrospective injury surveillance. NZ J Sports Med. 2022;48:46–51.
6. Goggins L, Peirce N, Ranson C, McCaig S, Newman D, Langley B, et al. Injuries in England and Wales elite

men's domestic cricket: a nine season review from 2010 to 2018. J Sci Med Sport. 2020;23(9):836–40. https://doi.org/10.1016/j.jsams.2020.03.009.
7. Warren A, Dale S, McCaig S, Ranson C. Injury profiles in elite women's T20 cricket. J Sci Med Sport. 2019;22(7):775–9. https://doi.org/10.1016/j.jsams.2019.01.018.
8. Walter S, King D, Hume P. New Zealand cricket injury analysis based on 12 years of accident compensation corporation data. BMJ Open Sport Exerc Med. 2022;8(3):e001340. https://doi.org/10.1136/bmjsem-2022-001340.
9. Jacobs J, Olivier B, Brandt C. Injury profiles in sub-elite women's cricket: exploring incidence, prevalence, nature, onset and body region. Phys Ther Sport. 2024;67:125–30. https://doi.org/10.1016/j.ptsp.2024.04.006.
10. Wilk KE, Arrigo CA, Andrews JR. Current concepts: the stabilizing structures of the glenohumeral joint. J Orthop Sports Phys Ther. 1997;25(6):364–79. https://doi.org/10.2519/jospt.1997.25.6.364.
11. Fleisig GS, Andrews JR, Dillman CJ, Escamilla RF. Kinetics of baseball pitching with implications about injury mechanisms. Am J Sports Med. 1995;23(2):233–9. https://doi.org/10.1177/036354659502300218.
12. Nebel AR, Fava AW, Bordelon NM, Oliver GD. Comparison of peak shoulder distraction forces between pain and pain-free youth baseball pitchers. Orthop J Sports Med. 2023;11(6):23259671231177320. https://doi.org/10.1177/23259671231177320.
13. Stuelcken M, Ferdinands RE, Ginn KA, Sinclair PJ. The shoulder distraction force in cricket fast bowling. J Appl Biomech. 2010;26(3):373–7.
14. Lesniak BP, Baraga MG, Jose J, Smith MK, Cunningham S, Kaplan LD. Glenohumeral findings on magnetic resonance imaging correlate with innings pitched in asymptomatic pitchers. Am J Sports Med. 2013;41(9):2022–7. https://doi.org/10.1177/0363546513491093.
15. Page P. Shoulder muscle imbalance and subacromial impingement syndrome in overhead athletes. Int J Sports Phys Ther. 2011;6(1):51–8.
16. Braun S, Kokmeyer D, Millett PJ. Shoulder injuries in the throwing athlete. J Bone Joint Surg Am. 2009;91(4):966–78. https://doi.org/10.2106/jbjs.H.01341.
17. Diercks R, Bron C, Dorrestijn O, Meskers C, Naber R, de Ruiter T, et al. Guideline for diagnosis and treatment of subacromial pain syndrome: a multidisciplinary review by the Dutch Orthopaedic association. Acta Orthop. 2014;85(3):314–22. https://doi.org/10.3109/17453674.2014.920991.
18. Jobe CM. Posterior superior glenoid impingement: expanded spectrum. Arthroscopy. 1995;11(5):530–6. https://doi.org/10.1016/0749-8063(95)90128-0.
19. Reinold MM, Gill TJ. Current concepts in the evaluation and treatment of the shoulder in overhead-throwing athletes, part 1: physical characteristics and clinical examination. Sports Health. 2010;2(1):39–50. https://doi.org/10.1177/1941738109338548.
20. Burkhart SS, Morgan CD, Kibler WB. The disabled throwing shoulder: spectrum of pathology part I: pathoanatomy and biomechanics. Arthroscopy. 2003;19(4):404–20.
21. Watson L, Balster S, Warby SA, Sadi J, Hoy G, Pizzari T. A comprehensive rehabilitation program for posterior instability of the shoulder. J Hand Ther. 2017;30(2):182–92. https://doi.org/10.1016/j.jht.2017.05.007.
22. Reinold MM, Curtis AS. Microinstability of the shoulder in the overhead athlete. Int J Sports Phys Ther. 2013;8(5):601–16.
23. Wilk KE, Meister K, Andrews JR. Current concepts in the rehabilitation of the overhead throwing athlete. Am J Sports Med. 2002;30(1):136–51.
24. Murphy M, Chivers P, Mahony K, Mosler A. Risk factors for dominant-shoulder injury in elite female Australian cricket players: a prospective study. Transl Sports Med. 2020;3:404–14.
25. Karasuyama M, Tsuruta T, Kawakami J, Oike T, Uchida K, Minamikawa T. Preventive interventions for throwing injuries in baseball players: a scoping review. J Shoulder Elb Surg. 2024;33:e451. https://doi.org/10.1016/j.jse.2023.12.008.
26. Møller M, Nielsen RO, Attermann J, Wedderkopp N, Lind M, Sørensen H, et al. Handball load and shoulder injury rate: a 31-week cohort study of 679 elite youth handball players. Br J Sports Med. 2017;51(4):231–7. https://doi.org/10.1136/bjsports-2016-096927.
27. Dutton M, Tam N, Brown JC, Gray J. The cricketer's shoulder: not a classic throwing shoulder. Phys Ther Sport. 2019;37:120–7. https://doi.org/10.1016/j.ptsp.2019.03.014.
28. Wilk KE, Andrews JR, Arrigo CA, Keirns MA, Erber DJ. The strength characteristics of internal and external rotator muscles in professional baseball pitchers. Am J Sports Med. 1993;21(1):61–6. https://doi.org/10.1177/036354659302100111.
29. Clarsen B, Bahr R, Andersson SH, Munk R, Myklebust G. Reduced glenohumeral rotation, external rotation weakness and scapular dyskinesis are risk factors for shoulder injuries among elite male handball players: a prospective cohort study. Br J Sports Med. 2014;48(17):1327–33. https://doi.org/10.1136/bjsports-2014-093702.
30. Walter S, Peterson C, Basu A. Are there any differences in the shoulder muscle strength and range of motion between cricket fast bowlers with and without shoulder pain? NZ J Sports Med. 2021;48(1):17–23.
31. Bowman TG, Hart JM, McGuire BA, Palmieri RM, Ingersoll CD. A functional fatiguing protocol and deceleration time of the shoulder from an internal rotation perturbation. J Athl Train. 2006;41(3):275–9.
32. Norton R, Honstad C, Joshi R, Silvis M, Chinchilli V, Dhawan A. Risk factors for elbow and shoulder injuries in adolescent baseball players: a systematic review. Am J Sports Med. 2019;47(4):982–90. https://doi.org/10.1177/0363546518760573.

33. Chaconas EJ, Kolber MJ, Hanney WJ, Daugherty ML, Wilson SH, Sheets C. Shoulder external rotator eccentric training versus general shoulder exercise for Subacromial pain syndrome: a randomized controlled trial. Int J Sports Phys Ther. 2017;12(7):1121–33. https://doi.org/10.26603/ijspt20171121.
34. Walter S, Moltchanova E, Petersen C. Effect of Indian clubbell exercises on cricket fast bowlers' shoulder kinematics. S Afr J Sports Med. 2023;35(1):v35i1a15103. https://doi.org/10.17159/2078-516X/2023/v35i1a15103.
35. Cools AM, Borms D, Castelein B, Vanderstukken F, Johansson FR. Evidence-based rehabilitation of athletes with glenohumeral instability. Knee Surg Sports Traumatol Arthrosc. 2016;24(2):382–9. https://doi.org/10.1007/s00167-015-3940-x.
36. Declève P, Van Cant J, Attar T, Urbain E, Marcel M, Borms D, et al. The shoulder endurance test (SET): a reliability and validity and comparison study on healthy overhead athletes and sedentary adults. Phys Ther Sport. 2021;47:201–7. https://doi.org/10.1016/j.ptsp.2020.12.005.
37. Sabick MB, Kim YK, Torry MR, Keirns MA, Hawkins RJ. Biomechanics of the shoulder in youth baseball pitchers: implications for the development of proximal humeral epiphysiolysis and humeral retrotorsion. Am J Sports Med. 2005;33(11):1716–22. https://doi.org/10.1177/0363546505275347.
38. Medina G, Bartolozzi AR 3rd, Spencer JA, Morgan C. The thrower's shoulder. JBJS Rev. 2022;10(3):e21.00194. https://doi.org/10.2106/jbjs.Rvw.21.00194.
39. Reinold M, Wilk K, Macrina L, Sheheane C, Dun S, Fleisig G, et al. Changes in shoulder and elbow passive range of motion after pitching in professional baseball players. Am J Sports Med. 2008;36(3):523–7.
40. Bailey LB, Thigpen CA, Hawkins RJ, Beattie PF, Shanley E. Effectiveness of manual therapy and stretching for baseball players with shoulder range of motion deficits. Sports Health. 2017;9(3):230–7. https://doi.org/10.1177/1941738117702835.
41. Hall K, Borstad JD. Posterior shoulder tightness: to treat or not to treat? J Orthop Sports Phys Ther. 2018;48(3):133–6. https://doi.org/10.2519/jospt.2018.0605.
42. Bahr R. Why screening tests to predict injury do not work-and probably never will...: a critical review. Br J Sports Med. 2016;50(13):776–80. https://doi.org/10.1136/bjsports-2016-096256.
43. Cools AM, Maenhout AG, Vanderstukken F, Declève P, Johansson FR, Borms D. The challenge of the sporting shoulder: from injury prevention through sport-specific rehabilitation toward return to play. Ann Phys Rehabil Med. 2021;64(4):101384. https://doi.org/10.1016/j.rehab.2020.03.009.
44. Achenbach L, Laver L, Walter SS, Zeman F, Kuhr M, Krutsch W. Decreased external rotation strength is a risk factor for overuse shoulder injury in youth elite handball athletes. Knee Surg Sports Traumatol Arthrosc. 2020;28(4):1202–11. https://doi.org/10.1007/s00167-019-05493-4.
45. Verhagen E, van Dyk N, Clark N, Shrier I. Do not throw the baby out with the bathwater; screening can identify meaningful risk factors for sports injuries. Br J Sports Med. 2018;52(19):1223–4. https://doi.org/10.1136/bjsports-2017-098547.
46. Pozzi F, Plummer HA, Shanley E, Thigpen CA, Bauer C, Wilson ML, et al. Preseason shoulder range of motion screening and in-season risk of shoulder and elbow injuries in overhead athletes: systematic review and meta-analysis. Br J Sports Med. 2020;54(17):1019–27. https://doi.org/10.1136/bjsports-2019-100698.
47. Keller RA, De Giacomo AF, Neumann JA, Limpisvasti O, Tibone JE. Glenohumeral internal rotation deficit and risk of upper extremity injury in overhead athletes: a meta-analysis and systematic review. Sports Health. 2018;10(2):125–32. https://doi.org/10.1177/1941738118756577.
48. Monti R, Fernandez-Fernandez A. The Kerlan-Jobe Orthopaedic Clinic Shoulder & Elbow Score used as a patient-reported outcome measure for the youth and high school aged baseball athlete. Int J Sports Phys Ther. 2022;17(5):879–86. https://doi.org/10.26603/001c.36634.
49. Painter DF, Quinn M, Dove JH, Testa EJ, Snow R, Byrne RA, et al. Arm health in elite collegiate summer league baseball players assessed by the Kerlan-Jobe Orthopaedic clinic score. J Athl Train. 2024;59(3):255–61. https://doi.org/10.4085/1062-6050-0123.23.
50. Franz JO, McCulloch PC, Kneip CJ, Noble PC, Lintner DM. The utility of the KJOC score in professional baseball in the United States. Am J Sports Med. 2013;41(9):2167–73. https://doi.org/10.1177/0363546513495177.
51. Saw R, Dennis RJ, Bentley D, Farhart P. Throwing workload and injury risk in elite cricketers. Br J Sports Med. 2011;45(10):805–8. https://doi.org/10.1136/bjsm.2009.061309.
52. Lyman S, Fleisig GS, Waterbor JW, Funkhouser EM, Pulley L, Andrews JR, et al. Longitudinal study of elbow and shoulder pain in youth baseball pitchers. Med Sci Sports Exerc. 2001;33(11):1803–10. https://doi.org/10.1097/00005768-200111000-00002.
53. McLaren SJ, Macpherson TW, Coutts AJ, Hurst C, Spears IR, Weston M. The relationships between internal and external measures of training load and intensity in team sports: a meta-analysis. Sports

Med. 2018;48(3):641–58. https://doi.org/10.1007/s40279-017-0830-z.
54. Mehta S, Tang S, Rajapakse C, Juzwak S, Dowling B. Chronic workload, subjective arm health, and throwing injury in high school baseball players: 3-year retrospective pilot study. Sports Health. 2022;14(1):119–26. https://doi.org/10.1177/19417381211055142.
55. Schwank A, Blazey P, Asker M, Møller M, Hägglund M, Gard S, et al. 2022 Bern consensus statement on shoulder injury prevention, rehabilitation, and return to sport for athletes at all participation levels. J Orthop Sports Phys Ther. 2022;52(1):11–28. https://doi.org/10.2519/jospt.2022.10952.
56. Seshadri DR, Li RT, Voos JE, Rowbottom JR, Alfes CM, Zorman CA, et al. Wearable sensors for monitoring the internal and external workload of the athlete. NPJ Digit Med. 2019;2:71. https://doi.org/10.1038/s41746-019-0149-2.
57. Windt J, Gabbett TJ. How do training and competition workloads relate to injury? The workload-injury aetiology model. Br J Sports Med. 2017;51(5):428–35. https://doi.org/10.1136/bjsports-2016-096040.
58. Lintner D, Noonan TJ, Kibler WB. Injury patterns and biomechanics of the athlete's shoulder. Clin Sports Med. 2008;27(4):527–51. https://doi.org/10.1016/j.csm.2008.07.007.
59. Chu SK, Jayabalan P, Kibler WB, Press J. The kinetic chain revisited: new concepts on throwing mechanics and injury. PM R. 2016;8(3 Suppl):S69–77. https://doi.org/10.1016/j.pmrj.2015.11.015.
60. Seroyer ST, Nho SJ, Bach BR, Bush-Joseph CA, Nicholson GP, Romeo AA. The kinetic chain in overhand pitching: its potential role for performance enhancement and injury prevention. Sports Health. 2010;2(2):135–46. https://doi.org/10.1177/1941738110362656.

Elbow Injuries in Cricket

34

Ben Langley, Elyse Potter, and Roger van Riet

34.1 Introduction

Elbow injuries in cricket are under-recognised [1]. A prevalence of 1.4 per 100 players per season has been published for elbow and forearm fractures [2] with elbow issues typically being non-time-loss in nature. This is somewhat surprising as elbow injuries are the signature injury in baseball, cricket's sister sport, and are primarily related to pitching which, unlike bowling in cricket, has a throwing motion. Recent experience suggests that incidence appears to be increasing in the elite male setting. Elbow injuries affect batters, bowlers and fielders but there are significant differences in the mechanism and pathology observed.

Elbow injuries can be broadly categorised into three main groups considering diagnostic and mechanism perspectives: (1) lateral elbow pain presentations, generally associated with batting; (2) medial elbow pain presentations, typically related to throwing/fielding; and (3) bowling-related elbow presentations, the most common of which is posterior impingement.

B. Langley (✉)
Global Head of Sports Science and Medicine, Mumbai Indians, Mumbai, India
e-mail: ben.langley@ril.com

E. Potter
Mumbai Indians WPL, Mumbai, India

R. van Riet
Department of orthopaedic surgery, AZ Monica, Orthoca, Antwerp, Belgium

Department of orthopaedic surgery, University Hospital Antwerp, Antwerp, Belgium
e-mail: drrogervanriet@azmonica.be

34.2 Common Presentation and Mechanism in Cricket

34.2.1 Batting-Related Elbow Pain

The most common presentation will demonstrate features of tendinopathy at the lateral elbow involving the Common Extensor Origin (CEO), widely referred to as the infamous 'tennis elbow' and previously described clinically as lateral epicondylitis. Ironically, tennis elbow has become less prevalent in tennis since the double-handed backhand technique has taken precedence.

Less frequently, a player will report similar symptoms at the medial elbow affecting the Common Flexor Origin (CFO). The same principles for lateral tendinopathy discussed below can be applied, but ulnar nerve involvement should be considered due to its proximity to the CFO. It is important to note that both lateral and medial elbow tendinopathy have been associated with subtle instability, so they should be thoroughly assessed [3, 4]. Both are far more common in athletes in the men's game than in the women's [2].

Tendon load relates to overall workload exposure, so both the volume of batting and intensity

B. Olivier, J. W. Orchard (eds.), *Cricket Sports Medicine*,
https://doi.org/10.1007/978-981-96-6321-7_34

of gripping of the bat accumulated across both training and matches must be considered. Lateral/CEO tendinopathy most frequently affects the 'top hand' of the batter (the hand closest to the end of the bat handle). The top hand is required to provide high levels of grip force to control the bat during the majority of batting shot techniques.

Different injury patterns have been identified across the different cricket formats [5]. In training for red ball cricket, such as Test and multi-day matches, batters typically undertake high volumes of batting training in preparation for long innings of unknown duration, the expectation being that they will bat 'all day', which may involve several hundred balls over a 7-h period.

In the evolving T20 format, a number of new shot techniques have evolved which require skill mastery, and the need to hit boundaries means that power-hitting practice (hitting the ball maximum distance) adds to the gripping load. Some shots, such as the reverse sweep and switch hit, have become a valuable stroke option and players are practising these in high volume to hone the skill. These are not traditional shots for the current generation of players, and so they may be exposed to unaccustomed movements and forces that they are not conditioned to.

The load is further influenced by a number of external factors, so consider changes in bat weight and handle/grip size and other gripping-related activity in the gym or other non-cricket activities (such as golf, tennis, padel) when managing these injuries.

Players often present as functional and play for an extended period with significant symptoms to maintain their availability and performance requires intensive management and significant input of time and resources from the medical team. Typically, these injuries will eventually require a protected block of time away from competitive cricket to manage workloads and better control symptoms to allow for adequate rehabilitation. However, surgery may be necessary in chronic injuries where rehabilitation and conservative management have failed. In 2023, Faf du Plessis withdrew from a franchise tournament to have surgery, stating that he had played with batting-related elbow pain for almost two years and had eight cortisone injections and felt like he was 'hitting at 80% power' [6].

Diagnosis involves typical clinical signs that may include varying degrees of tenderness at lateral epicondyle, pain with resisted extension of the wrist which is more pronounced with the arm in extension, pain on resisted extension of wrist/third and fourth fingers, reduced grip strength +/− pain especially in extended elbow positions but also in functional positions. Imaging can assist with confirming diagnosis and excluding other pathology.

Early detection is important, and active management should begin at the first sign or suspicion of injury. The obvious challenge is modifying a player's workload when they are preparing for or are in competition. A reduction in workload may not necessarily result in improvement in their symptoms, given the short-term impact of relative rest is variable.

34.2.2 Management Approaches

34.2.2.1 Conservative

- Focus on longer term workload management as this is typically a self-limiting issue.
- Strength work for the lower arm and stretching/release of the extensor muscle groups can modify symptoms. Assess the response to isometric and eccentrics loads when applied to the tendon to assist with short and longer term symptom management.
- 'Off-loading the tendon' with a counterforce brace/strap, compression sleeve and/or taping whilst undertaking batting activity appears more effective than local treatment (soft tissue massage, joint mobilisation, dry needling acupuncture), which usually offers only temporary relief.

34.2.2.2 Medical

- Symptom management including but not limited to oral analgesia and NSAIDs should be limited. Consider local NSAID gel or lidocaine patches to assist in keeping the player active in addition to cryotherapy/heat modalities.

34.2.2.3 Interventions

- Corticosteroid injections (CSI) for elbow tendinopathies should be avoided where possible. If a decision is made to utilise CSI to assist in managing critical periods, such as reaching the final of a tournament, it must be prescribed in the knowledge that outcomes in the medium-term are typically less favourable [7, 8].
- Consider the use of biologic therapy such as Platelet Rich Plasma (PRP) injection if an injection must be used, as these have superior results to CSI [9, 10].
- Surgery is rare in professional athletes and should be undertaken only in chronic, recalcitrant cases, and this can be done arthroscopically or via mini-open procedures [11].

34.2.3 Throwing-Related Elbow Pain

Cricket has long considered fielding as the 'third discipline' behind batting and bowling. Throwing in cricket has not received the same attention that pitching and throwing have received in baseball. Throwing-related elbow pain (TEP) in cricket is usually a performance-limiting issue, but time-loss injury does occur. TEP is less common in the women's game, where the majority of throwing-related issues are seen more proximally at the shoulder [12].

More recently, the growth of the T20 format and associated franchise competitions has produced increased demand for a high-performing throw (and not just a functional one) in all fielding positions. A player with a poor throwing arm would previously have been 'hidden' in a less demanding fielding position, and this is no longer an acceptable option for coaches.

Ulnar collateral ligament (UCL) injuries (often described as the baseball pitcher's elbow) are typically of lower severity than observed in baseball, and surgical repair of the UCL ('Tommy John' procedure [13]) is infrequent. Most cases require a more dedicated approach to throwing preparation following comprehensive rehabilitation. Strengthening the surrounding wrist-finger flexors and pronators should be a key component of the programme if ligament laxity is present. If a rupture of the UCL is diagnosed acutely, direct repair may be possible, but the Tommy John reconstructive procedure usually requires 12 months or more of season-ending rehabilitation [14].

A common presentation of TEP in cricket is of an insidious and non-specific nature that often relates to a throwing arm that has not been adequately prepared for the demands. A player may describe generalised soreness/ache through the elbow joint, a tired/tight bicep muscle and a reduced ability to generate throwing intensity or cover longer distances. A reassuring sign is that they can undertake all other cricket-related activities without significant restriction. Clinical examination may reveal mild symptoms and reduction of end-range flexion and extension. This is suggestive of joint inflammation and irritation relating to load rather than any serious mechanical or pathological issue.

Practitioners should be aware of and consider Valgus Extension Overload Syndrome [15–17] (VEOS) that, again, is more commonly seen in baseball, especially when symptoms are reported as being postero-medial in location. The presentation in cricket, where throwing stress is generally a lot lower than that seen in baseball pitchers, is often more mixed, so consider VEOS as part of the overall clinical picture.

34.2.4 Management Approaches

34.2.4.1 Conservative

- The number one tip is to focus on workload management, as this plays a large role in driving TEP in cricket. Many players are inconsistent in how frequently they throw, often reporting low loads during breaks before returning to competitive periods and then are exposed to large lifts in volume and intensity when performance demands it.

- Throwing should be performed regularly and be treated like any other exercise in a player's physical preparation programme to maintain range, strength and co-ordination of the movement.
- Players should be encouraged and supported to take responsibility for their throwing arm and maintain consistent base workloads (taking into consideration volume and intensity) between series from which they can transition to performance levels of preparation.
- The key consideration is high-intensity throwing that replicates that experienced in a match. Exposure to sudden increases of load at this level is when you can expect a heightened risk of elbow pain.
- Sports science and medicine (SSM) staff should work with coaches in a positive manner and not be seen to be restricting throwing exposure unless clearly indicated.
- Collaborate with the coaching staff to progress a squad of players towards high-intensity, competitive fielding drills rather than making this part of their first throwing session after a break period.
- With respect to throwing technique, this should only be modified or adjusted after thorough consideration of a player's biomechanics, and this process would involve the wider SSM team, coaching staff and the player themselves. As is the case with fast bowling, the older and more established a player is, the more engrained their existing technique and physical features will be. Technical changes may have other effects that may impact on performance and even contribute to secondary injury issues.
- An example would be a throw with a low-arm slot where the shoulder is well below 90-degree of abduction when in the fully cocked position. This allows the player to release the ball more quickly but would likely generate increased load and possibly produce symptoms at the medial aspect of the elbow. The immediate reaction is to 'improve' the throw and offload the elbow by raising their arm slot. This may inadvertently aggravate a player's shoulder and/or reduce their performance with a longer load-up period.
- Recurrent or ongoing generalised TEP, as described earlier, does require greater focus on preparing the player's 'arm' for throwing demands. Workload management is a given, but consider the whole player, especially when the cause and clinical examination are not conclusive. Refer to the Throwing Arm Screen below as a starting point.

34.2.4.2 Interventions

- Most UCL injuries are not severe and resolve with conservative management, but the symptoms of chronic injuries may be improved with biologic therapy such as PRP injection if not responding to rehabilitation.
- UCL reconstructive surgery is uncommon in cricket but must be considered in higher-grade injuries/ligament rupture.

Throwing Arm Screen

With the growth of T20 franchise cricket and the critical requirement of throwing as a distinct discipline in the format, an abbreviated screen relating to immediate performance is beneficial to highlight the potential impact on performance and injury risk.

This could consist of:

- Recent workload history (ideally 4 weeks): consider training loads and competitive matches played, and gain an understanding of the exposure to throwing intensity [18].
- Recent 'throwing arm pain' (including shoulder, elbow or elsewhere) or reduction in perceived throwing performance (reduced power, loss of distance).
- Total range of shoulder rotation: the sum of internal (IR) and external rotation (ER) ranges (Figs. 34.1a and b) at 90-degree shoulder abduction. Assess and check for asymmetry in these totals and consider hyper vs. hypomobility presentations.
- 'Full can' strength test (Fig. 34.2): using dynamometry to provide an objective mea-

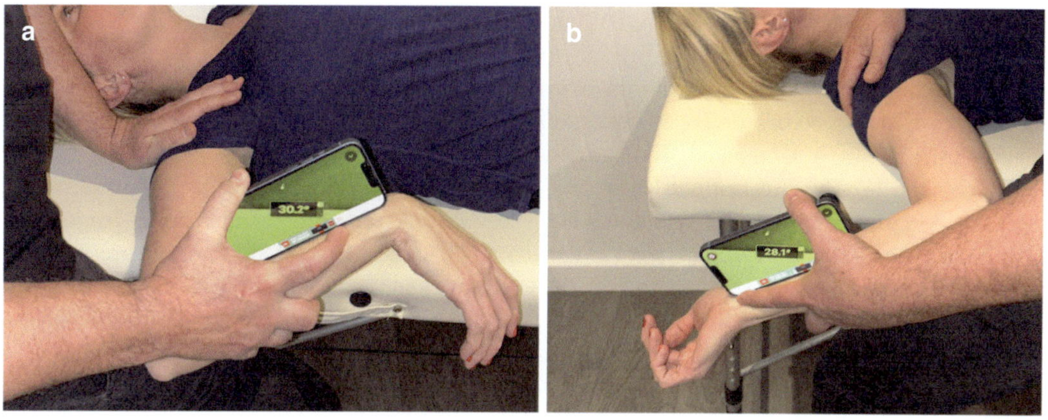

Fig. 34.1 Measuring passive (**a**) internal rotation and (**b**) ER range of the shoulder in supine

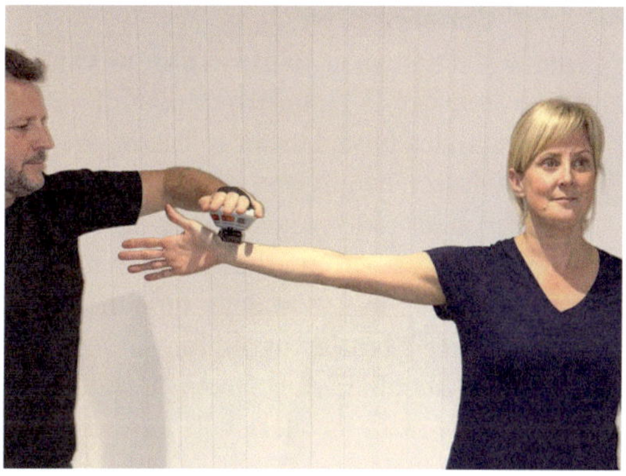

Fig. 34.2 'Full can' test measured with a hand-held dynamometer

surement, symmetry or greater strength in the throwing arm is expected.

- Internal and external rotator strength (tested at 90 ° abduction): ER:IR strength ratios may be helpful when there is hypermobility of the glenohumeral joint, such as in female players or observed in the range tests above. There are a number of protocols to achieve these measures that can utilise a hand-held or fixed-position dynamometer [19]. There are challenges of variable inter-rater reliability when using most of these protocols so choose a test that is most appropriate to the player and the practitioner to reliably undertake testing.

If any of the above screening tests flag a concern, further clinical examination and physical testing should be considered to develop a clear understanding of the issue with a targeted programme of management.

34.2.5 Bowling-Related Elbow Pain

The action of fast bowling requires the player to load the elbow in an extended and often hyperextended position to generate a high pace of the ball on release.

Most bowling-related elbow pain occurs after re-introduction of bowling after a period of no/minimal training or competitive cricket. It may also relate to the volume of the match workload, especially when effort balls (maximum-intensity deliveries) are required in a match situation. Interestingly, bowling fuller-length balls (i.e. yorkers where the ball lands close to the batter's feet) may induce greater symptoms than shorter-length balls (i.e. bouncers), where the ball is bowled with an effort to have it bounce up at the level of the batter's head. This relates to the longer length of time that the bowler's elbow spends in full extension before the ball is released.

Bowling-related elbow pain can present with many variations. Return-to-bowling pain often presents as posterior elbow ache/soreness primarily aggravated by elbow extension. There can be apparent irritation/inflammation of the fat pad in the olecranon fossa as it adapts to the extension movement created leading to ball release. This presentation will usually settle with conservative treatment and load management, but persistent symptoms should be investigated to understand if there is any hard tissue involvement, such as loose bodies or bone formation. Figure 34.3 shows a Computed Tomography (CT) image of the elbow of fast bowler presenting with posterior impingement symptoms and clear bone formation in the olecranon fossa. This player was managed conservatively and continues to play international level cricket.

If a player experiences persistent elbow pain whilst bowling that is not improving with conservative management, irrespective of the location of symptoms, then a differential diagnosis should be sought to exclude the involvement of intra-articular issues, loose bodies and the presence of impingement injury.

Though not common, there have been instances where chronic elbow pain has resulted in prematurely ended playing careers due to the impact on performance, such as Australian fast bowler Shaun Tait. Tait's high bowling pace was renowned but was directly impacted by his elbow injury, and he stated on retirement, 'when you're not contributing on the field as much as you'd like to, it's time to finish up' [20]. There are also recent cases of ulnar stress fracture reported in male elite fast bowlers. Practitioners are unlikely to be challenged with the differential diagnosis and management of these injuries in the non-elite setting where players are unlikely to bowl at very high paces of 90mph (145kmh) and above.

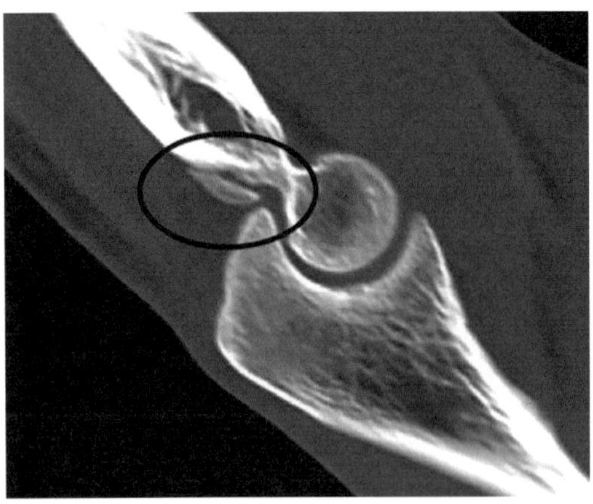

Fig. 34.3 CT image of the elbow of a fast bowler presenting with posterior impingement symptoms and clear bone formation in the olecranon fossa

It is important to investigate these injuries with early detection of symptoms during and post-bowling (may be non-specific/generalised), reduction in bowling speeds and/or avoidance of certain deliveries (often will be fuller-length balls and off-cutters which require wrist-forearm supination) and clinical features may include pain at end of range extension and/or flexion and on resisted biceps contraction.

34.2.6 Management Approaches

34.2.6.1 Conservative

- One of the first areas to explore is proximally at the shoulder as reduced shoulder elevation range may lead to a bowler releasing the ball from a lower height and can increase load in other areas. Any added force that can be diverted away from the elbow through improvement in shoulder mobility will likely reduce a bowler's symptoms.
- Overhead shoulder (OHS) range should be assessed as many bowlers will have reduced mobility that relates to tightness in their accelerator muscles (such as pec major, lat dorsi and subscapularis), glenohumeral joint range and cervico-thoracic movement. Even relatively small improvements in range and end-feel can alter force transmission and affect a noticeable difference in symptom awareness.
- There are several methods to measure active and passive OHS range objectively, with one method shown in Fig. 34.4 there will be significant variation in this range between bowlers dependent on many factors, including age, gender, ethnicity and physical development.
- Compare the bowling arm to the contralateral side and consider how this influences their bowling technique and may impact on the elbow. This is useful not only for elbow issues

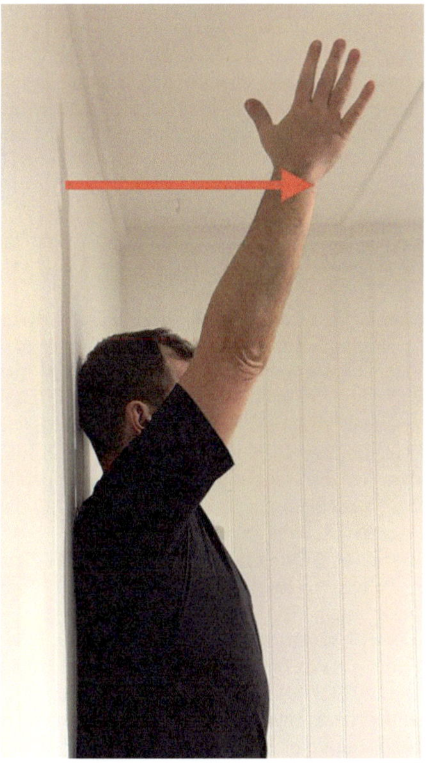

Fig. 34.4 A method of assessing active overhead shoulder range:measure distance from wall to the ulnar styloid at the wrist.

but also for shoulder and spinal issues, including lumbar bone stress injury (LBSI).

- Consider radiological investigation for persistent elbow soreness relating to bowling, especially fast bowlers.
- Remember that stress fracture of the elbow in cricket is not common, so consider other differential diagnoses before this.
- Treat high suspicion of bone involvement similarly to suspected LBSI and proceed quickly to radiological investigation. In this case, an Magnetic Resonance Imaging (MRI) is needed to check for bone oedema and other potential pathology.

34.2.6.2 Interventions

- As per general principles, CSI should be avoided where possible though targeting areas of impingement may assist in reducing symptoms, including in the presence of bony change.
- Arthroscopic surgery may be required to alleviate the symptoms through the removal of loose bodies or debriding bony areas of impingement. Screw fixation of stress fractures may be necessary to achieve union and healing in the face of ongoing high forces from fast bowling.

34.3 Radiology: A Guide for Imaging the Elbow

In athletes, MRI has rightly become the standard imaging modality. Tendon or ligament injury and intra-articular pathology (such as increased fluid, synovitis, cartilage lesions or bone oedema) are best diagnosed with MRI.

Imaging of the injured elbow may start with plain antero-posterior and lateral radiographs, but in most players, these will be of little clinical value. They may show (subtle) signs of degenerative change, previous trauma or sequelae of osteochondritis dissecans (OCD).

If bony injury is prevalent or suspected, a CT scan is helpful to quantify the pathology further. CT is always indicated if the player experiences locking or clicking, indicative of an intra-articular loose body. In later stages of an impingement-related injury, including Valgus Extension Overload Syndrome (VEOS), osteophytes can be found at the posteromedial tip of the olecranon, together with bone at the medial side of the olecranon fossa which is indicative of bony impingement.

Ultrasound (US) may be useful especially in cases involving tendinopathy. MRI is very sensitive for soft tissue and cartilage lesions, whereas US has the advantage of being a dynamic technique. This will allow the ultrasonographer to examine tissues whilst contracted or stretched. Subtle instability, (sub)luxation of the ulnar nerve, snapping triceps or snapping annular ligament may be identified with dynamic US techniques in more complicated cases where differential diagnosis is challenging.

34.4 Indications for Surgery

- All surgery at the elbow should be considered as a last resort given the impact the procedure can have on range of motion, proprioception and strength. This is especially true for fast bowlers in whom any reduction in these areas would contribute to a significant loss in performance.
- That said, when function of the elbow is not allowing desired performance and clinical presentation indicates, surgery may be necessary.
- Due to the potential impact on performance, engage with surgeons who specialise in surgery of the elbow/upper limb and have experience/understanding of the relation and impact of any procedure on their sport.
- The most common indication for surgery in overhead athletes is arthroscopy for decreased range of motion, instability or locking of the elbow. Open surgery should be considered in the more rare cases that may necessitate primary reconstruction of the UCL rupture and fixation of stress fractures.

34.5 Areas for Future Research Consideration

As in other professional sports, such as baseball or tennis, epidemiological studies are necessary in cricket. Data can be used to develop prevention strategies. This is especially helpful in guiding the management of developing players.

There is little specific biomechanic or motion analysis data available for the elbow in cricket players. Insights from this data could be used to improve our understanding of injury as well as performance and technique.

Developments in wearable technology may soon provide valuable insights into the kinetics involved in throwing as well as workload data.

References

1. Felton PJ, McCaig S, King MA. Cricket fast bowling: the relationship between range of motion and key performance and injury technique characteristics. J Sports Sci. 2023;41(2):112–20. https://doi.org/10.1080/02640414.2023.2200520.
2. Orchard JW, Inge P, Sims K, et al. Comparison of injury profiles between elite Australian male and female cricket players. J Sci Med Sport. 2023;26(1):19–24. https://doi.org/10.1016/j.jsams.2022.12.002.
3. Kholinne E, Liu H, Kim H, Kwak JM, Koh KH, Jeon IH. Systematic review of elbow instability in association with refractory lateral epicondylitis: myth or fact? Am J Sports Med. 2021;49(9):2542–50. https://doi.org/10.1177/0363546520980133.
4. Kwak SH, Lee SJ, Jeong HS, Do MU, Suh KT. Subtle elbow instability associated with lateral epicondylitis. BMC Musculoskelet Disord. 2018;19(1):136. https://doi.org/10.1186/s12891-018-2069-8.
5. Goggins L, Williams S, Griffin S, Langley B, Newman D, Peirce N. English and welsh men's domestic cricket injury risk by activity and cricket type: a retrospective cohort study from 2010 to 2019. J Sci Med Sport. 2024;27(1):25–9. https://doi.org/10.1016/j.jsams.2023.07.013.
6. Faf du Plessis ruled out from remainder of CPL 2023 due to tennis elbow injury. https://www.royalchallengers.com/rcb-cricket-news/news/faf-du-plessis-ruled-out-from-remainder-of-cpl-2023-due-to-tennis-elbow
7. Bisset L, Beller E, Jull G, Brooks P, Darnell R, Vicenzino B. Mobilisation with movement and exercise, corticosteroid injection, or wait and see for tennis elbow: randomised trial. BMJ. 2006;333(7575):939. https://doi.org/10.1136/bmj.38961.584653.AE.
8. Smidt N, van der Windt DA, Assendelft WJ, Deville WL, Korthals-de Bos IB, Bouter LM. Corticosteroid injections, physiotherapy, or a wait-and-see policy for lateral epicondylitis: a randomised controlled trial. Lancet. 2002;359(9307):657–62. https://doi.org/10.1016/S0140-6736(02)07811-X.
9. Mi B, Liu G, Zhou W, et al. Platelet rich plasma versus steroid on lateral epicondylitis: meta-analysis of randomized clinical trials. Phys Sportsmed. 2017;45(2):97–104. https://doi.org/10.1080/00913847.2017.1297670.
10. Arirachakaran A, Sukthuayat A, Sisayanarane T, Laoratanavoraphong S, Kanchanatawan W, Kongtharvonskul J. Platelet-rich plasma versus autologous blood versus steroid injection in lateral epicondylitis: systematic review and network meta-analysis. J Orthop Traumatol. 2016;17(2):101–12. https://doi.org/10.1007/s10195-015-0376-5.
11. Pierreux P, Caekebeke P, van Riet R. The role of arthroscopy in instability of the elbow. JSES Int. 2023;7(6):2594–9. https://doi.org/10.1016/j.jseint.2022.12.001.
12. Jacobs J, Olivier B, Brandt C. Injury profiles in sub-elite women's cricket: exploring incidence, preva-

lence, nature, onset and body region. Phys Ther Sport. 2024;67:125–30. https://doi.org/10.1016/j.ptsp.2024.04.006.
13. Willemot L, Hendrikx FR, Byrne AM, van Riet RP. Valgus instability of the elbow: acute and chronic form. Obere Extrem. 2018;13(3):173–9. https://doi.org/10.1007/s11678-018-0465-1.
14. Verstuyft L, Caekebeke P, van Riet R. Postoperative rehabilitation in elbow surgery. J Clin Orthop Trauma. 2021;20:101479. https://doi.org/10.1016/j.jcot.2021.101479.
15. Ahmad CS, Conway JE. Elbow arthroscopy: valgus extension overload. Instr Course Lect. 2011;60:191–7.
16. Ahmad CS, ElAttrache NS. Valgus extension overload syndrome and stress injury of the olecranon. Clin Sports Med. 2004;23(4):665–76, x. https://doi.org/10.1016/j.csm.2004.04.013.
17. Wilson FD, Andrews JR, Blackburn TA, McCluskey G. Valgus extension overload in the pitching elbow. Am J Sports Med. 1983;11(2):83–8. https://doi.org/10.1177/036354658301100206.
18. Schwank A, Blazey P, Asker M, et al. 2022 Bern consensus statement on shoulder injury prevention, rehabilitation, and return to sport for athletes at all participation levels. J Orthop Sports Phys Ther. 2022;52(1):11–28. https://doi.org/10.2519/jospt.2022.10952.
19. VALD Knowledge Base. https://support.vald.com/hc/en-au/articles/14564824963481-DynaMo-Plus-Test-Shoulder-Strength-Protocol
20. Shaun Tait: Former Australia pace bowler retires from cricket. https://www.bbc.co.uk/sport/cricket/39404083

Wrist and Hand Injuries in Cricket

35

Douglass Wheen

35.1 Causes of Hand Injuries in Cricket

The hands and wrists are one of the most common sites of injury in cricket, accounting for approximately 10% of all injuries, independent of age, format and level of competition [1–4]. This is hardly surprising as the hand and fingers are uniquely exposed in cricket and are constantly moving and functioning in danger zones. The game involves control of a hard, high-speed projectile (the ball) by either poorly padded or completely unpadded hands. Furthermore, there is frequent contact of the hands with the ground when catching, or running and diving. Brooks et al [1] found that fielders, excluding wicketkeepers, had the highest rate of hand fractures during matches (1 fracture per 1338 balls) compared to both batters and wicketkeepers. In summary, the causes of injury are usually due to either balls or falls.

35.1.1 Falls

During catching the thrusting, outstretched hand and fingers may sustain both a direct impact into the ground and being sandwiched between the high-speed ball and the ground, both with little protection. When running and diving while batting, the outstretched hand may have some protection from the batting glove and support of the bat handle, although the ground of the wicket surface will be harder than the outfield. Impacts may, of course, also occur with any accidental fall, including during training and drills.

35.1.2 Balls

(i) Catching: The hands of all members of the fielding team are constantly involved in catching. Wicketkeepers are a special case, being involved in some way in the result of almost every ball bowled. They at least have glove protection. However, for all fielders small misjudgements and miscatches may result in high direct impact forces or high axial forces on the digits. Axial loading of a digit may result in the particularly difficult comminuted, depressed intra-articular disruption of the base of either the distal phalanx (DIP joint) or middle phalanx (PIP joint), known as Pilon fractures. These fractures can be very difficult to treat. Cricket is the most frequent sport that I have seen to cause double-level Pilon injuries (DIPJ and PIPJ Pilon fractures in the same digit).

(ii) Batting: Injuries usually occur due to a direct impact injury on a digit or metacarpal.

D. Wheen (✉)
Sydney Hospital, Sydney, Australia
e-mail: dwheen@handsurgery.com.au

B. Olivier, J. W. Orchard (eds.), *Cricket Sports Medicine*,
https://doi.org/10.1007/978-981-96-6321-7_35

Because the bone is crushed between the ball and the relatively fixed, hard bat handle closed, comminuted fractures are a common outcome.

Furthermore, the cricket environment has changed. Athletes are more professional and are fitter and stronger than ever. Batters are stronger and wield heavier bats, imparting greater force on the ball. Fielders have become more athletic and attempt catches of great difficulty when moving at speed, particularly in the short forms of the game. Such games occur with great regularity, allowing for only short recovery times. Players are highly motivated but impatient, and there is great and sometimes conflicting stress on all the coaches, physiotherapists, sports physicians and treating surgeons to move quickly. Unfortunately, tissue healing has not sped up commensurately.

35.2 Assessment of Hand Injuries

35.2.1 History of Injury

It is important to understand the history and mechanism of an injury to gain an appreciation of the forces and energy involved as this will help guide the prognostic expectations. In acute injuries, the mechanism will often be obvious, and during high-level games, the injury may have been captured on video images. In chronic injuries, it is vital to assess any pre-existing injuries or conditions, prior treatments including steroid injections and future expectations.

35.2.2 Examination

There are few other parts of the body where so many vital structures are packed together into such a confined volume. Although imaging of an injury is important, informed examination of the hand and wrist rapidly yields an enormous amount of useful information. Assessment of wrist instability, small joint ligament injuries and tendon issues is primarily clinical. The better one's knowledge of hand and wrist anatomy, the more valuable the examination will be, and time spent improving anatomical knowledge is very well spent.

In acute injuries, the site(s) of swelling, bruising and direct local tenderness will give useful guidance to the underlying injured structures. Fractures will usually cause quite diffuse swelling and bruising, whereas in ligament injuries, these will usually be more localised. Deformities, particularly rotational deformities, are best appreciated clinically and with flexion & extension. Fractures with rotational malalignment never self-correct with time. Open injuries, such as lacerations, open dislocations and open fractures, will require more urgent operative treatment with meticulous surgical debridement to minimise infection. The status of the digital nerves, arteries and tendons should be assessed and documented.

35.2.3 Imaging

(a) Plain X-rays

Good quality standard plain radiographs are vital for all bone and joint injuries and should not be neglected. Despite the role of other imaging modalities, good plain radiographs are all that is required for most injuries, and non-complex fractures. It is important to pay attention to the soft tissues, as well as the more obvious bony detail.

(b) CT scans

CT scans are excellent for fractures and bone pathology. They are particularly indicated for comminuted and intra-articular fractures, scaphoid fractures and PIPJ & DIPJ injuries. CT scans are usually widely and easily available, even after hours.

(c) MRI scans

MRI scans are appropriate for difficult soft tissue injuries including tendon & ligamentous injuries and they have become almost mandatory for detailed assessment of wrist injuries. MRIs are the earliest imaging modality that can detect scaphoid fractures, but they are not usually available urgently or in most emergency departments of public hospitals.

(d) Ultrasound

Ultrasound is particularly useful for soft tissue imaging. It is the only dynamic modality and can therefore assess structures as they move, which can be very useful in tendon and ligament injuries. It can also be used to accurately localise sites of tenderness and to perform image-guided injections. Small ultrasound machines are portable and, with appropriate training, can easily be used by sports physicians.

35.3 Specific Injuries and the Approaches to Treatment of Hand Fractures

In an epidemiological study of surgeries performed in professional Australian male cricketers by Orchard et al [4], 21 of the 33 surgical hand procedures were for acute injuries, of which the majority (16/21) were for fracture fixation.

The foundation of any treatment is to quickly and accurately diagnose the injury, and then to plan a course of treatment which will enable the most rapid primary healing possible, while also incorporating injury rehabilitation and return to use of the injured part for training and then on-field play. The initial triage should include assessment of any open component of the injury, whether the injury is stable or unstable, and whether there is displacement or joint involvement, if the injury involves a fracture. Nerves, arteries, tendons and other soft tissues must also be assessed as the soft tissue injury may determine the time to recovery.

In sport, many fractures benefit from surgical open reduction & internal fixation (ORIF). The principles and methods of this are well understood [5]. Acute surgical fixation must be considered for unstable fractures in which reduction cannot otherwise be achieved or maintained; for displaced, rotated and intra-articular fractures; and for open joint injuries and fractures which require surgical debridement to prevent infection. However, it is essential that surgery does not unthinkingly become the default treatment option. Although adequate ORIF may assist early movement of the injured part and earlier rehabilitation, improved strength and an earlier return to training and play, surgery itself also causes a degree of swelling, scarring and stiffness which may diminish the expected gains. There can also be complications of surgery, such as infection, which can completely annul any expected advantage.

Many fractures heal very adequately with closed treatment and splintage, and with careful therapy, this may be the preferred course of treatment [6]. Expert closed fracture treatment is superior to poor internal fixation, and the worst situation occurs when a poor ORIF case needs to be treated with static immobilisation or casting post-operatively. An early assessment and treatment plan should ideally be made in consultation with surgeons of adequate skill, experience and wisdom. To this end, it has been very helpful over many years in my practice to have had a close liaison between many of the Cricket Australia sports physicians and members of the Sydney Hospital Hand Unit so that the injury history, imaging and diagnosis can be shared quickly, treatment plans can be formulated, and any necessary surgery can be undertaken promptly by experienced surgeons in suitable facilities.

When ORIF of fractures is indicated, the aim of surgery is to anatomically reduce, stabilise (fix) and essentially eliminate the fracture such that early movement and functional use of the part can be commenced as soon as possible. Surgical approaches and incisions should be carefully planned to minimise surgical injury to the tendons. Mid-lateral digital incisions and percutaneous techniques are advantageous when possible. Reducing surgical soft tissue trauma will reduce swelling, tendon adhesions and joint stiffness, encouraging earlier resolution of the soft tissue components of both the original injury and the surgery. These aims will not always be achievable. The actual surgical outcome and therefore the post-operative therapy and rehabilitation plan should be objectively, honestly and clearly communicated to the player and to the involved (hand) therapists and sports physicians. The detailed programme for return to sport will then be formulated by the team doctors and physios working alongside the athlete, with appropriate adjustments as healing progresses.

Although most fractures will unite after appropriate treatment, on occasions there may be delayed union or even non-union of a fracture. This is particularly common in scaphoid fractures [7], and in other fractures where surgical fixation has been inadequate or resisted movements have been commenced too early, causing fixation to loosen and fail. Secondary capsular, ligamentous and joint stiffness usually ensues. This situation is a disaster for the player and causes significant delays in return to the field. It is easy to say that the situation is best avoided if possible, usually by doing the best procedure first, with appropriately strong initial surgical fixation. However, when non-union has occurred, it should be treated by the principles outlined by Buchler et al [8] including resection of the non-union, revision with strong internal fixation and supplementary autologous bone graft, necessary capsuloligamentous joint releases and early hand therapy (Fig. 35.1).

Fracture examples: As reported by Brooks et al [1], the 'exterior' bones of the hand are more frequently fractured in cricket. The examples below illustrate surgical principles and techniques for these fractures.

35.3.1 Distal Phalangeal Fractures and Fingertips

The fingertips take the brunt of impact injuries. Tuft fractures of the distal phalanx are common and often comminuted. The vast majority do not need surgical fixation, but do need routine ice, elevation, swelling reduction tape and splint protection. A thimble splint or moulded thermoplastic cylinder is usually helpful. These fractures are often accompanied by a subungual haematoma, which can be particularly painful. Traditional emergency management is to decompress the tense haematoma through the nail plate with a heated paperclip or 19-gauge hollow bore needle used as a drill. However, drainage may be inadequate, and infection can be introduced. Larger haematomas may be accompanied by a nail bed tear communicating with the fracture. These are

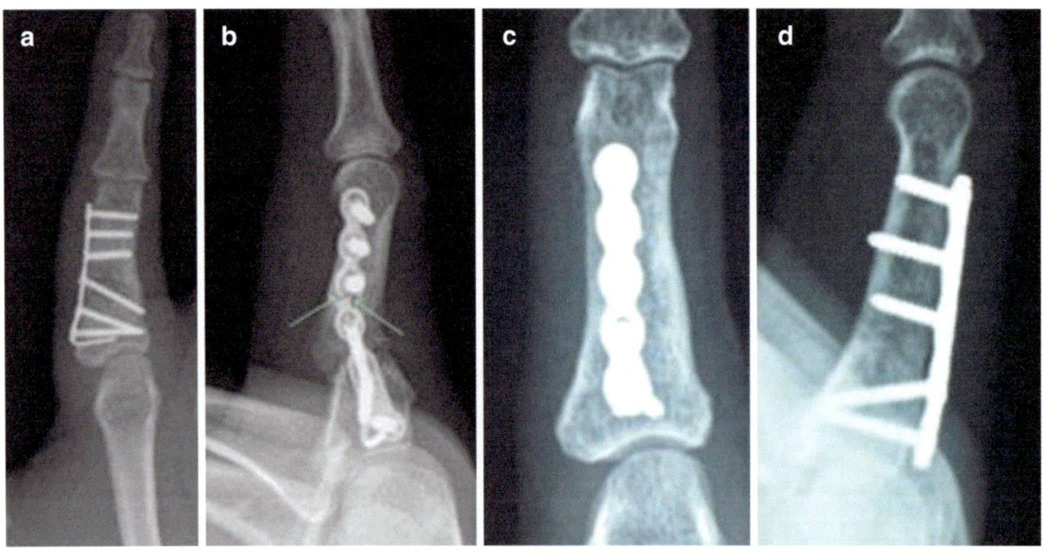

Fig. 35.1 (**a**)-(**d**) This player experienced failure (breakage) of fixation due to fracture non-union. Successful reconstruction involved resection of the non-union, wide soft tissue releases, autologous bone grafting, refixation and a considerable time away from cricket

better treated by formal elevation of the nail plate under anaesthesia, and accurate nail bed repair. Fractures of the neck and body of the distal phalanx are often unstable and slow to heal, particularly if they are displaced. Closed reduction and percutaneous K-wire fixation under fluoroscopy are usually required. The distal phalanx and DIPJ should be statically splinted for as long as the K-wire is in situ. Tendinous mallet finger injuries and mallet fractures are usually treated with cylinder splints, and mallet fractures may be treated with splints, k-wires or internal fixation dependent on the fragment size and any degree of DIPJ subluxation. Intra-articular impaction fractures of the base of the distal phalanx can be considered like Pilon fractures and are discussed below (see also Fig. 35.2).

35.3.2 Fractures of the Metacarpals and Proximal and Middle Phalanges

Many of these fractures will benefit from surgical fixation and the standard principles apply [5]. Oblique and spiral shaft fractures usually do well with lag screw fixation, with or without a supplementary neutralisation plate. The latter gives greater stability and early strength but usually requires a longer incision, and there may cause greater interference with the soft tissues and tendon function. There is also a greater likelihood that a later secondary surgery will be needed to remove the hardware. Transverse fractures of the neck and shafts have been conventionally fixed with plates and screws. Following the work of del Pinal [9], there has been an explosion of interest in fixation using longitudinal intra-osseous screws. This technique aims to reduce tendon adhesions and increase ease and range of early movement and use, consistent with our aims (Fig. 35.3). Custom screws have been specifically designed for these applications.

Volar plate avulsion fractures are common. After assessment of PIPJ congruity and stability, most of these can be treated non-operatively with a dorsal block splint and movement exercises. Larger avulsion fractures may require surgical fixation to restore joint congruity. Surgical fixation of intra-articular and condylar fractures of the phalanges requires careful planning and delicate techniques for exposure and fixation. Tendons may need to be retracted or split and stabilising ligaments similarly elevated or split. It is vital to preserve enough capsular and collateral ligament attachments to maintain vascularity of fracture fragments and avoid avascular necrosis of the condyles. If a joint is to be opened, accurate anatomical condylar reduction must be achieved to justify the surgical intrusion. If ana-

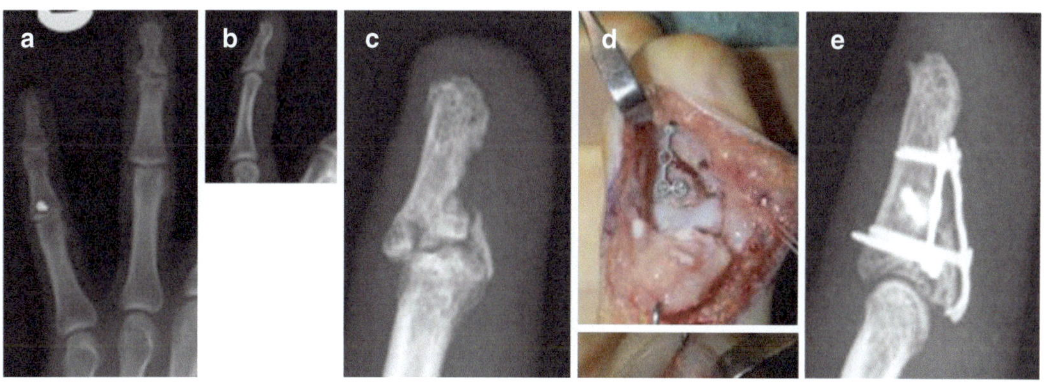

Fig. 35.2 (**a**)-(**f**) This player had simple fixation of a PIPJ fracture of the little finger, then later non-operative treatment of a base of distal phalanx of ring finger fracture, followed by delayed restoration of a highly comminuted Pilon fracture of another distal phalanx, all with good results and return to play. The hybrid fixation is shown

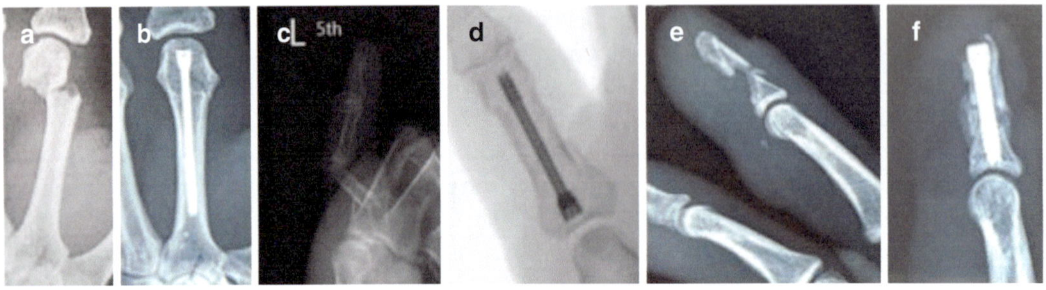

Fig. 35.3 (**a**)-(**f**) Examples of intramedullary (IM) fixation of fractures. *1*. The index metacarpal. *2*. Proximal phalanx of the little finger and *3*. Non-union of a fracture of the distal phalanx. This technique minimises soft tissue scarring, adhesions and stiffness. All Fig. 35.3 images courtesy of Dr Damian Ryan, with permission

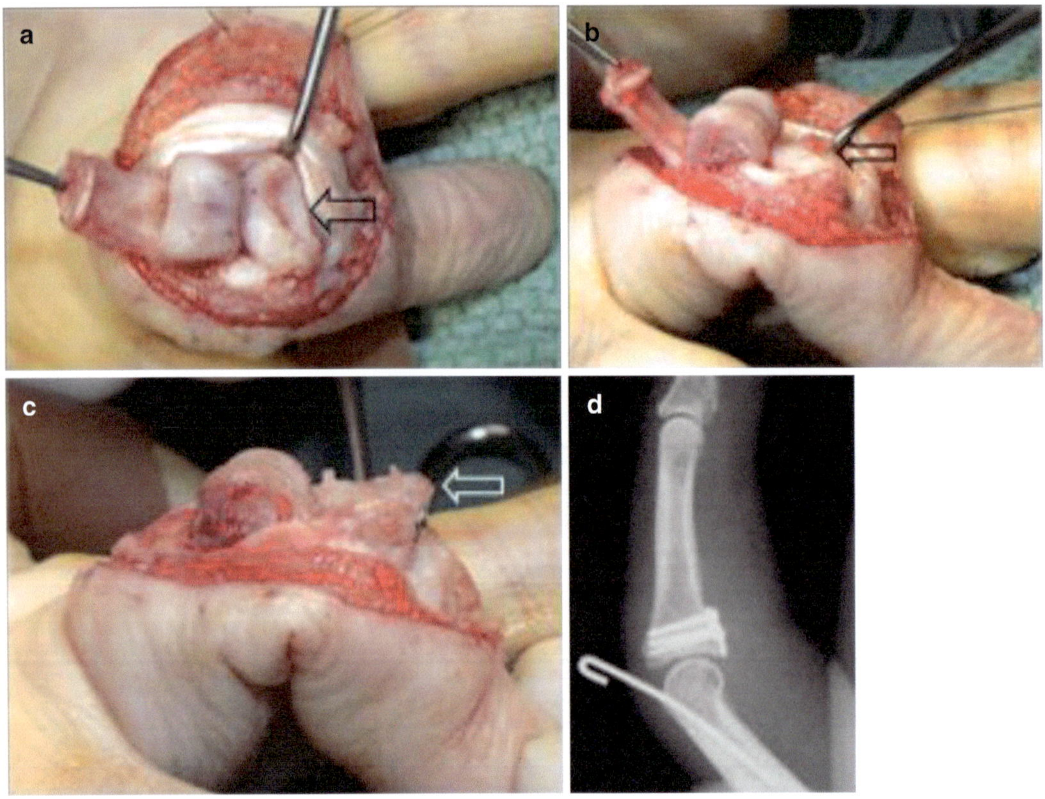

Fig. 35.4 (**a**)-(**d**): Shotgun approach to a Pilon fracture, with anatomic reduction and rigid fixation. The volar lip (arrowed) is carefully restored. Post-operative hand therapy is essential

tomical reduction is unlikely to be achieved, it may be better not to operate at all. Fixation in this situation demands 1.0 mm or 1.2 mm screws and plates, or fine buried k-wires. Hardware in this position usually requires later removal to assist maximising ROM.

Pilon fractures (Fig. 35.4) are caused by direct axial impaction forces on the digits leading to fractures of the bases of the middle and distal phalanges. The rigid head of the more proximal phalanx (the hammer) is driven into the opposing articular surface and supporting metaphyseal bone, which can become like a 'bag of chips'.

The cartilage of both joint surfaces is usually injured, and articular fragments can be driven several millimetres inside the phalanx. The resultant joint disruption causes long-term pain, swelling, stiffness and loss of function of the vital PIP and DIPJ.

These Pilon fractures are the most challenging of all hand fractures. As previously discussed, the specific high-speed axial ball impactions in cricket predispose to this type of fracture. The PIPJ is more commonly affected, but in cricket, the DIPJ may be similarly injured, and cricket is the only sport in which I have encountered double-level (PIPJ and DIPJ) Pilon fractures in the same digit. Careful and informed X-ray evaluation, with the addition of fine-cut CT scans through the injured joint(s), will allow initial treatment planning. However, these fractures are usually more comminuted than is seen on pre-operative imaging and plans need to be adaptable. The assessment, planning, operative approaches, reduction, fixation and necessary splintage all require experience, skill and a degree of obsessiveness. The aim is to restore joint alignment, movement and function, by restoration of accurate articular congruity.

For small, confined, stable articular defects, simple early protected ROM or dynamic traction devices may be appropriate. For highly comminuted articular fractures where operative fixation would be difficult or impossible, dynamic traction splints or fixators may again be used to commence joint movement while maintaining digital alignment as the fracture moulds and heals. This is not an easy process.

If there is a single depressed articular fragment in a fresh injury, percutaneous fluoroscopic fragment manipulation and reduction using a blunt k-wire passed through a distal drill hole can give excellent results. This technique can be particularly useful at the DIPJ. Early protected movement can be commenced, but the fracture must be allowed to heal before training is recommenced.

For cases suitable for open reduction and fixation, the surgical approach may be either dorsal, lateral or the volar Shotgun approach (Fig. 35.4). Lateral exposure is suitable only for limited unilateral fractures but it may allow easier post-operative movement and rehabilitation. Dorsal joint approaches are considered when the dorsum of the middle phalanx is already fractured.

After exposure of the dorsal fragment between the lateral bands, and with preservation of the attachment of the central slip of the extensor tendon, the articular surface may be exposed by elevating and hinging the dorsal fracture fragment proximally—almost a reverse Chamay exposure. After correcting the joint surface, some of the stabilising subarticular fixation and buttressing will be provided by the final cortical screw fixation of the dorsal cortex fragment on the way out. Larger defects may require autologous bone graft or synthetic substitute.

When a volar 'Shotgun' approach is used, the joint is completely hinged open by incision of the flexor sheath, retraction of the flexor tendons, release of the distal insertion of the volar plate and accessory collateral ligaments, and complete elevation of the origin of both collateral ligaments. This is quite an intrusive approach which gives unparalleled exposure to the entirety of both joint surfaces. However, the Shotgun approach may also open and displace associated longitudinal fractures of the middle phalanx. Once the joint is open, the fractures are assessed, and then without any unnecessary further bony disruption, the impacted fragments are reduced, and the curved volar lip of the phalangeal base is carefully restored. This usually requires more reduction than is initially apparent and can be a very exacting process.

Subarticular defects should be filled with cancellous bone graft, bone graft substitutes or screws. Definitive fixation is delicate and often creative, frequently using a combination of 1 mm screws, 0.6 mm K-wires, fine cerclage wire, bone anchors and small buttress plates. In unfortunate cases where the volar rim of the middle phalanx is unreconstructable, either a volar plate advancement arthroplasty or a hemi-hamate arthroplasty (below) is an option. These will hopefully have been considered preoperatively and discussed with the patient.

Although such PIPJ injuries cause pain, swelling and stiffness, professional cricketers are habituated to a regular degree of finger joint injury and pain and Pilon fractures may not always be initially recognised or investigated. The diagnosis may only be made after the articular surface is no longer able to be restored. In this situation, a hemi-hamate arthroplasty may be considered [10–12]. A volar Shotgun approach is again used. If the volar basal articular defect is less than 50% of the total joint surface, that part of the joint is excised. A carefully measured non-vascularised osteochondral graft is harvested from the ipsilateral dorsal hamate into the 4-5th carpometacarpal joints. The distal articular surface of the hamate closely replicates the bicondylar fossae of the volar base of the middle phalanx, with a central ridge. The defect is carefully remeasured and cut, and then, a matching graft is measured and mapped onto the distal hamate. The ridge on the graft coincides with the 4–5 intermetacarpal joint. The graft is meticulously cut using sharp osteotomes and a beaver blade, with the deeper 'undercut' made using a curved osteotome. With experience, the side cuts may be made a little obliquely if the graft ridge is not perpendicular. The graft is then solidly fixed into the defect with 2–3 x 1.2 mm or 1.3 mm screws. The joint is reduced, and passive ROM and PIPJ stability is assessed. The fixation is checked with fluoroscopy, and after wound closure, early active ROM can usually be commenced, with a dorsal blocking splint at approximately 0–10 degrees of flexion (Fig. 35.5).

35.4 Wrist Injuries

The wrist is the most complex joint in the body due to its eight intra-articular carpal bones and its complex of stabilising ligaments and musculotendinous motor units and the adjacent distal radioulnar joint (DRUJ). Together, these allow wrist flexion, extension, radial and ulnar deviation, circumduction of the hand on the forearm and forearm rotation. A myriad of injuries may occur, the most common being fractures of the scaphoid, injuries to the scapholunate ligament (SLL) and the triangular fibrocartilage complex (TFCC). Diagnosis and treatment are continually in evolution, and entire books have been written on these and other wrist injuries [7, 13]. Diagnosis depends on careful clinical examination to localise tenderness and assess instability, high-quality standard X-rays and then either or both of CT scan (primarily for bone assessment such as for scaphoid fractures) or MRI scan (primarily to assess ligament injuries and the TFCC). In professional athletes, X-ray-guided percutaneous screw fixation is indicated for most acute scaphoid fractures. Many major wrist ligament injuries, such as of the SLL and TFCC, require additional diagnostic assessment by wrist arthroscopy, combined with arthroscopic-assisted or open ligament reconstructions dependent on the findings [14]. Surgical techniques are in constant evolution, and sub-specialist expertise is required to appropriately match the kinematic problem,

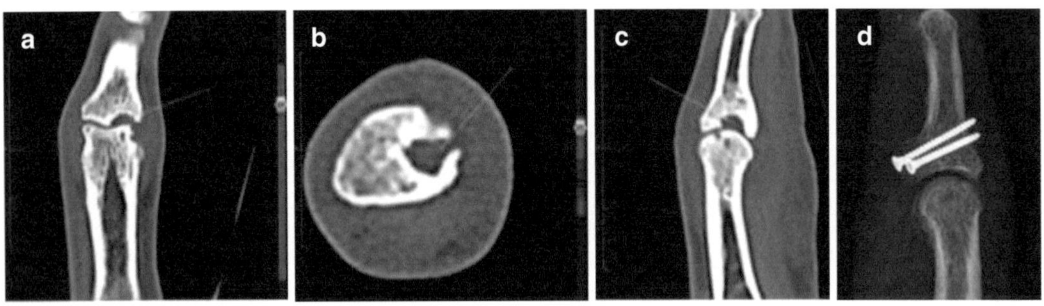

Fig. 35.5 (**a**)-(**d**): Hemi-hamate arthroplasty. PIPJ Pilon fracture of the right index finger in a wicketkeeper. The site was reinjured 1 year later after continuing to play. Conventional fixation and synthetic graft did not resolve the issue. The joint remained painful. Hemi-hamate arthroplasty was undertaken with a very good outcome and return to play

the ligament pathology and the operative treatment.

In summary, hand injuries in cricketers require early, accurate diagnosis. An endlessly fascinating variety of injuries occur. The experienced hand surgeon requires a large toolkit of techniques and tricks, the most important being wisdom, skill and a surrounding team of therapists, sports physicians and support staff to assist the injured player to recover and return to play.

References

1. Brooks K, Orchard JW, Saw AE, Kountouris A. Hand fractures and return to play in elite Australian cricketers. J Orthop. 2020 Mar 26;22:100–3. https://doi.org/10.1016/j.jor.2020.03.039.
2. Ahearn N, Bhatia R, Griffin S. Hand and wrist injuries in professional county cricket. Hand Surg 2015;20(1):89–92. https://doi.org/10.1142/S0218810415500124. PMID: 25609280.
3. Orchard J, James T, Alcott E, Carter S, Farhart P. Injuries in Australian cricket at first class level 1995/1996 to 2000/2001. Br J Sports Med 2002 Aug;36(4):270–274; discussion 275. https://doi.org/10.1136/bjsm.36.4.270. PMID: 12145117; PMCID: PMC1724521.
4. Orchard JW, Down S, James TG, Hoy GA, Young DA, Farhart P, Ryan MA, Wheen D, Kontouris A. Surgeries performed in professional Australian male cricketers. NZ J Sports Med. 2015;42:8–12.
5. AO Principles of Fracture Management, 2nd expanded ed, Thieme, New York, 2007.
6. Geoghegan L, Scarborough A, Rodrigues JN, Hayton MJ, Horwitz MD. Return to sport after metacarpal and phalangeal fractures: a systematic review and evidence appraisal. Orthop J Sports Med 2021 Feb 23;9(2):2325967120980013. https://doi.org/10.1177/2325967120980013. PMID: 33709003; PMCID: PMC7907947.
7. The Fractured Scaphoid, Herbert TJ, Quality Medical Publishing, St Louis, 1990.
8. Buchler U, Gupta A, Ruf S. Corrective osteotomy for post-traumatic malunion of the phalanges in the hand. J Hand Surg (Br). 1996;21(1):33–42. https://doi.org/10.1016/s0266-7681(96)80009-x.
9. del Piñal F, Moraleda E, Rúas JS, de Piero GH, Cerezal L. Minimally invasive fixation of fractures of the phalanges and metacarpals with intramedullary cannulated headless compression screws. J Hand Surg Am 2015 Apr;40(4):692–700. https://doi.org/10.1016/j.jhsa.2014.11.023. Epub 2015 Feb 7. PMID: 25661294.
10. Hastings H, Capo J, Steinberg B, Stern P. Hemicondylar hamate replacement arthroplasty for proximal interphalangeal joint fracture/dislocations (abstr) Presented at the 54th annual meeting of the American Society for Surgery of the Hand, Boston, 1999. https://doi.org/10.1016/j.jhsa.2008.01.012. PMID: 18590857.
11. Williams RM, Kiefhaber TR, Sommerkamp TG, Stern PJ. Treatment of unstable dorsal proximal interphalangeal fracture/dislocations using a hemi-hamate autograft. J Hand Surg Am 2003 Sep;28(5):856–865. https://doi.org/10.1016/s0363-5023(03)00304-6. PMID: 14507519.
12. Calfee RP, Kiefhaber TR, Sommerkamp TG, Stern PJ. Hemi-hamate arthroplasty provides functional reconstruction of acute and chronic proximal interphalangeal fracture-dislocations. J Hand Surg Am 2009 Sep;34(7):1232–1241. https://doi.org/10.1016/j.jhsa.2009.04.027. PMID: 19700071.
13. Buijze GA, Jupiter J, editors. Scaphoid fractures: evidence-based management. St Louis: Elsevier; 2018.
14. Mathoulin C. Treatment of dynamic scapholunate instability dissociation: contribution of arthroscopy. Hand Surg Rehabil 2016 Dec;35(6):377–392. https://doi.org/10.1016/j.hansur.2016.09.002. Epub 2016 Oct 7. PMID: 27890246.

Side and Abdominal Strains in Cricket

36

Andrew Nealon, Patrick Farhart, and James M. Linklater

36.1 Introduction and Epidemiology

'Side strains' are common in cricketers, with over half of Australian and English elite fast bowlers sustaining at least one in their careers [1]. Side and abdominal strains were second to hamstring injuries in terms of match incidence in Australian male elite cricket from 1994 to 2022 [2, 3] and in Australian female elite cricket from 2015 to 2021 [4]. In males, approximately 1 side strain injury occurs per season in State and National teams [1]. Abdominal wall injuries are 10 times more common in fast than spin bowlers and 20 times more common than in batters or wicketkeepers [1].

Side and abdominal strains also cause considerable player unavailability, and from 2016 to 2022, in male Australian elite cricketers, were the third highest cause of missed matches (0.8%), just behind hamstring injuries (0.9%) [3]. Similarly, side strains were the fifth highest cause of missed matches in female Australian elite cricket [4].

36.2 Risk Factors

There is no prospective research investigating potential risk factors for side strain. Standing height, trunk height, bowling arm [1], active trunk lateral flexion range of motion (ROM) [5] either toward or away from the bowling arm and side bridge endurance test [6] capacity have been shown to not be associated with a past history of side strain. However, some associations have been reported.

36.2.1 Young Age

A survey of 207 Australian and English elite fast bowlers reported that 77% of first-time side strains occurred in bowlers aged 24 and under, with bowlers aged 25 and older comprising less than 25% of primary injuries. Ages 22 and 23 combined comprised 30% of primary injuries [1], and an MRI study of 39 elite fast bowlers reported that 49% were aged 23 or younger [7]. Australian elite cricket data reported that bowlers aged 24 or younger were 3 times more likely to incur a side strain than bowlers aged 30 years or older and twice as likely as bowlers aged 25–29 [8]. Over

A. Nealon (✉)
Aspire Physiotherapy Centre, Erina, NSW, Australia

P. Farhart
School of Sport, Exercise and Rehabilitation, Faculty of Health, Human Performance Research Centre, University of Technology Sydney, Ultimo, NSW, Australia
e-mail: patrick.j.farhart@student.uts.edu.au

J. M. Linklater
Castlereagh Radiology, Sydney, NSW, Australia
e-mail: JamesLinklater@casimaging.com

B. Olivier, J. W. Orchard (eds.), *Cricket Sports Medicine*,
https://doi.org/10.1007/978-981-96-6321-7_36

Table 36.1 Weekly match bowling workloads preceding injury [12]

	Overs	Notes
Day of injury	5	78% of cases: less than 10 overs
Day before injury	2	85% of cases: less than 10 overs Only 1 case: more than 20 overs
Week of injury	16 overs 2 bowling days	45% of cases: less than 10 overs 19% of cases: more than 30 overs
2 Weeks leading to injury	13 overs/week 1.5 bowling days/week	43% of cases: less than 10 overs/week
3 Weeks leading to injury	12 overs/week 1.5 bowling days/week	48% of cases: less than 10 overs/week
4 Weeks leading to injury	12 overs/week 1.5 bowling days/week	48% of cases: less than 10 overs/week

50% of muscle injuries suffered by bowlers aged 22 and under were to the lumbar spine and trunk region, with side strain constituting 93% of these [9]. With increasing age, this steadily reduced to 14% for bowlers aged 31 and over [9].

36.2.2 Exposure to Highest Levels of Competition

Over 90% of fast bowlers that had played a minimum of 5 first class or 10 list A or 10 state, county or international T20 matches ('first class volume') had suffered at least 1 side strain during their career. Only 60% of elite bowlers that had not suffered a side strain had reached 'first class volume'. This difference in injury history may be associated with higher level competition demanding higher intensities to sustain bowling pace and performance. It could also be related to longer durations of the elite game, higher match and training volumes, compression of fixtures and variability between forms of the game. Higher injury rates with higher levels of competition have also been demonstrated for hamstring injury in football codes [10, 11].

36.2.3 Time of Season and Bowling Workload

Australian data indicate that side strains occur most commonly in the first months of the competitive season [8]. High early season incidence suggests that transitions in intensity from off-season deconditioning to the highly specific task of competitive fast bowling is not sufficiently countered by preparation for a forthcoming season. Prospective data of 56 side strain injuries (Table 36.1) in Australian and English elite fast bowlers demonstrate low competition mean bowling workloads immediately preceding injury [12].

More than twice the number of bowlers who delivered less than 10 competition overs in the 7 days prior to injury sustained a side strain in comparison to bowlers who delivered more than 30 competition overs in the same time frame. For weeks 1–4 leading up to injury, over 40% of bowlers averaged less than 10 competition overs per week. This suggests that cumulative fatigue is not a likely factor in this injury.

Season match bowling workloads prior to injury demonstrate that the highest proportion of injuries occurred at the lowest number of overs bowled. There were 52% of injuries within the first 100 overs and 10 match days (Table 36.2). Only 21% were injured after more than 200 overs with only 26% after 30 match bowling days (Table 36.3).

Table 36.2 Season match bowling overs preceding injury [12]

0–50 overs	38%
51–100 overs	14%
101–150 overs	16%
151–200 overs	11%
201–250 overs	7%
251–300 overs	5%
300+ overs	9%

Table 36.3 Season match bowling days preceding injury [12]

0–10 days	52%
11–20 days	21%
21–30 days	14%
31–40 days	7%
41–50 days	5%
50+ days	0%

These data suggest that accumulating match bowling workloads also accrue protection against side strain. Preparation for competition fast bowling should strive for injury protection and performance and include fast bowling at match speeds in training environments. The use of speed guns for monitoring bowling speeds consistent with matches is recommended so that the transition to matches only adds the element of competition and not also an increase in physical intensity.

36.3 Clinical Features

All cases in the cricket literature are reported on the side contralateral to the bowling arm in fast bowlers [1] but ipsilateral injuries have been reported in spin bowlers and the lead side of batters. Injury onset may be acute, with intense pain developing during or immediately after delivery or over several deliveries. The pain usually renders the bowler unable to continue, can vary from mild discomfort to excruciating and is generally located over the lateral aspect of the lower ribcage [13–16]. There may be significant pain with deep breathing and extreme pain with coughing and sneezing [17]. Pain is often reproduced by palpation and movements that place demands on the trunk musculature, such as rolling over in bed, rising from sitting, getting into and out of a car, and even stabilising the trunk to maintain an upright sitting position whilst driving a car [17]. Diagnosis is clinical; however, imaging is often performed [17].

> I've never had a side strain before but when I bowled the ball that caused the low-grade tear, it must be what surgery without the anaesthetic feels like, it was agony. Ben Stokes [18]

36.4 Clinical Assessment

Physiotherapists are typically the primary practitioners for players with side strain injuries. Clinical assessment includes objective measures regarding respiratory function, ROM, contractile tests and imaging.

36.4.1 Respiratory Function

Respiratory function is assessed with the following:

* Ability to take a full deep breath
* Pain intensity * / 10 with full deep breath
* Pain intensity * / 10 with maximal cough from full deep breath (without expectant aggravation of injury)

36.4.2 Range of Motion

Measurement of active trunk lateral flexion ROM for side strain is common practice [5] using a simple method (Fig. 36.1) for which intra-rater and inter-rater reliability has been demonstrated [5]. Minimum detectable change was shown to be 41 mm toward and 28 mm away from the bowling arm. 1736 monthly measurements of 238 uninjured fast bowlers over 3 years showed ROM was consistent, both toward and away from the bowling arm. This demonstrates that a single ROM measure taken at any time of the year is a valid baseline.

Unpublished prospective data shows the proportion of elite fast bowlers measured on days 1, 3 and 7 following side strain with significant ROM reductions (Table 36.4). This suggests that side strain more commonly causes significant reductions in active trunk lateral flexion range away from the bowling arm rather than toward it. Although daily life rarely commands extreme lateral flexion ROM [19], kinematic analysis has shown that fast bowling induces 30% greater lateral flexion during the front-foot phase of the delivery stride than measured in standing [20]. This movement is an essential component of the fast bowling action. Measurement is simple and

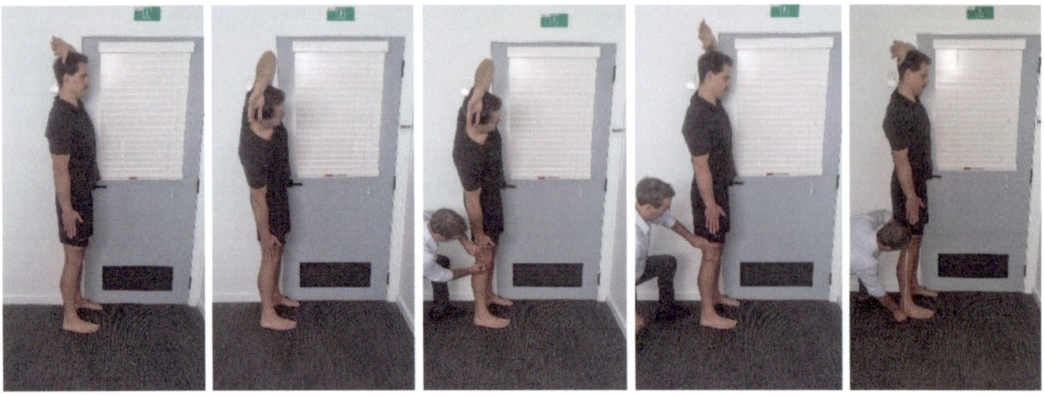

Fig. 36.1 Active trunk lateral flexion ROM measurement

Table 36.4 Significant reduction in active trunk lateral flexion ROM post-injury [12]

Day (# Bowlers)	Toward (%)	Away (%)
Day 1 (34)	41	59
Day 3 (29)	34	52
Day 7 (36)	14	33

Table 36.5 ROM limiting symptoms for all uninjured measurements [12]

	Away	Toward
Normal Stretch	52%	69%
Stretch/Pull	6%	10%
Jam/Squash	41%	21%
Dull Pain	<1% (3 measures)	0
Sharp Pain	0	0

reliable and should be included within clinical assessment.

End range symptoms also provide useful information. Baseline ROM range limiting symptoms were reported as follows (Table 36.5) [12]:

In uninjured bowlers, no player reported dull or sharp pain when laterally flexing toward the bowling arm. Only three were limited by dull pain when moving away from the bowling arm. The injury side limited ROM in 79% of uninjured measurements toward and 58% away from the bowling arm. The injured player's limiting symptoms, as well as ROM, should be compared to baselines during clinical assessment.

Trunk rotation, flexion and extension movement patterns should also be assessed, and when found to be suboptimal, may benefit from being addressed. However, there is no empirical information about these movements in uninjured fast bowlers or in the instance of side strain.

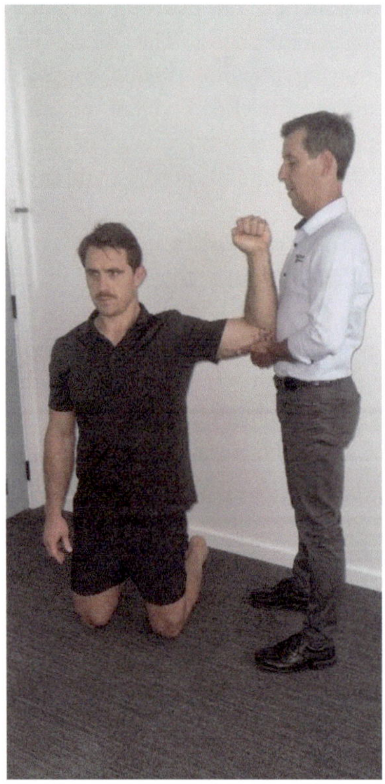

Fig. 36.2 Front arm pull

36.4.3 Contractile Tests

Generation and tolerance of force of the lateral trunk musculature should be tested.

The 'Front Arm Pull' (Fig. 36.2) is an isometric shoulder adduction test at 90° of shoulder abduc-

Table 36.6 Pain intensity on front arm pull test [12]

Day 1 post-injury (42 bowlers)		Day 3 post-injury (34 bowlers)		Day 7 post-injury (35 bowlers)	
Pain intensity/10	Proportion of bowlers (%)	Pain intensity/10	Proportion of bowlers (%)	Pain intensity/10	Proportion of bowlers (%)
0	21	0	26	0	46
1–3	19	1–3	26	1–3	37
4–6	24	4–6	24	4–6	14
7–10	36	7–10	24	7–10	3

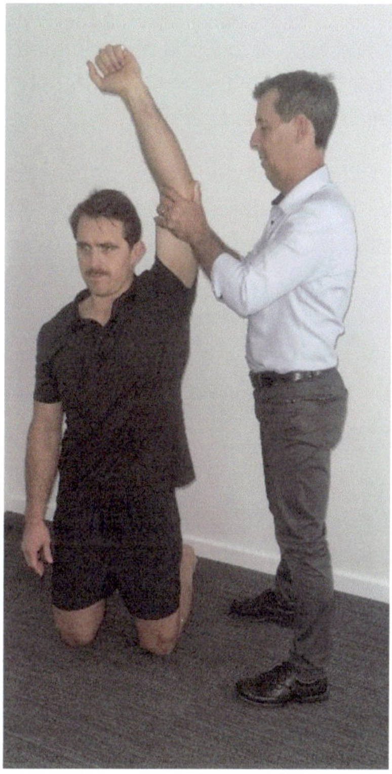

Fig. 36.3 Front side pull

tion and elbow flexion, performed with the player kneeling to enable the practitioner to readily oppose this force and increase the stabilising demands on the trunk musculature. The clinician may record the force generated at pain onset using a hand-held dynamometer and/or ask the player to report their proportion of maximum effort at pain onset. During rehabilitation, this can be a progress indicator.

Prospective injury data (Table 36.6) [12] on day 1 post-injury indicates that bowlers reported mean pain intensity of 4.4/10, with 79% reporting pain. By Day 7, mean pain intensity had reduced to 1.6/10, with 54% still reporting pain.

The 'Front Side Pull' (Fig. 36.3) differs only in that the shoulder adduction contraction is from

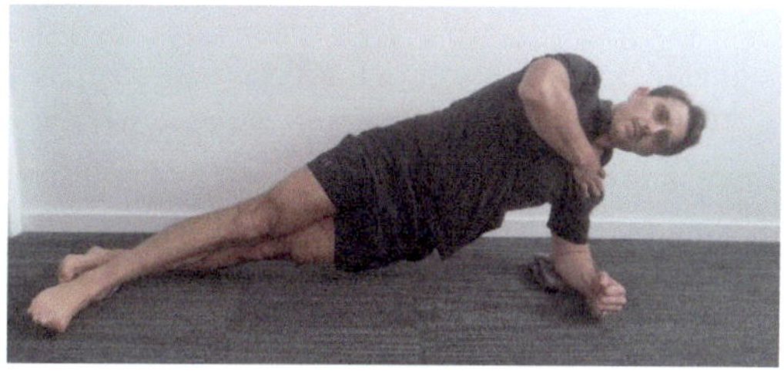

Fig. 36.4 Side bridge endurance hold

maximal arm elevation. In our experience, this test rarely adds more clinical information than the 'Front Arm Pull'.

The 'Side Bridge Hold' (Fig. 36.4) [6] for 30 seconds may be considered a more endurance demanding test.

Prospective injury data (Table 36.7) [12] on day 1 post-injury indicates that 6 bowlers were unable to get into position, 31% had 7–10/10 pain getting into position, and 52% were unable to sustain 30 seconds. By day 7, 2 bowlers were unable to get into position, 4% had 7–10/10 pain getting into position, and 81% could sustain 30 seconds with 34% pain free.

36.4.4 Imaging and the Varied Pathology of Side Strain

Side strain is typically imaged in elite cricketers [17] with ultrasound [16] and MRI [7, 13, 14]. Imaging side strain can be difficult, and reporting MRI scans of side strain has been shown to be of variable reliability [7]. Therefore, it is recommended that it is performed by imaging facilities with radiologists experienced with this specific injury present [7].

A prospective series [7] of 39 MRI scans in elite fast bowlers defined a muscle tear as 'architectural disruption' and was reported in 77% of injured bowlers. Internal oblique muscle injury

Table 36.7 Pain intensity on side bridge endurance test [12]

Day 1 post-injury (33 bowlers)		Day 3 post-injury (34 bowlers)		Day 7 post-injury (35 bowlers)	
Pain intensity/10	Proportion of bowlers (%)	Pain intensity/10	Proportion of bowlers (%)	Pain intensity/10	Proportion of bowlers (%)
Unable	52	Unable	47	Unable	19
0	21	0	26	0	34
1–3	18	1–3	20	1–3	38
4–6	9	4–6	7	4–6	3
7–10	0	7–10	0	7–10	6

(signal hyperintensity or defect) was demonstrated in 79% of cases and external oblique in 13%. There was no muscle pathology in 8% of injuries. Haematoma, or blood fluid products, was reported in 56% of injuries. Periosteal stripping only occurred with a muscle tear and was reported in 33% of cases and with 29% of internal oblique injuries and 80% of external oblique injuries. Rib oedema is a rare finding, reported in only 5% of cases, and only in the 12th rib.

The following are examples of different types of side strain injuries demonstrated on MRI (Figs. 36.5, 36.6, and 36.7):

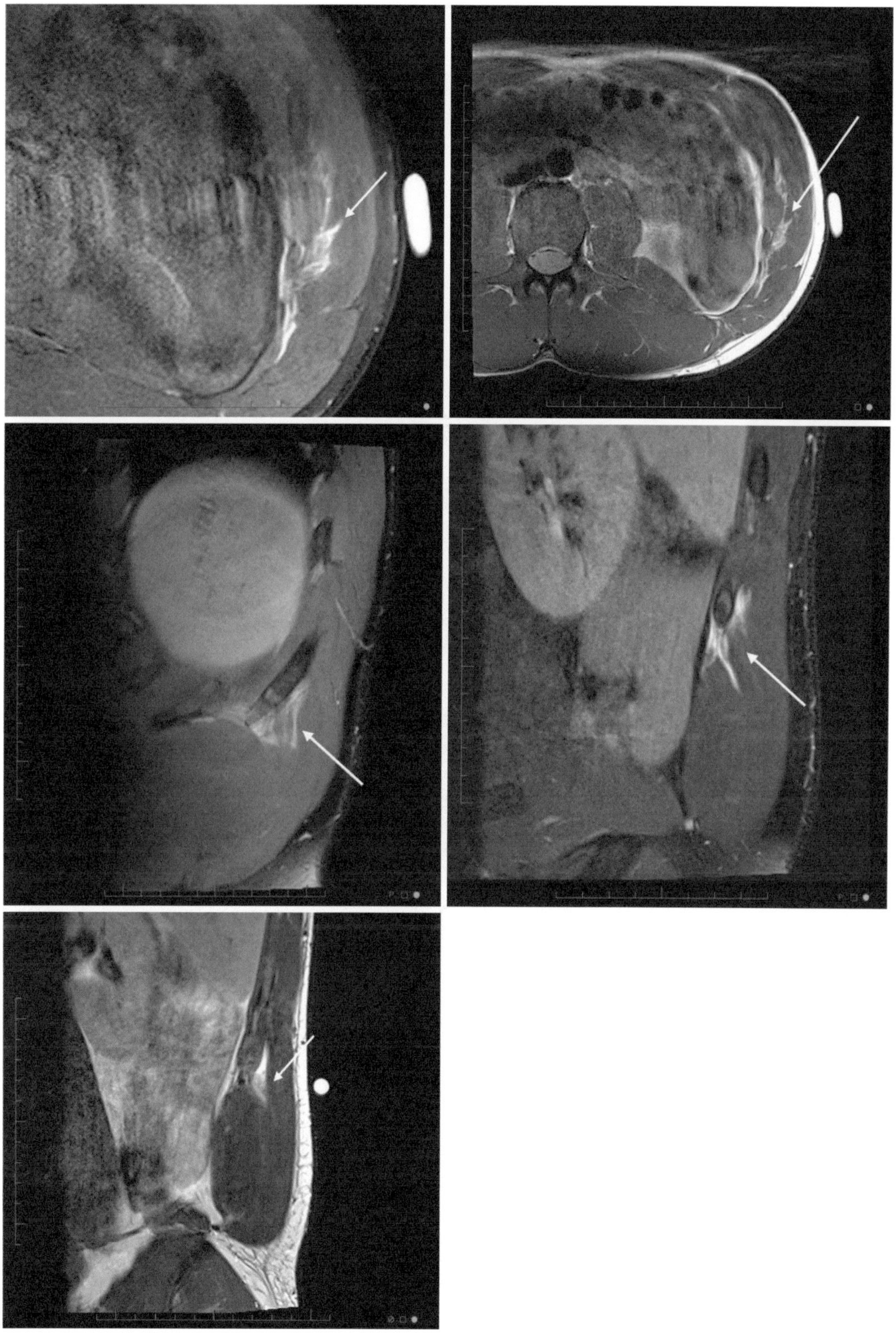

Fig. 36.5 A 25-year-old cricket player with left-sided lateral abdominal pain. MRI performed with skin marker placed over the site of symptoms. PD and PD fat suppressed sequences demonstrating small non-retracted partial tear at the origin of the left internal oblique off the anterior aspect of the left 11th rib with associated intramuscular oedema and perifascial fluid compatible with internal oblique strain injury

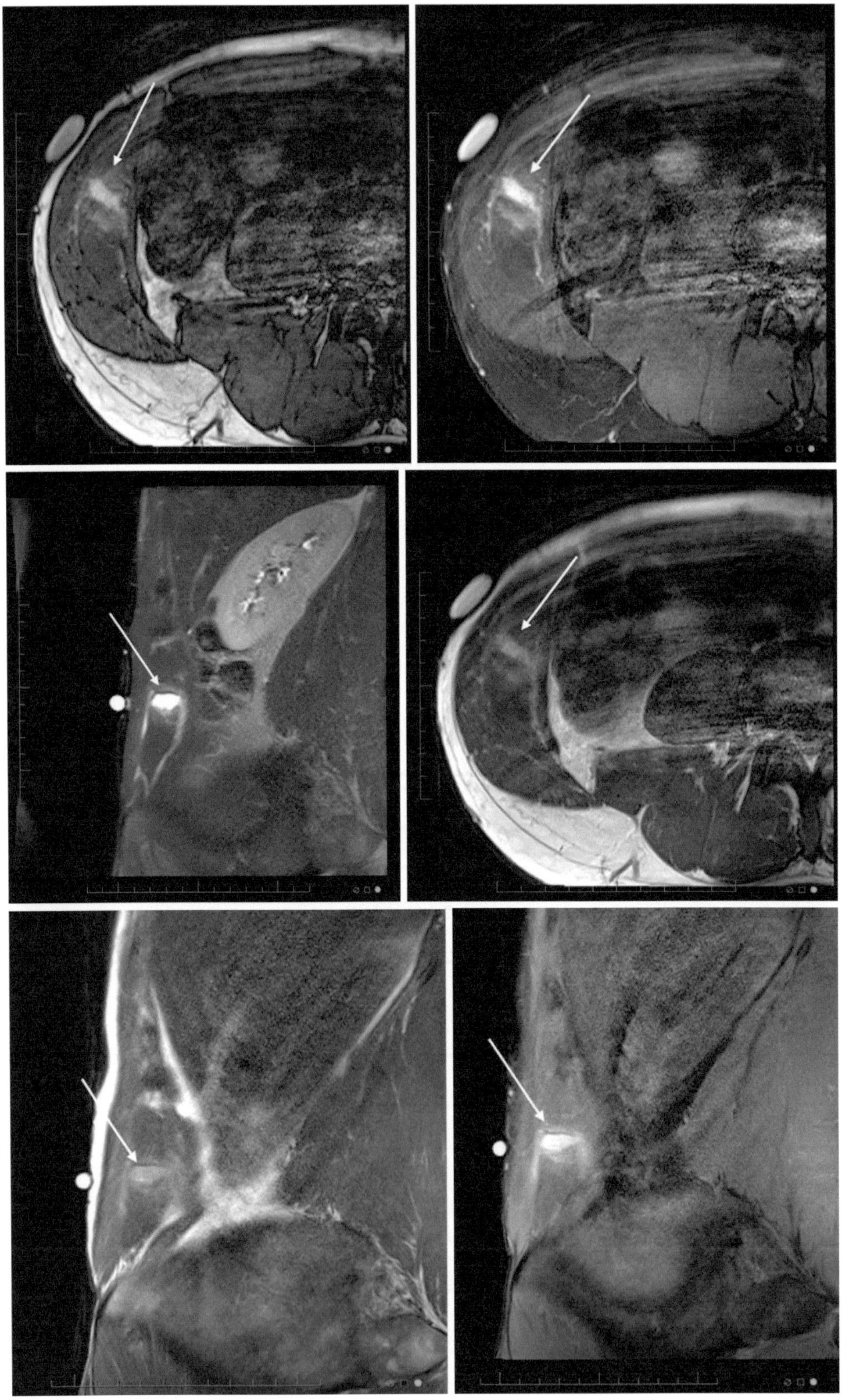

Fig. 36.6 A 17-year-old cricket player with right lateral abdominal wall pain. MRI performed with skin marker over the site of symptoms. PD and PD fat-suppressed sequences demonstrating tear of the right internal oblique muscle above the iliac crest with mild adjacent intramuscular oedema

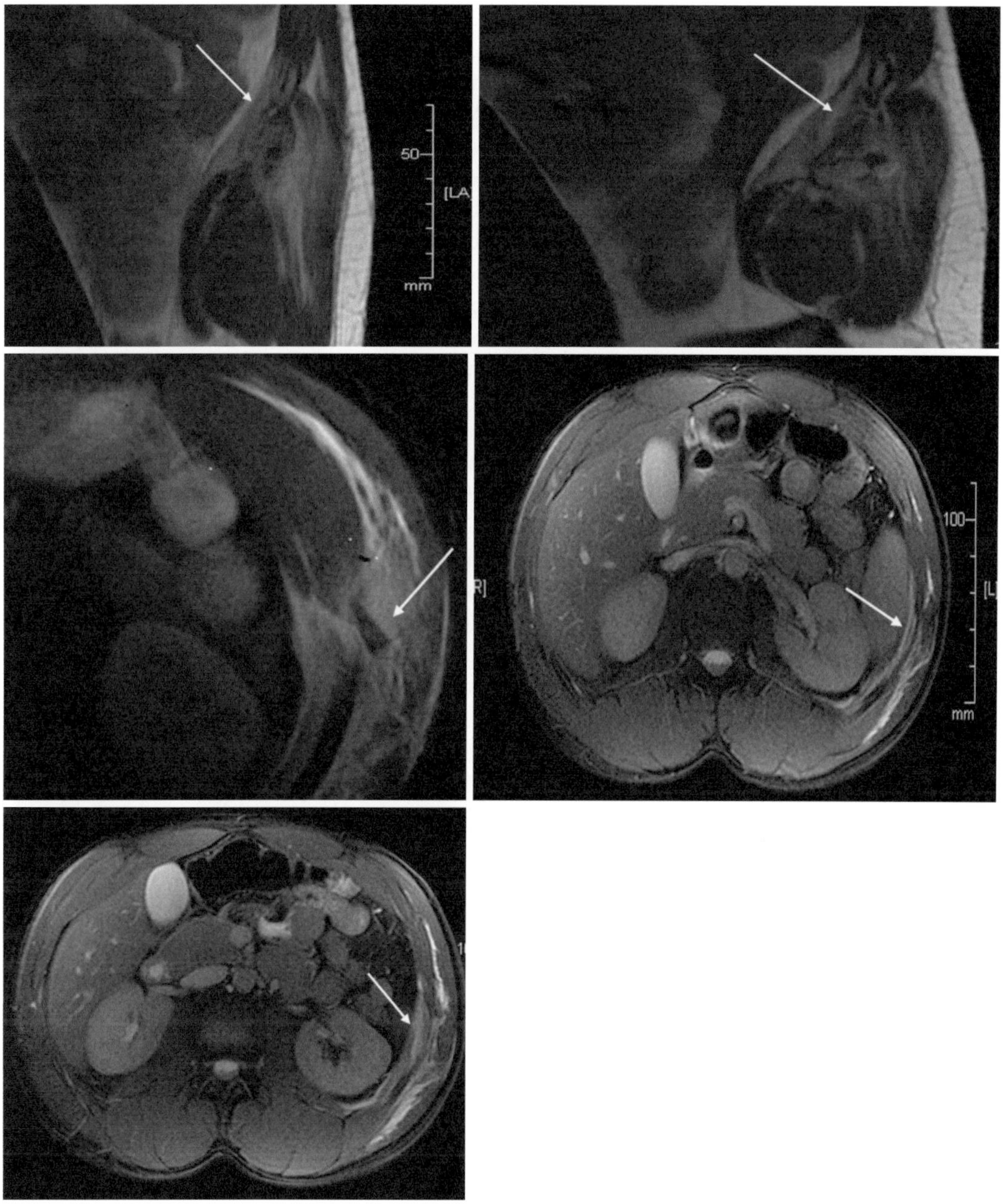

Fig. 36.7 A 22-year-old male cricket player with left lower lateral abdominal wall pain. MRI performed with PD and PD fat-suppressed sequences demonstrating an acute displaced costal cartilage fracture of the left 11th rib with moderate intramuscular oedema of the left internal oblique muscle with shallow perifascial fluid collection

36.5 Costoiliac Impingement and Other Diagnoses

Costoiliac (or side) impingement occurs in a similar location to side strain but is typically of insidious onset [17, 21]. It can develop as an isolated entity or during the return to bowling phase in over 30% of elite bowlers recovering from side strain. Costoiliac impingement can be persistent in 20% of bowlers at time of return to play (RTP) [17], and symptomatic bone and hypertrophic scar can cause ongoing symptoms and inability to bowl. There are two reported [15] cases of English elite fast bowlers who suffered this for 6 and 8 months respectively. Imaging demonstrated oedema of the tip of the 11th rib in both cases with hypertrophic soft tissue arising from the rib in one case. Both players underwent surgical resection of the distal 2 cm of the hypertrophied 11th rib. Within 4 months both players were bowling and by 6 months both were playing competitively and symptom free.

Other causes of lateral trunk pain can include costal cartilage injury, referred pain from the thoracic spine or costovertebral joints, upper lumbar bone stress injuries and non-musculoskeletal causes such as gastrointestinal illnesses, kidney disorders and shingles. Clinicians shouldn't automatically assume that lateral trunk pain in their symptomatic player is a 'side strain'. A thorough and systematic clinical assessment is paramount to determine the cause of symptoms, which may have contractile and/or non-contractile elements, and then plan and implement the required investigations and rehabilitation.

36.6 Recovery Time

One prospective study reported 39 cases of side strain to elite cricket fast bowlers with RTP at elite level within the same season [7]. Time to RTP averaged 39 days (range: 12–67). Only 10% of players returned in less than 3 weeks, whilst 46% required 4–6 weeks. Over 6 weeks was required by 44% of bowlers.

The only MRI parameter associated with time to RTP is the presence of a muscle tear. Fast bowlers with a muscle tear on MRI required a mean 43 days (range: 16–67) to RTP. The 78% of bowlers with a muscle tear were 8 times more likely to require more than 6 weeks than those without a muscle tear, with RTP at a mean 26 days (range: 12–47). Of the 36% of bowlers with RTP in under 5 weeks, 78% had no muscle tear.

It is notable that 8% of this sample exhibited no reported pathology on MRI but had a clinically diagnosed side strain and were unavailable to play due to symptoms. This is a similar proportion to the 13% of professional footballers reported as 'MRI negative' that required a mean of only 8 days to RTP from 'hamstring' injury [22]. However, 'MRI negative' side strain bowlers required 22, 46 and 47 days to RTP. Thus, the pain generating structures of a bowler with 'MRI negative' side strain may differ from those with the MRI parameters that have been described. In contrast to posterior thigh pain, the absence of MRI findings does not assume a shorter time to RTP.

Side strain time to RTP is prolonged compared to many other injuries. The injury needs time to heal; it requires a bowler to regain running fitness and strength, experience a graded return to bowling, restore bowling intensity and loads to levels to return to competition, and demonstrate a high likelihood of sustaining this to prevent recurrence, whilst returning to performance levels warranting selection. This is different for a footballer with a hamstring injury, as once they can sprint, repeat sprint and demonstrate readiness to play in training, the demands of returning to play are essentially achieved. The unique stress of bowling adds time to the recovery period.

36.7 Recurrence

The likelihood of recurrence should be considered during rehabilitation planning. Unfortunately, 30% of bowlers have been reported to sustain at least one recurrence following primary side strain, comprising 16% of all elite fast bowlers. About half of recurrences occurred within the first 2 years and a further 27% within the third year. One third of bowlers that sustain one recurrence proceed to suffer at least one more [1].

36.8 Rehabilitation

Planning requires an appreciation of the available research regarding likely recovery timeframes, objective clinical assessment and an understanding of the demands of fast bowling. Fast bowling is a complicated, high speed, high force, repetitive activity and is the most common mechanism of injury in cricket. Resolution of clinical markers will indicate readiness for loading injured structures with the purpose of restoring function and resilience. Rehabilitation should include exercises and conditioning that mimic the various roles of injured structures at levels of demand that are tolerable at the stages that they are implemented, with demand increasing towards the ultimate task of fast bowling that is required to RTP.

The following stages and time frames are a guide only and based on the player requiring the mean time of RTP of 5–6 weeks, remaining mindful that almost half of elite bowlers require more than 6 weeks.

36.8.1 Stage 1: Resolving Chest Wall Signs

Muscles that are typically injured in side strain have roles in respiration and visceral support for the trunk [17]. However, internal and external obliques also link the pelvis to the torso and are key during tasks that demand trunk stabilisation and axial torque, flexion and side flexion. They must be capable of performing their role in respiration whilst also generating and tolerating high abdominal pressure forces during coughing and sneezing, as well as high-intensity upper and lower limb force-generating movements during which the trunk remains static.

Most players will report resolution of symptoms with normal breathing within 2–3 days and with a full deep breath within 3–5 days. Players will then typically tolerate exercises that require the abdominal oblique muscles to fulfil their isometric roles as trunk wall stabilisers at relatively low pressures, using the upper and/or lower limbs to apply load. Such exercises could be performed in standing, supine or 4-point kneeling. The clinician should also be mindful of the player maintaining cardiovascular fitness during this stage, and they will likely tolerate non- to low-impact activity such as stationary biking, elliptical/cross-training and walking.

Asymptomatic cough from a full deep breath can take 5–10 days, varying with injury severity. Front arm pull test may take 10–15 days to resolve. During this time, the player can usually tolerate more demanding exercises that require sustaining asymptomatic high abdominal pressures with a static trunk. Examples include sub-maximal front arm pull (Fig. 36.8), supine

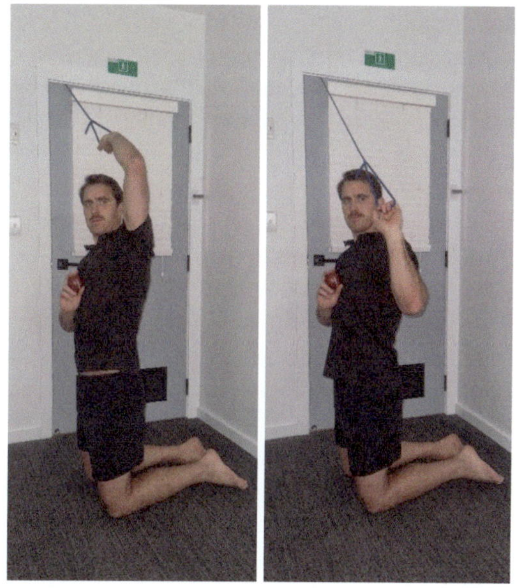

Fig. 36.8 Front arm pull exercise

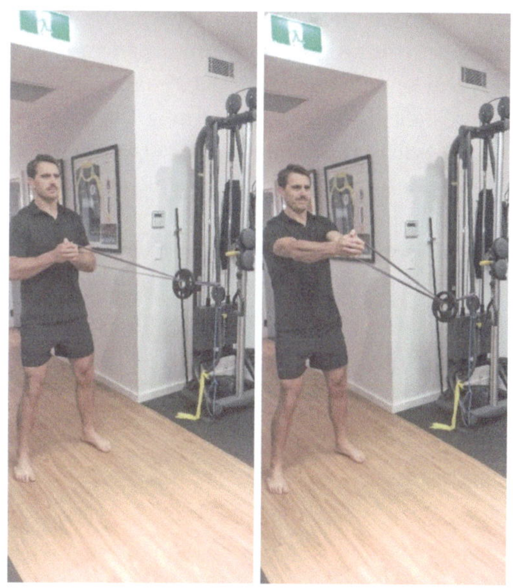

Fig. 36.9 Pallof press with band and plate

single and double leg lowers, dead bugs, trunk extensions in prone and Pilates reformer exercises in supine and kneeling. Most players can return to lower limb resistance training at 7–10 days and upper limb resistance training with a neutral trunk position at 10–14 days. Exercises could include side bridge hold for short durations (less than 30 seconds), lat pulldowns, squats, Pallof press (Fig. 36.9), med ball core drills in supine and kneeling, bent over rows and dead lifts. Cardiovascular training can progress to rowing, swimming and returning to running as able, with speed increasing to sprinting at about 2 weeks post-injury.

36.8.2 Stage 2: Restoring Trunk Range of Motion

Once tolerance of the roles of the oblique musculature in a neutral trunk position has been achieved, ROM needs to be restored. Usually, the only affected movement is trunk lateral flexion. Given that this has been shown not to vary in uninjured fast bowlers and is reduced in most injured bowlers, it follows that given the inherent requirements of this movement for bowling, ROM is restored to baseline and undesirable end range symptoms are resolved. When moving away from the injured side, a 'stretch/pull' at end range may be worked into providing symptoms are not aggravated. However, when moving towards the injured side, pushing into a jam/squash, which is a common end range symptom, is not helpful. It needs to be remembered that 21% of uninjured fast bowlers reported 'jam/squash' as their limiting symptom when moving away from the bowling arm and this may be the injured bowler's own baseline, or prevailing, symptom.

It is during this stage that manual therapy is likely to be of greatest benefit. The injury area may be desensitised and haematoma addressed with soft tissue techniques, muscle spasm eased and muscle recruitment optimised. Thoracic spine mobilisation and manipulation may assist the restoration of lateral flexion range. As it is likely that the injured bowler won't have been able to move freely for some time, all other priority areas for bowling, such as lumbar extension and hip ROM, also require restoration.

36.8.3 Stage 3: Regaining Dynamic Trunk Motion and Strength

The highly repetitive demands of fast bowling and power hitting in batting invoke unilateral, asymmetrical, explosive and repetitive actions. Following the resolution of chest wall signs, restoration of trunk ROM and demonstration of tolerance of exercises and activities requiring the lateral chest wall musculature to withstand high-pressure isometric contractions, the player should be progressed to induce the dynamic roles of this region at low loads and speeds. This includes other roles and skills within the game, such as high-intensity running progressing to sprinting, agility training, catching, fielding and batting. Batters should initially avoid cross-bat and more explosive shots following progressions through defensive and straight bat strokes.

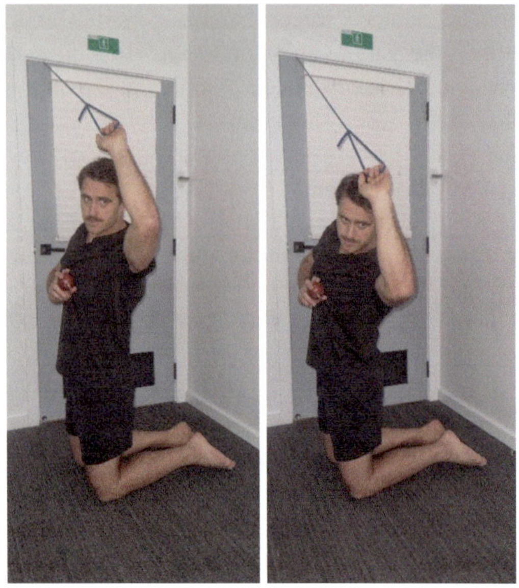

Fig. 36.10 Front side pull exercise

Dynamic trunk exercises that load the lateral chest wall should be performed at relatively low speed and high volumes, then increasing to higher speeds to mimic the demands of bowling. Some trunk loading exercises may be performed in kneeling. This removes the balance provided by the lower limbs, thus increasing the demands on the trunk musculature to stabilise the chest wall whilst simultaneously generating movement and speed. Examples include the front side pull (Fig. 36.10) and delivery pull, which may commence using rubber tubing attached overhead, building up to using a cable pulley with a weight stack, to using medicine balls. Exercises should

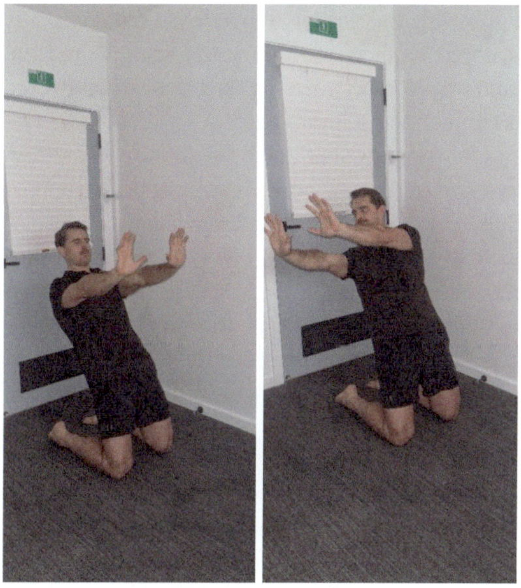

Fig. 36.11 Reverse Nordic plus trunk twist

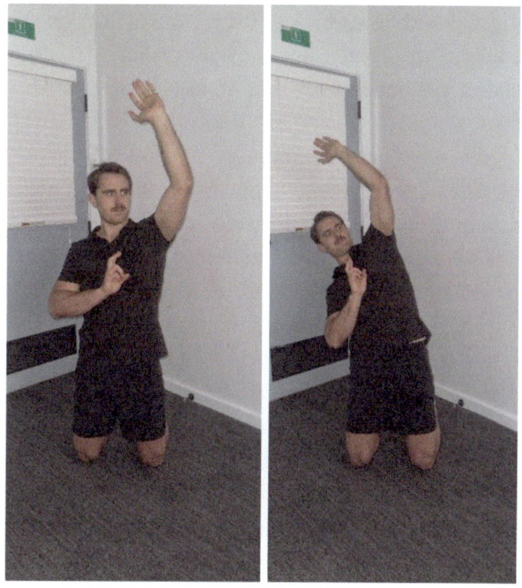

Fig. 36.12 Reverse Nordic delivery

include combinations of higher resistance at slower speeds, mixed with lower resistance at higher speeds. It is uncommon for muscle to be reinjured at lower speeds, and so higher forces may be utilised earlier on, and then forces reduced as speed of force generation is increased. In the case of a fast bowler side strain, the bowler has been injured propelling a ball that only weighs 156 g, and this is the task for which they are preparing. Exercises should progress to demand force generation through the full range of trunk motion and in the movement planes of the bowler's own action. For example, dynamic strengthening exercises shouldn't remain purely 'side on' when the bowler's own action is 'semi-open'. Exercises should be customised to the bowler's own movement pathways, such as Reverse Nordics with various ranges of trunk rotation (Fig. 36.11) and Reverse Nordic delivery (Fig. 36.12).

36.8.4 Stage 4: Returning to Bowling

Bowlers are usually ready to return to throwing at 2–3 weeks and bowling in training environments at 3–4 weeks post-injury. However, all side strains are different, and progressions must be based on achieving clinical and functional milestones including restoration then maintaining baseline trunk lateral flexion ROM with comfortable end range symptoms. The risk of costoiliac impingement and recurrence must be considered when determining readiness to return to bowling.

Returning to bowling is a nervous time for the bowler after side strain. The pitch often feels much longer. Bowlers often tend to 'put the ball there' rather than 'pull through'. This apprehension is natural, akin to someone increasing running speed towards sprinting after hamstring injury. However, this alters bowling mechanics and can cause complications. For example, avoiding 'pulling through' with the front arm in their natural plane causes 'falling away' into higher magnitudes of lateral flexion during delivery. Forceful extension of the front arm during delivery is not only a key force generator to engage the lateral trunk to generate speed for pace bowling, but the front arm also acts as the 'rudder of the trunk'. With the rudder 'falling away', aside from compromising pace, wrist position, delivery release height and consistent performance, the increased magnitude of trunk lateral flexion further approximates the lower ribcage and the iliac crest.

Following side strain, there is likely to be hypersensitive scar tissue from the repairing muscle and/or sensitive costal periosteum (especially if the injury involved periosteal stripping and/or rib oedema), which then directly impacts against the much larger iliac crest. This is the likely cause of the significant portion of bowlers that develop a stage of costoiliac impingement during their return to bowling. The resultant pain can be difficult for the bowler and clinician to differentiate from a low-grade recurrence of the original muscle injury and can also prolong the return to bowling process as it takes a brave clinician to advise the bowler to continue to increase their bowling volume, and especially, speed.

Reassessing contractile signs using tests such as front arm pull, and side bridge hold and dip is valuable. Although these tests can induce high levels of force generation, they are performed with the trunk in neutral or inner ranges of trunk lateral flexion towards the injured side. Therefore, if the contractile structures remain intact and the bowler does not report symptoms on these tests, it is most likely that the pain experienced whilst bowling is costoiliac impingement and not a recurrence of muscle injury. The pain or discomfort of bowling may be reproduced at end range active trunk lateral flexion towards the injury side, albeit commonly at a much lower intensity given that this is a controlled, non-impact and slow movement compared to bowling. The clinician should remain mindful that whilst this test may induce and later be clear of symptoms, the bowler's action won't be a pure lateral flexion movement. This stage of symptoms may be transient, or it can persist and become problematic.

The symptom pattern of this condition is often similar to other impingement syndromes that are suffered by fast bowlers, such as posterior ankle or elbow impingement. The first few balls of a spell are usually the most painful, often sharp, but then tend to ease and may resolve. One could argue that the pain of initial deliveries eases as the painful tissue desensitises. Alternatively, the pain may occur during initial deliveries because the bowler isn't yet sufficiently 'warmed up' and/or confident to 'pull through' with their typical force and, therefore, in their typical 'plane'. Following the initial deliveries, their action is restored to their pre-injury kinematics, and the pain resolves because the sensitive structures are no longer being impinged.

One strategy that has been found to be effective is returning to bowling on a shorter pitch so that the bowler doesn't feel they have to 'muscle' the ball along the full length of the pitch. It is also recommended that although delivery effort will initially be sub-maximal, the bowler generates their usual momentum into delivery from their typical run up speed, which has earlier been restored. This may feel unusual at low bowling speeds. However, failure to generate normal run up momentum shifts demand to generate force to the delivery. The delivery is where the bowler will have 'memory' of the injury occurring, and it is where they will understandably be most hesitant and even afraid. Approaching delivery with momentum minimises force generation at delivery at lower ball speeds, and shortening the pitch reduces the distance of ball propulsion.

A second useful strategy is increasing bowling intensity via the use of short-pitched deliveries before returning to fuller lengths. Although this might seem counterintuitive, bowling a short-pitched delivery necessitates 'pulling through' and 'finishing off' the bowling action, restoring the bowler's usual kinematics as soon as possible. This practice can prevent and resolve the common stage of costoiliac impingement whilst returning to bowling in rehabilitation or competition. This highlights that anxiety can sometimes only be induced by the performance demands of competition and can manifest as compromising bowling mechanics.

> If I'd had a normal (side strain), a big injury and you know you're going to be out, then you can deal with it all at once. But it just kept teasing, kept teasing, I might be able to play this one, I might be able to play that one… I've certainly had a typical side strain, where you tear your oblique, you can't bowl another ball and are out for at least six or seven weeks. This one was different … the strength came back really quickly, and I could do a lot of things in the gym. It was just bowling, that dynamic movement, that caused a bit of grief. It was an unusual one.
> Josh Hazlewood [23]

36.8.5 Stage 5: Returning to Play

Clinicians must be sensitive to non-physical factors of injury and remain mindful of the natural emotions of their bowlers. Only once competitive instincts are challenged will the returning bowler feel the anxiety of the contest with the batter. Some will cope with this better than others. However, such emotions are not limited to the mind in their consequences. Fear and trepidation, especially following a painful and expensive injury such as side strain, can impact kinematics, and altered kinematics can cause other physical issues.

Following side strain, this may be costoiliac impingement, but failure to generate usual forces from the trunk places greater demands for force generation elsewhere, with potential victims being the elbow and shoulder of the bowling arm. Fast bowling is unique, and ultimately the best preparation for and accumulation of protection against injury is by fast bowling itself. This should include the variations of deliveries that are now commonplace, especially in white ball cricket. Slower balls, straight and wide yorkers, bouncers, slower ball bouncers, length, bowling over and around the wicket are deliveries now delivered in various combinations, and all exert different demands on the fast bowler. They all need to be practiced for both skill and physical resilience and should be included in the rehabilitation plan.

Reaccumulating workload contributes significant time to recovery. RTP at a mean of 5–6 weeks is similar to recommencing the season, which is the most common time of side strain and a likely factor in recurrence. Speed guns are recommended to ensure that bowling intensity is replicating match conditions so that only mental and performance aspects of competition are added upon RTP. Once the injured bowler has returned to play, workload management is essential to manage factors that may have contributed to the injury and aim to prevent recurrence.

References

1. Nealon AR, Cook JL. Trunk side strain has a high incidence in first-class cricket fast bowlers in Australia and England. Clin J Sport Med. 2018;28(3):284–8.
2. Orchard J, Kountouris A, Sims K, Orchard J, Beakley D, Brukner P. Injury report 2014: Cricket Australia. Sports Health. 2014;32(4):14–8.
3. Orchard JW, Inge P, Sims K, Kountouris A, Saw AE, Saw R, Beerworth K. Comparison of injury profiles between elite Australian male and female cricket players. J Sci Med Sport. 2023;26(1):19–24.
4. Orchard J, Kountouris A, Inge P, Beakley D, Beerworth K, Golding L, Saw A. Cricket Australia: injury report 2021.
5. Nealon A, Cook J, Docking S. A novel method of assessing trunk lateral-flexion range of movement in first-class cricket players. J Athl Train. 2021;56(12):1355–61.
6. McGill SM, Childs A, Liebenson C. Endurance times for low back stabilization exercises: clinical targets for testing and training from a normal database. Arch Phys Med Rehabil. 1999;80(8):941–4.
7. Nealon AR, Docking SI, Lucas PE, Connell DA, Koh ES, Cook JL. MRI findings are associated with time to return to play in first class cricket fast bowlers with side strain in Australia and England. J Sci Med Sport. 2019;22(9):992–6.
8. Humphries D, Orchard J, Kountouris A. Abdominal wall injuries at the elite level in Australian male professional cricketers. J Postgrad Med Educ Res. 2017;49(4):155–8.
9. Blanch P, Orchard J, Kountouris A, Sims K, Beakley D. Different tissue type categories of overuse injuries to cricket fast bowlers have different severity and incidence which varies with age. S Afr J Sports Med. 2015;27(4):108–13.
10. Woods C, Hawkins RD, Maltby S, Hulse M, Thomas A, Hodson A. The Football Association Medical Research Programme: an audit of injuries in professional football—analysis of hamstring injuries. Br J Sports Med. 2004;38(1):36–41.
11. Verrall GM, Slavotinek JP, Barnes PG, Fon GT, Spriggins AJ. Clinical risk factors for hamstring muscle strain injury: a prospective study with correlation of injury by magnetic resonance imaging. Br J Sports Med. 2001;35(6):435–9.
12. Nealon A. Side strain injury in first class cricket bowlers. Dissertation, Latrobe University, Melbourne. 2018.
13. Connell DA, Jhamb A, James T. Side strain: a tear of internal oblique musculature. Am J Roentgenol. 2003;181(6):1511–7.
14. Humphries D, Jamison M. Clinical and magnetic resonance imaging features of cricket bowler's side strain. Br J Sports Med. 2004;38(5):e21.

15. Cam NB, Muthukumar N, Boyle S, Lawton JO. Rib impingement in first class cricketers: case reports of two patients who underwent rib resection. Br J Sports Med. 2006;40(8):732–3.
16. Obaid H, Nealon A, Connell D. Sonographic appearance of side strain injury. Am J Roentgenol. 2008;191(6):W264–7.
17. Nealon AR, Kountouris A, Cook JL. Side strain in sport: a narrative review of pathomechanics, diagnosis, imaging and management for the clinician. J Sci Med Sport. 2017;20(3):261–6.
18. Stokes B. Injury felt like surgery without anaesthetic but I want to play through pain in Hobart. Daily Mirror UK [Internet 11 January 2022]. Accessed 1 Nov 2024. https://www.mirror.co.uk/sport/cricket/injury-felt-like-surgery-without-25912195?1
19. Mellin G. Physical therapy for chronic low back pain: correlations between spinal mobility and treatment outcome. Scand J Rehabil Med. 1985;17(4):163–6.
20. Ranson C, King M, Burnett A, Worthington P, Shine K. The effect of coaching intervention on elite fast bowling technique over a two-year period. Sports Biomech. 2009;8(4):261–74.
21. Orchard J, James T, Kountouris A, Blanch P, Sims K, Orchard J. Injury report 2011: cricket Australia. Sports Health. 2011;29(4):16–29.
22. Ekstrand J, Healy JC, Waldén M, Lee JC, English B, Hägglund M. Hamstring muscle injuries in professional football: the correlation of MRI findings with return to play. Br J Sports Med. 2012;46(2):112–7.
23. Healy C. Understandably flat: Aussie star sidelined with same injury that derailed Ashes summer. Fox Sports [Internet 8 December 2022]. Accessed 15 Nov 2024. https://www.foxsports.com.au/cricket/understandably-flat-aussie-star-sidelined-with-same-injury-that-derailed-ashes-summer/news-story/03dc26a8d0fe31acc62bc457b3ff3464

37 Lower Limb Muscle Strains in Cricket

John W. Orchard, Ben Langley, Thomas Cooney, Elyse Potter, Paul Chapman, Ashton Reeve, Eugene Ng, and James M. Linklater

37.1 Overall Pattern of Lower Limb Muscle Strains in Cricket

Muscle strains are an overall injury category where, in cricket, males suffer higher rates of injury than females (Table 37.1) [1]. In particular, hamstring strains are more common in males. Although males also suffer slightly more quadriceps strains than females, there are relatively more quadriceps strains in female cricket as a percentage of all lower limb muscle strains (Table 37.1). This trend (towards more muscle strains, particularly hamstring strains in males) has also been noted in sports in the USA such as soccer, track and field and field hockey [2, 3].

Calf strains are strongly associated with increasing player age (older players are much more likely to suffer calf strains), whereas hamstring muscle strains have a weak correlation with increasing age [4]. There is no significant relationship between age and quadriceps and groin strains. Younger players may be more likely to suffer the relatively uncommon iliopsoas strain [5] (and also younger fast bowlers are more likely to suffer side strains) [6].

In men's cricket, hamstring strains are most common in batters in the shorter formats of the game, associated with running between the wickets, and fast bowlers in red ball (multi-day) cricket [7]. Historically, most hamstring and running-related research has been related to male cricketers and athletes, and further studies are required to better understand the female cricketer.

37.2 Utility of MRI in Determining Prognosis

At the community level, MRI is rarely required for diagnosis of a muscle strain injury as the clinical examination findings make the diagnosis obvious. There is a marginal utility in using MRI scans

J. W. Orchard (✉)
School of Public Health, University of Sydney, Sydney, NSW, Australia
e-mail: john.orchard@sydney.edu.au

B. Langley · E. Potter
Mumbai Indians, Mumbai, Maharashtra, India
e-mail: ben.langley@ril.com

T. Cooney
Stadium Sports Medicine Centre, Sydney, Australia

P. Chapman
Queensland Cricket, Brisbane, Australia
e-mail: Paul.Chapman@qldcricket.com.au

A. Reeve · E. Ng · J. M. Linklater
Castlereagh Imaging, Sydney, Australia
e-mail: AshtonReeve@casimaging.com; EugeneNg2@casimaging.com; JamesLinklater@casimaging.com

B. Olivier, J. W. Orchard (eds.), *Cricket Sports Medicine*,
https://doi.org/10.1007/978-981-96-6321-7_37

Table 37.1 Incidence of muscle strain injuries (causing missed playing time) per 100 players per season in elite Australian cricket

Males	2015-16	2016-17	2017-18	2018-19	2019-20	2020-21	2021-22	Average M
Groin injuries	*3.9*	*2.1*	*3.7*	*2.0*	*3.5*	*3.1*	*1.0*	*2.8*
Hamstring strains	*8.3*	*8.3*	*4.2*	*6.6*	*7.5*	*9.4*	*7.3*	*7.4*
Quadriceps strains	*2.2*	*2.6*	*3.7*	*4.6*	*2.0*	*3.7*	*2.6*	*3.0*
Calf strains	*6.1*	*2.6*	*1.0*	*1.5*	*2.5*	*3.7*	*6.3*	*3.3*
Females	**2015-16**	**2016-17**	**2017-18**	**2018-19**	**2019-20**	**2020-21**	**2021-22**	**Average F**
Groin injuries	*0.0*	*0.0*	*2.2*	*1.5*	*1.4*	*0.7*	*0.7*	*0.9*
Hamstring strains	*3.9*	*4.3*	*3.0*	*2.2*	*2.9*	*2.9*	*2.8*	*3.1*
Quadriceps strains	*0.8*	*0.7*	*1.5*	*2.2*	*2.9*	*3.6*	*4.9*	*2.4*
Calf strains	*1.6*	*1.4*	*0.0*	*0.0*	*1.4*	*0.7*	*0.7*	*0.8*

Adapted from [1]

to grade injuries in professional players. Perhaps the greatest benefit of an MRI scan at an elite level, when positive, is to remind the player, coaching and medical staff that there is a structural injury so that all stakeholders are less tempted to rush the player back as quickly as possible [8]. Figures 37.1 and 37.2 (hamstring muscle group), Figs. 37.3 and 37.4 (quadriceps muscle group) and Figs. 37.5 and 37.6 (calf muscle group) show the ability of MRI scans to give very detailed imaging of severity of muscle and tendon injury in a strain. Images such as these are now obtained routinely at professional level.

37.3 Radiological Severity of Hamstring Strains in Cricket Is Related to Clinical Severity

A recent review of 141 hamstring strain injuries in elite Australian male and female cricketers [9] found increased time to return to play for injuries graded 2 or 3 (more severe) under the BAMIC (British Athletics muscle injury classification) system [10]. Similarly, injuries which involved tendon disruption (grade C) on MRI also had longer return-to-play times [9].

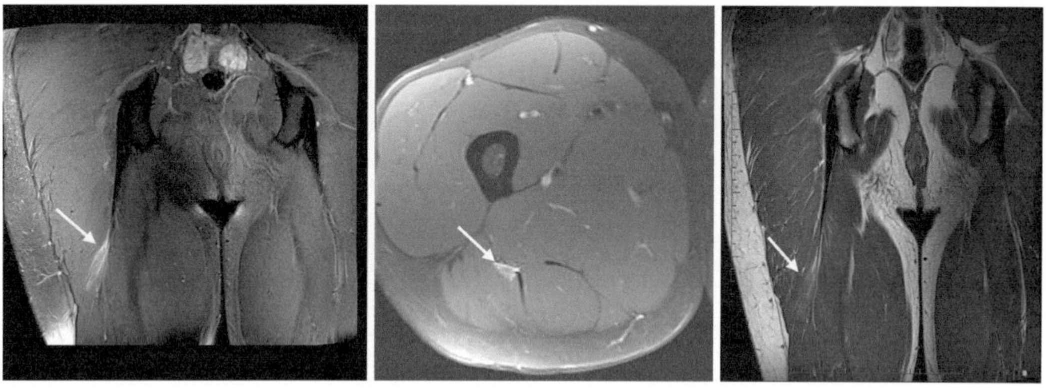

Fig. 37.1 (**a**)–(**c**) A 25-year-old male with low-grade strain injury of the right biceps femoris proximal muscle-tendon junction

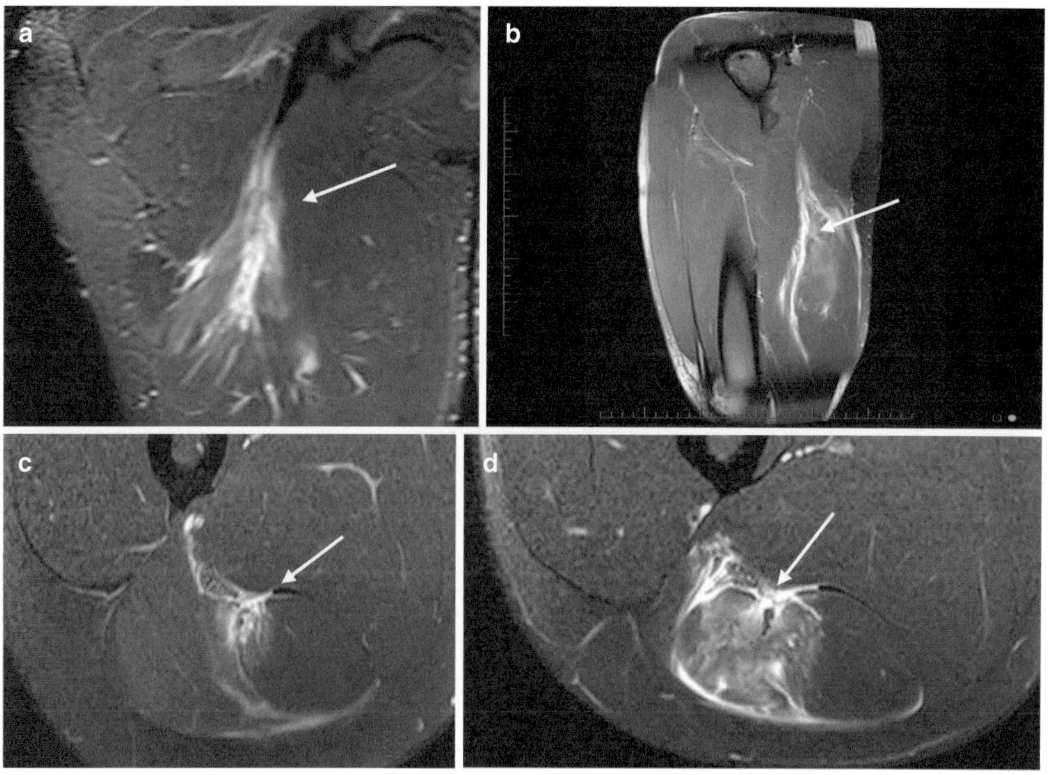

Fig. 37.2 (**a**)–(**d**) A 22-year-old male with partial tear of the proximal muscle-tendon junction of the biceps femoris-semitendinosus complex at the conjoint tendon

BAMIC size of injury was related to length of time to return to play in all players (Fig. 37.7) [9]. For injuries of higher severity in terms of architecture disruption, return to play was particularly slow in pace bowlers (Fig. 37.8). In other sports, intramuscular tendon disruption is associated with prolonged return-to-play times [11].

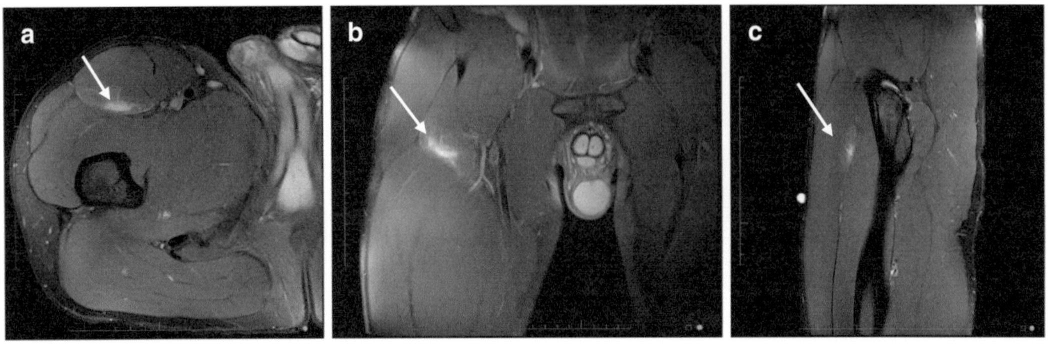

Fig. 37.3 (**a**)–(**c**) A 20-year-old male with low-grade small myofascial tear of the right rectus femoris muscle posteriorly

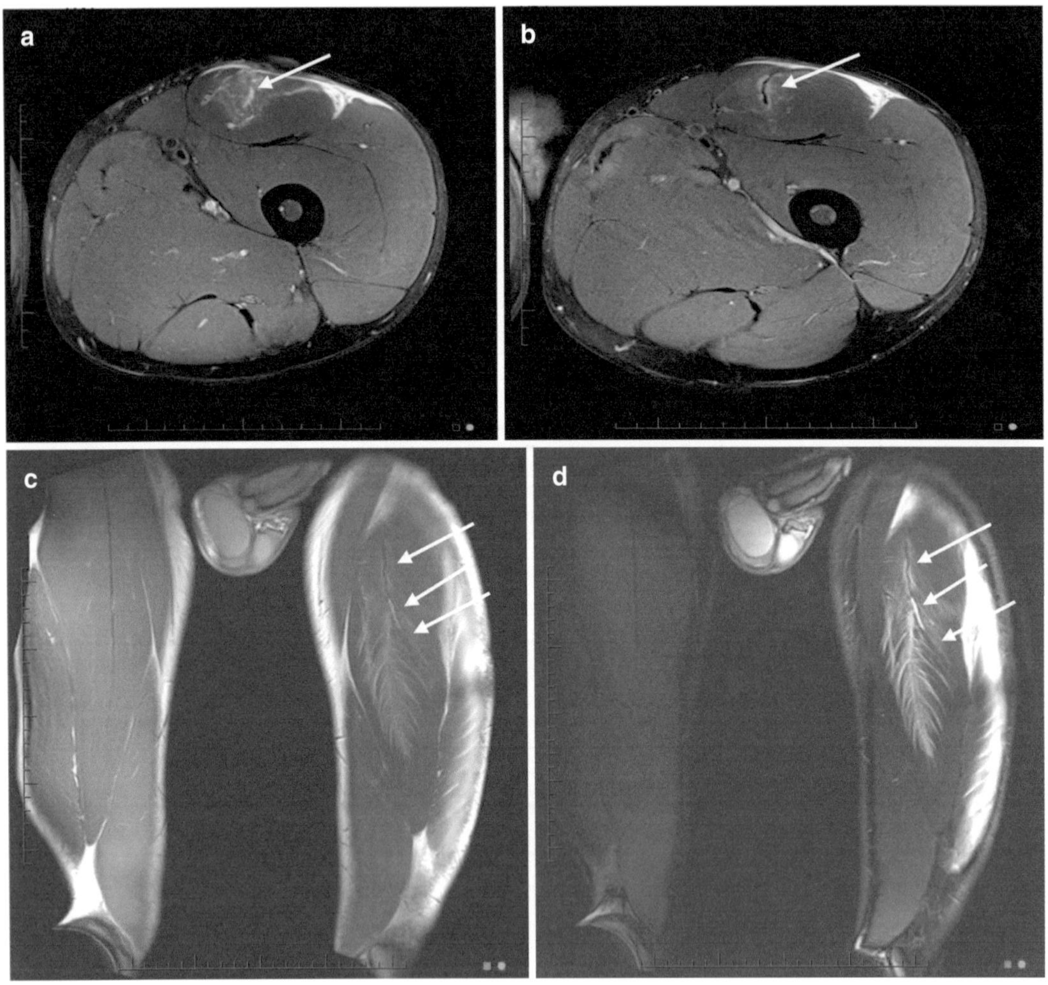

Fig. 37.4 (**a**)–(**d**) A 28-year-old male with recent tear of the central-proximal tendon of rectus femoris with tendon fibre discontinuity, extensive adjacent feathery intramuscular oedema and overlying subfascial fluid beneath the investing fascia of the rectus femoris and vastus lateralis

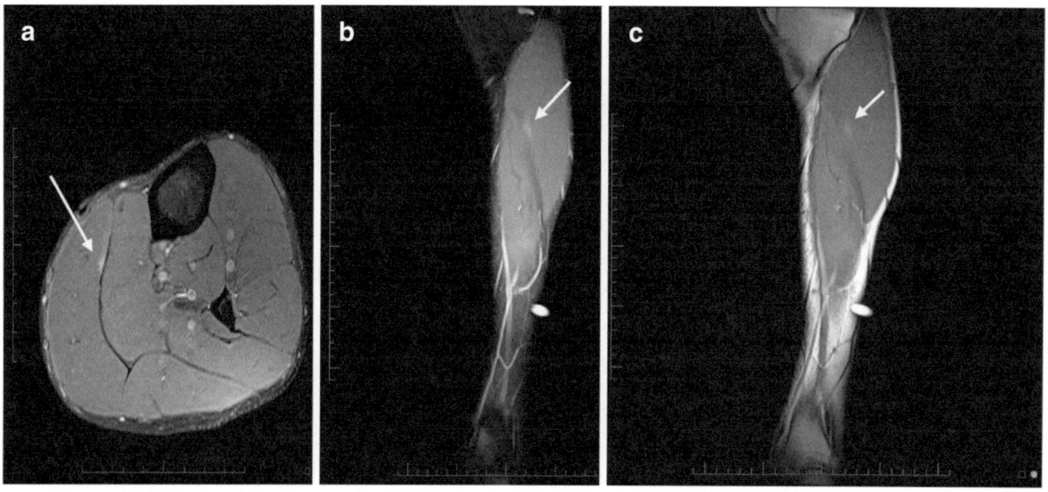

Fig. 37.5 (**a**)–(**c**) A 21-year-old male with low-grade injury of the medial head of gastrocnemius immediately superficial to the mid-aspect of its aponeurotic insertion. No associated muscle fibre discontinuity or tendon injury is evident

37.4 Biomechanics of Muscle Strains

Hamstring muscle strains generally occur during sprinting at high speed [12], which in cricket means during fast bowling, running between the wickets when batting, and when chasing a ball in the field. They are also quite common during cricket conditioning training when players are both trying to improve speed and become conditioned to the regular sprinting they will require when batting and fielding in elite cricket. Matches in Australia have higher rates of hamstring strains than in other countries [13], almost certainly related to the larger size of the playing field, meaning that both batters and fielders run more often. Although formal data has not been presented anywhere, anecdotally, visiting teams suffer high rates of muscle strains when touring Australia because of the additional running required on the larger grounds that they may not be conditioned to. This increased risk possibly also applies to international player signings in the BBL and WBBL T20 leagues.

Quadriceps strains typically occur during deceleration movements [12]. In fielding this is most common when chasing a ball to the boundary and then needing to slow down rapidly to avoid touching the boundary rope when the ball is close to passing over it. In fast bowling, it is the quadriceps muscle on the bowling side that tends to be at most at risk, from the deceleration of the bowling side leg just before delivery. In this sense, quadriceps strains follow the opposite rule to most lower body fast bowling injuries (which are generally more common on the non-bowling side due to higher force on the front foot). This mechanism of quadriceps strains in fast bowling is probably similar to the deceleration involved on the kicking side leg during 'kicking on the run' in the football codes [12].

Calf injuries are more common either when immediately taking off from a standing start (gastrocnemius) [14] or during prolonged running (soleus).

Groin injuries are often related to change of direction activities but can simply be overuse injuries as well, particularly in fast bowlers.

37.5 Risk of Recurrence

Recurrence of muscle strains is common in all sports [8]. There are fewer studies on recurrence in cricketers [15], perhaps because of the lack of a consistent schedule (also a logistical problem in track and field sprinting) makes studying the

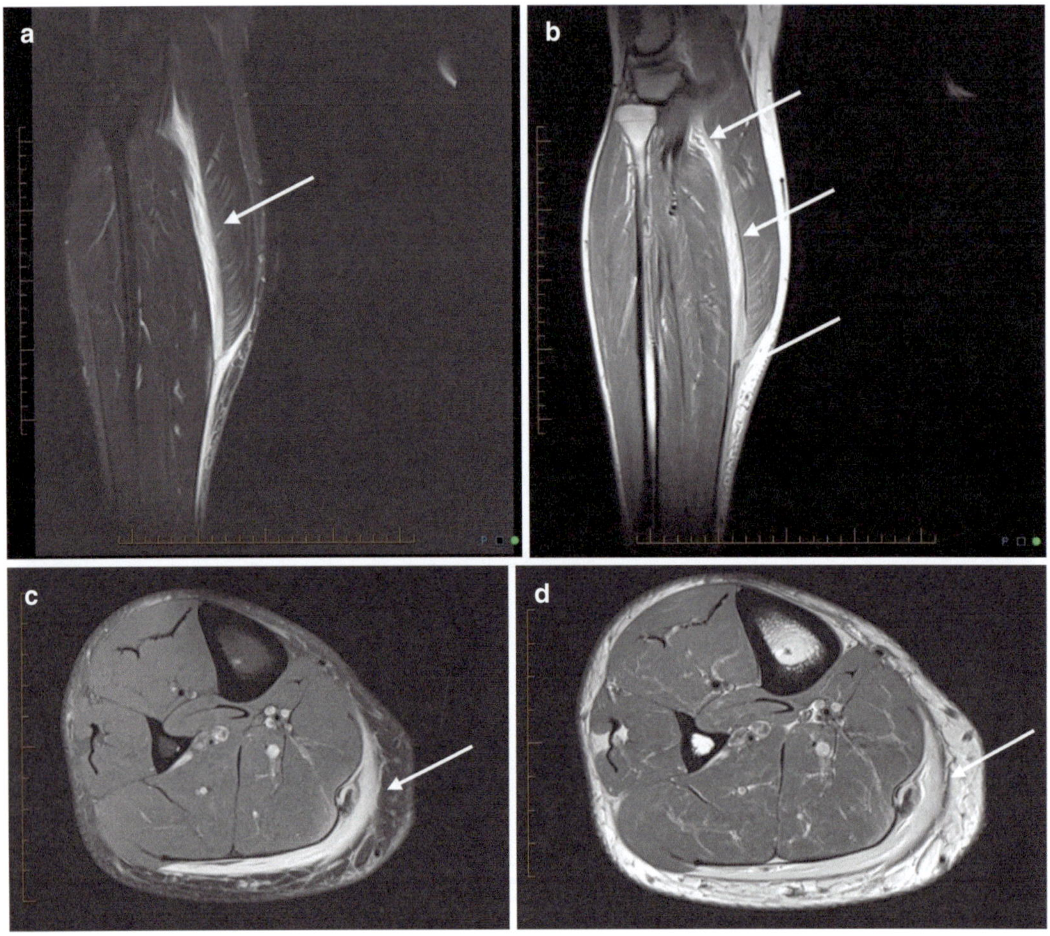

Fig. 37.6 (**a**)–(**d**) A 38-year-old male with recent tear of the aponeurotic tendon insertion of the medial head of gastrocnemius, at approximately the level of the distal muscle-tendon junction with distal tendon retraction, minimal muscle retraction and moderately extensive associated haematoma

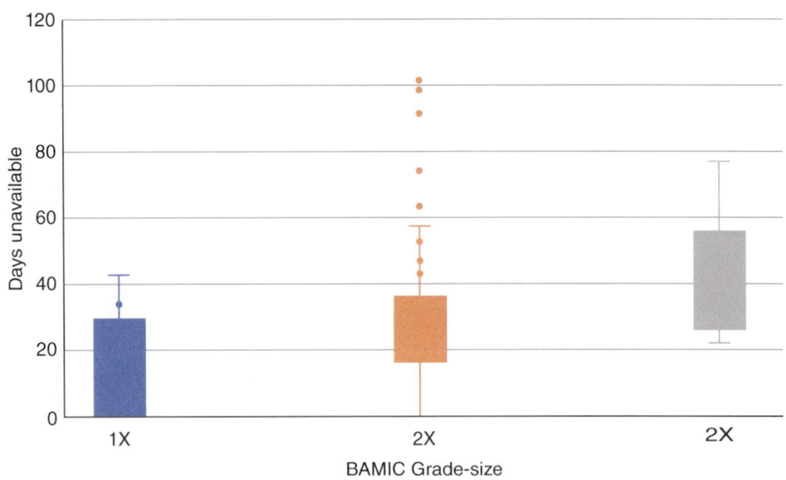

Fig. 37.7 Return-to-play times as a function of hamstring muscle strain size [9]

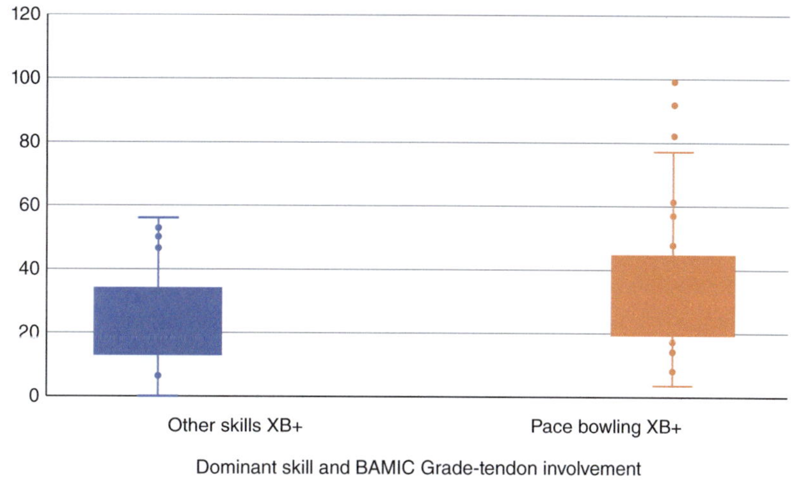

Fig. 37.8 Return-to-play time for B or C grade injuries in pace bowlers versus other skilled groups [9]

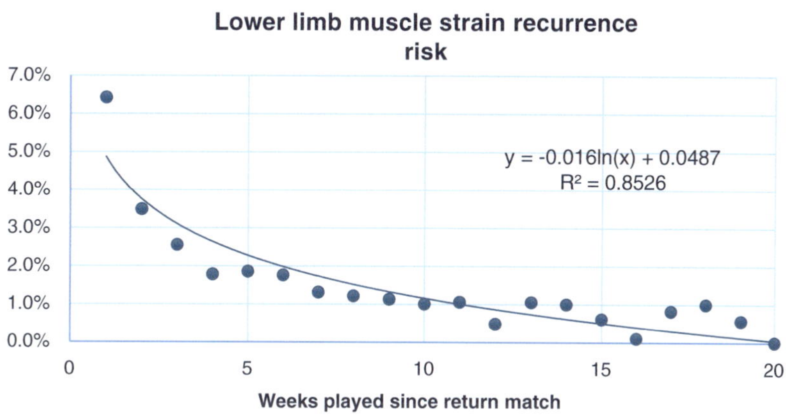

Fig. 37.9 Recurrence rates for all muscle strains for each week after return from the index injury [4]

recurrence rates more challenging than in the football codes, where games are played generally once per week. Studies from Australian Rules Football show that muscle strains have the highest risk of recurrence in the first match back from injury, with recurrence rate dropping slightly each week but remaining above baseline for up to 15 weeks (Fig. 37.9) [4]. The trend for recurrence, which improved dramatically from the 1990s to the early 2010s [16], does not seem to be improving over the last decade [17]. Recent data from the Australian Football League suggests a recurrence rate of 20% for hamstring strains with half of these occurring within 2 months of the original injury [18].

37.6 Hamstring Tears...the Problem That Isn't Going Away

Hamstring injury warrants a deeper discussion given the consistent high incidence and recurrence observed in cricket as described earlier [7]. This is despite injury surveillance stimulating focussed attention on prevention strategies and rehabilitation processes. It is evident across other sports that numerous factors can be considered and there is no guaranteed recipe for success. The key principles to improve chances of a satisfactory return are outlined below. These can be considered and applied to each injury.

37.7 Understand the Demands of the Sport...

The bulk of available information regarding the physical demands that may influence hamstring injury is generated from research in other sports, typically more running-based such as soccer and AFL football. Cricket is clearly a unique sport that was previously viewed as predominantly skill-based but its evolution now places far more physical demands on players [19]. These are variable within the game itself depending on the player type and their primary disciplines (batting, fast and spin bowling, and wicket-keeping/fielding position). There are studies that have utilised Global Positioning Satellite (GPS) to assess the running and acceleration-deceleration loads seen in the different formats of cricket [20]. Awareness of the differences assists practitioners charged with preparing players who may specialise in white or red ball formats.

Running in cricket can't be directly compared to running-based sports, and it can be divided into sub-categories. When fielding in the outfield, high-speed running may be reached for a ball chase of 40 metres or more. A fast bowler's run-up involves running with a ball in hand and aiming to achieve a 'rhythm' before a jump and gather that leads into delivery with a hard deceleration at the crease. Another variation involves batters sprinting between the wickets over '22 yards' wearing pads and protective equipment before changing direction at 180° and accelerating back down the wicket. Some players will experience all of these running demands in a single game so need to be prepared with a multifaceted approach. Running, including drills and any technical work-ons, should form a large component of a player's rehabilitation programme from the earliest possible opportunity.

Understanding the running speed a player reaches is necessary to balance this with their hamstring muscle strength requirements which increase significantly as speed increases. Most hamstring injuries occur in matches when the intensity, complexity and volume of the load are at their highest so it is important to replicate this as closely as possible in training to determine readiness.

37.8 ...and Understand the Player

It is then important to know how the player matches up and then adequately prepare to meet these demands. What is the apparent gap and do they exhibit sufficient physical qualities to allow them to execute performance without exposing themselves to risk? Consider fitness outputs such as running speed, power and strength qualities, as well as mobility of local areas (the hamstring unit itself, the hip joint and the lumbar spine) and more general body motion. Movement competency and control are important, especially regarding cricket-specific running mentioned above. Identify the areas you want to target and include in their overall physical preparation programme that drives readiness to perform as well as maximising availability.

37.9 Clinical Presentation

Hamstring injury is more common and usually of higher grade in male players. As discussed above, radiology provides accurate and helpful prognostic indicators to assist guidance of management timelines [9]. It is important to correlate the radiological signs with other valuable clinical markers.

A longer return to play can be expected when a player reports a popping sensation, shows demonstrable bruising and describes significant pain (VAS scores of >6) on ADLs such as walking. Slower recovery and higher recurrence risk are anticipated with a post-injury passive Straight Leg Raise (SLR) test of <60° and/or significant pain and restriction on the Maximal Hip Flexion Active Knee Flexion (MHFAKE) test [21].

Reliable initial tests that assist in monitoring improvement include:

- Length of palpatory tenderness
- Resisted eccentric hamstring strength measured at 90–90 hip and knee flexion measured with a hand-held dynamometer/HHD [22]
- Resisted hamstring strength at 15° knee flexion in prone with neutral hip position measured with an HHD (see Fig. 37.10).

The involvement of the lumbar spine should always be considered even in the absence of local

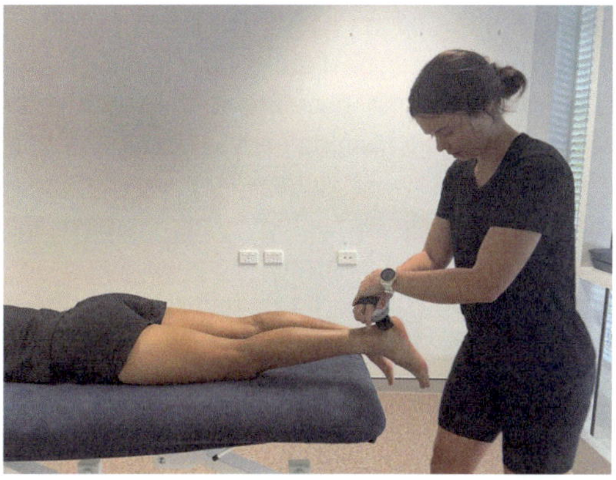

Fig. 37.10 Resisted hamstring strength at 15° knee flexion

symptoms. Batting can generate discogenic issues due to the flexed nature of the lumbar spine, and the high forces involved in bowling may produce acute and chronic changes in the joints and bones of the posterior column. Either present may lead to local mechanical issues as well as secondary neural signs that may affect the hamstring. Assessment involves palpation, range, strength, neural mobility and movement control of the associated areas.

37.10 'Return to Play Is Only Half Way'

It is a common observation that players returning to play after hamstring injury exhibit ongoing muscle atrophy and strength deficits when compared to the contralateral side. This can be the case many months after their return to competitive sport, and this is why the phrase above was coined. Ongoing, targeted rehabilitation exercises must continue to be part of the player's programme irrespective of a lack of symptoms or re-attainment of high-level output or skill performance. It has been noted that the eccentric loads that increase fascicle length in the shortened, injured muscle tissue will quickly revert when exposure to that type of exercise stops. Knowing that past history is the greatest risk factor, it is imperative that any post-injury deficits are addressed with a long-term plan and ideally returned to pre-morbid levels.

37.11 Surgery May Occasionally Be the Best Option

It was only recently that sending a player for surgery to repair a hamstring tear was almost unheard of. For starters, high-grade injuries were unusual in cricket and these were almost always managed conservatively in the first instance. The T20 format now sees 'more athletic' players with higher maximal running speeds and power attributes (amongst others) that place them at greater risk because of the forces they produce and are exposed to. In many elite settings nowadays, surgical repair is considered immediately for the highest grade injuries to ensure optimal return-to-play time and to reduce the chances of recurrence. Those hamstring tears that involve tendons and a demonstrable gap (BAMIC grade 3c) with resultant loss of muscle tension are elements of the presentation that require specialist opinion to advise best primary management [23]. As you would expect, surgery is going to be more prevalent in the elite setting where access to the resources of specialist care and rehabilitation support is more accessible.

37.12 Prevention Is Better Than the Cure...But Are Our Prevention Strategies Working?

Hamstring injury incidence in cricket is not reducing, and increasing rates have been reported in other sports, such as football (soccer) [17]. There are a number of factors to consider when discussing why sport isn't winning the war on hamstring strains. The implementation and execution of science-based prevention strategies have merit and remain a valuable addition to a holistic physical performance programme for cricket. The challenges faced revolve around an inability to effectively execute these programmes due to numerous factors impacting schedules, increasing player migration across teams and the evolving environment of autonomous athletes.

The increasing density of match fixtures in international, domestic and franchise cricket schedules results in increasing exposure to match workloads, travel, disrupted recovery and reduced training and prevention exposure. The moves between formats of the game associated with a change in positional demands are becoming increasingly apparent, such as a wicketkeeper in multi-day cricket who may transition to an outfielder in short-format cricket. Likewise, a fielder in multi-day cricket may assume a stationary catching position for weeks on end before quickly moving into high-frequency match exposures involving high-intensity outfield positions. Players are often transitioning regularly between teams and franchises, often competing in multiple tournaments throughout the year with inconsistent training exposure and support structures. These environments have short competition cycles and tend to have high-frequency schedules with primary focus on competition outcomes. Consistently switching through these environments can only result in an ever-decreasing exposure to appropriate training and prevention stimulus which only increases the risk factors associated with lower limb injury.

As discussed with rehabilitation of an injury, prevention strategies must be applied individually and consider a player's specific needs. A generic approach being applied to a squad of players with varying disciplines is unlikely to yield the desired results. However, there are key principles that practitioners can use to base their physical programming:

- Exposure to well-planned and progressive high-speed running is protective
- Hamstring strength is also protective
- Programme mechanical exposure to optimise tissue adaptation and minimise fatigue
- Manage transition periods between formats during in-season schedules

An area to discuss in greater detail would be high-speed running. The demands of cricket as a sport are incredibly variable in nature and matches are unpredictable in their physical demands. Exposure to increasing weekly sprint distances (90–120 m above 95% maximum velocity) and exposures (6–10 efforts) in team-based running sports has been shown to have a protective effect against lower limb muscle injury [24]. However, the planning and execution of acute high-speed running should be applied progressively and avoid sudden increases in exposure [25]. GPS technology has enabled the varying match and positional demands to be captured and found that sprinting increases in shorter format match exposure across most positions [26]. Specificity is important when considering high-speed running demands in cricket and appropriate preparation models. Often the interaction with a ball is the most common scenario during which an athlete will be required to sprint, and this will commonly include lateral movement, change of direction, acceleration, deceleration and diving. Coaching a technical running model that focuses on upright posture mechanics and utilising mechanical drills is commonly used; however, it is also important to consider the positional demands associated with the game. An example would be running with a bat in hand whilst being outstretched in full hip flexion and knee extension. Similarly, fielders are regularly exposed to high-intensity accelerations in varying body positions.

With respect to the protective role that strength can play in hamstring injury prevention, it is clear that eccentric strengthening reduces injury incidence and improves hamstring strength, fascicle length, hamstring/quadriceps ratio and limb asymmetry [27]. A holistic strength approach is required to acknowledge the role of the hamstrings with respect to knee flexion and hip extension. The Nordic hamstring exercise has been popularised and can provide a useful indicator of medial hamstring strength. However, it is important to objectively consider the lateral hamstring and its role in hip extension. The development of novel prone hip extension strength assessments is an important consideration when assessing and monitoring hamstring strength (Fig. 37.11). From a functional strength perspective, the use of Glute-Ham Developer (GHD) device (Fig. 37.12) and supine barbell eccentric hamstring bridges (Fig. 37.13) are examples of exercise selection that will preferentially recruit the lateral hamstrings.

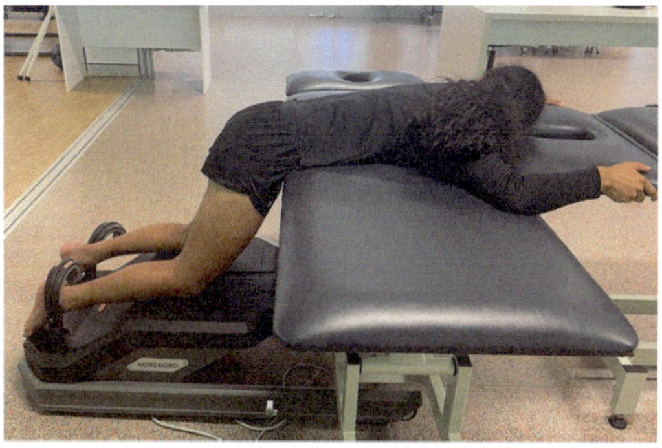

Fig. 37.11 Prone hamstring assessment using Nordboard (45-degree hip and knee flexion)

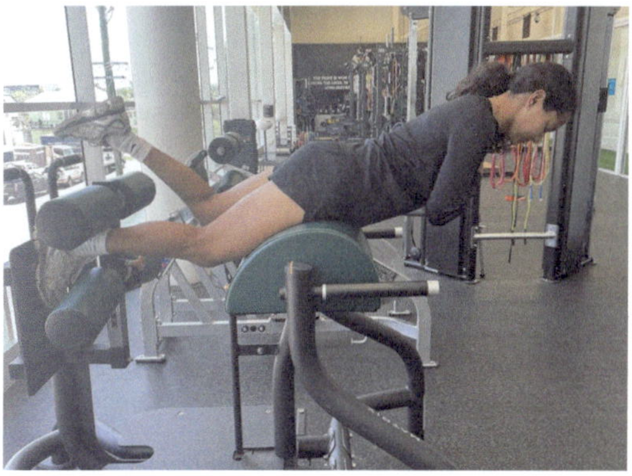

Fig. 37.12 Glute-Ham Developer (GHD) device

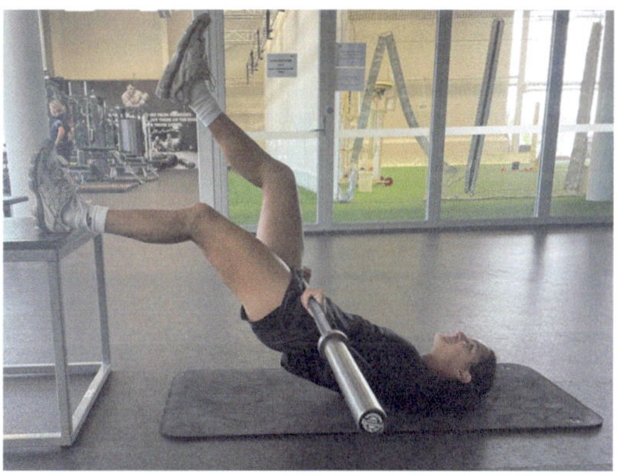

Fig. 37.13 Supine barbell eccentric hamstring bridges

These exercises can be prescribed with a load based on bodyweight percentage to provide some objective feedback on unilateral strength and comparison to the contralateral side.

References

1. Orchard JW, Inge P, Sims K, Kountouris A, Saw AE, Saw R, et al. Comparison of injury profiles between elite Australian male and female cricket players. J Sci Med Sport. 2023;26(1):19–24. https://doi.org/10.1016/j.jsams.2022.12.002.
2. Cross KM, Gurka KK, Conaway M, Ingersoll CD. Hamstring strain incidence between genders and sports in NCAA athletics. Athl Train Sports Health Care. 2010;2(3):124–30.
3. O'Sullivan L, Tanaka M. Sex-based differences in hamstring injury risk factors. J Women's Sports Med. 2021;1(1):20–9.
4. Orchard JW, Chaker Jomaa M, Orchard JJ, Rae K, Hoffman DT, Reddin T, et al. Fifteen-week window for recurrent muscle strains in football: a prospective cohort of 3600 muscle strains over 23 years in professional Australian rules football. Br J Sports Med. 2020;54(18):1103–7. https://doi.org/10.1136/bjsports-2019-100755.
5. Magistrali M, Stefanini L, Abate M, Biancalana G, Stegagno A, Cugia P, et al. Epidemiology of noncontact muscle injuries in the Italian male elite Under-19 football (soccer) championship. Sports Med Open. 2024;10(1):75. https://doi.org/10.1186/s40798-024-00738-0.
6. Nealon AR, Cook JL. Trunk side strain has a high incidence in first-class cricket fast bowlers in Australia and England. Clin J Sport Med. 2018;28(3):284–8. https://doi.org/10.1097/JSM.0000000000000450.
7. Goggins L, Langley B, Griffin S, Peirce N, McKay C, Stokes K, et al. Hamstring injuries in England and Wales elite men's domestic cricket from 2010 to 2019. J Sci Med Sport. 2022;25(6):474–9. https://doi.org/10.1016/j.jsams.2022.02.001.
8. Orchard J, Best TM. The management of muscle strain injuries: an early return versus the risk of recurrence. Clin J Sports Med. 2002;12(1):3–5. https://doi.org/10.1097/00042752-200201000-00004.
9. Cooney T, Reeve A, Saw A, Kountouris A, Orchard J, Linklater J. Hamstring strain grade on MRI and return to play in elite Australian cricket players. MedRxiv. 2024; https://www.medrxiv.org/content/10.1101/2024.11.07.24316885v1
10. Pollock N, James SL, Lee JC, Chakraverty R. British athletics muscle injury classification: a new grading system. Br J Sports Med. 2014;48(18):1347–51. https://doi.org/10.1136/bjsports-2013-093302.
11. Kerin F, O'Flanagan S, Coyle J, Farrell G, Curley D, McCarthy Persson U, et al. Intramuscular tendon injuries of the hamstring muscles: a more severe variant? A narrative review. Sports Med Open. 2023;9(1):75. https://doi.org/10.1186/s40798-023-00621-4.
12. Orchard J. Biomechanics of muscle strain injury. N Z J Sports Med. 2002;30(4):92–8.
13. Orchard JW, Kountouris A, Sims K. Risk factors for hamstring injuries in Australian male professional

cricket players. J Sport Health Sci. 2017;6(3):271–4. https://doi.org/10.1016/j.jshs.2017.05.004.
14. Orchard JW, Alcott E, James T, Farhart P, Portus M, Waugh SR. Exact moment of a gastrocnemius muscle strain captured on video. Br J Sports Med. 2002;36(3):222–3. https://doi.org/10.1136/bjsm.36.3.222.
15. Orchard J, James T, Kountouris A, Portus M. Changes to injury profile (and recommended cricket injury definitions) based on the increased frequency of Twenty20 cricket matches. Open Access J Sports Med. 2010;1:63–76. https://doi.org/10.2147/oajsm.s9671.
16. Orchard JW, Seward H, Orchard JJ. Results of 2 decades of injury surveillance and public release of data in the Australian football league. Am J Sports Med. 2013;41(4):734–41. https://doi.org/10.1177/0363546513476270.
17. Ekstrand J, Waldén M, Hägglund M. Hamstring injuries have increased by 4% annually in men's professional football, since 2001: a 13-year longitudinal analysis of the UEFA elite Club injury study. Br J Sports Med. 2016;50(12):731–7. https://doi.org/10.1136/bjsports-2015-095359.
18. Breed R, Opar D, Maniar N, Pizzari T. Epidemiology of hamstring strain injuries in elite male Australian football players: an analysis of 773 injuries over 7 seasons. JOSPT Open. 2024;2(4):289–96.
19. Orchard JJ, Orchard JW, La Gerche A, Raju H, Semsarian C. Misclassification of cricket in the American College of Cardiology (ACC) Task Force classification of sports. Br J Sports Med. 2020;54(8):491–2. https://doi.org/10.1136/bjsports-2018-099865.
20. Bliss A, Ahmun R, Jowitt H, Scott P, Jones TW, Tallent J. Variability and physical demands of international seam bowlers in one-day and Twenty20 international matches across five years. J Sci Med Sport. 2021;24(5):505–10. https://doi.org/10.1016/j.jsams.2020.11.012.
21. Aspetar: Assessment – Maximal Hip Flexion Active Knee Extension (MHFAKE) Test. https://youtu.be/KEMj1oYGFEg?si=bBRcao_dCXeu5pAd. (2017). Accessed December 1, 2024.
22. Aspetar: Assessment – Eccentric Outer-Range Strength Test. https://youtu.be/ly7DzZkgba4?si=bso9LBm0u-f8UI6J. (2017). Accessed December 1, 2024.
23. Yetter TR, Halvorson RT, Wong SE, Harris JD, Allahabadi S. Management of Proximal Hamstring Injuries: non-operative and operative treatment. Curr Rev Musculoskelet Med. 2024;17(9):373–85. https://doi.org/10.1007/s12178-024-09911-0.
24. Malone S, Roe M, Doran DA, Gabbett TJ, Collins K. High chronic training loads and exposure to bouts of maximal velocity running reduce injury risk in elite Gaelic football. J Sci Med Sport. 2017;20(3):250–4. https://doi.org/10.1016/j.jsams.2016.08.005.
25. Duhig S, Shield AJ, Opar D, Gabbett TJ, Ferguson C, Williams M. Effect of high-speed running on hamstring strain injury risk. Br J Sports Med. 2016;50(24):1536–40. https://doi.org/10.1136/bjsports-2015-095679.
26. Petersen CJ, Pyne D, Dawson B, Portus M, Kellett A. Movement patterns in cricket vary by both position and game format. J Sports Sci. 2010;28(1):45–52. https://doi.org/10.1080/02640410903348665.
27. Rudisill SS, Varady NH, Kucharik MP, Eberlin CT, Martin SD. Evidence-based hamstring injury prevention and risk factor management: a systematic review and meta-analysis of randomized controlled trials. Am J Sports Med. 2023;51(7):1927–42. https://doi.org/10.1177/03635465221083998.

38 Knee Injuries and Pain Related to Cricket

Mandeep S. Dhillon, Himmat Dhillon,
Sidak Dhillon, Aman Hooda,
and Prasoon Kumar

38.1 Introduction

Knee injuries in sports significantly affect the athlete; despite being a non-contact sport, knee problems are seen in many cricketers. Knee pain could have an acute onset, when it is related to injury, or could present as chronic pain related to overload situations. A significant factor is the repetitive stress placed on the knee joint during batting, bowling, and fielding, leading to overuse injuries such as patellar tendinopathy or patellofemoral pain syndrome (PFPS) [1]. Additionally, the biomechanics of cricket movements, including sudden changes in direction, jumping and squatting, further strain the knee joint, increasing the risk of ligamentous injuries such as anterior cruciate ligament (ACL) tears or meniscal damage. The prevalence of knee pain in cricket varies across age groups and levels of play, with younger players often experiencing growth-related issues like Osgood-Schlatter disease, whereas older players are more prone to degenerative conditions like osteoarthritis.

38.2 Epidemiology of Knee Pain in Cricket

The exact data about knee problems in cricket is not readily available, but studies from different countries giving an overview reveal a significant incidence of the problem (Table 38.1).

M. S. Dhillon (✉) · A. Hooda
Regenerative & Sports Medicine & Orthopaedics, Fortis Hospital Mohali, Mohali, Punjab, India

H. Dhillon
Sports Health Physio & Sports Injury Clinic, Melbourne, Australia

S. Dhillon
Sports Physician, Roundglass Football Club, Mohali, Punjab, India

P. Kumar
Department of Orthopaedics, PGIMER, Chandigarh, India

B. Olivier, J. W. Orchard (eds.), *Cricket Sports Medicine*,
https://doi.org/10.1007/978-981-96-6321-7_38

Table 38.1 Published data on epidemiology of knee problems in cricketers

Country data	No & type of players	Player age (years)	Sex	% knee problems	Player type
Munir et al. [2], Pakistan	89, Domestic clubs	19.4+/–3.12	Males	34.8%	Specific data not available
Jacobs et al. [3] Meta-analysis	23 studies Elite & Community players	All ages	Females	7–13% from evaluated data	Children had 75% pain incidence
Orchard [4] Australia Data for 2014–2015	Elite	Not defined	Males	Cartilage 0.3% Other knee injury 0.3%, Quads strain 0.6%	Pace bowlers had highest overall Injury rates
Dhillon et al. [5] India	95, Domestic, Punjab state	23.24 (19–34)	Males	4 of 94 All ligament injuries	
Mansingh et al. [6] West Indies	All Matches 2003–4, Test & One day	Not defined	Males	4 of 50	2 batsmen, 1 wicketkeeper

38.3 Anterior Knee Pain

Anterior knee pain is often seen in cricketers, especially in the bowlers of age group 15–30 years. The commonest cause is patellar tendinitis/tendinopathy with bursitis, chondromalacia and stress fractures also being reported. Bowling involves repeated high extensor load on the knee due to jumping and landing, with complex movements of both the upper and lower limbs along with the trunk. It has been well documented that even in asymptomatic elite athletes, calcifications in the patellar tendon along with hypoechoic areas signifying tears of its fibres are seen on ultrasonography, which on prolonged use can become symptomatic and cause anterior knee pain [7].

Repeated strain on the patellar tendon due to periodic overuse in bowling can lead to tendinopathy, wherein the tendon fibres weaken and can tear up. It has been reported that the tendon tears most commonly at its proximal attachment onto the patella [8]. Initially, there is inflammation which occurs at the tendon-bone interface, which causes symptoms during bowling and fielding as it involves running and jumping; this is known as jumper's knee. However, as the problem persists and progresses the bowlers start getting symptoms even after the matches or practice sessions, affecting his/her daily activities [7].

Patellar tendinitis or tendinopathy is seen more commonly in recreational fast bowlers than the professional ones; better training and conditioning in the latter may be the reason for this [9]. It has strong male preponderance and affects adolescents and young fast bowlers in their twenties. Associated factors described include inadequate training leading to muscle stiffness or weakness and postural malalignment during bowling.

Clinically, the presenting symptom is pain at the lower pole of the patella, where tenderness can also be elicited. Plain radiographs may show signs of calcification; however, ultrasound and MRI are superior tools for diagnosis, which can show areas of fibre tears [8].

The first line of management involves rest, icing, compression/taping and NSAIDs/anti-inflammatory medications. Severe cases may require electrotherapy or extracorporeal shock wave therapy in addition to local steroid injection. Surgery may be needed if there is complete tear or avulsion of the patellar tendon.

Rehabilitation involves physiotherapy and individualised training programmes for better conditioning and acclimatisation of the knee extensors to eccentric loading.

38.4 ITB Syndrome and Knee Pain

The ITB is a fibrous continuation of the tensor fascia lata (TFL) and some fibres from the gluteus Maximus. It runs longitudinally along the lateral side of the thigh and attaches at the Gerdy's tubercle on the lateral aspect of the proximal tibia. As it crosses the two joints, it helps in stabilising the hip and knee joints in the frontal plane during walking and running [10]. As it is a fibrous band, over time due to the tension that it undergoes after repetitive stress from running, the athlete starts to develop a sharp pain or burning over the lateral aspect of the knee, called ITB syndrome.

ITB syndrome is the most common cause of lateral knee pain in runners or athletes with high running load, contributing between 5% and 14% of knee injuries [11]. During the front foot contact phase of fast bowling the Gluteus muscle group and the TFL prevent the hip from going into hyper-adduction. If these muscles are weak, there is hyper-adduction at the hip which causes the ITB to stretch and compress the lateral femoral condyle resulting in pain [12].

Fast bowlers can present with lateral sided knee pain, which increases with increased running intensity. The pain may be reproduced while sitting for prolonged periods of time with knee in a flexed position [13]. Local tenderness and mild swelling may be present on the lateral aspect of the knee, above the joint line where the band slides over the lateral femoral condyle.

The Noble's compression test (Fig. 38.1) is the best confirmatory test for ITB syndrome [14]. The knee is placed in 90° flexion, compression is applied about 2 cm above the lateral joint line and the knee is then gradually extended; this reproduces the same intense pain felt during running.

The Renne test (Fig. 38.2) is another confirmatory test in which the athlete is made to do single leg squats up to 30–40° of knee flexion which reproduces the pain. Additionally, flexibility tests like Ober's test and modified Thomas test are done to confirm the tightness of the ITB, which is a contributing factor to ITB syndrome.

The immediate management is to reduce pain and inflammation. Oral NSAIDs, cryotherapy and local modalities are very helpful in the acute phase. All aggravating activities need to be stopped. Once inflammation and pain are controlled, stretching exercises are started. Swimming is encouraged to maintain cardiovascular fitness. Most athletes return to play by 6 weeks post-injury, but some can return sooner depending on when they can perform all strengthening exercises without pain. Surgical intervention is only required when conservative management fails.

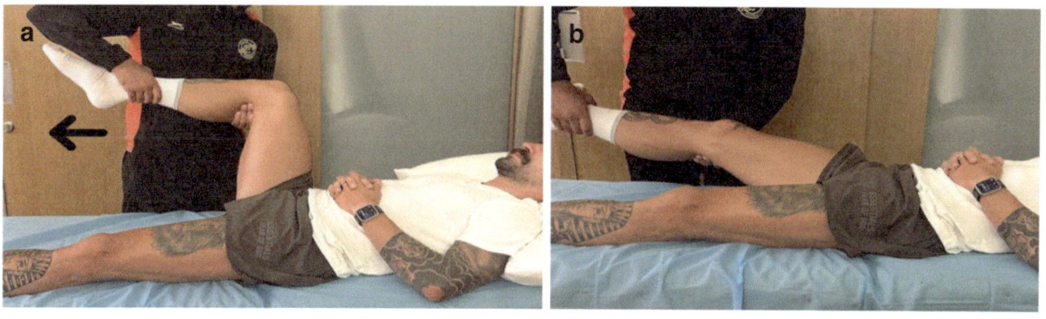

Fig. 38.1 Performing Noble test

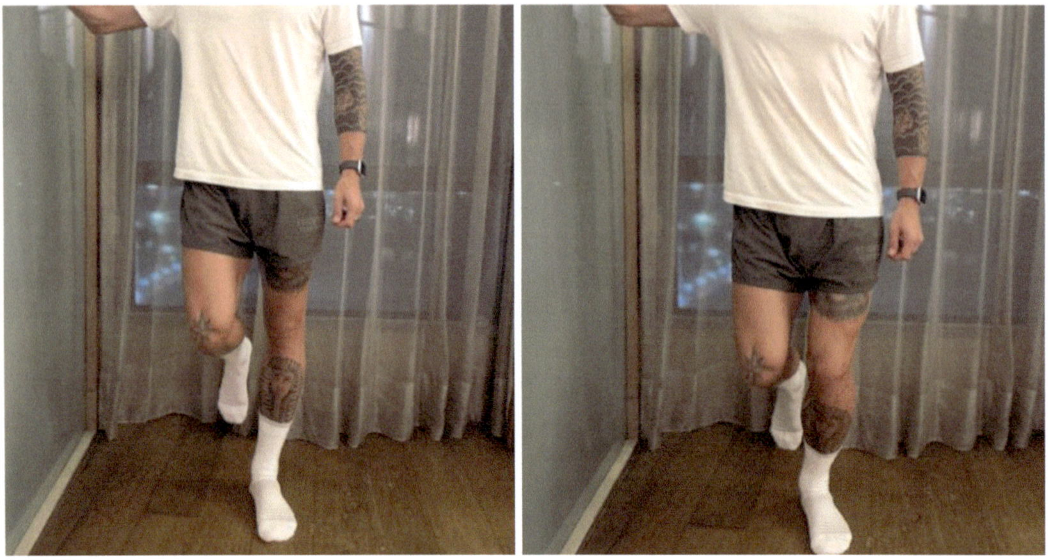

Fig. 38.2 Demonstrating Renne test

38.5 Meniscus Injuries

Associated with twisting of the knee, meniscal injuries often occur during fielding; a problem unique to cricket has been a report associated with 'the sliding stop' method *(the fielder intercepts the ball by sliding at speed on the hip and knee and then standing and throwing the ball, all in 1 smooth manoeuvre)* [15]. Most meniscus injuries are easy to diagnose, and delays should be avoided; early MRI after clinical suspicion is the key for this. A double bucket handle tear of both menisci has also been documented in a Pakistani player, associated with an ACL tear [16].

Unstable meniscal tears require early arthroscopic intervention, with good outcomes and early return to sport (Fig. 38.3).

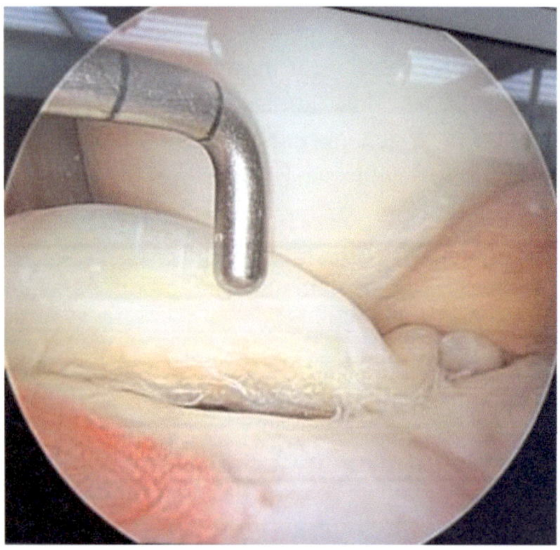

Fig. 38.3 Arthroscopic view of a displaced bucket handle tear of meniscus

38.6 Ligament Injuries

Knee ligament injuries are somewhat uncommon in cricket and are most often reported in cricketers playing football as part of cross-training drills [17]. Fast bowlers with unconventional follow-through actions and fielders while sliding or landing are prone to medial collateral ligament (MCL) and ACL tears [18]. Swelling associated with an acute knee injury is usually a sign of significant intra-articular ligament damage, and early MRIs should be planned (Fig. 38.4).

Isolated MCL injuries (even when grade 3) are amenable to non-operative treatment; ACL tears should ideally be treated by arthroscopic reconstruction, as many are associated with meniscal injuries. The choice of graft varies, autograft or allograft, depending on availability. For autografts, most centres use the hamstrings to reconstruct the ACL; this is better in female players, but heavier male cricketers may be better served by the more robust patellar tendon reconstruction; some surgeons are reinforcing soft tissue autografts with '*internal bracing*' albeit with limited evidence in support of this.

Posterior cruciate (PCL) and lateral collateral ligament (LCL) injuries are rare and infrequently documented in cricket.

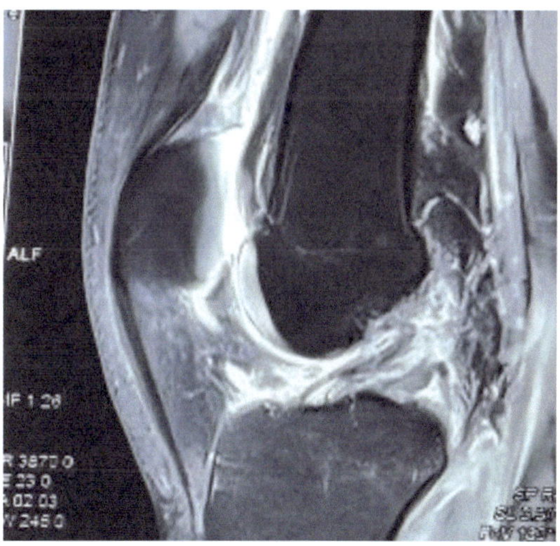

Fig. 38.4 ACL tear as seen on MRI

Aggressive post-operative rehabilitation protocols have now been developed for the knee, which allow earlier return to sports, both after non-operative and operative treatment of knee ligament injuries.

38.7 Cartilage Injuries

Knee cartilage injuries in cricketers present a significant challenge due to the sport's dynamic and high-impact nature; these may involve the articular cartilage of the tibio-femoral articulation or the patella-femoral joint.

The repetitive stress of sudden stops and pivoting movements in cricket can lead to gradual wear and tear of the cartilage, resulting in conditions like chondromalacia patellae or focal cartilage defects. Additionally, acute trauma from falls, collisions, or sudden twists can cause more immediate cartilage injuries such as osteochondral fractures or loose bodies within the joint.

Anteromedial articular impingement injury specific to fast bowlers has been recently documented [19]. Seven international fast bowlers (*mean age 26 years*) developed anteromedial pain in their lead leg; MRI revealed oedema in medial femoral condyle in all, with 4 having associated cartilage loss, emphasising that this lesion should be suspected in this sub-group of players. A case of Juvenile Osteochondritis Dissecans in a 16-year-old fast bowler has also been documented, which was treated by arthroscopy and aggressive rehabilitation [20] (Fig. 38.5).

Diagnosing cartilage injuries in cricket players often involves a combination of clinical evaluation, imaging studies like radiographs, MRI and sometimes arthroscopy for precise assessment [21].

Management strategies range from conservative treatments like rest, physical therapy and anti-inflammatory medications in mildly symptomatic patients to surgical interventions such as arthroscopic debridement, microfracture, or autologous chondrocyte implantation for more severe cases.

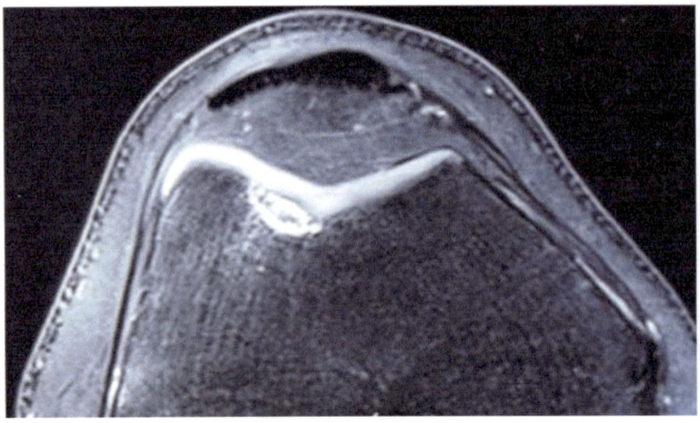

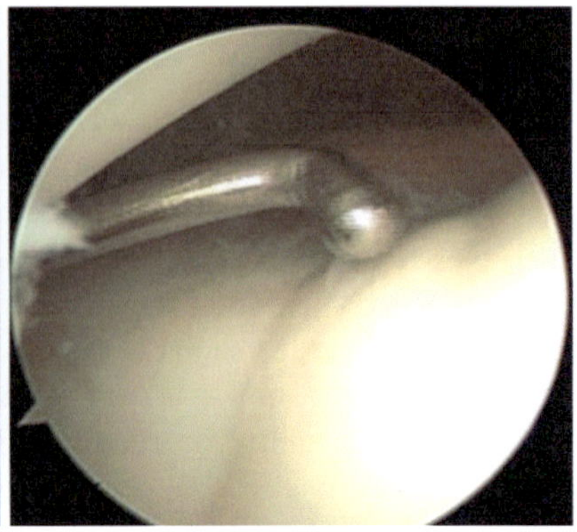

Fig. 38.5 Osteochondritis Dissecans of femoral trochlea; MRI shows separated fragment, but arthroscopy reveals intact cartilage

38.8 Knee Degeneration

The prevalence of osteoarthritis among the general population aged 50 and above is 13% [22]. However, due to the rigorous demands of cricket, former elite players can experience joint degeneration at a much higher rate, reported to be up to 44% [23]. Bowlers commonly face shoulder issues and spinal degeneration, while knee osteoarthritis is frequently observed in all-rounders; studies have documented knee replacement rates nearing 11% among former cricketers [23]. The biomechanical stresses on joints during bowling, including sprinting and knee extension upon delivery, result in peak vertical forces up to 9 times the body weight, increasing injury risk and potential joint degeneration [24].

Although knee osteoarthritis is more prevalent in females in general, a comparison of former male and female elite cricketers found no significant differences, albeit with only 3% female representation in their dataset [25]. When comparing professional and recreational former cricketers, rates of knee degeneration do not vary significantly, nor do they correlate with career longevity; however, studies have identified higher incidences of hand injuries and arthritis among the former [25].

Overall, former cricketers commonly experience chronic knee issues that can impact their quality-of-life post-retirement. Strategies should be implemented to ensure they lead physically active lives after retirement. During their playing careers, efforts to prevent injuries through strength and endurance training, along with early diagnosis, treatment and rehabilitation, are crucial. Players should be encouraged to report injuries promptly rather than dismissing them as minor issues, as neglecting proper care could have long-term consequences.

38.9 Rehabilitation

Rehabilitation for knee pain related to cricket depends on whether the problem is of acute onset or something of a chronic overload situation.

Preventative measures include proper warm-up routines, strengthening exercises and biomechanical assessments to correct any imbalances or weaknesses that could predispose players to such knee injuries [26]. Vigilant monitoring and early intervention are crucial to prevent the progression of cartilage damage, which can significantly impact a cricket player's performance and long-term joint health.

Coaches should be aware of the potential for knee injury, especially in younger players with inadequate training. The sliding stop should be discouraged as a means of fielding in cricket unless appropriately coached.

Return to sports after a major knee injury has been discussed by many authors; some key factors identified for return to sports after ACL injury have been player motivation and fear of re-injury, especially in younger players. A systematic review of 10 studies found equivocal gender-related findings, with competitive male athletes more likely to return to sports than their female counterparts [27]. An interesting finding was that good knee function was not always associated with a higher probability of return to sports; this data, however, is not specific to cricket.

References

1. Houghton K, Button L, Horsley I, et al. Knee injuries in cricket: a review of current concepts. J Sci Med Sport. 2019;22(6):656–60.
2. Munir A, Akhtar M, Khalid A, Khan HF, Kiran F, Bahar G. Assessment of musculoskeletal disorders among cricketers playing in domestic clubs of Lahore. J Pak Med Assoc. 2022;72(5):878–81.
3. Jacobs J, Olivier B, Dawood M, Perera NKP. Prevalence and incidence of injuries among female cricket players: a systematic review and meta-analysis. JBI Evid Synth. 2022;20(7):1741–90.
4. Orchard JW, Kountouris A, Sims K. Incidence and prevalence of elite male cricket injuries using updated consensus definitions. Open Access J Sports Med. 2016;7:187–94.
5. Dhillon MS, Soni RK, Aggarwal S, Dhillon H, Prabhakar S. Epidemiology of orthopedic injuries in Indian cricket: a prospective one year observational study. J Postgrad Med Edu Res. 2015;49(4):168–72.
6. Mansingh A, Harper L, Headley S, King-Mowatt J, Mansingh G. Injuries in West Indies cricket 2003–2004. Br J Sports Med. 2006;40(2):119–23; discussion 119–23.
7. Cook JL, Khan KM, Harcourt PR, Kiss ZS, Fehrmann MW, Griffiths L, Wark JD. Patellar tendon ultrasonography in asymptomatic active athletes reveals hypoechoic regions: a study of 320 tendons. Victorian Institute of Sport Tendon Study Group. Clin J Sport Med. 1998;8(2):73–7.
8. Shafi M. Cricket injuries: an orthopaedist's perspective. Orthop Surg. 2014;6(2):90–4.
9. Thaigarajan KA, Parikh T, Sayed A, Gnanavel MB, Arumugam S. Cricket biomechanics analysis of skilled and amateur fast bowling techniques. J Postgrad Med Edu Res. 2015;49(4):173–81.
10. Hutchinson LA, Lichtwark GA, Willy RW, Kelly LA. The iliotibial band: a complex structure with versatile functions. Sports Med. 2022;52(5):995–1008.
11. van der Worp MP, van der Horst N, de Wijer A, Backx FJ, Nijhuis-van der Sanden MW. Iliotibial band syndrome in runners: a systematic review. Sports Med. 2012;42(11):969–92.
12. Noehren B, Davis I, Hamill J. ASB clinical biomechanics award winner 2006. Clin Biomech. 2007;22(9):951–6.
13. Fredericson M, Wolf C. Iliotibial band syndrome in runners: innovations in treatment. Sports Med. 2005;35(5):451–9.
14. Noble CA. The treatment of iliotibial band friction syndrome. Br J Sports Med. 1979;13(2):51–4.
15. Von Hagen K, Roach R, Summers B. The sliding stop: a technique of fielding in cricket with a potential for serious knee injury. Br J Sports Med. 2000;34:379–81.
16. Sohail MA, Bashir A, Hassan UU. Combined medial and lateral bucket handle meniscus tears with associated complete anterior cruciate ligament tear: a case report. J Pak Med Assoc. 2023;73(11):2257–9.
17. Orchard JW, James T. Australian cricket board injury report 2001–02. Melbourne: Australian Cricket Board; 2002.
18. Pardiwala DN, Rao NN, Varshney AV. Injuries in cricket. Sports Health. 2018;10(3):217–22.
19. Reid MJ, Alva A, Thompson SM, et al. Fast bowler's knee—anteromedial articular impingement. J Exp Ortop. 2020;7:20. https://doi.org/10.1186/s40634-020-00237-7.
20. Dhillon MS, Prabhakar S, Bhushan C, Swaminathan S. Juvenile Osteochondritis Dissecans of the femoral trochlea in a cricket fast bowler. N Z J Sports Med. 2014;41(2):54–5.
21. Khan M, Osman K, Green G, Haddad F. The management of articular cartilage defects in the knee. J Bone Joint Surg Br. 2010;92(10):1429–36.
22. Steptoe A, Breeze E, Banks J, Nazroo J. Cohort profile: the English longitudinal study of ageing. Int J Epidemiol. 2013;42(6):1640–8.
23. Jones ME, Davies MAM, Leyland KM, Delmestri A, Porter A, Ratcliffe J, Peirce N, Newton JL, Arden NK. Osteoarthritis and other long-term health conditions in former elite cricketers. J Sci Med Sport. 2018;21(6):558–63.
24. Hurrion PD, Dyson R, Hale T. Simultaneous measurement of back and front foot ground reaction forces during the same delivery stride of the fast-medium bowler. J Sports Sci. 2000;18(12):993–7.
25. Cai H, Bullock GS, Sanchez-Santos MT, Peirce N, Arden NK, Filbay SR. Joint pain and osteoarthritis in former recreational and elite cricketers. BMC Musculoskelet Disord. 2019;20(1):596.
26. Dhillon H, Dhillon S, Dhillon MS. Current concepts in sports injury rehabilitation. Indian J Orthop. 2017;51(5):529–36. Erratum in: Indian J Orthop. 2017;51(6):724.
27. Ross CA, Clifford A, Louw QA. Intrinsic factors associated with return to sport after anterior cruciate ligament reconstruction: a systematic review. S Afr J Physiother. 2015;71(1):230.

Foot and Ankle Injuries in Cricket

39

Bikram Pratap Karmakar and Michael Symes

39.1 Foot and Ankle Introduction

The foot and ankle serve crucial roles in both stability and mobility. In cricket, fast bowlers place significant loads through their ankles, particularly on landing at the point of delivery. Fielders inside the circle are required to change direction suddenly. Fielders on the boundary often must delicately navigate boundary ropes. Batters achieve stability through the footwork, allowing them to stay balanced at the crease. Cricket's high impact and dynamic nature predispose players to various foot and ankle injuries. The differences in ground surfaces between grass and the turf wicket may also be a factor. Foot and ankle injuries can occur in an acute incident or develop from overuse. Understanding the mechanism of injuries and associated contributing factors is required to manage and prevent chronicity effectively. This chapter will explore the epidemiology of foot and ankle injuries in cricket, provide a clinical approach to assessment, and discuss specific foot and ankle injuries that are prevalent in cricket.

39.1.1 Epidemiology of Foot and Ankle Injuries in Cricket

A 4-year study of South African elite cricketers reported 104 foot and ankle injuries, with ankle injuries more common than foot injuries. Lateral ankle ligament injuries accounted for 35% of the total injuries, often occurring on the non-dominant side and mostly in fielders and bowlers [1]. In Australia, a 10-year analysis revealed that injuries to the shin, foot and ankle accounted for 16.9% of all injuries per squad per season [2]. Lower limb injuries represented up to 49.8% of all cricket injuries, with foot and ankle injuries making up 8.7%. Most foot and ankle injuries are contusions or haematomas (41%) and ligamentous injuries or sprains (29%) [3]. The average incidence of new below-knee injuries per 100 players measured across 10 years was 10.7 [4]. In cricket, bowling-related injuries account for the highest proportion of foot and ankle injuries. However, injuries occur with other non-cricket skill-related activities, including running for con-

B. P. Karmakar (✉)
Balmain Sports Medicine, Rozelle, NSW, Australia

School of Psychiatry, UNSW Medicine, Sydney, NSW, Australia

Cricket New South Wales, Sydney Olympic Park, NSW, Australia

M. Symes
Department of Orthopaedics and Trauma Surgery, Royal North Shore Hospital, St Leonards, NSW, Australia

Department of Orthopaedic Surgery, St George Hospital, Kogarah, NSW, Australia

St. George and Sutherland Clinical School, UNSW Medicine, Sydney, NSW, Australia

B. Olivier, J. W. Orchard (eds.), *Cricket Sports Medicine*,
https://doi.org/10.1007/978-981-96-6321-7_39

dition and warm-up activities like soccer [1]. Gender differences may exist between injuries with an incidence rate ratio of match time loss of 0.6 for lower leg, foot and ankle stress fractures, indicating a lower risk for males than females [5].

39.1.2 Clinical Approach

Clinical evaluation requires a detailed history of previous lower limb injuries, treatments and rehabilitation outcomes. In the setting of prior ankle ligament injuries, persistent instability is an important consideration for ongoing management. It is critical to note the player's skill set as this may impact their availability or impose limitations to return to play. Recent changes to workload can contribute to overuse, with fast bowlers at particular risk for lower limb injuries [4]. Acute injuries must be assessed through careful inspection for swelling, bruising, deformity and weight-bearing capacity. In the ankle, limited dorsiflexion range may predispose to altered load distribution and affect bowling mechanics [6]. This can be assessed with a knee-to-wall test. Periodic assessment during the season, with particular attention to a reduction in baseline knee-to-wall range, can help identify the at-risk athlete. Improvement in the range is an important indicator of improvement with rehabilitation. Plantar flexion range can be assessed in the standing position and may be compromised in posterior impingement. Passive plantar flexion with overpressure can diagnose more subtle cases of posterior impingement. Repetitive single-leg calf raises can assess muscle strength and endurance and may be sensitive in Achilles tendinopathy. Single-Leg Balance and Hop Tests can aggravate pain from lower limb stress injuries and help evaluate functional stability where deficits may contribute to injury risk. In cases of lateral ligament pain, the anterior draw and talar tilt tests can indicate the integrity of the anterior talofibular and calcaneofibular ligaments. Valgus or eversion stress test can identify laxity or injury to the deltoid ligament. Instability tests should be assessed for an endpoint, and laxity should be compared to the contralateral ankle. The ankle syndesmosis can be tested with compression of the fibula and tibia above the level of the ankle joint. Pain elicited with external rotation and dorsiflexion of the foot with the knee flexed indicates syndesmosis injury. Palpation of the entire fibula length is important to identify the Maisonneuve fracture.

39.1.3 Biomechanics

Specific movement patterns across different cricket skills can contribute to injury patterns in the foot and ankle. Bowling, especially fast bowling, is associated with a high incidence of lower limb injuries due to the repetitive high-impact forces and torsional stresses on the lower extremities. Fielding can contribute to these injuries through sudden speed, jumping and abrupt directional changes. The prevalence of non-contact gradual onset injuries, such as those resulting from high workload or impairments in balance, flexibility and strength, indicates the importance of training loads and biomechanical factors in injury prevention [7].

Understanding the key phases of fast bowling helps identify factors contributing to foot and ankle injury patterns in this group.

Run-up phase
Bowlers aim to build momentum through high linear acceleration. The biomechanics during this phase focus on optimising run-up speed to generate kinetic energy to transfer in the subsequent phases [8]
Delivery stride
The bowler's back-foot contacts (BFC) the ground, helping initiate momentum transfer. This is followed by front foot contact (FFC), helping absorb and redirect energy transfer to facilitate ball release [9]
Follow-through phase
After the ball is released, high eccentric loads occur in the lower limb and paraspinal muscles to help the body decelerate [10]

Fast bowlers experience significant ground reaction forces (GRF) during the delivery stride, particularly at front foot contact (FFC). The GRF at

FFC can be up to eight or nine times the bowler's body weight [11, 12]. These forces are particularly high during the initial ankle plantarflexion phase, where velocities can reach up to 1200°/s, coinciding with peaks in the abduction and external rotation angles and plantarflexion and adduction moments [13]. Eccentric contraction of the anterior compartment muscles, including the tibialis anterior, extensor digitorum longus and extensor hallucis longus, followed by eccentric contraction of the posterior compartment muscles, especially the gastrocnemius and soleus, during dorsiflexion, is required for energy absorption and force dissipation at ball release.

During fast bowling, the ankle joint undergoes extensive movement and experiences high internal loads, which increase with stride length. A longer stride length places the body's centre of mass (COM) further behind the front ankle joint, increasing the negative work and plantarflexion experienced by the ankle [13]. The bowling action may also alter stressors, with mixed action types demonstrating higher back-foot ankle inversion at the time of FFC [14].

39.1.4 Podiatric Assessment

Appropriate footwear selection and sometimes customisation are essential for providing stability and mitigating the high GRF experienced by fast bowlers during the delivery stride. This is achieved with specially designed cricket shoes with reinforced toe caps, additional cushioning, and spikes for traction when landing on the turf surface. Conventional cricket shoes significantly reduce front foot lateral shear force and front knee joint external rotation moment compared to custom-modified cross-trainers [15]. Cricketers often wear high-top shoes due to a perceived increase in stability. Increased plantarflexion and adduction loads at FFC in the delivery stride can contribute to heightened injury risk, including posterior impingement [16]. Custom modifications are often applied to provide further durability or support, including with orthotics. Fast bowlers often remove the toe-box over the first toe, which otherwise slides in the shoe and is associated with bruising, pain and nail bed trauma.

39.2 Ankle

39.2.1 Lateral Ligament Injuries

Lateral ankle ligament injuries are particularly prevalent among fast bowlers. Injuries to the lateral ligament often manifest as acute sprains. Lateral ankle ligament injuries primarily involve the anterior talofibular ligament (ATFL) and the calcaneofibular ligament (CFL). Acute injuries occur due to sudden inversion of the ankle, leading to partial or complete tears of these ligaments. A unique risk factor in cricket is the boundary rope, on which an outfielder may inadvertently step and invert their ankle. Chronic lateral ankle instability can result from repeated acute injuries or inadequate rehabilitation, leading to persistent symptoms and functional instability [17]. Chronic instability is a particularly challenging problem affecting player availability, performance and career longevity. Furthermore, it heightens the risk of other injuries, including a predisposition to hindfoot injuries [18].

Several risk factors contribute to the high incidence of lateral ankle ligament injuries in cricketers:

High GRF
Significant GRF during the fast bowler delivery stride
A sudden change of direction
Pivoting and directional changes in bowling and fielding place pressure on lateral ligaments, particularly in resisting inversion
Previous ankle injuries
Previous injuries may result in ligament laxity and proprioceptive deficits that prevent the ankle from resisting forces that would normally be prevented. Chronic instability increases the risk of recurrent ankle injuries [19]

Most lateral ankle injuries, acute and chronic, can be managed non-surgically with structured rehabilitation. Surgery may be considered in persistent instability cases that do not respond to conservative measures. Persistent pain or insta-

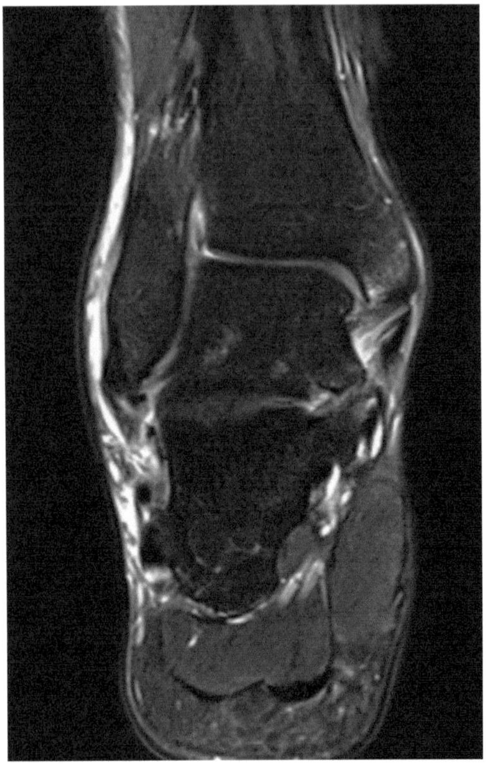

Fig. 39.1 Disruption of both ATFL and CFL components of the lateral ligament complex

bility after 3 months of conservative treatment should also prompt the clinician to consider other concomitant injuries, including peroneal tendon tear or dysfunction, syndesmosis sprain, ankle impingement or osteochondral lesion of the talus [20] (Fig. 39.1).

Acute management
The 'POLICE' acronym denotes protection, optimal loading, ice, compression and elevation, forming the initial management principle. This approach emphasises early mobilisation to retain function
Rehabilitation
A structured rehabilitation programme emphasises recovering range of motion, proprioception and strength [21]. Before returning to cricket, assessing the ability to partake in specific movement patterns the player will face in match situations without pain and with good stability is crucial. Rehabilitation also encompasses preventative measures, which involve exercises that emphasise balance to recover proprioceptive deficits that develop post-injury
Adjuncts
Ankle bracing and taping can be used to provide additional support. These are often used long term in situations of recurrent instability
Surgical management
Anatomical reconstruction: Brostrom repair is the most common of these procedures and involves direct repair of the torn ligaments to maintain normal anatomic kinematics. Modifications to this procedure include using suture anchors and fibre tape to confer additional support to the lateral ligaments [22] Non-anatomical reconstruction: These procedures involve reinforcing the lateral ligament without direct repair. They include tendon grafts, such as the Chrisman-Snook procedure, which may be used in more severe cases of recurrent instability or revision procedures [20]

39.2.2 Medial Ligament Injuries

Although less prevalent than lateral ligament injuries, medial ankle ligament/deltoid injuries can significantly impact an athlete's performance and recovery. The deltoid ligament consists of superficial and deep fibres. Together, they provide stability against valgus and external rotation forces at the ankle [17]. Injuries typically result from excessive eversion or external rotation forces. Pre-existing deformities like valgus-flat foot may predispose athletes to pronation-eversion injuries [23]. Injury to the deltoid ligament should raise suspicion for concomitant injury to the lateral ligament, syndesmosis or ankle fracture.

Similar principles to acute lateral ligament injury management are applied with POLICE and structured rehabilitation. Custom orthotics to support the medial arch may reduce valgus loading and better support the deltoid ligament [24]. Surgical intervention should be considered for complete deltoid ligament tears due to the risk of persistent instability. Biomechanical cadaveric studies indicate complete deltoid ligament tear associated with a 23° increase in plantarflexion eversion angle [25]. Surgical management includes open and arthroscopic techniques to directly repair the torn deltoid ligament or recon-

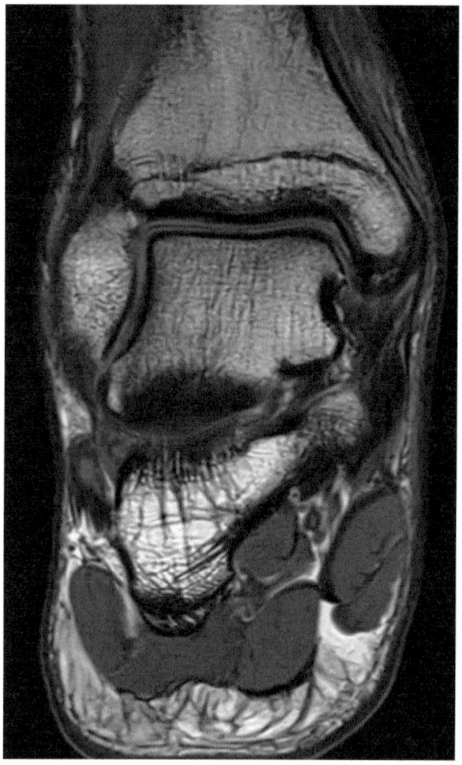

Fig. 39.2 Non-retracted tibial avulsion of the tibiocalcaneal component of the deltoid ligament

struction with tendon grafts to restore function (Fig. 39.2).

39.2.3 Syndesmosis Injuries

Ankle syndesmosis injuries are commonly referred to as high ankle sprains. The ankle syndesmosis comprises the anterior inferior tibiofibular ligament (AITFL), posterior inferior tibiofibular ligament (PITFL) and the interosseous ligament (IOL) [26]. The syndesmosis confers stability to the distal tibiofibular joint. Combined injury with the deltoid is associated with increased talar instability [24]. Syndesmosis injuries account for 1 18% of ankle sprains in athletic populations. This figure is likely understated due to many missed or underreported injuries and limited use of advanced imaging such as MRI. This is problematic due to the risk of developing chronic ankle dysfunction and delayed return to high-level activity [27]. Mechanisms of injury include excessive or forced external rotation and dorsiflexion, which may occur in fast bowlers in the delivery stride [28]. Inversion injuries may cause concomitant injury to the lateral ligaments but typically only involve the AITFL component of the syndesmosis [29].

Acute syndesmosis injuries typically require a period of immobilisation in a cast or walking boot with protected weight bearing. Surgical fixation is indicated if instability is noted at the distal tibiofibular joint. This is indicated if there is evidence of diastasis on a weight bearing or stress X-ray or static widening on an MRI scan. Arthroscopy may be required to assess stability if diagnostic doubt remains. A grading system using MRI can assist with management options.

Grade	Description	Management consideration
I	Injury to the AITFL only	Stable injury can be managed conservatively
II	Injury to AITFL and IOL	Potentially unstable, requires further assessment
III	Injury to AITFL, IOL and PITFL with diastasis	Unstable injury that requires definitive stabilisation

Athletes who exhibit higher impact loads on their ankle, such as a fast bowler in the delivery stride, may experience functional instability with lower grades of injury and require a more graded return to play. Surgical options include stabilisation of the distal tibiofibular joint with a suture-button device and, less frequently, with screws. Arthroscopy can assess the integrity of the syndesmosis and ensure anatomical reduction. Rehabilitation focuses on restoring range of motion, strength and proprioception. Return-to-play considerations are like lateral ligament injuries, but identical-grade injuries can take twice as long to return to the pre-injury level [26] (Fig. 39.3).

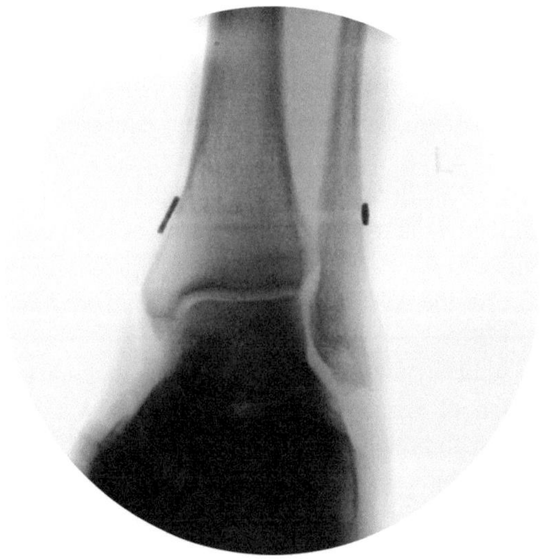

Fig. 39.3 Syndesmosis injury stabilised with a tightrope

39.2.4 Peroneal Tendinopathy

The peroneal tendons are located on the lateral side of the ankle. Peroneal tendinopathy in cricketers occurs due to overuse. It occurs in fast bowlers and fielders due to repetitive stress and high-impact and repetitive lateral movements. Again, the high-GRF during the delivery stride predispose fast bowlers to this condition. Management may require a short rest period from the offending activities, rehabilitation focusing on strengthening the tendon through a gradual loading programme and using orthotics to provide additional support and reduce stress on the tendons. In severe cases, surgical intervention can involve repair or debridement of the involved peroneal tendon [19].

39.2.5 Achilles Tendinopathy

Repetitive plantar flexion with a high GRF leads to high mechanical loading of the Achilles tendon and, subsequently, pain and degeneration. This is most evident in fast bowlers in the delivery stride. Additional risk factors include sudden increases in training intensity, poor footwear, inadequate warm-up routines and pre-existing biomechanical abnormalities such as overpronation or limited ankle dorsiflexion. Inadequate recovery and rehabilitation contribute to chronicity.

Conservative treatment is the cornerstone for managing Achilles tendinopathy. Key strategies include:

Eccentric loading exercises
Eccentric exercises promote collagen synthesis, tendon remodelling and pain relief [30]. However, they may also instigate pain, particularly in severe cases. Isometric exercises can be a bridge before gradually integrating eccentric components into the rehabilitation
Activity modification
Aggravating exercises, including running, may need to be reduced before gradually increasing the load. Warming up before activity can be beneficial for symptoms
Orthotics
Biomechanical issues, including overpronation and pes planus, may contribute to the overloading of the Achilles tendon. Orthotics can help reduce the dynamic load during activities. A heel lift may provide symptomatic relief for insertional tendinopathy
Platelet-rich plasma (PRP)
Injecting a patient's concentration of platelets for Achilles tendinopathy has shown mixed results. There is evidence to demonstrate improved pain and function, while other studies do not show significant benefits [31]. The differences in PRP preparation are important, as higher PRP concentrations or platelet counts are more likely to be efficacious
Extracorporeal Shockwave Therapy (ESWT)
ESWT is an effective adjunct treatment option to reduce pain and improve function in mid-portion Achilles tendinopathy but not insertional tendinopathy [32]. The sound waves are thought to assist by promoting blood flow and triggering cellular repair

Returning to play with symptomatic Achilles tendinopathy can be delicate due to pain and loss of confidence. The cricketer should ideally be able to perform sport-specific tasks with minimal to no pain. Good markers of functional ability include restoration of normal range of motion, calf flexibility and strength compared to the contralateral sides. Other functional manoeuvres, including single-leg hop tests, are also useful determinants of readiness for plyometric demands [33].

39.2.6 Posterior Ankle Impingement

Posterior ankle impingement syndrome (PAIS) develops due to repetitive loaded ankle plantar flexion. Fast bowlers are particularly susceptible at the delivery stride due to the rapid transition from dorsiflexion to plantarflexion. High GRFs generated at FFC are followed by sudden deceleration [9]. Anatomical variants, including an Os trigonum and Stieda process, when present, are susceptible to compression in plantar flexion and can be a source of pain and inflammation [34]. Soft tissue impingement can occur secondary to scarring or inflammation of the posterior capsule, PITFL or posterior deltoid fibres [35]. Clinical assessment is critical, as associating factors on imaging do not always equate to impingement or pain syndromes and, in symptomatic cases, may not necessarily be the primary pain driver [36].

PAIS is particularly important to manage in fast bowlers, as pain in the delivery stride can impact performance and confidence. Pain is typically felt on FFC during bowling but not necessarily when running [37]. PAIS also debilitates elite ballet dancers, with studies comparing them to athletes demonstrating that both may present with posterior talocrural and subtalar joint effusion-synovitis on imaging. However, athletes had a higher prevalence of either Os trigonum or Stieda process than dancers [34]. Ballet dancers may experience PAIS due to their significantly higher-than-average plantar flexion range. In contrast, athletes like fast bowlers experience it due to repetitive load and plantar flexion.

In cricketers and particularly fast bowlers, managing PAIS effectively requires addressing symptoms and the underlying biomechanical factors contributing to the condition. Conservative management is the first line.

Rest and activity modification
Reduce or modify activities that exacerbate symptoms to allow the inflammation to subside. Subsequent graded increase of activity after initial symptoms subside
Rehabilitation
Strengthening and flexibility exercises for the ankle and calf muscles are essential. Eccentric strengthening of the calf muscles and proprioception exercises help improve strength and ankle stability. Single-leg endurance has been demonstrated to be less in patients with PAIS and should be addressed in rehabilitation [38]
Anti-inflammatory
Nonsteroidal anti-inflammatory drugs (NSAIDs) can help reduce pain and inflammation
Injection therapy
Corticosteroid injections can reduce inflammation and provide temporary relief [37]
Adjuncts
Orthotics and taping can help support the ankle better and resist excessive motion. Cryotherapy or ultrasound may reduce inflammation and pain

Surgical intervention is indicated when conservative treatments fail to relieve symptoms. Given their functional demands, fast bowlers are less likely to tolerate the symptoms of PAIS, and a lower threshold for intervention may be necessary. Surgical intervention targets individual-specific factors that may be implicated in the posterior impingement. Arthroscopic debridement can be used to remove bony or soft tissue causing pain. In severe cases, posterior ankle release is indicated to relieve pressure and allow greater plantar flexion range.

Treatment of a fast bowler with PAIS must further include strategies to prevent recurrence. This involves biomechanical analysis of the bowling action and subsequent modifications. A multidisciplinary collaborative approach is required between the physician, physiotherapist, sports scientist and bowling coaches. Modifications to the bowler's action, training and rehabilitation that may be necessary to reduce posterior stresses on the ankle include [13]:

Stride length adjustment
Longer stride length may be associated with higher ankle joint load. Adjustments should be subtle so as not to disturb other aspects of the bowling mechanics
Foot placement
Front foot contact (FFC) in a square position can reduce external rotation and abduction forces
Load management
Monitoring the total number of balls or overs bowled can reduce repetitive loads and ensure adequate rest between sessions
Kinematic corrections
Attending to overall alignment, balance and stability through follow-through can assist in distributing the total load more evenly and reduce excess stress in the ankle joint

39.3 Foot

39.3.1 Stress Injuries of the Lower Leg

Stress reactions in the lower leg most commonly involve the tibia due to its predominant role in weight-bearing and shock absorption. Other sites of the lower leg can develop stress reactions due to biomechanic or kinematic factors. The fibula may develop stress if the lateral side is preferentially loaded. Stress reactions in the medial malleolus may occur due to excessive rotational forces on weight bearing. The navicular may be vulnerable due to excessive foot pronation. Other sites may be loaded on impact, such as the calcaneus on heel strike during FFC in the delivery stride or on jumping and the loading of the metatarsals during propulsion or change of direction [39]. Fast bowlers are particularly susceptible to medial sesamoid stress injuries due to the repetitive dorsiflexion and impact forces on the hallux during delivery strides. The fibular sesamoid can also develop stress fractures in fast bowlers, although less commonly [40]. Adolescent athletes may experience periphyseal stress injuries, which can impact the proximal or distal tibia, fibula, first or second metatarsal or proximal phalanges of the toes [41]. The medial malleolus, talus, navicular, fifth metatarsal base, anterior tibia, medial malleolus and sesamoid are considered high risk given the greater propensity to develop non-union and require more aggressive management [39], likely meaning boot or even plaster immobilisation and occasionally surgical fixation. Some common stress fractures (middle metatarsals, posterior tibia and fibula) can be treated symptomatically and may not require lengthy immobilisation.

Repetitive impact during the delivery stride and high training volumes, particularly with running loads, contribute significantly to stress reactions in the foot and ankle. Running loads incorporate cumulative running distances during training and matches. As with other overuse injuries, increases in running peaks can be assessed with the acute-to-chronic workload ratio. Other factors include overstriding or incorrect foot placement, contributing to increased lower leg load. Low energy availability can occur due to high training volume relative to caloric intake. This can impair bone mineralisation and increase the risk of stress reactions with female athletes at particular risk [42].

Effective management involves reducing bone stress and addressing underlying factors to reduce the risk of recurrence. The management is primarily conservative, with surgical intervention only considered for complete fractures or if there is potential for earlier return with fixation.

Load management
Activity modification is required to offload the site of stress. A period of non-weight bearing may be required, depending on the athlete's pain profile and if the stress reaction is in a weight-bearing zone. Progressive loading should occur in a pain-free manner. Adjuncts, including Alter-G treadmills, can facilitate an earlier return to running
Rehabilitation
Particular attention should be on strengthening regional muscles, particularly the calf muscles, improving the range of motion of surrounding joints to aid the distribution of load and improving functional strength through the kinematic chain, with particular attention on improving balance and stability to provide a stable base for energy transfer
Biomechanical modifications
Gait analysis and pressure plate analysis can help understand patterns of load distribution. Modifications to running technique, including optimising stride length or landing position, are best addressed by specialised coaches. Orthotics are a useful adjunct to support the medial arch better or distribute the load
Nutrition
Athletes may underestimate the caloric requirements for their level of training. Education helps empower the athlete and ensure that total caloric intake is optimised relative to the energy demands of training and recovery. A dietitian is best placed to ensure ongoing education and adherence

Return to play after a stress reaction should occur gradually with a structured plan. Regular monitoring, including GPS loads, can track total running loads and ensure no sudden increases in peak loads occur. A common return-to-running regimen is to increase distance and intensity by no more than 10% per week [43]. Regular clinical assessment for clinical tenderness and pain on functional tests, such as single-leg hop, and cal-

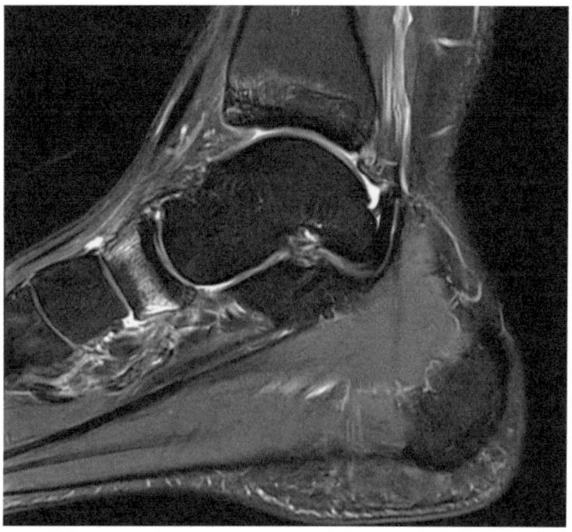

Fig. 39.4 Stress reaction through the body of the navicular

culated use of imaging can help guide the progression of load (Fig. 39.4).

39.3.2 Turf Toe

Turf toe is commonly observed in rugby, American football and soccer. It occurs when hyperextension at the first metatarsophalangeal (MTP) joint causes injury to the plantar plate. In the acute setting, it may occur due to forced dorsiflexion when suddenly pushing off to start. It can also develop chronically due to repetitive stopping and starting or direction changes. In cricket, these mechanisms are more likely to occur in fast bowlers and fielders. Artificial surfaces are considered a risk factor in American football and soccer, though there is limited data to prove this. In cricket, it could be hypothesised that the differences in the hardness of the turf wickets and occasionally in some outfields may lead to higher impact forces transmitted to the MTP joint [44].

Turf toe may present with pain, swelling and a limited range of motion at the first MTP joint, particularly pain-limited hyperextension. Instability can be tested with a vertical Lachman test at the 1st MTP. A combination of imaging, typically an MRI, and clinical findings can be used to grade the injury [45].

Grade 1
Stretching of the plantar complex with mild tenderness
Grade 2
Partial tearing of the plantar complex with moderate swelling and restricted range
Grade 3
Complete tearing of the plantar complex with significant swelling and marked loss of range

Most turf toe injuries can be managed conservatively. An initial period of rest and ice is recommended to reduce inflammation in acute injuries. Immobilisation of the 1st MTP joint may be required to manage pain with a walker boot or stiff-soled shoe. Taping to limit hyperextension at the 1st MTP joint is often employed when re-introducing toe push-off activities. Rehabilitation aims to improve 1st MTP range of motion, regional muscle strength and proprioception. Return-to-play criteria include restoring the range of motion and strength required to perform sport-specific activities without pain or limitation. Recovery time can vary between management options and grading. Grade 1 injuries may be able to keep playing, whereas extended time off may occur in higher-grade injuries. NFL players treated non-operatively for high-grade turf toe injuries had an RTP rate of 100% with a mean time of 75.8 days, whereas those undergoing surgery had an 80% RTP rate with a mean time of 221.4 days [46]. Surgery is best reserved for when conservative management fails. It is more likely in complete tears, particularly in the setting of large capsular avulsions or overt instability that may occur with concomitant sesamoid fractures or persistent instability [45] (Fig. 39.5).

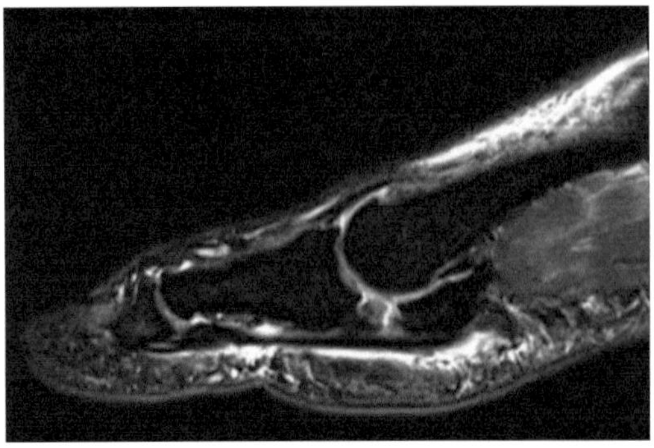

Fig. 39.5 Acute sesamoid avulsion of the tibial sesamoid phalangeal ligament extending into the plantar plate

39.3.3 Plantar Fasciitis

Plantar fasciitis is a common overuse injury in the athletic and general populations. The plantar fascia is a thick connective tissue band most susceptible to irritation at its origin at the calcaneus. It supports the plantar arch and acts as a shock absorber. Plantar fasciitis in cricket is most likely related to repetitive running and jumping movements, eventually leading to microtears in the plantar fascia. Fast bowlers are most susceptible in the delivery stride and landing phases, where maximal force is exerted onto the heel. Other risk factors include high body mass index, prolonged standing, pes planus and pes cavus [47]. Calf muscle tightness may also increase tension on the plantar fascia and contribute to more load in the region. Cricketers may also add to their risk because of improper footwear and insufficient conditioning of the lower limb muscles.

Plantar fasciitis is a significant issue as it can limit the ability to move without pain and detrimentally impact performance. Treatment for plantar fasciitis typically begins with conservative measures. In the acute setting, this includes relative rest, ice, nonsteroidal anti-inflammatory drugs (NSAIDs) and physical therapy with stretching and strengthening exercises for the plantar fascia and calf muscles. A progressive upgrade of the load is essential to prevent further degeneration. PRP injections to the plantar fascia have been more efficacious in the long term in reducing pain and disability than corticosteroid injections [48]. Shockwave therapy stimulates healing by promoting neovascularisation and tissue regeneration [49]. Other treatments are considered adjuncts, including night splints and orthotic devices to support the arch and reduce strain on the plantar fascia. Surgery should only be considered for recalcitrant cases and may include open or endoscopic partial or complete plantar fascia release to reduce tension. Surgery involves long recovery periods and significant game time missed (Fig. 39.6).

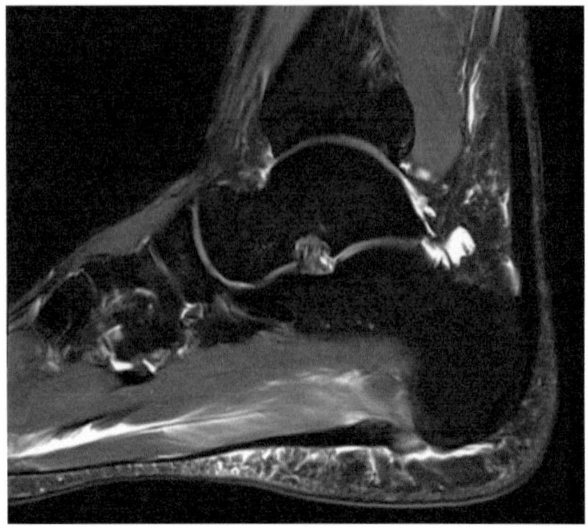

Fig. 39.6 Thickened appearance of the plantar fascia with surrounding perifascial oedema secondary to recent injection

39.3.4 Sesamoiditis

Sesamoid injuries occur due to repetitive stress in the forefoot. The sesamoid bones are embedded within the two tendons of the flexor hallucis brevis muscle. They provide a smooth surface for the tendons to glide, helping to distribute weight transfer and allow shock absorption in high-impact activities. In bowling, significant loading of the forefoot occurs during the delivery stride. During bowling and batting, the repetitive dorsiflexion and plantarflexion of the big toe can lead to inflammation, bone stress and fractures of the sesamoid bones. As with other lower leg stress-related injuries, additional risk may occur due to playing on hard surfaces and improper footwear. Presentation occurs with pain, swelling and tenderness at the sesamoids and the first metatarsophalangeal (MTP) joint. Imaging, including X-rays, MRI, or CT scans, is essential to assess the severity of the injury and differentiate between sesamoiditis and sesamoid fracture. Comparative radiographs of the opposite foot can also help differentiate bipartite sesamoids from fractures [50].

Management aims to unload the sesamoid and provide symptom relief. A period of rest from offending activities is recommended. Immobilisation in a walking boot may be required if there is pain with walking. A stiff-soled shoe can also help resist excessive dorsiflexion loads. Custom orthotics or taping can be made to either offload pressure on the sesamoid or to correct the malposition of the sesamoid [51]. Rehabilitation exercises are to strengthen the calf and foot muscles involved in propulsion. Surgical options are reserved for persistent pain despite rehabilitation. This can involve partial or complete sesamoid excision. Return to play at the same level as pre-surgery has been reported in up to 67% of competitive athletes following sesamoid excision, with an average return to play of approximately 5 months [52].

Return to play after sesamoid injuries should be gradual and based on the athlete's recovery progress. Key considerations that allow a successful return to play following sesamoid injuries include pain-free sport-specific activities, restoration of strength and stability comparable to the contralateral side, and the ability to perform functional tests such as single-leg hop tests that translate to other additional demands that can occur in gameplay (Fig. 39.7).

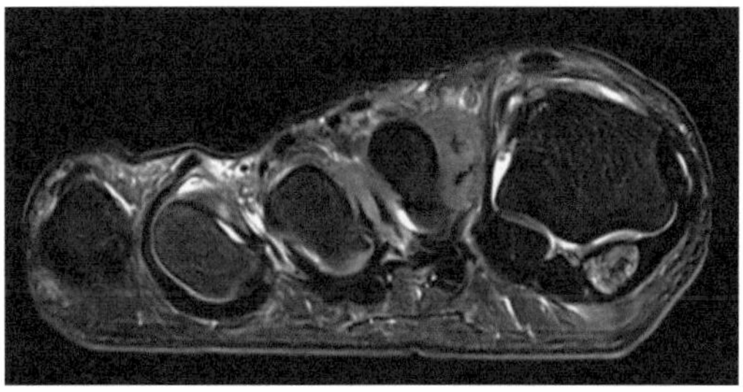

Fig. 39.7 Stress reaction within the tibial sesamoid of the forefoot

39.3.5 Subungual Haematoma

Subungual haematoma is a common nail injury characterised by the accumulation of blood underneath a toenail or fingernail. This injury typically occurs in cricket due to direct trauma to the toe, such as being struck by a cricket ball or from repetitive pressure and friction within tight footwear. Fast bowlers are particularly susceptible to repetitive friction, which can occur when the foot slides in their shoe on FFC during the delivery stride. The sudden impact can cause the blood vessels under the nail to rupture, leading to a painful, swollen and discoloured nail [53].

Clinical assessment involves thoroughly examining the affected toe to evaluate the extent of the haematoma. Pain intensity and discolouration of the nail may correlate with the level of haematoma. Significant pain should prompt consideration for an underlying fracture, particularly in the setting of direct trauma. It is crucial to distinguish subungual haematoma from subungual melanoma, a rare but aggressive skin cancer. A key differentiating feature is Hutchinson's sign in subungual melanoma, where pigmentation extends onto the surrounding nail folds. Definitive diagnosis of subungual melanoma requires biopsy and histological evaluation [54].

Treatment of subungual haematoma is required in the setting of significant pain and to reduce the risk of nail deformity. Trephination involves creating a small hole in the nail to drain accumulated blood. It is best performed with a heated needle and ideally done within 48 h of onset and can provide immediate relief [55]. Correct-fitting shoes are essential to reduce repetitive friction forces. Some bowlers may opt to increase cushioning for their toes in their footwear or cut open an area to allow their 1st toe to slide without causing friction with their shoe. A shoe with firm support around the heel and a heel-lock shoelace tying method may assist in reducing foot slide within the shoe. Batters should have adequate toe protection to reduce direct impact from a ball (Fig. 39.8).

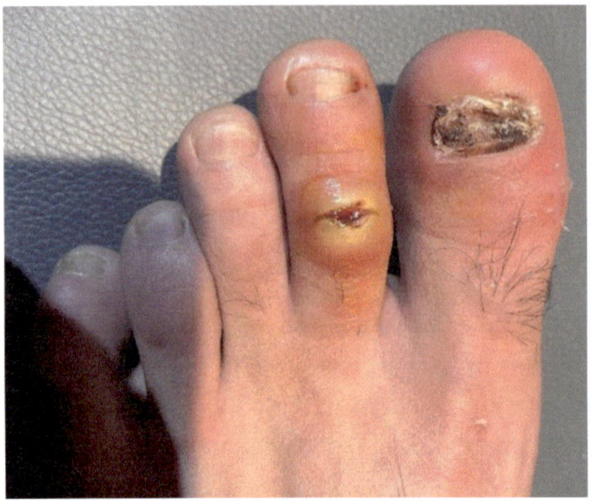

Fig. 39.8 Long-term appearance of a fast bowler's toe

References

1. Olivier B, Naude J, Mnguni N, Thotse M, Phalandwa P, Ferrao P, Saragas NP. Foot and ankle injuries in elite south African cricketers: a descriptive analysis of injury surveillance data. Indian J Orthop. 2023;57(10):1592–9. https://doi.org/10.1007/s43465-023-00934-2. PMID: 37766951; PMCID: PMC10519890.
2. Orchard JW, James T, Portus MR. Injuries to elite male cricketers in Australia over a 10-year period. J Sci Med Sport. 2006;9(6):459–67. https://doi.org/10.1016/j.jsams.2006.05.001.
3. Dhillon MS, Patel S, Arora SS, Bachhal V, Rajnish RK. Foot and ankle injuries in cricket players: the current state of our knowledge. J Postgrad Med Edu Res. 2016;50(2):95–102. https://doi.org/10.5005/jp-journals-10028-1647.
4. Orchard JW, Kountouris A, Sims K. Incidence and prevalence of elite male cricket injuries using updated consensus definitions. Open Access J Sports Med. 2016;7:187–94. https://doi.org/10.2147/OAJSM.S117497. PMID: 28008292; PMCID: PMC5167453.
5. Orchard JW, Inge P, Sims K, Kountouris A, Saw AE, Saw R, Beerworth K. Comparison of injury profiles between elite Australian male and female cricket players. J Sci Med Sport. 2023;26(1):19–24. https://doi.org/10.1016/j.jsams.2022.12.002. Epub 2022 Dec 5. PMID: 36522249.
6. Dennis RJ, Finch CF, McIntosh AS, Elliott BC. Use of field-based tests to identify risk factors for injury to fast bowlers in cricket. Br J Sports Med. 2008;42(6):477–82. https://doi.org/10.1136/bjsm.2008.046698. Epub 2008 Apr 7. PMID: 18390922.
7. Olivier B, Taljaard T, Burger E, Brukner P, Orchard J, Gray J, Botha N, Stewart A, Mckinon W. Which extrinsic and intrinsic factors are associated with non-contact injuries in adult cricket fast bowlers? Sports Med. 2016;46(1):79–101. https://doi.org/10.1007/s40279-015-0383-y.
8. Felton PJ, Yeadon MR, King MA. Optimising the front foot contact phase of the cricket fast bowling action. J Sports Sci. 2020;38(18):2054–62. https://doi.org/10.1080/02640414.2020.1770407. Epub 2020 May 31. PMID: 32475221.
9. Epifano DJ, Ryan S, Clarke AC, Huynh M, Anderson H, Middleton KJ. Comparing tibial accelerations between delivery and follow-through foot strikes in cricket pace bowling. Sports Biomech. 2022:1–14. https://doi.org/10.1080/14763141.2022.2136582. Epub ahead of print. PMID: 36266941.
10. Forrest MRL, Scott BR, Hebert JJ, Dempsey AR. Injury prevention strategies for adolescent cricket pace bowlers. Sports Med. 2018;48(11):2449–61. https://doi.org/10.1007/s40279-018-0981-6.
11. Portus M, Mason BR, Elliott BC, Pfitzner MC, Done RP. Technique factors related to ball release speed and trunk injuries in high performance cricket fast bowlers. Sports Biomech. 2004;3(2):263–84. https://doi.org/10.1080/14763140408522845. PMID: 15552585.
12. Elliott BC, Hardcastle PH, Burnett AE, Foster DH. The influence of fast bowling and physical factors on radiologic features in high performance young fast bowlers. Sports Med Train Rehabil. 1992;3(2):113–30. https://doi.org/10.1080/15438629209517008.
13. Spratford W, Hicks A. Increased delivery stride length places greater loads on the ankle joint in elite male cricket fast bowlers. J Sports Sci. 2014;32(12):1101–9. https://doi.org/10.1080/02640414.2014.886130. Epub 2014 Feb 28. PMID: 24576107.
14. Schaefer A, Ferdinands RED, O'Dwyer N, Edwards S. A biomechanical comparison of conventional classifications of bowling action-types in junior fast bowlers. J Sports Sci. 2020;38(10):1085–95. https://doi.org/10.1080/02640414.2020.1741972. Epub 2020 Apr 12. PMID: 32281483.
15. Bishop C, Thewlis D. Footwear in cricket: issues facing podiatrists treating fast bowlers. J Foot Ankle Res. 2011;4(Suppl 1):P5. https://doi.org/10.1186/1757-1146-4-S1-P5. PMCID: PMC3103027.
16. Bishop C, Bartold S, Thewlis D. Effects of footwear on lead limb knee and ankle joint kinematics in a fast bowler with a history of posterior ankle joint impingement-a case report. Clin J Sport Med. 2013;23(6):491–3. https://doi.org/10.1097/JSM.0b013e318291d154. PMID: 23657121.
17. Pereira H, Guillo S, Glazebrook M, Takao M, Calder J, Van Dijk N, Karlsson J. Lateral ankle instability: an international approach by the Ankle Instability Group. 1st ed. Berlin: Springer Berlin Heidelberg; 2021. https://doi.org/10.1007/978-3-662-62763-1.
18. Pardiwala DN, Rao NN, Varshney AV. Injuries in Cricket. Sports Health. 2018;10(3):217–22. https://doi.org/10.1177/1941738117732318. Epub 2017 Oct 3. PMID: 28972820; PMCID: PMC5958448.
19. Dhillon MS, Rajnish RK, Sharma S. Foot and ankle injuries in cricket players: the current state

of our knowledge. J Postgrad Med Edu Res. 2023;57(4):186–90.
20. Camacho LD, Roward ZT, Deng Y, Latt LD. Surgical Management of Lateral Ankle Instability in athletes. J Athl Train. 2019;54(6):639–49. https://doi.org/10.4085/1062-6050-348-18. PMID: 31238016; PMCID: PMC6602388.
21. van den Bekerom MP, Kerkhoffs GM, McCollum GA, Calder JD, van Dijk CN. Management of acute lateral ankle ligament injury in the athlete. Knee Surg Sports Traumatol Arthrosc. 2013;21(6):1390–5. https://doi.org/10.1007/s00167-012-2252-7. Epub 2012 Oct 30. PMID: 23108678.
22. Li X, Killie H, Guerrero P, Busconi BD. Anatomical reconstruction for chronic lateral ankle instability in the high-demand athlete: functional outcomes after the modified Broström repair using suture anchors. Am J Sports Med. 2009;37(3):488–94. https://doi.org/10.1177/0363546508327541. PMID: 19251684.
23. Lötscher P, Hintermann B. Medial ankle ligament injuries in athletes. Oper Tech Sports Med. 2014;22(4):290–5. https://doi.org/10.1053/j.otsm.2014.09.009.
24. Massri-Pugin J, Lubberts B, Vopat BG, Wolf JC, DiGiovanni CW, Guss D. Role of the deltoid ligament in syndesmotic instability. Foot Ankle Int. 2018;39(5):598–603. https://doi.org/10.1177/1071100717750577. Epub 2018 Jan 10. PMID: 29320936.
25. Brady AW, Bryniarski A, Brown JR, Waltz R, Stake IK, Kreulen CD, Haytmanek CT, Clanton TO. The biomechanical role of the deltoid ligament on ankle stability: injury, repair, and augmentation. Am J Sports Med. 2023;51(10):2617–24. https://doi.org/10.1177/03635465231181082. Epub 2023 Jul 14. PMID: 37449714.
26. Press CM, Gupta A, Hutchinson MR. Management of ankle syndesmosis injuries in the athlete. Curr Sports Med Rep. 2009;8(5):228–33. https://doi.org/10.1249/JSR.0b013e3181b7ec0c. PMID: 19741349.
27. McCollum GA, van den Bekerom MP, Kerkhoffs GM, Calder JD, van Dijk CN. Syndesmosis and deltoid ligament injuries in the athlete. Knee Surg Sports Traumatol Arthrosc. 2013;21(6):1328–37. https://doi.org/10.1007/s00167-012-2205-1. Epub 2012 Oct 7. PMID: 23052109.
28. Waterman BR, Belmont PJ Jr, Cameron KL, Svoboda SJ, Alitz CJ, Owens BD. Risk factors for syndesmotic and medial ankle sprain: role of sex, sport, and level of competition. Am J Sports Med. 2011;39(5):992–8. https://doi.org/10.1177/0363546510391462. Epub 2011 Feb 2. PMID: 21289274.
29. Uys HD, Rijke AM. Clinical association of acute lateral ankle sprain with syndesmotic involvement: a stress radiography and magnetic resonance imaging study. Am J Sports Med. 2002;30(6):816–22. https://doi.org/10.1177/03635465020300061101. PMID: 12435647.
30. Maquirriain J. Leg stiffness changes in athletes with Achilles tendinopathy. Int J Sports Med. 2012;33(7):567–71. https://doi.org/10.1055/s--0032-1304644. Epub 2012 Apr 12. PMID: 22499572.
31. Sneed D, Wong C. Platelet-rich plasma injections as a treatment for Achilles tendinopathy and plantar fasciitis in athletes. PM R. 2023;15(11):1493–506. https://doi.org/10.1002/pmrj.12965. Epub 2023 May 11. PMID: 36929699.
32. Paantjens MA, Helmhout PH, Backx FJG, van Etten-Jamaludin FS, Bakker EWP. Extracorporeal shockwave therapy for mid-portion and insertional Achilles tendinopathy: a systematic review of randomized controlled trials. Sports Med Open. 2022;8(1):68. https://doi.org/10.1186/s40798-022-00456-5. PMID: 35552903; PMCID: PMC9106789.
33. Habets B, van den Broek AG, Huisstede BMA, Backx FJG, van Cingel REH. Return to sport in athletes with Midportion Achilles tendinopathy: a qualitative systematic review regarding definitions and criteria. Sports Med. 2018;48(3):705–23. https://doi.org/10.1007/s40279-017-0833-9. PMID: 29249084; PMCID: PMC5808052.
34. Baillie P, Cook J, Ferrar K, Smith P, Lam J, Mayes S. Magnetic resonance imaging findings associated with posterior ankle impingement syndrome are prevalent in elite ballet dancers and athletes. Skeletal Radiol. 2021;50(12):2423–31. https://doi.org/10.1007/s00256-021-03811-x. Epub 2021 May 19. PMID: 34013446.
35. Lavery KP, McHale KJ, Rossy WH, Theodore G. Ankle impingement. J Orthop Surg Res. 2016;11(1):97. https://doi.org/10.1186/s13018-016-0430-x. PMID: 27608626; PMCID: PMC5016963.
36. Baillie P, Ferrar K, Cook J, Smith P, Lam J, Mayes S. Posterior ankle impingement syndrome clinical features are not associated with imaging findings in elite ballet dancers and athletes. Clin J Sport Med. 2022;32(6):600–7. https://doi.org/10.1097/JSM.0000000000001021. Epub 2022 Feb 21. PMID: 36315819.
37. Mansingh A. Posterior ankle impingement in fast bowlers in cricket. West Indian Med J. 2011;60(1):77–81. PMID: 21809717.
38. Baillie P, Cook J, Ferrar K, Mayes S. Single-leg heel raise capacity is lower, and perceived ankle instability is greater, in dancers and athletes with posterior ankle impingement syndrome. Clin J Sport Med. 2024;34(4):376–80. https://doi.org/10.1097/JSM.0000000000001217. Epub 2024 Mar 20. PMID: 38507243.
39. Mayer SW, Joyner PW, Almekinders LC, Parekh SG. Stress fractures of the foot and ankle in athletes. Sports Health. 2014;6(6):481–91. Erratum in: Sports Health. 2015;7(6):557. 10.1177/1941738115609304. PMID: 25364480; PMCID: PMC4212349.
40. Dhillon H, Behera P, Prabhakar S, Dhillon S, Dhillon MS. Stress fracture of the fibular sesamoid bone of the foot in cricket: an unusual injury in bowlers. J Foot Ankle Surg (Asia-Pacific). 2016;3(1):59–62. https://doi.org/10.5005/jp-journals-10040-1050.

41. Caine D, Meyers R, Nguyen J, Schöffl V, Maffulli N. Primary Periphyseal stress injuries in young athletes: a systematic review. Sports Med. 2022;52(4):741–72. https://doi.org/10.1007/s40279-021-01511-z. Epub 2021 Aug 9. PMID: 34370212.
42. Tenforde AS, Carlson JL, Chang A, Sainani KL, Shultz R, Kim JH, Cutti P, Golden NH, Fredericson M. Association of the Female Athlete Triad Risk Assessment Stratification to the development of bone stress injuries in collegiate athletes. Am J Sports Med. 2017;45(2):302–10. https://doi.org/10.1177/0363546516676262. Epub 2016 Dec 30. PMID: 28038316.
43. Coslick AM, Lestersmith D, Chiang CC, et al. Lower extremity bone stress injuries in athletes: an update on current guidelines. Curr Phys Med Rehabil Rep. 2024;12:39–49. https://doi.org/10.1007/s40141-024-00429-7.
44. Frimenko RE, Lievers W, Coughlin MJ, Anderson RB, Crandall JR, Kent RW. Etiology and biomechanics of first metatarsophalangeal joint sprains (turf toe) in athletes. Crit Rev Biomed Eng. 2012;40(1):43–61. https://doi.org/10.1615/critrevbiomedeng.v40.i1.30. PMID: 22428798.
45. Vopat ML, Hassan M, Poppe T, Tarakemeh A, Zackula R, Mulcahey MK, Mullen S, Burkholder R, Schroeppel JP, Vopat BG. Return to sport after turf toe injuries: a systematic review and meta-analysis. Orthop J Sports Med. 2019;7(10):2325967119875133. https://doi.org/10.1177/2325967119875133. PMID: 31663005; PMCID: PMC6792281.
46. Lindsey BB, Bakshi NK, Walton DM, Holmes JR, Talusan PG. Return to play following high-grade turf toe injuries in National Football League Athletes. Foot & Ankle Orthopaedics. 2020;5(4) https://doi.org/10.1177/2473011420S00055.
47. Luffy L, Grosel J, Thomas R, So E. Plantar fasciitis: a review of treatments. JAAPA. 2018;31(1):20–4. https://doi.org/10.1097/01.JAA.0000527695.76041.99.
48. Peerbooms JC, Lodder P, den Oudsten BL, Doorgeest K, Schuller HM, Gosens T. Positive effect of platelet-rich plasma on pain in plantar fasciitis: a double-blind multicenter randomized controlled trial. Am J Sports Med. 2019;47(13):3238–46. https://doi.org/10.1177/0363546519877181. Epub 2019 Oct 11. PMID: 31603721.
49. Rompe JD, Decking J, Schoellner C, Nafe B. Shock wave application for chronic plantar fasciitis in running athletes. A prospective, randomized, placebo-controlled trial. Am J Sports Med. 2003;31(2):268–75. https://doi.org/10.1177/03635465030310021901. PMID: 12642264.
50. Stracciolini A, Dahlberg BW, Quinn B, Sugimoto D, Stein C. Sesamoid injuries in pediatric and adolescent athletes presenting to sports medicine clinic. Orthop. J Sports Med. 2019;7(3 Suppl):2325967119S00183. https://doi.org/10.1177/2325967119S00183. PMCID: PMC6447960
51. Carroll LA, Paulseth S, Martin RL. Forefoot injuries in athletes: integration of the movement system. Int J Sports Phys Ther. 2022;17(1):81–9. https://doi.org/10.26603/001c.30021. PMID: 35024208; PMCID: PMC8720253.
52. Dean RS, Coetzee JC, McGaver RS, Fritz JE, Nilsson LJ. Functional outcome of sesamoid excision in athletes. Am J Sports Med. 2020;48(14):3603–9. https://doi.org/10.1177/0363546520962518. Epub 2020 Oct 23. PMID: 33095661.
53. Akella A, Daniel AR, Gould MB, Mangal R, Ganti L. Subungual Hematoma. Cureus. 2023;15(11):e48952. https://doi.org/10.7759/cureus.48952. PMID: 38111403; PMCID: PMC10726102.
54. Amin K, Edmonds K, Fleming A, Powell B. Subungual malignant melanoma–re-learning the lesson. BMJ Case Rep. 2011;2011:bcr1020103422. https://doi.org/10.1136/bcr.10.2010.3422. PMID: 22701073; PMCID: PMC3063313.
55. Tanzi EL, Scher RK. Managing common nail disorders in active patients and athletes. Phys Sportsmed. 1999;27(9):35–47. https://doi.org/10.3810/psm.1999.09.976. PMID: 20086743.

MIX
Papier aus verantwortungsvollen Quellen
Paper from responsible sources
FSC® C105338

If you have any concerns about our products,
you can contact us on
ProductSafety@springernature.com

In case Publisher is established outside the EU,
the EU authorized representative is:
Springer Nature Customer Service Center GmbH
Europaplatz 3, 69115 Heidelberg, Germany

Printed by Libri Plureos GmbH
in Hamburg, Germany